BROWN'S ATLAS OF REGIONAL
ANESTHESIA

BROWN'S ATLAS OF REGIONAL ANESTHESIA

Sixth Edition

Ehab Farag MD, FRCA, FASA
Professor of Anesthesiology
Cleveland Clinic Lerner College of Medicine
Case western University
Director of Clinical Research,
Department of General Anesthesia and Outcomes
Research, Anesthesiology Institute,
Cleveland Clinic
Cleveland, Ohio

Loran Mounir-Soliman, MD
Staff Anesthesiologist
Director, Acute Pain Service
Director, Regional Anesthesiology and Acute Pain Medicine Fellowship
Institute of Anesthesia, Critical Care & Comprehensive Pain Management
Cleveland Clinic
Cleveland, Ohio

With David L. Brown
Emeritus Professor of Anesthesiology
Cleveland Clinic Lerner College of Medicine
Former Chairman of Anesthesiology Institute
Cleveland Clinic
Cleveland, Ohio

ILLUSTRATIONS BY
Joe Kanasz (fifth and sixth edition)
Jo Ann Clifford (fourth edition)

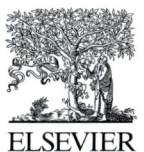

ELSEVIER

Elsevier
1600 John F. Kennedy Blvd.
Ste 1800
Philadelphia, PA 19103-2899

BROWN'S ATLAS OF REGIONAL ANESTHESIA, SIXTH EDITION   ISBN: 978-0-323654357

Copyright © 2021 by Elsevier, Inc. All rights reserved.

No part of this publication may be reproduced or transmitted in any form or by any means, electronic or mechanical, including photocopying, recording, or any information storage and retrieval system, without permission in writing from the publisher. Details on how to seek permission, further information about the Publisher's permissions policies and our arrangements with organizations such as the Copyright Clearance Center and the Copyright Licensing Agency, can be found at our website: www.elsevier.com/permissions.

This book and the individual contributions contained in it are protected under copyright by the Publisher (other than as may be noted herein).

Notice

Practitioners and researchers must always rely on their own experience and knowledge in evaluating and using any information, methods, compounds or experiments described herein. Because of rapid advances in the medical sciences, in particular, independent verification of diagnoses and drug dosages should be made. To the fullest extent of the law, no responsibility is assumed by Elsevier, authors, editors or contributors for any injury and/or damage to persons or property as a matter of products liability, negligence or otherwise, or from any use or operation of any methods, products, instructions, or ideas contained in the material herein.

Previous editions copyrighted 2017, 2010, 2006, 1999, and 1992

Library of Congress Control Number: 2020936134

Content Strategist: Sarah Barth
Content Development Specialist: Laura Klein
Publishing Services Manager: Shereen Jameel
Project Manager: Rukmani Krishnan
Design Direction: Brian Salisbury

Printed in China

Last digit is the print number: 9 8 7 6 5 4 3 2 1

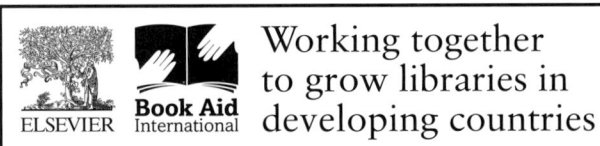

Dedicated to

To my wonderful wife, Abeer, and daughters, Monica and Rebecca, for their constant support, encouragement, and comfort.
Ehab Farag

I dedicate this book to an amazing woman, my wife Dalia, whose relentless support is my real strength; to Natalie, Krista, and Nicole, the true joys of my life; and last but not least, my mom whose prayers bless my steps.
Loran Mounir-Soliman

Contributors

Sanchit Ahuja, MD
Department of Anesthesiology
Pain Management and Perioperative Medicine
Henry Ford Health System
Detroit, Michigan

Wael Ali Sakr Esa, MD, PhD, MBA
Assistant Professor of Anesthesiology and Pain Management
CCLCM, Case Western Reserve University
General Anesthesiology, Pain Management
Section Head Orthopedic Anesthesia
Staff Outcome Research Anesthesiology Institute
Cleveland Clinic
Cleveland, Ohio

Kenneth C. Cummings III, MD, MS, FASA
Associate Professor of Anesthesiology
CCLCM, Case Western Reserve University
General Anesthesiology, Pain Management
Staff Outcome Research Anesthesiology Institute
Cleveland, Ohio

Rajeev Krishnaney Davison, MD
Anesthesiology Institute
Cleveland Clinic
Cleveland, Ohio

Hesham Elsharkawy, MD, MBA, MSc
Associate Professor of Anesthesiology
Case Western Reserve University
Outcomes Research Consortium
Anesthesiology Institute
Cleveland Clinic
Cleveland, Ohio

Jacob Ezell, MD
Fellow
Pain Management
University of California - San Diego
La Jolla, California

Ibrahim Farid, MD, FASA
Professor of Anesthesia, NEOMED
Director, Pediatric Pain Center
Pediatric Anesthesiologist
Akron Children's Hospital
Akron, Ohio

Mauricio Forero, MD, FIPP
Associate Professor
Department of Anesthesia
McMaster University
Hamilton, Ontario, Canada

Rami Edward Karroum, MD
Staff, Department of Pediatric Anesthesiology
Akron Children's Hospital
Assistant Professor of Anesthesiology, NEOMED
Akron, Ohio

Sree Kolli, MD
Assistant Professor
Department of General Anesthesiology & Regional Anesthesiology
Cleveland Clinic
Cleveland, Ohio

Kamal Maheshwari, MD, MPH
Anesthesiologist
Department of General Anesthesiology and Outcomes Research
Anesthesiology Institute
Cleveland Clinic Foundation
Cleveland, Ohio

Mohammed Faysal Malik, MD
Clinical Fellow
Regional Anesthesia & Acute Pain Management
Cleveland Clinic
Cleveland, Ohio

Junaid Mukhdomi, MD, MS
Resident
Pain Management
Cleveland Clinic Foundation
Cleveland, Ohio

Vicente Roqués-Escolar, MD
Anesthesiologist
Anesthesia and chronic pain treatment,
Hospital Universitario Virgen de la Arrixaca
Murcia, Spain

Ana Isabel Sànchez-Amador, MD
Anesthesiologist
Anesthesia and chronic pain treatment
Hospital Universitario Virgen de la Arrixaca
Murcia, Spain

John Seif, MD
Department of General Anesthesiology
Department of Pediatric Anesthesiology
Anesthesiology Institute
Cleveland Clinic
Cleveland, Ohio

Samantha Stamper, MD
Associated Professor
Anesthesiology and Acute Pain Management
Cleveland Clinic Foundation
Cleveland, Ohio

Chihiro Toda, MD
Clinical Fellow
Regional Anesthesia & Acute Pain Management,
Cleveland Clinic,
Cleveland, Ohio

Cynthia A. Wong, MD
Professor and Chair
Department of Anesthesia
University of Iowa
Iowa City, Iowa

Maria Yared, MD
Assistant Professor
Anesthesiology and Perioperative Medicine
Medical University of South Carolina (MUSC)
Charleston, South Carolina

Foreword

Richard W. Rosenquist, MD

It is a special privilege to be asked to write this foreword by the editors of *Brown's Atlas of Regional Anesthesia*, Drs. Ehab Farag and Loran Mounir-Soliman, with whom I have been working for the past 8.5 years. I met Dr. David L. Brown in 1988 when I attended my first ASRA meeting. Little did I know at that time that he would become a colleague, mentor, and friend in the years to come and have a tremendous impact on my academic and medical career choices and personal development. I have endeavored over the years to collect autographs from the primary authors of influential textbooks and one of the most treasured of these is the first edition of the *Atlas of Regional Anesthesia* signed with a note by David Brown. It has been an extremely useful textbook, and in the years following the publication of the first edition, I have watched the various iterations with interest, both as a consumer and author.

The first edition of the *Atlas of Regional Anesthesia* was written entirely by David L. Brown, MD while he was an Associate Professor of Anesthesiology at Mayo Medical School in Rochester, MN, and published in 1992. At a time when regional anesthesia was a blend of art and science and practitioners across the country were divided into various camps depending on where they had trained or who they believed, there were significant variations in practice and many lively discussions at ASRA meetings. Those who were heavily influenced by Dr. Daniel Moore frequently advocated for the use of multiple injections and paresthesias to confirm correct needle placement and did not ascribe to the fascial sheath approaches being promoted by Dr. Alon Winnie. Dr. Brown's goal in creating this *Atlas of Regional Anesthesia* was to "utilize a heavy proportion of art (i.e., illustrations) in the 'mix'", with the thought that "these images will provide physicians with an improved understanding of the anatomy and the technical details necessary for the successful use of regional anesthesia".

The first edition had 40 chapters, of which one was about local anesthetics and equipment, 6 were about anatomy, and 33 were about blocks. It was widely used and recognized as successful in its mission to improve understanding of the relevant anatomy and its application to regional anesthesia and care for patients with chronic and cancer pain at a time when visualizing the relevant anatomy by memory when performing blocks was critical.

The second edition in 1999 was also a single author publication that included one chapter about local anesthetics and equipment, six chapters of anatomy, and ten new chapters that included a chapter on Chronic and Cancer Pain Care: An Introduction and Perspective and nine new block chapters and modifications including continuous peripheral nerve blocks, infraclavicular block, the addition of saphenous block to the popliteal block chapter, paravertebral blocks, facet block, sacroiliac block, superior hypogastric plexus block cervical, and lumbar transforaminal injection, implantation of spinal drug delivery systems, and spinal cord stimulation.

The third edition in 2006 was the first multi-author publication with the addition of Drs. André P. Boezaart, James P. Rathmell, and Richard W. Rosenquist as authors as well as a new artist, Joanna Wild. The text had the same number of chapters as the second edition with modifications to the existing chapters to introduce new chapters including cervical and lumbar transforaminal injections.

The fourth edition in 2010 brought additional changes including three more contributors—Ursula A. Galway, Brian D. Sites, and Brian C. Spence. This edition was the first to address the rapidly growing use of ultrasound guidance for the performance of regional blocks. It increased the total number of chapters to 51 with a new chapter on transversus abdominis plane block and provided access to an online version with educational videos to demonstrate the role and use of ultrasound in the performance of regional anesthesia.

The fifth edition in 2016 brought extensive changes to the text and focus and a change in title to *Brown's Atlas of Regional Anesthesia*. The primary authors Ehab Farag and Loran Mounir-Soliman collaborated with David L. Brown as well as seven new contributors. The total number of chapters was expanded to 56 to incorporate new chapters on the pharmacology of local anesthetics in pediatrics, adductor canal block, trigeminal (Gasserian) ganglion block, subcostal transversus abdominal plane block, quadratus lumborum block, and four chapters on pediatric regional anesthesia using ultrasound: caudal block, ilioinguinal and iliohypogastric block, superficial cervical plexus block and rectus sheath block in pediatrics. Existing chapters on anatomy were supplemented with additional images from commonly used cross-sectional techniques such as computed tomography (CT) and magnetic resonance imaging (MRI), all of the chapters related to chronic and cancer pain were removed, and a second illustrator Joe Kanasz was added. Finally, the videos were updated to include blocks on real patients to provide additional insights to the reader.

This quote from Leonardo da Vinci was included in the first four editions of the book:

"And you who think to reveal the figure of a man in words, with his limbs arranged in all their different attitudes, banish the idea from you, for the more minute your description the more you will confuse the mind of the reader and the more you will lead him away from the knowledge of the thing described. It is necessary therefore for you to represent and describe."

Leonardo da Vinci
(1452-1519)
The Notebooks of Leonardo da Vinci, Vol. I, Ch. III

Despite the centuries that have passed since this quote was first penned, the truth of its admonition is just as relevant today as it was then. The primary goal of this book to "utilize a heavy proportion of art (i.e., illustrations) in the 'mix'", with the thought that "these images will provide physicians with an improved understanding of the anatomy and the technical details necessary for the successful use of regional anesthesia" has been maintained with focused improvements incorporated into each successive edition. The sixth edition scheduled for publication in 2020 has 10 new contributors and a reduction in the total number of chapters to 48 maintaining its focus on regional anesthesia and analgesia. This includes expansion of the types of blocks incorporating ultrasound guidance and the introduction of a section on obstetric regional anesthesia. As I review the list of new contributors and see those who have had the opportunity to work with Dr. Brown and those whose careers have been fostered and impacted by the new editors as well, I am confident that the tradition begun by Dr. Brown remains on sound footing. I am certain that this text will continue to be a valuable resource that incorporates the "art and science" of regional anesthesia into a single source that improves the successful use of regional anesthesia for generations to come. I look forward to adding this new edition to my library and collecting the autographs from the primary authors.

Preface to the Sixth Edition

What nobler employment or more advantageous to mankind than that of the man who correctly instructs the rising generation?

Cicero

In this new edition of *Brown's Atlas of Regional Anesthesia* we have tried our best to make those words of Cicero our motto. Since the last edition, several new blocks, specifically interfascial plane blocks, have been added to our clinical practice, including serratus anterior, PECS, erector spinae blocks, and many more. Therefore, in this edition we tried our best to delve deeper and to add all the nuances in the field of regional anesthesia. Furthermore, we added a new chapter for regional anesthesia written by a world-renowned obstetric anesthesiologist, Dr. Cynthia Wong. We have recruited well-versed authors in the field of regional anesthesia from both the United States and Europe to enrich the content of the text. In this edition, we tried to maintain the theme that characterizes *Brown's Atlas* from its first edition, which is the simplicity and easily performed techniques that can be routinely adopted in everyday clinical practice. All the videos in this edition, as in the previous one, have been performed on real patients in order to transform the atlas into a virtual workshop that can be used by physicians in their clinical practices. Moreover, we not only included the largest library of videos covering virtually every block in the atlas, but we also added an introductory video by Dr. Seif that discusses in detail commonly performed blocks. We hope this new edition will be useful to everyone interested in regional anesthesia from the novice to the master in the field.

We would like to express our gratitude to Drs. John Seif and Vicente Roqués-Escolar for their invaluable help in making the videos of the new edition. We would like to thank Mr. Joe Kanasz and Brandon Stelter for their extraordinary medical illustrations and video production, as well as Mrs. Tanya Smith, our editorial assistant, and Laura Klein and Sarah Barth from Elsevier for their generous help and support during the production process of this new edition.

Editors
Ehab Farag, MD, FRCA, FASA
Loran Mounir-Soliman, MD

Preface to the Fifth Edition

Regional anesthesia is one of the fundamental pillars of modern anesthesia. *The Atlas of Regional Anesthesia* by Dr. David Brown has become a classic textbook for regional anesthesia since its first edition in 1991. Since the last edition published in 2010, the use of ultrasound has changed the map of the practice of regional anesthesia. In this new edition, now *Brown's Atlas of Regional Anesthesia*, we combined the classical techniques from the original atlas with updated techniques and blocks using ultrasound. We believe the eyes do not see what the brain does not recognize. Therefore we felt it was important to include a number of ultrasound images and figures that identify the optimal position of the needle, as well as the best position of the patient and the anesthesiologist during the procedure. We have tried to retain the simplicity of the original atlas through self-explanatory figures and a few purposeful pearls to demonstrate the block performance. We tried to limit the techniques to the most commonly used and routinely adopted in our practice. Moreover, we have added videos of real patients for better clarification, showing real-time blocks performance in addition to advanced techniques using peripheral nerve catheters. Our aim is to transform the atlas into a virtual workshop that enables the reader to feel comfortable with the procedures after reading the text and watching the video. In this new edition we did rewrite all the blocks using ultrasound and added new blocks like subcostal, quadratus lumborum, paravertebral, adductor canal, and many more. We have added new chapters on regional anesthesia pharmacology and on regional anesthesia using ultrasound in pediatric patients. We hope this new edition will be useful to anyone interested in learning regional anesthesia or in mastering regional anesthesia.

We would like to thank Mr. Joe Kanasz for his extraordinary medical illustrations; Mrs. Mariela Madrilejos, our editorial assistant; Ms. Carole McMurray and Mr. William Schmitt from Elsevier for their help and incessant support during the production process of this edition.

Editors
Ehab Farag, MD, FRCA
Loran Mounir-Soliman, MD

Introduction to the Fourth Edition

The necessary, but somewhat artificial, separation of anesthetic care into regional or general anesthetic techniques often gives rise to the concept that these two techniques should not or cannot be mixed. Nothing could be further from the truth. To provide comprehensive regional anesthesia care, it is absolutely essential that the anesthesiologist be skilled in all aspects of anesthesia. This concept is not original: John Lundy promoted this idea in the 1920s when he outlined his concept of "balanced anesthesia." Even before Lundy promoted this concept, however, George Crile had written extensively on the concept of anociassociation.

It is often tempting, and quite human, to trace the evolution of a discipline back through the discipline's developmental family tree. When such an investigation is carried out for regional anesthesia, Louis Gaston Labat, MD, often receives credit for being central in its development. Nevertheless, Labat's interest and expertise in regional anesthesia were nurtured by Dr. Victor Pauchet of Paris, France, to whom Dr. Labat was an assistant. The real trunk of the developmental tree of regional anesthesia consists of the physicians willing to incorporate regional techniques into their early surgical practices. In Labat's original 1922 text, *Regional Anesthesia: Its Technique and Clinical Application,* Dr. William Mayo in the foreword stated:

The young surgeon should perfect himself in the use of regional anesthesia, which increases in value with the increase in the skill with which it is administered. The well-equipped surgeon must be prepared to use the proper anesthesia, or the proper combination of anesthesias, in the individual case. I do not look forward to the day when regional anesthesia will wholly displace general anesthesia; but undoubtedly it will reach and hold a very high position in surgical practice.

Perhaps if the current generation of both surgeons and anesthesiologists keeps Mayo's concept in mind, our patients will be the beneficiaries.

It appears that these early surgeons were better able to incorporate regional techniques into their practices because they did not see the regional block as the "end all." Rather, they saw it as part of a comprehensive package that had benefit for their patients. Surgeons and anesthesiologists in that era were able to avoid the flawed logic that often seems to pervade application of regional anesthesia today. These individuals did not hesitate to supplement their blocks with sedatives or light general anesthetics; they did not expect each and every block to be "100%." The concept that a block has failed unless it provides complete anesthesia without supplementation seems to have occurred when anesthesiology developed as an independent specialty. To be successful in carrying out regional anesthesia, we must be willing to get back to our roots and embrace the concepts of these early workers who did not hesitate to supplement their regional blocks. Ironically, today some consider a regional block a failure if the initial dose does not produce complete anesthesia; yet these same individuals complement our "general anesthetists" who utilize the concept of anesthetic titration as a goal. Somehow, we need to meld these two views into one that allows comprehensive, titrated care to be provided for all our patients.

As Dr. Mayo emphasized in Labat's text, it is doubtful that regional anesthesia will "ever wholly displace general anesthesia." Likewise, it is equally clear that general anesthesia will probably never be able to replace the appropriate use of regional anesthesia. One of the principal rationales for avoiding the use of regional anesthesia through the years has been that it was "expensive" in terms of operating room and physician time. As is often the case, when examined in detail, some accepted truisms need rethinking. Thus it is surprising that much of the renewed interest in regional anesthesia results from focusing on health care costs and the need to decrease the length and cost of hospitalization.

If regional anesthesia is to be incorporated successfully into a practice, there must be time for anesthesiologist and patient to discuss the upcoming operation and anesthetic prescription. Likewise, if regional anesthesia is to be effectively used, some area of an operating suite must be used to place the blocks before moving patients to the main operating room. Immediately at hand in this area must be both anesthetic and resuscitative equipment (such as regional trays), as well as a variety of local anesthetic drugs that span the timeline of anesthetic duration. Even after successful completion of the technical aspect of regional anesthesia, an anesthesiologist's work is really just beginning: it is as important to use appropriate sedation intraoperatively as it was preoperatively while the block was being administered.

Contents

Section I: Introduction

Chapter 1: Pharmacology 3
Kamal Maheshwari and David L. Brown with contributions from Brian D. Sites and Brian C. Spence

Chapter 2: Pharmacology of Local Anesthetics in Pediatrics 7
Ibrahim Farid and Rami Edward Karroum

Chapter 3: Equipment and Ultrasound 13
Kamal Maheshwari and Loran Mounir-Soliman

Section II: Upper Extremity Blocks

Chapter 4: Upper Extremity Block Anatomy 25
David L. Brown

Chapter 5: Interscalene Block 33
Ehab Farag with David L. Brown

Chapter 6: Supraclavicular Block 45
Ehab Farag and David L. Brown

Chapter 7: Suprascapular Block 55
Wael Ali Sakr Esa

Chapter 8: Infraclavicular Block 59
Kenneth C. Cummings III and Ehab Farag

Chapter 9: Axillary Block 69
Wael Ali Sakr Esa and David L. Brown

Chapter 10: Distal Upper Extremity Blocks 77
Sree Kolli and Sanchit Ahuja

Chapter 11: Intravenous Regional Block 85
David L. Brown

Section III: Lower Extremity Blocks

Chapter 12: Lower Extremity Block Anatomy 91
David L. Brown

Chapter 13: Lumbar Plexus Block 99
Loran Mounir-Soliman and David L. Brown

Chapter 14: Sciatic Block 107
Ehab Farag and David L. Brown

Chapter 15: Femoral Block 115
Ehab Farag and David L. Brown

Chapter 16: Ultrasound for Fascia Iliaca and Inguinal Region Blocks 127
Mohammed Faysal Malik and Chihiro Toda

Chapter 17: Lateral Femoral Cutaneous Nerve Block 131
Sanchit Ahuja and Sree Kolli

Chapter 18: Obturator Block 135
Loran Mounir-Soliman and David L. Brown

Chapter 19: Popliteal and Saphenous Block 141
Maria Yared and David L. Brown

Chapter 20: Adductor Canal Block 151
Ehab Farag

Chapter 21: Ankle Block 157
Maria Yared and David L. Brown

Section IV: Head and Neck Blocks

Chapter 22: Retrobulbar (Peribulbar) Block 167
David L. Brown

Chapter 23: Cervical Plexus Block 171
Jacob Ezell and Samantha Stamper

Chapter 24: Stellate Ganglion Block 177
Vicente Roqués-Escolar and Ana Isabel Sánchez-Amador

Section V: Airway Blocks

Chapter 25: Airway Block Anatomy 183
David L. Brown

Chapter 26: Glossopharyngeal Block 189
David L. Brown

Chapter 27: Superior Laryngeal Block 193
David L. Brown

Chapter 28: Translaryngeal Block 195
David L. Brown

Section VI: Truncal Blocks

Chapter 29: Truncal Block Anatomy 199
David L. Brown

Chapter 30: PECS and Pecto-Intercostal Blocks 203
Loran Mounir-Soliman

Chapter 31: Serratus Anterior Block 207
Loran Mounir-Soliman

Chapter 32: Ultrasound for Intercostal Block 211
Ehab Farag and Rajeev Krishnaney Davison

Chapter 33: Paravertebral Block 215
Ehab Farag

Chapter 34: Erector Spinae Plane Block 221
Vicente Roqués-Escolar and Mauricio Forero

Chapter 35: Rectus Sheath Block and Catheter in Adults 227
Jacob Ezell, Junaid Mukhdomi, Samantha Stamper, and John Seif

Chapter 36: Transversus Abdominis Plane Block (Classic Approach) 231
Loran Mounir-Soliman

Chapter 37: Subcostal Transversus Abdominal Plane Block 233
Ehab Farag

Chapter 38: Quadratus Lumborum Block 237
Hesham Elsharkawy and Ehab Farag

Section VII: Neuraxial Blocks

Chapter 39: Ultrasound-Assisted Neuraxial Blocks 243
Loran Mounir-Soliman

Chapter 40:	Spinal Block..................................249	Chapter 47:	Paravertebral Catheters in Pediatrics............293
	David L. Brown		John Seif
Chapter 41:	Epidural Block................................261		
	David L. Brown		
Chapter 42:	Caudal Block 273		
	David L. Brown		

Section IX: Obstetrics Regional Anesthesia

Chapter 48: Regional Techniques During Pregnancy and Delivery......................................297
Cynthia A. Wong

Section VIII: Pediatric Regional Using Ultrasound

Chapter 43:	Caudal Block in Pediatrics 281	
	John Seif	
Chapter 44:	Ilioinguinal and Iliohypogastric Block..........283	
	John Seif	
Chapter 45:	Superficial Cervical Plexus Block 287	
	John Seif	
Chapter 46:	Pudendal Nerve Block 291	
	John Seif	

Index..303

The videos accompanying this text can be accessed at www.expertconsult.com and includes over 40 ultrasound scans of procedures discussed in the book. The videos should be used in conjunction with the text and not as a standalone product.

SECTION 1
Introduction

Pharmacology

Kamal Maheshwari and David L. Brown
with contributions from Brian D. Sites and Brian C. Spence

Regional anesthesia is a fast-growing field with application in a wide range of surgical procedures. Better technique with the help of ultrasound, better and safer local anesthetics, and better drug delivery systems for continuous anesthesia all helped in gaining the current status. Far too often, those unfamiliar with regional anesthesia regard it as complex because of the long list of local anesthetics available and the varied techniques described. The goal throughout this book is to simplify regional anesthesia by providing specific information about various elements involved in decision making.

One of the first steps in simplifying regional anesthesia is to understand the two principal decisions necessary in prescribing a regional technique. First, the *appropriate technique* needs to be chosen for the patient, the surgical procedure, and the physicians involved. Second, the *appropriate local anesthetic and potential additives* must be matched to patient, procedure, regional technique, and physician. This book will detail how to integrate these concepts into your practice.

DRUGS

Numerous local anesthetic drugs are used in varied concentrations and with different additives. The decision to choose one particular local anesthetic is influenced by patient factors, surgical factors, and the available resources (cost factors). Not all procedures are created equal in terms of the amount of time needed to complete an operation, and the severity or nature of pain will be different. If anesthesiologists are to use regional techniques effectively, they must be able to choose a local anesthetic that lasts the right amount of time and provides effective anesthesia and analgesia. To do this, they need to understand the local anesthetic timeline from the shorter-acting to the longer-acting agents (Fig. 1.1) and the effect of additives. Also, they need to understand the factors associated with successful continuous nerve block management.

All local anesthetics share the basic structure of aromatic end, intermediate chain, and amine end (Fig. 1.2). This basic structure is subdivided clinically into two classes of drugs: the amino esters and the amino amides. The *amino esters* possess an ester linkage between the aromatic end and the intermediate chain. These drugs include cocaine, procaine, 2-chloroprocaine, and tetracaine (Figs. 1.3 and 1.4). The *amino amides* contain an amide link between the aromatic end and the intermediate chain. These drugs include lidocaine, prilocaine, etidocaine, mepivacaine, bupivacaine, and ropivacaine (see Figs. 1.3 and 1.4).

AMINO ESTERS

Cocaine was the first local anesthetic used clinically, and it is used today primarily for topical airway anesthesia. It is unique among the local anesthetics in that it is a vasoconstrictor rather than a vasodilator. Some anesthesia departments have limited the availability of cocaine because of fears of its abuse potential. In those institutions, mixtures of lidocaine and phenylephrine rather than cocaine are used to anesthetize the airway mucosa and shrink the mucous membranes.

Procaine was synthesized in 1904 by Einhorn, who was looking for a drug that was superior to cocaine and other solutions in use. Currently, procaine is seldom used for peripheral nerve or epidural blocks because of its low potency, slow onset, short duration of action, and limited power of tissue penetration. It is an excellent local anesthetic for skin infiltration, and its 10% form can be used as a short-acting (i.e., lasting <1 hour) spinal anesthetic.

Chloroprocaine has a rapid onset and a short duration of action. Its principal use is in producing epidural anesthesia for short procedures (i.e., lasting <1 hour). Its use declined during the early 1980s after reports of prolonged sensory and motor deficits resulting from unintentional subarachnoid administration of an intended epidural dose. The adverse effects were related to low pH and the use of sodium metabisulfite as a preservative. However, newer drug formulation has used EDTA as the preservative. Still, short-lived yet annoying back pain may develop after large (>30 mL) epidural doses of 3% chloroprocaine, presumably due to calcium binding by the EDTA. For spinal anesthesia, a dose of 30 and 60 mg 1%–2% 2-chloroprocinae can last up to 60 minutes, however its use is still limited.

	Procaine	Chloroprocaine	Lidocaine	Mepivacaine	Tetracaine	Ropivacaine	Etidocaine	Bupivacaine
Infiltration	45–60		75–90					180–360
+ epi	60–90		90–180					200–400
Peripheral			90–120	100–150		360–480		480–780
+ epi			120–180	120–220		480–600		600–900
SAB*	60–75		60		70–90			90–110
+ epi	75–90		75–100		100–150			100–150
phenylephrine†	90–120				200–300			
Epidural		45–60	80–120	90–140		140–200	120–200	165–225
+ epi		60–90	120–180	140–200		160–220	150–225	180–240

*Subarachnoid block.
†For lower extremity surgery.

Fig. 1.1 Local anesthetic timeline (length in minutes of surgical anesthesia). *Epi,* epinephrine.

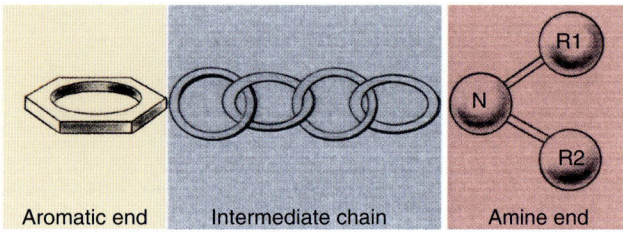

Fig. 1.2 Basic local anesthetic structure.

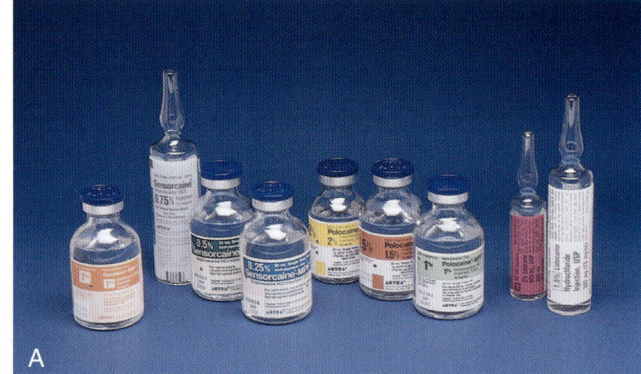

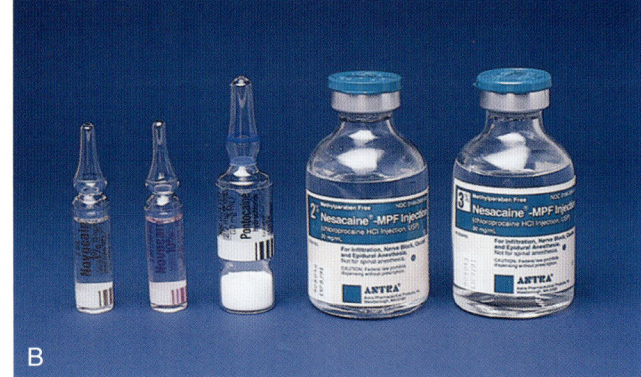

Fig. 1.3 Local anesthetics commonly used in the United States. (A) Amides. (B) Esters.

Tetracaine, first synthesized in 1931, has become widely used in the United States for spinal anesthesia. It may be used as an isobaric, hypobaric, or hyperbaric solution for spinal anesthesia. Without epinephrine, it typically lasts 1.5 to 2.5 hours, and with the addition of epinephrine, it may last up to 4 hours for lower extremity procedures. Tetracaine is also an effective topical airway anesthetic, although caution must be used because of the potential for systemic side effects. Tetracaine is available as a 1% solution for intrathecal use or as anhydrous crystals that are reconstituted as tetracaine solution by adding sterile water immediately before use. Tetracaine is not as stable as procaine or lidocaine in solution, and the crystals undergo deterioration over time. Nevertheless, when a tetracaine spinal anesthetic is ineffective, one should question technique before "blaming" the drug.

AMINO AMIDES

Lidocaine was the first clinically used amide local anesthetic, having been introduced by Lofgren in 1948. Lidocaine has become the most widely used local anesthetic in the world because of its inherent potency; rapid onset; tissue penetration; and effectiveness during infiltration, peripheral nerve block, and both epidural and spinal blocks. During peripheral nerve block, a 1% to 1.5% solution is often effective in producing an acceptable motor blockade, whereas during epidural block, a 2% solution seems most effective. In spinal anesthesia, a 5% solution in dextrose is most commonly used, although it may also be used as a 0.5% hypobaric solution in a volume of 6 to 8 mL. Others use lidocaine as a short-acting 2% solution in a volume of 2 to 3 mL. The suggestion that lidocaine causes an unacceptable frequency of neurotoxicity with spinal use needs to be balanced against its long history of use. We believe that the basic science research may not

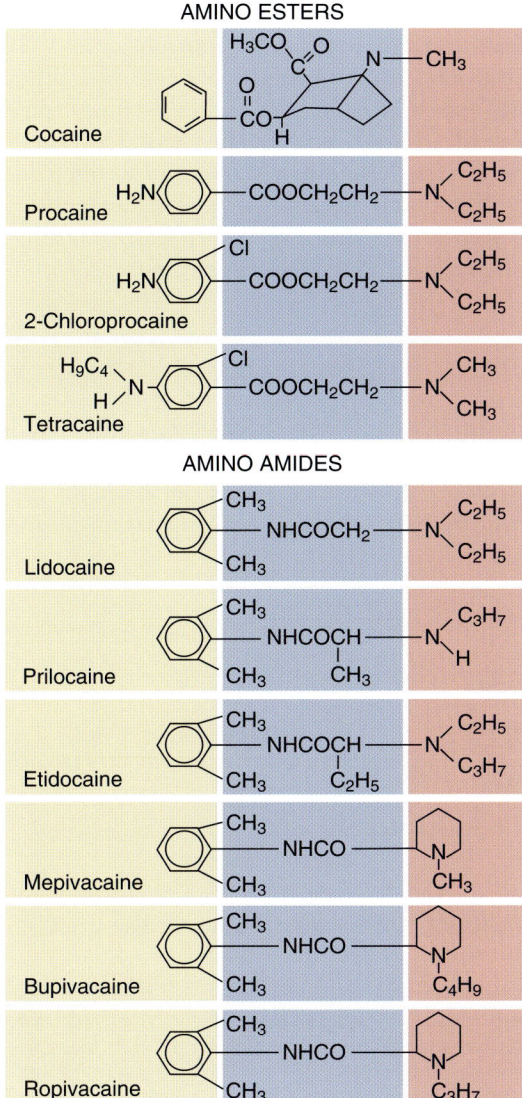

Fig. 1.4 Chemical structure of commonly used amino ester and amino amide local anesthetics.

anesthesia. Prilocaine is not more widely used because, when metabolized, it can produce both orthotoluidine and nitrotoluidine, agents in methemoglobin formation.

Etidocaine is chemically related to lidocaine and is a long-acting amide local anesthetic. Etidocaine is associated with profound motor blockade and is best used when this attribute can be of clinical advantage. It has a more rapid onset of action than bupivacaine, but is used less frequently. Those clinicians using etidocaine often use it for the initial epidural dose and then use bupivacaine for subsequent epidural injections.

Mepivacaine is structurally related to lidocaine, and the two drugs have similar actions. Overall, mepivacaine is slightly longer acting than lidocaine, and this difference in duration is accentuated when epinephrine is added to the solutions.

Bupivacaine is a long-acting local anesthetic that can be used for infiltration, peripheral nerve block, and epidural and spinal anesthesia. Useful concentrations of the drug range from 0.125% to 0.75%. By altering the concentration of bupivacaine, sensory and motor blockade can be separated. Lower concentrations provide sensory blockade principally, and as the concentration is increased, the effectiveness of motor blockade increases with it. If an anesthesiologist had to select a single drug and a single drug concentration, 0.5% bupivacaine would be a logical choice because at that concentration it is useful for peripheral nerve block, subarachnoid block, and epidural block. Cardiotoxicity during systemic toxic reactions with bupivacaine became a concern in the 1980s. Although it is clear that bupivacaine alters myocardial conduction more dramatically than lidocaine, the need for appropriate and rapid resuscitation during any systemic toxic reaction cannot be overemphasized. Levobupivacaine is the single enantiomer (L-isomer) of bupivacaine and appears to have a systemic toxicity profile similar to that of ropivacaine, and clinically it has effects similar to those of racemic bupivacaine.

Ropivacaine is another long-acting local anesthetic, similar to bupivacaine; it was introduced in the United States in 1996. It may offer an advantage over bupivacaine because experimentally it appears to be less cardiotoxic.

completely reflect the typical clinical situation. In any event, we have reduced the total dose of subarachnoid lidocaine we administer to less than 75 mg per spinal procedure, inject it more rapidly than in the past, and no longer use it for continuous subarachnoid techniques. Patients often report that lidocaine causes the most common local anesthetic allergies. However, many of these reported allergies are simply epinephrine reactions resulting from intravascular injection of the local anesthetic epinephrine mixture, often during dental injection.

Prilocaine is structurally related to lidocaine, although it causes significantly less vasodilation than lidocaine and thus can be used without epinephrine. Prilocaine is formulated for infiltration, peripheral nerve block, and epidural anesthesia. Its anesthetic profile is similar to that of lidocaine, although in addition to producing less vasodilation, it has less potential for systemic toxicity in equal doses. This attribute makes it particularly useful for intravenous regional

Initial studies also suggest that ropivacaine may produce less motor block than that produced by bupivacaine, with similar analgesia. Ropivacaine may also be slightly shorter acting than bupivacaine, with useful drug concentrations ranging from 0.25% to 1%. Many practitioners believe that ropivacaine may offer particular advantages for postoperative analgesic infusions and obstetric analgesia.

Levobupivacaine is a pure S enantiomer of bupivacaine with lower cardiac toxicity profile but similar pharmacokinetic profile. Levobupivacaine potency is less than bupivacaine and more than ropivacaine. It can be used for all peripheral nerve blocks and neuraxial blocks.

Exparel (bupivacaine liposome injectable suspension) is a new drug that utilizes the DepoFoam technology developed by Pacira Pharmaceuticals, Inc. (Parsippany, NJ, USA). The bupivacaine is encapsulated in multivesicular liposomes, from which sustained release of the drug happens in the infiltrated areas for up to 72 hours. Exparel is indicated for single-dose infiltration in adults to produce postsurgical local analgesia and as an interscalene brachial plexus nerve block to produce postsurgical regional analgesia. The 20 ml Exparel can be mixed with saline or plain bupivacaine, if larger infiltration volume is required.

VASOCONSTRICTORS

Vasoconstrictors are often added to local anesthetics to prolong the duration of action and improve the quality of the local anesthetic block. Although it is still unclear whether vasoconstrictors actually allow local anesthetics to have a longer duration of block or are effective because they produce additional antinociception through α-adrenergic action, their clinical effect is not in question.

Epinephrine is the most common vasoconstrictor used; overall, the most effective concentration, excluding spinal anesthesia, is a 1:200,000 concentration. When epinephrine is added to local anesthetic in the commercial production process, it is necessary to add stabilizing agents because epinephrine rapidly loses its potency on exposure to air and light. The added stabilizing agents lower the pH of the local anesthetic solution into the 3 to 4 range and, because of the higher pKa values of local anesthetics, slow the onset of effective regional block. Thus if epinephrine is to be used with local anesthetics, it should be added at the time the block is performed, at least for the initial block. In subsequent injections made during continuous epidural block, commercial preparations of local anesthetic–epinephrine solutions can be used effectively.

Phenylephrine also has been used as a vasoconstrictor, principally with spinal anesthesia; effective prolongation of block can be achieved by adding 2 to 5 mg of phenylephrine to the spinal anesthetic drug. Norepinephrine also has been used as a vasoconstrictor for spinal anesthesia, although it does not appear to be as long lasting as epinephrine or to have any advantages over it. Because most local anesthetics are vasodilators, the addition of epinephrine often does not decrease blood flow as many fear it will; rather, the combination of local anesthetic and epinephrine results in tissue blood flow similar to that before injection.

LOCAL ANESTHETIC TOXICITY

Local anesthetic can cause direct nerve injury and/or systemic toxicity. If systemic toxicity is suspected, it should be treated swiftly with Intralipid. See Table 1.1 for the local anesthetic systemic toxicity (LAST) management protocol.

Table 1.1

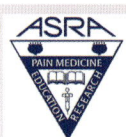

AMERICAN SOCIETY OF REGIONAL ANESTHESIA AND PAIN MEDICINE

Checklist for Treatment of Local Anesthetic Systemic Toxicity

The pharmacologic treatment of Local Anesthetic Systemic Toxicity (LAST) is different from other cardiac arrest scenarios.

- **Get Help**
- **Initial Focus**
  - **Airway management:** ventilate with 100% oxygen
  - **Seizure suppression:** benzodiazepines are preferred; **AVOID propofol** in patients having signs of cardiovascular instability
  - **Alert** the nearest facility having **cardiopulmonary bypass** capability
- **Management of Cardiac Arrhythmias**
  - **Basic and Advanced Cardiac Life Support (ACLS)** will require adjustment of medications and perhaps prolonged effort
  - **AVOID vasopressin, calcium channel blockers, beta blockers, or local anesthetic**
  - **REDUCE individual epinephrine doses to <1 µg/kg**
- **Lipid Emulsion (20%) Therapy** (values in parentheses are for 70 kg patient)
  - **Bolus 1.5 mL/kg** (lean body mass) intravenously over 1 minute (~100 mL)
  - **Continuous infusion 0.25 mL/kg/min** (~18 mL/min; adjust by roller clamp)
  - Repeat bolus once or twice for persistent cardiovascular collapse
  - Double the infusion rate to 0.5 mL/kg/min if blood pressure remains low
  - **Continue infusion** for at least 10 minutes after attaining circulatory stability
  - Recommended upper limit: Approximately 10 mL/kg lipid emulsion over the first 30 minutes
- **Post LAST events at** www.lipidrescue.org and report use of lipid to www.lipidregistry.org

Data from: American Society of Regional Anesthesia and Pain Medicine Checklist for Managing Local Anesthetic Systemic Toxicity: 2012 Version.

Pharmacology of Local Anesthetics in Pediatrics

Ibrahim Farid and Rami Edward Karroum

Key Points

Neonates and infants are more prone to developing systemic toxicity to local anesthetics (LAs), particularly amide LAs, compared with older children and adults. This is due to reduced plasma concentration of α_1-acid glycoprotein with higher unbound fraction and decreased clearance of amide LAs.

Higher baseline heart rates in neonates and infants predispose them to increased sensitivity for bupivacaine-induced cardiotoxicity compared with adults. This is due to the strong affinity of bupivacaine for the fast sodium channels, resulting in prolonged blockade of these channels in the cardiac conduction system and a profound decrease in ventricular conduction velocity.

Chloroprocaine is the LA of choice for epidural infusion in neonates and small infants due to its very low risk of systemic toxicity and accumulation compared with amide LAs in this age group as well as easier dosing and pump programming.

Regional anesthesia is usually performed under general anesthesia, which may mask the earliest signs of systemic toxicity, particularly central nervous system (CNS) signs. Therefore refractory cardiovascular collapse may be the first and only sign in pediatric patients.

It is recommended that an epinephrine-containing test dose be used in all regional blocks before giving the full bolus dose. Order of sensitivity for detection of unintentional intravascular injection in pediatric patients when a test dose of LAs mixed with epinephrine is given, from most to least sensitive, is:

> Increase T wave amplitude and ST segment changes > increase in systolic blood pressure more than 10% > increase in heart rate 10% to 15% above baseline heart rate before administration of test dose.

Total doses of LAs should not exceed the maximum allowable dose under any circumstances. The dose should be based on the lean body weight rather than the actual body weight, particularly in obese patients.

INTRODUCTION

LAs are divided into two main chemical compounds: the amides and the esters.

Amide LAs are metabolized exclusively in the liver by cytochrome P450 enzymes. These enzymes reach adult activity level by 9 months to 1 year of age. Therefore neonates and infants have a decreased clearance of amide LAs. Amide LAs bind to serum proteins. α_1-acid glycoprotein is the major serum protein that binds amide LAs. Albumin has a very low affinity to bind amide LAs. However, being the most abundant protein in serum, albumin binding capacity to amide LAs is not insignificant.

Infants have a decreased level of α_1-acid glycoprotein and albumin. Adult levels of protein binding are reached at about 1 year of age. Therefore neonates and infants are more prone to developing toxicity from amide LAs due to a higher serum-free fraction and lower clearance rate. The susceptibility to cardiac toxicity is amplified by increased heart rates. Due to their higher baseline heart rates neonates and infants are more sensitive than adults to amide LA-induced cardiotoxicity.

Neonates and infants have a relatively larger volume of distribution (VD) of amide LAs compared with adults. Toxicity will be more likely to occur following repeated doses and/or continuous infusion. This can be explained by the fact that larger VD prevents high serum drug concentrations from occurring after a slow incremental injection of a single dose of amide LAs.

Commonly used amide LAs in children include lidocaine, ropivacaine, bupivacaine, its L-enantiomer levobupivacaine, and eutectic mixture of local anesthetics (EMLA) cream.

Ester LAs are degraded in plasma by cholinesterases. Although neonates and infants have a lower level of cholinesterases, this has not been shown to be of clinical significance. Commonly used ester LAs in children include tetracaine and 2% to 3% chloroprocaine. Chloroprocaine use for continuous epidural analgesia in neonates and infants has been on the rise due to its rare incidence of systemic toxicity.

AMIDE LOCAL ANESTHETICS

BUPIVACAINE

This is the most commonly used amide LA for regional blockade in pediatric anesthesia. Its long duration of action is related to its high binding to plasma proteins. Adding epinephrine will not result in further prolongation of the duration of action. However, epinephrine will reduce the rate of systemic absorption and the peak plasma concentration of bupivacaine. Its relatively slow onset of action is due to its high pKa of 8.1. It is a racemic mixture of levorotatory (L) and dextrorotatory (D) enantiomers; the L-enantiomer is the bioactive form, and the D-enantiomer is responsible for its toxicity. Toxicity from bupivacaine can be serious, ranging from CNS excitation to cardiovascular collapse. Direct cardiac toxicity is due to prolonged blockade of the sodium channels in the cardiac conduction system, resulting in a profound decrease in ventricular conduction velocity. This phenomenon is markedly amplified by tachycardia due to the strong affinity of bupivacaine for the fast sodium channels. Stereoselectivity of the sodium channel in the open state, however, has not been demonstrated.

The threshold for toxicity occurs at a bupivacaine level of 2 to 4 µg/mL. The maximum dose of bupivacaine is 2.5 to 3 mg/kg. The most commonly used concentration for single-shot peripheral nerve block and caudal epidural is 0.25% (Table 2.1). After a single administration, analgesia usually lasts for 3 to 4 hours. For an epidural catheter the loading dose is 0.05 mL/kg/spinal segment or between 0.5 and 1 mL/kg, not to exceed the maximum dose of 2.5 mg/kg. For continuous epidural infusion a concentration ranging from 0.0625% to 0.125% is used and usually runs at a dose of 0.2 to 0.4 mg/kg/h (Table 2.2).

LIPOSOMAL BUPIVACAINE

Recently, a liposome bupivacaine has been approved by the Food and Drug Administration (FDA) for use in adults as a local anesthetic injected into the surgical site for postsurgical pain relief. The liposome bupivacaine formulation incorporates liposome-encapsulated bupivacaine (DepoFoam) and a small amount of extraliposomal bupivacaine. The liposome-encapsulated component permits bupivacaine release over an extended period. The extraliposomal component allows for rapid release and relatively rapid onset of action. There are some recent studies evaluating its use in the epidural space in adults as an alternative to continuous bupivacaine infusion through an indwelling epidural catheter. Liposomal bupivacaine is not currently approved for use in children. If approved, it may offer an attractive alternative for children in whom an indwelling catheter is not an option, but in whom prolonged regional blockade provided by liposome bupivacaine formulation may be beneficial.

LEVOBUPIVACAINE (L-ENANTIOMER OF BUPIVACAINE)

Levobupivacaine has almost the same blocking properties and pharmacokinetics as its racemic counterpart bupivacaine. The effect on the cardiac conduction system is stereospecific, with the L-enantiomer having much less of an effect than the D-enantiomer present in the racemic mixture of bupivacaine. As a result, levobupivacaine carries a reduced risk of cardiac toxicity compared with bupivacaine. It is currently unavailable in the United States.

ROPIVACAINE

This exists as an L-enantiomer. It is chemically similar to bupivacaine, but differs from it structurally having a propyl (three-carbon) side chain rather than a butyl (four-carbon) side chain. In an equipotent dose it carries a lower risk of cardiac and neurological toxicities compared with bupivacaine. This makes ropivacaine an attractive alternative to bupivacaine in pediatric patients. The data available from studies on infants and children do not report greater

Table 2.1 Single-Shot Caudal Epidural Dose of Local Anesthetics

Local anesthetic	Concentration	Dose (mg/kg)	Dose (mL/kg)
Bupivacaine	0.25% (2.5 mg/mL)	2.5	1
Ropivacaine	0.2% (2 mg/mL)	2	1

Table 2.2 Suggested Epidural Infusion Concentrations and Rates for Pediatric Patients

Local anesthetic	Maximum rate of infusion and suggested infusion concentration (conc.)		
	Neonates and infants up to 6 months	Infants (6 months to 1 year)	Children older than 1 year
Chloroprocaine[a]	Conc. of 2%. Rate of 5 to 15 mg/kg/h.	N/A[c]	N/A[c]
Bupivacaine	Conc. of 0.0625%. Rate of 0.2 mg/kg/h for no more than 48 hours.	Conc. of 0.0625% to 0.125%. Rate of 0.3 to 0.4 mg/kg/h. Reduce the infusion rate 30% after 48 hours and discontinue after 72 hours.	Conc. of 0.0625% to 0.125%. Rate of 0.4 mg/kg/h.
Ropivacaine[b]	Conc. of 0.1%. Rate of 0.2 mg/kg/h for no more than 72 hours. Reduce the infusion rate 30% after 48 hours.	Conc. of 0.1% to 0.2%. Rate of 0.3 to 0.4 mg/kg/h. Reduce the infusion rate 30% after 48 hours.	Conc. of 0.1% to 0.2%. Rate of 0.4 mg/kg/h.

[a]Chloroprocaine is the first choice for epidural infusion in neonates due to reduced risk of systemic toxicity compared with amide LAs.
[b]Ropivacaine is the second choice for epidural infusion in neonates due to its better toxicity profile compared with bupivacaine.
[c]N/A, nonapplicable. Chloroprocaine is not usually used in this age group and is replaced by amide LAs.

sparing of motor function following ropivacaine blockade compared with bupivacaine. Adult studies are conflicting in this regard.

The most commonly used concentration for single-shot caudal and single-shot peripheral nerve block is 0.2% (see Table 2.1). For an epidural catheter, the loading dose is 0.05 mL/kg/spinal segment or between 0.5 and 1 mL/kg, not to exceed the maximum dose of 3 mg/kg. For continuous infusion, the concentration range is from 0.1% to 0.2% and usually runs at a dose of 0.2 to 0.5 mg/kg/h (see Table 2.2).

LIDOCAINE

Lidocaine is not commonly used in pediatrics due to its short duration of analgesia. The amides ropivacaine and bupivacaine are more commonly used instead.

EMLA CREAM

This is a eutectic mixture of equal quantities of lidocaine 2.5% and prilocaine 2.5%. It is commonly used to provide transdermal local anesthesia in pediatric patients. Methemoglobinemia has been reported with the use of EMLA cream. Therefore the maximum total surface area to which the cream is applied should be calculated in advance, and the maximum allowable dose should never be exceeded (Table 2.3). This is particularly important in neonates. However, close attention should also be paid to the dose used in infants and toddlers. EMLA cream should be applied only to intact skin, and the dose should be reduced in case it is applied to mucous membranes. Other reported side effects include blanching and rash at the site of application. The duration of action is 1 to 2 hours.

LIDOCAINE AND TETRACAINE (SYNERA) TRANSDERMAL PATCH

This is a combination of lidocaine, an amide LA, and tetracaine, an ester LA. The drug formulation is an emulsion in which the oil phase is a 1:1 eutectic mixture of lidocaine 7% and tetracaine 7%. Each patch contains 70 mg lidocaine and 70 mg tetracaine and has a total skin contact area of 50 cm, and an active drug-containing area of 10 cm². The eutectic mixture has a melting point below room temperature, and therefore both LAs exist as a liquid oil rather than as crystals. The patch has a heating component that begins to heat once the patch is removed from the pouch and is exposed to oxygen in the air. It increases skin temperature slightly to increase blood flow into the area and speeds up delivery of LAs to provide anesthesia to a depth of almost 7 mm. It is used to facilitate venipuncture, intravenous cannulation, and some superficial dermatological procedures. It should be applied only to intact skin. Methemoglobinemia has been reported, and caution should be exercised in patients with congenital or idiopathic methemoglobinemia. Caution should be exercised in patients with pseudocholinesterase deficiency, as they are at greater risk of tetracaine toxicity.

If being used with other products containing an LA consider the potential for additive effects. The heating component contains iron powder and must be removed before magnetic resonance imaging (MRI). Application of the patch for a longer duration than recommended, or simultaneous or sequential application of multiple patches, is not recommended because of the risk for increased drug absorption and possible adverse reactions. Cutting the patch or removing the top cover could cause the patch to heat to temperatures that could result in thermal injury. On the other hand, covering the holes on the top side of the patch could cause the patch not to heat. The most common side effects are local skin reactions such as redness of the skin and swelling; these reactions are generally mild and resolve spontaneously after discontinuation of the patch. Safety and effectiveness of the patch have been established in patients 3 years of age and older. Apply the patch for 20 to 30 minutes prior to venipuncture or intravenous cannulation. For superficial dermatological procedures such as superficial excision or shave biopsy, apply the patch for 30 minutes prior to the procedure. A topical cream of lidocaine and tetracaine (Pliaglis) also exists, but is indicated only for adult use.

ESTER LOCAL ANESTHETICS

TETRACAINE

Tetracaine is the most commonly used LA for spinal anesthesia in children. Some centers use spinal anesthesia with tetracaine as the sole anesthetic for inguinal hernia repair in premature or expremature neonates. This practice is most relevant for those premature neonates who are less than 60 weeks postconceptual age at the time of surgery. This population is at risk for developing postoperative apnea, and the use of spinal anesthesia may decrease the incidence of this complication.

Neonates have a larger total volume of cerebrospinal fluid (CSF) compared with adults (4 mL/kg compared with 2 mL/kg, respectively). In addition, 50% of the total CSF volume is in the spinal portion of the subarachnoid space compared with only 25% of the total CSF volume in adults. Neonates also have a more rapid turnover of CSF than adults. As a result, neonates require larger doses of LAs for spinal anesthesia, and the duration of the spinal block is shorter.

Tetracaine is used in a concentration of 1% (10 mg/mL), and the calculated dose is mixed in an equivalent volume of dextrose 10% to make the solution hyperbaric. The final concentration of tetracaine is 0.5% (5 mg/mL). For inguinal

Table 2.3 Maximum Recommended Doses and Application Areas for EMLA Cream

Body weight and age	Maximum total dose (g)	Maximum surface area (cm²)
0 to 3 months or <5 kg	1	10
3 to 12 months and 5 to 10 kg	2	20
1 to 6 years and 10 to 20 kg	10	100 1
7 to 12 years and >20 kg	20	200

Table 2.4 Tetracaine Dose for Spinal Anesthesia for Inguinal Hernia Repair

Local anesthetic	Age and weight	Dose (mg/kg)	Duration of action
Tetracaine 1% in 10% dextrose (1:1 dilution) (hyperbaric)	Neonates and less than 5 kg[a] Infants and 5 to 15 kg Children and greater than 15 kg	0.5 to 0.6 0.3 to 0.4 0.2 to 0.3	90 to 120 minutes[b]

[a]Maximum dose of 1 mg/kg can be used to achieve mid to high thoracic level dermatomes.
[b]Duration can be extended by 30% with the addition of epinephrine.

hernia repair neonates less than 5 kg require the largest dose of 0.5 to 0.6 mg/kg. For infants 5 to 15 kg, the dose is 0.3 to 0.4 mg/kg, and for children greater than 15 kg, the dose is 0.2 to 0.3 mg/kg (Table 2.4).

The duration of the block is 90 to 120 minutes. This can be extended by 30% with the addition of epinephrine 1:100,000. If a higher block level is desired in neonates the dose can be increased up to a maximum of 1 mg/kg. This dose can result in a block that extends to a dermatome height in the mid to upper thoracic region.

CHLOROPROCAINE

Chloroprocaine is increasingly used to provide continuous epidural infusion for postoperative pain control in neonates. It is rapidly metabolized by cholinesterases, with an elimination half-life of a few minutes. Although neonates have a reduced level of plasma esterases compared with adults this is clinically insignificant. Therefore the incidence of systemic toxicity is rare and the risk of accumulation is minimal. This safety profile allows better analgesia in neonates as it allows the use of higher infusion rates and thus wider dermatomal coverage compared with amide LAs. Chloroprocaine has a rapid onset of action (5 to 10 minutes) because of its high tissue penetrance. It has a short duration of action (45 minutes) that can be prolonged to 70 to 90 minutes with the addition of epinephrine. Its potency is 25% that of bupivacaine or tetracaine. Epidural anesthesia is achieved by administering up to 1 mL/kg of 2% to 3% chloroprocaine with epinephrine 1:200,000 (maximum dose of chloroprocaine: 20 to 30 mg/kg). For continuous epidural analgesia rates refer to Table 2.2.

TOXICITY OF LOCAL ANESTHETICS

DIRECT NEUROTOXICITY

All LAs are potentially capable of producing direct neurotoxicity. This complication is rare and conclusive human studies are still lacking in this field. However, animal studies show that the risk is higher on the developing nervous system and is directly related to the concentration of the LA. Therefore neonates and infants are at higher risk since their nervous system is still developing. The recommendation is to avoid the use of a high concentration of LAs in this age group.

SYSTEMIC TOXICITY

Predisposing Factors

Neonates and infants are more prone to developing systemic toxicity to LAs, particularly amide LAs, compared with older children and adults. This is due to:

- Reduced plasma concentration of α_1-acid glycoprotein in this age group, resulting in higher unbound fraction of amide LAs, which is responsible for toxicity.
- Decreased clearance of amide LAs in neonates and infants due to decreased metabolism in the liver by cytochrome P450 enzymes.
- Regional anesthesia is usually performed under general anesthesia, which may mask the earliest signs of systemic toxicity, particularly CNS signs. Therefore refractory cardiovascular collapse may be the first and only sign.
- Higher baseline heart rates in neonates and infants predispose them to increased sensitivity for bupivacaine-induced cardiotoxicity compared with adults.

Clinical Picture

- Systemic toxicity can result from accidental intravascular injection of LAs or secondary to systemic absorption of LAs from the regional block site, particularly when maximum recommended doses are exceeded.
- Systemic toxicity is consistent with signs of CNS and cardiac toxicity.
- Regional anesthesia is usually performed under general anesthesia in pediatric patients. Although general anesthesia with inhalational agents raises the threshold for seizure, it will also lower the threshold for cardiac toxicity. Therefore, general anesthesia may confound the diagnosis of systemic toxicity, and the first sign may be cardiovascular collapse.
- The bupivacaine threshold for cardiac toxicity is lower than its CNS toxicity in pediatrics. Therefore in pediatrics signs of cardiac toxicity may precede signs of CNS toxicity, or may be the only sign of systemic toxicity. This is different from adults where signs of CNS toxicity usually precede cardiac toxicity.
- Signs of systemic toxicity under general anesthesia may be nonspecific and consist of muscle rigidity,

- unexplained hypoxemia, unexplained tachycardia, dysrhythmias, and cardiovascular collapse.
- When bupivacaine is mixed with epinephrine (usually in a 1:200,000 dilution), the earliest and most reliable sign of unintentional intravascular injection is increase in the T wave amplitude of more than 50% compared with the baseline, with associated ST segment changes. These electrocardiogram (EKG) changes are very sensitive. They occur within 60 seconds of injection. If only a small test dose is given, these changes are transient and brief and do not progress into cardiovascular collapse.
- Following a test dose of bupivacaine and epinephrine, tachycardia is not a sensitive sign for unintentional intravascular injection in pediatrics.
- Order of sensitivity for detection of unintentional intravascular injection in pediatrics, from most to least sensitive, is:

  Increase T wave amplitude and ST segment changes > increase in systolic blood pressure more than 10% > increase in heart rate 10% to 15% above baseline heart rate before administration of test dose.

- After the age of 8 years, T wave changes are less sensitive for the detection of intravascular injection.
- If a bolus dose of bupivacaine is unintentionally injected intravascularly, cardiac arrhythmias and subsequent cardiovascular collapse develop rapidly.

Prevention/Reducing the Risk

- Careful calculation of total doses of LAs administered.
- Total doses of LAs should not exceed the maximum allowable dose under any circumstances (Table 2.5).
- The dose should be based on the lean body weight rather than the actual body weight, particularly in obese patients. Lean body weight can be extrapolated by knowing actual body weight and ideal body weight.
- The dose should be reduced in pediatric patients with associated comorbidities such as patients with liver failure or congestive heart failure (CHF).
- Decrease bolus dose of amide LAs by 30% for all infants younger than 6 months of age.
- Limit the duration of amide LA infusion to no more than 48 hours for bupivacaine and 72 hours for ropivacaine for all infants and neonates less than 6 months of age (see Table 2.2).

Table 2.5 Maximum Recommended Doses of Commonly Used Local Anesthetics

Local anesthetic	Dose (mg/kg)
Bupivacaine	2.5 to 3
Ropivacaine	3
Levobupivacaine	3
Lidocaine/lidocaine + epinephrine	4/7
2-Chloroprocaine	20

- Chloroprocaine is the LA of choice for epidural infusion in neonates and small infants due to its very low risk of systemic toxicity and accumulation compared with amide LAs in this age group.
- When mixing two different LAs, toxicity is additive. Thus when mixing equivalent amounts of two different LAs the maximum dose for each should be reduced by 50%.
- Using ropivacaine or levobupivacaine instead of bupivacaine may reduce the risk of cardiotoxicity.
- When performing an epidural block, aspiration of blood or CSF through the needle or catheter may indicate that the tip is within a vessel or subarachnoid space, respectively. However, a false negative aspiration test tends to occur frequently in pediatric patients. This is related to the fact that even the smallest applied negative pressure can result in collapse of the thin-walled vessels.
- The recommendation is to use an epinephrine-containing test dose in all regional blocks before giving the full bolus dose. This will help detect unintentional intravascular injections as mentioned earlier.
- The only exception for the use of an epinephrine-containing test dose is the block that involves an end artery, such as penile and digital blocks.
- Slow and intermittent injection of all bolus doses should occur over several minutes. Rapid injection can result in systemic toxicity, even if the maximum allowable dose is not exceeded and the injection is not intravascular. This results from a rapid surge of LAs in the blood beyond the protein-carrying capacity of neonates and infants.
- Absorption of LAs from the site of regional block from higher to lower is:

  Intercostal > caudal > lumbar epidural > thoracic epidural brachial > femoral > sciatic.

- Ilioinguinal/iliohypogastric nerve blocks, particularly in children less than 15 kg, are associated with alarming levels of bupivacaine in the blood, even when half the maximum recommended dose is used. Therefore this block should be performed under ultrasound guidance, as it can limit the required volume needed to perform the block. A volume of 0.2 mL/kg of ropivacaine 0.2% is used in an ultrasound-guided block compared with the anatomic landmark method that may require the use of up to 1 mL/kg.
- Whenever a regional block is performed in pediatric patients all resuscitation equipment should be immediately available.

Treatment

Effective CPR

- This is the first line of treatment in conjunction with Intralipid administration.
- This includes securing the airway and ensuring adequate breathing and circulation through the performance of quality chest compression.

Intralipid 20%

- This is recommended as the next line of treatment for cardiotoxicity induced by bupivacaine and ropivacaine.
- Give immediately and without delay *in conjunction* with cardiopulmonary resuscitation (CPR).
- Acts as a "lipid sink" by promoting dissociation of bupivacaine from the myocardium and therefore shortens the duration of bupivacaine-induced asystole.
- Pediatric dose is similar to adult doses and consists of a bolus of 1.5 mL/kg over 1 minute. Repeat bolus dose can be given in 3 to 5 minutes with a maximum of 3 mL/kg. This is followed by a maintenance infusion of 0.25 mL/kg/min until the circulation is restored.

Prevention and Treatment of Seizure

- Should only occur after securing the airway and ensuring adequate breathing and oxygenation, because the majority of cases of morbidity that occurs with seizure are related to airway complications such as aspiration and hypoxia.
- Midazolam 0.05 to 0.2 mg/kg IV (intravenous) is the agent of choice.
- Propofol 1 to 2 mg/kg may be also used to control seizure; however, this should be used with caution and in the absence of hypotension or cardiovascular instability.
- Mild hyperventilation can help raise the seizure threshold by inducing respiratory alkalosis.
- Some case reports suggest the use of Intralipid 20% to treat CNS toxicity of LAs, even in the absence of cardiotoxicity, and suggest its use as a first line of treatment in this context.

Support the Circulation

- Intravenous fluid bolus with 10 to 20 mL/kg of isotonic fluids such as lactated Ringer's.
- Phenylephrine infusion starting at a rate of 0.1 µg/kg/min to support the vascular tone antagonizes the LA-induced vasodilatation.
- Successful use of cardiopulmonary bypass has been also reported.

Suggested Reading

Amory C, Mariscal A, Guyot E, et al. Is ilioinguinal/iliohypogastric nerve block always totally safe in children? *Paediatr Anaesth*. 2003;13:164–166.

Bardsley H, Gristwood R, Baker H, et al. A comparison of the cardiovascular effects of levobupivacaine and rac-bupivacaine following intravenous administration to healthy volunteers. *Br J Clin Pharmacol*. 1998;46:245–249.

Berde CB. Toxicity of local anesthetics in infants and children. *J Pediatr*. 1993;122:S14–S20.

Cook DR. Paediatric anaesthesia: pharmacological considerations. *Drugs*. 1976;12:212–221.

Coté CJ, Lerman J, Todres ID. Regional anesthesia. In: *A Practice of Anesthesia for Infants and Children*. 5th ed. Philadelphia: Saunders Elsevier; 2013.

Gorfine SR, Onel E, Patou G, Krivokapic ZV. Bupivacaine extended-release liposome injection for prolonged postsurgical analgesia in patients undergoing hemorrhoidectomy: a multicenter, randomized, double-blind, placebo-controlled trial. *Dis Colon Rectum*. 2011;54:1552–1559.

Gourrier E, Karoubi P, el Hanache A, et al. Use of EMLA cream in a department of neonatology. *Pain*. 1996;68:431–434.

Hodgson PS, Neal JM, Pollock JE, Liu SS. The neurotoxicity of drugs given intrathecally (spinal). *Anesth Analg*. 1999;88:797–809.

Krane EJ, Haberkern CM, Jacobson LE. Postoperative apnea, bradycardia, and oxygen desaturation in formerly premature infants: prospective comparison of spinal and general anesthesia. *Anesth Analg*. 1995;80:7–13.

Litz RJ, Roessel T, Heller AR, Stehr SN. Reversal of central nervous system and cardiac toxicity after local anesthetic intoxication by lipid emulsion injection. *Anesth Analg*. 2008;106:1575–1577.

Mauch JY, Spielmann N, Hartnack S, Weiss M. Electrocardiographic and haemodynamic alterations caused by three different test solutions of local anaesthetics to detect accidental intravascular injection in children. *Br J Anaesth*. 2012;108:283–289.

McCloskey JJ, Haun SE, Deshpande JK. Bupivacaine toxicity secondary to continuous caudal epidural infusion in children. *Anesth Analg*. 1992;75:287–290.

Mirtallo J. State of the art review: intravenous fat emulsions: current applications, safety profile, and clinical implications. *Ann Pharmacother*. 2010;44:688–700.

Rice LJ, DeMars PD, Whalen TV, et al. Duration of spinal anesthesia in infants less than one year of age. Comparison of three hyperbaric techniques. *Reg Anesth*. 1994;19:325–329.

Ward RM, Mirkin BL. Perinatal/neonatal pharmacology. In: Brody TM, Larner J, Minneman KP, eds. *Human Pharmacology: Molecular to Clinical*. 3rd ed. St Louis: Mosby-Year Book; 1998:873–883.

Weinberg GL. Treatment of local anesthetic systemic toxicity (LAST). *Reg Anesth Pain Med*. 2010;35:188–193.

Weinberg G, Lin B, Zheng S, et al. Partitioning effect in lipid resuscitation: further evidence for the lipid sink. *Crit Care Med*. 2010;38:2268–2269.

Willschke H, Marhofer P, Bosenberg A, et al. Ultrasonography for ilioinguinal/iliohypogastric nerve blocks in children. *Br J Anaesth*. 2005;95:226–230.

Equipment and Ultrasound

Kamal Maheshwari and Loran Mounir-Soliman

EQUIPMENT

NEEDLES, CATHETERS, AND SYRINGES

Effective regional anesthesia requires comprehensive knowledge of equipment—that is, the needles, syringes, and catheters that allow the anesthetic to be injected into the desired area. In early years, regional anesthesia found many variations in the method of joining needle to syringe. Around the turn of the century, Schneider developed the first all-glass syringe for Hermann Wülfing-Luer. Luer is credited with the innovation of a simple conical tip for easy exchange of needle to syringe, but the "Luer-Lok" found in use on most syringes today is thought to have been designed by Dickenson in the mid-1920s. The Luer fitting became virtually universal, and both the Luer slip tip and the Luer-Lok were standardized in 1955.

In almost all disposable and reusable needles used in regional anesthesia, the bevel is cut on three planes. The design theoretically creates less tissue laceration and discomfort than the earlier styles did, and it limits tissue coring. Many needles that are to be used for deep injection during regional block incorporate a security bead in the shaft so that the needle can be easily retrieved on the rare occasions when the needle hub separates from the needle shaft. Fig. 3.1 contrasts a blunt-beveled, 25-gauge needle with a 25-gauge "hypodermic" needle. Traditional teaching holds that the short-beveled needle is less traumatic to neural structures. There is little clinical evidence that this is so, and experimental data about whether sharp or blunt needle tips minimize nerve injury are equivocal.

Fig. 3.2 shows various spinal needles. The key to their successful use is to find the size and bevel tip that allow one to cannulate the subarachnoid space easily without causing repeated unrecognized puncture. For equivalent needle size, rounded needle tips that spread the dural fibers are associated with a lesser incidence of headache than are those that cut fibers. The past interest in very-small-gauge spinal catheters to reduce the incidence of spinal headache, with controllability of a continuous technique, faded during the controversy over lidocaine neurotoxicity.

Fig. 3.3 depicts epidural needles. Needle tip design is often mandated by the decision to use a catheter with the epidural technique. Fig. 3.4 shows two catheters available for either subarachnoid or epidural use. Although each has advantages and disadvantages, a single–end-hole catheter appears to provide the highest level of certainty of catheter tip location at the time of injection, whereas a multiple–side-hole catheter may be preferred for continuous analgesia techniques.

Continuous Infusion Dosage With the advent of ultrasound and better training, more and more continuous nerve block catheters are performed to help patients. Current practice is to limit continuous infusion at 0.4/mg/kg/h (bupivacaine/ropivacaine). See Table 3.1 for specific block recommendations.

NERVE STIMULATORS

In recent years, use of nerve stimulators has increased from occasional use to common use and is often of critical importance. The growing emphasis on techniques that use either multiple injections near individual nerves or placement of stimulating catheters has provided impetus for this change. The primary impediment to successful use of a nerve stimulator in a clinical practice is that it is at least a three-handed or two-individual technique (Fig. 3.5), although there are devices allowing control of the stimulator current using a foot control, eliminating the need for a third hand or a second individual. In those situations, requiring a second set of hands, correct operation of contemporary peripheral nerve stimulators is straightforward and easily taught during the course of the block. There are a variety of circumstances in which a nerve stimulator is helpful, such as in children and adults who are already anesthetized, when a decision is made that regional block is an appropriate technique, in individuals who are unable to report paresthesias accurately, in performing local anesthetic administration on specific nerves, and in placement of stimulating catheters for anesthesia or postoperative analgesia. Another group that may benefit from the use of a nerve stimulator is patients with chronic pain, in whom accurate needle placement and reproduction of pain with electrical stimulation or elimination of pain with accurate administration of small volumes of local anesthetic may improve diagnosis and treatment.

When nerve stimulation is used during regional block, insulated needles are most appropriate because the current from such needles results in a current sphere around the needle tip, whereas uninsulated needles emit current at the tip as well as along the shaft, potentially resulting in less precise needle location. A peripheral nerve stimulator should allow between 0.1 and 10 milliamperes (mA) of

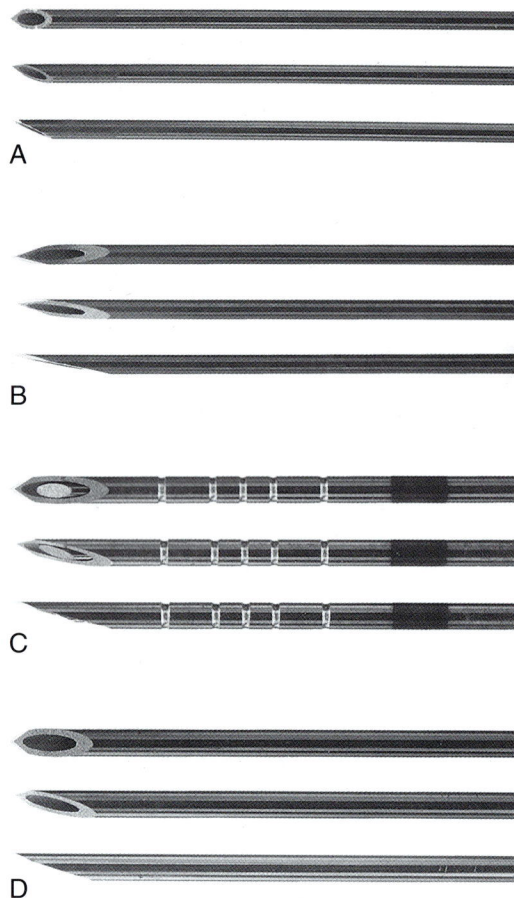

Fig. 3.1 Frontal, oblique, and lateral views of regional block needles. **(A)** Blunt-beveled, 25-gauge axillary block needle. **(B)** Long-beveled, 25-gauge ("hypodermic") block needle. **(C)** 22-gauge ultrasonography "imaging" needle. **(D)** Short-beveled, 22-gauge regional block needle. *(From Brown DL: Regional Anesthesia and Analgesia. Philadelphia, WB Saunders, 1996. "Used with permission of Mayo Foundation for Medical Education and Research. All rights reserved.")*

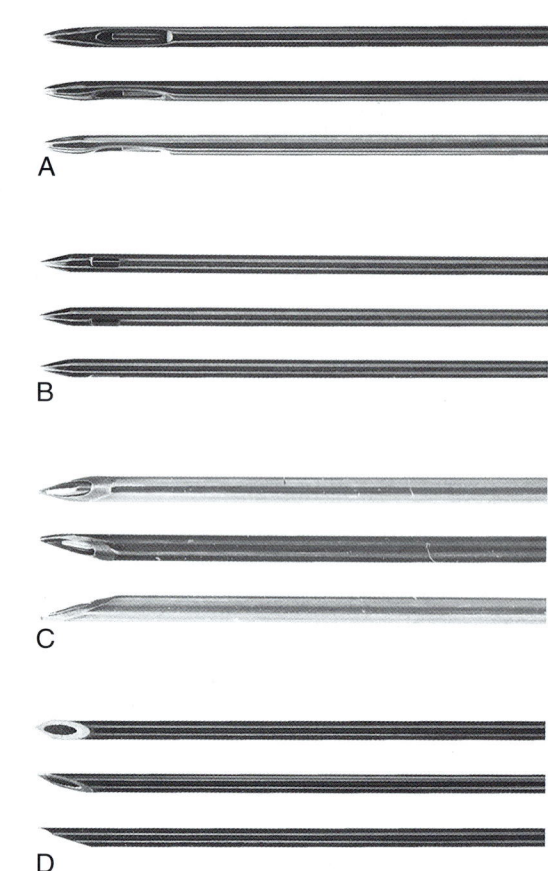

Fig. 3.2 Frontal, oblique, and lateral views of common spinal needles. **(A)** Sprotte needle. **(B)** Whitacre needle. **(C)** Greene needle. **(D)** Quincke needle. *(From Brown DL: Regional Anesthesia and Analgesia. Philadelphia, WB Saunders, 1996. "Used with permission of Mayo Foundation for Medical Education and Research. All rights reserved.")*

current in pulses lasting approximately 200 ms at a frequency of 1 or 2 pulses per second. The peripheral nerve stimulator should have a readily apparent readout of when a complete circuit is present, a consistent and accurate current output over its entire range, and a digital display of the current delivered with each pulse. This facilitates generalized location of the nerve while stimulating at 2 mA and allows refinement of needle positioning as the current pulse is reduced to 0.5–0.1 mA. The nerve stimulator should have the polarity of the terminals clearly identified because peripheral nerves are most effectively stimulated by using the needle as the cathode (negative terminal). Alternatively, if the circuit is established with the needle as anode (positive terminal), approximately four times as much current is necessary to produce equivalent stimulation. The positive lead of the stimulator should be placed in a site remote from the site of stimulation by connecting the lead to a common electrocardiographic electrode (see Fig. 3.5).

The use of a nerve stimulator is not a substitute for a complete knowledge of anatomy and careful site selection for needle insertion; in fact, as much attention should be paid to the anatomy and technique when using a nerve stimulator as when not using it. Large myelinated motor fibers are stimulated by less current than are smaller unmyelinated fibers, and muscle contraction is most often produced before patient discomfort. The needle should be carefully positioned to a point where muscle contraction can be elicited with 0.5–0.1 mA. If a pure sensory nerve is to be blocked, a similar procedure is followed; however, correct needle localization will require the patient to report a sense of pulsed "tingling or burning" over the cutaneous distribution of the sensory nerve. Once the needle is in the final position and stimulation is achieved with 0.5–0.1 mA, 1 mL of local anesthetic should be injected through the needle. If the needle is accurately positioned, this amount of solution should rapidly abolish the muscle contraction or the sensation with pulsed current.

ULTRASOUND

In the last decade, image-guided peripheral nerve blocks have become the norm for anesthesiologists at the forefront of regional anesthesia innovation. The dominant method of imaging is ultrasonography. Ultrasonographic imaging devices are noninvasive, portable, and moderately priced. Most work has been done using scanning probes with frequencies in the range of 5–10 megahertz (MHz). These devices are capable of identifying vascular and bony structures but not nerves. Contemporary devices using high-resolution probes (12–15 MHz) and compound imaging allow clear visualization of nerves, vessels, catheters, and local anesthetic injection and can potentially improve the techniques of ultrasonography-assisted peripheral nerve

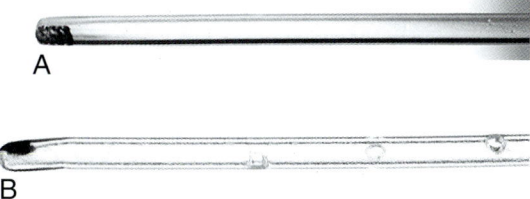

Fig. 3.4 Epidural catheter designs. (A) Single distal orifice. (B) Closed tip with multiple side orifices. (From Brown DL: Regional Anesthesia and Analgesia. Philadelphia, WB Saunders, 1996. "Used with permission of Mayo Foundation for Medical Education and Research. All rights reserved.")

block. Use of these devices is limited by their cost, the need for training in their use and familiarity with ultrasonographic image anatomy, and the extra set of hands required. They work best with superficial nerve plexuses and can be limited by excessive obesity or anatomically distant structures. One of the keys to using this technology effectively is a sound understanding of the physics behind ultrasonography. A corollary to understanding the physics is the need for study and appreciation of the relevant human anatomy.

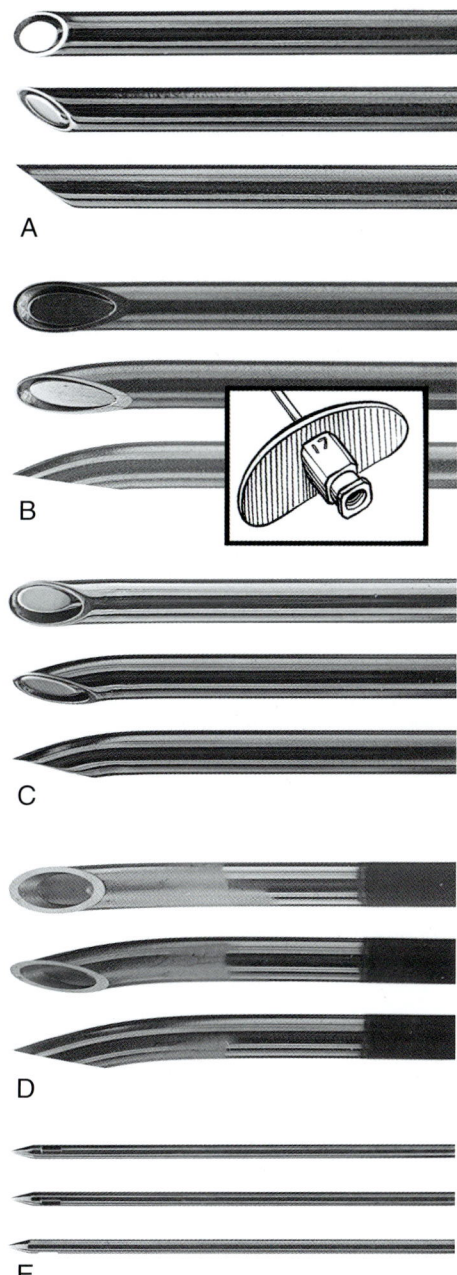

Fig. 3.3 Frontal, oblique, and lateral views of common epidural needles. (A) Crawford needle. (B) Tuohy needle; the *inset* shows a winged hub assembly common to winged needles. (C) Hustead needle. (D) Curved, 18-gauge epidural needle. (E) Whitacre, 27-gauge spinal needle. (From Brown DL: Regional Anesthesia and Analgesia. Philadelphia, WB Saunders, 1996. "Used with permission of Mayo Foundation for Medical Education and Research. All rights reserved.")

> **American Society of Regional Anesthesiologists Recommendations**
>
> The following are the American Society of Regional Anesthesiologists recommendations for performing an ultrasonography-guided block:
>
> 1. Visualize key landmark structures, including muscles, fascia, blood vessels, and bone.
> 2. Identify the nerves or plexus on short-axis imaging, with the depth set 1 cm deep to the target structures.
> 3. Confirm normal anatomy or recognize anatomic variation(s).
> 4. Plan for the safest and most effective needle approach.
> 5. Use the aseptic needle insertion technique.
> 6. Follow the needle under real-time visualization as it is advanced toward the target.
> 7. Consider a secondary confirmation technique, such as nerve stimulation.
> 8. When the needle tip is presumed to be in the correct position, inject a small volume of a test solution.
> 9. Make necessary needle adjustments to obtain optimal perineural spread of local anesthesia.
> 10. Maintain traditional safety guidelines of frequent aspiration, monitoring, patient response, and assessment of resistance to injection.

Table 3.1 Commonly Used Dose and Pump Setting for Continuous Peripheral Nerve Block Infusion

Block type	Local anesthetic*	Continuous rate (mL/hr)	Bolus dose (mL)	Lock-out interval (min)	Number of bolus per hour
Interscalene	0.25 % Bupivacaine or 0.2 % ropivacaine	8-10	8-12	60	1
Supraclavicular	0.25 % Bupivacaine or 0.2 % ropivacaine	8-10	8-12	60	1
Popliteal	0.25 % Bupivacaine or 0.2 % ropivacaine	8-10	8-12	60	1
Femoral or Adductor canal^	0.12 % Bupivacaine or 0.1 % ropivacaine	6-8	0	—	—

*Overall cumulative dose of local anesthetic for any 4 hours period should be less than the toxic dose. Conservative dosage is recommended for elderly and frail patients.

^Lower dose is recommended to avoid quadriceps weakness

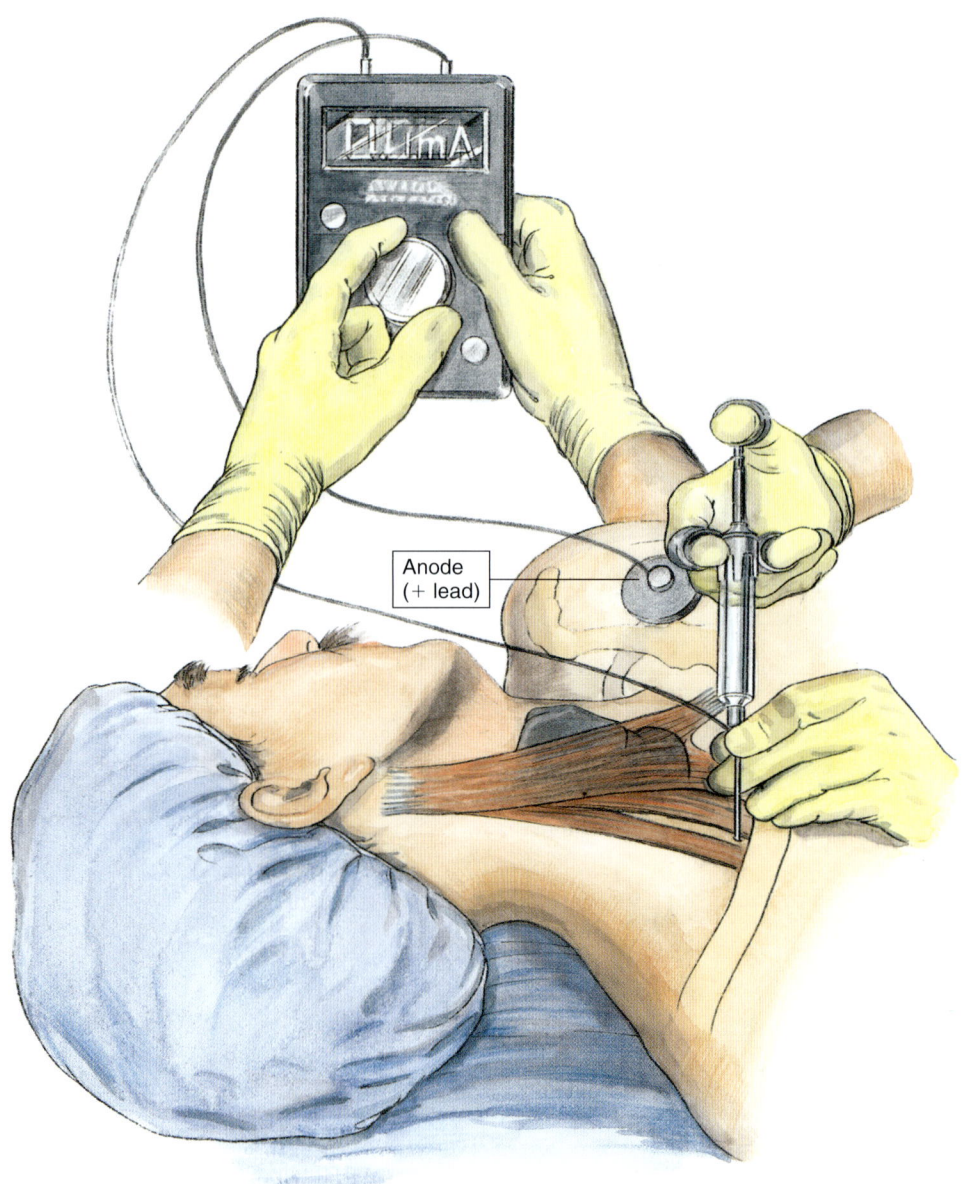

Fig. 3.5 Nerve stimulator technique.

WAVELENGTH AND FREQUENCY

Ultrasound is a form of acoustic energy defined as the longitudinal progression of pressure changes (Fig. 3.6). These pressure changes consist of areas of compression and relaxation of particles in a given medium. For simplicity, an ultrasound wave is often modeled as a sine wave. Each ultrasound wave is defined by a specific wavelength (λ) measured in units of distance, amplitude (h) measured in decibels (dB), and frequency (f) measured in hertz (Hz) or cycles per second. Ultrasound is defined as a frequency of more than 20,000 Hz. Current transducers used for ultrasonography-guided regional anesthesia generate waves in the 3- to 13-MHz range (or 30,000–130,000 Hz).

ULTRASOUND GENERATION

Ultrasound is generated when multiple piezoelectric crystals inside a transducer rapidly vibrate in response to an alternating electric current. Ultrasound then travels into the body where, on contact with various tissues, it can be reflected, refracted, and scattered (Fig. 3.7).

To generate a clinically useful image, ultrasound waves must reflect off tissues and return to the transducer. The transducer, after emitting the wave, switches to a receive mode. When ultrasound waves return to the transducer, the piezoelectric crystals will vibrate once again, this time transforming the sound energy back into electrical energy. This process of transmission and reception can be repeated over 7000 times per second, and when coupled with computer processing results in the generation of a real-time, two-dimensional image that appears seamless. By convention, whiter (hyperechoic) objects represent a larger degree of reflection and higher signal intensities, whereas darker (hypoechoic) images represent less reflection and weaker signal intensities.

CLINICAL ISSUES RELATED TO PHYSICS

Resolution. Resolution refers to the ability to clearly distinguish two structures lying beside one another.

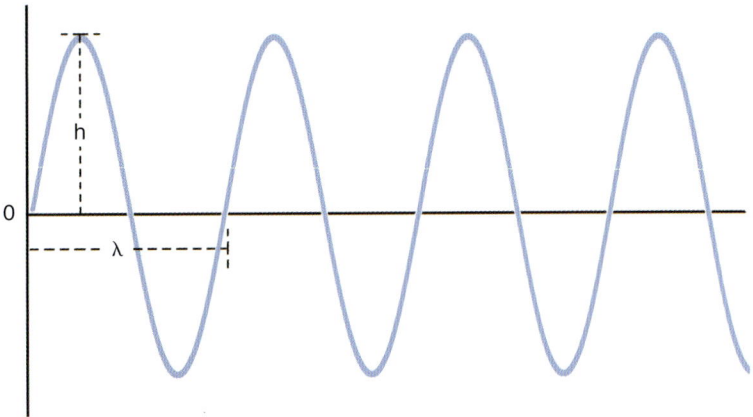

h = height of the wave, or amplitude
λ = wavelength

$$f = \frac{\text{velocity of ultrasound}}{\lambda}$$

Fig. 3.6 Ultrasound wave basics.

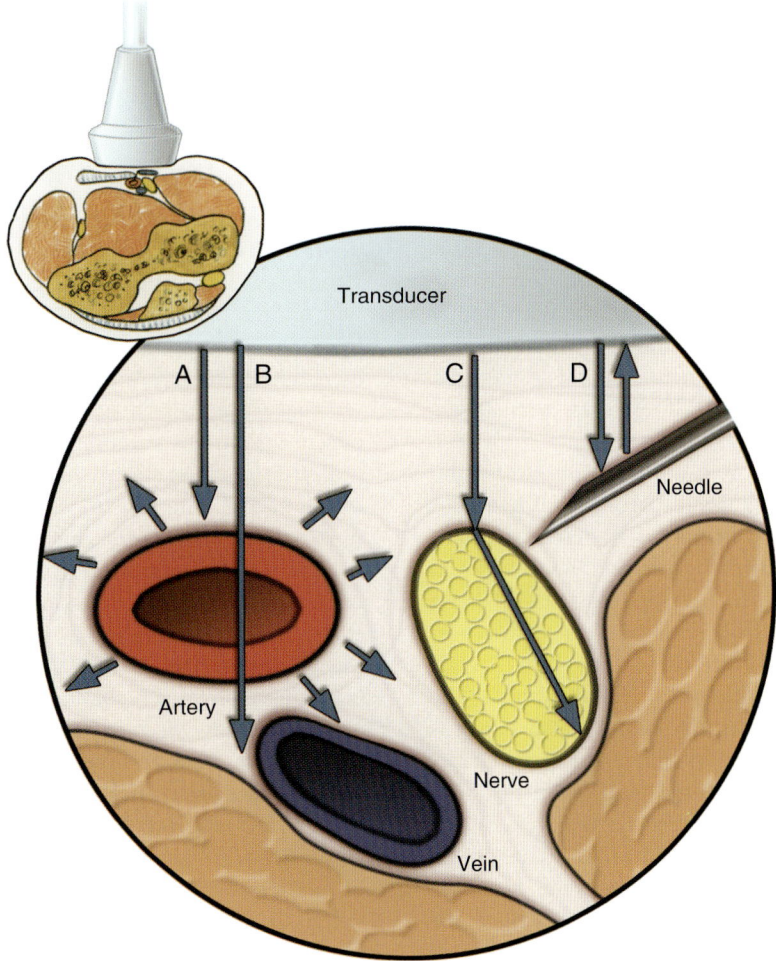

Fig. 3.7 Production of an ultrasonographic image. This figure demonstrates the many responses that an ultrasound wave produces when traveling through tissue. (A) Scatter reflection: the ultrasound wave is deflected in several random directions both toward and away from the probe. Scattering occurs with small or irregular objects. (B) Transmission: the ultrasound wave continues through the tissue away from the probe. (C) Refraction: when an ultrasound wave contacts the interface between two media with different propagation velocities, the wave is refracted (bent) to an extent depending on the difference in velocities. (D) Specular reflection: a large, smooth object (e.g., the needle) returns (reflects) the ultrasound wave toward the probe when it is perpendicular to the ultrasound beam.

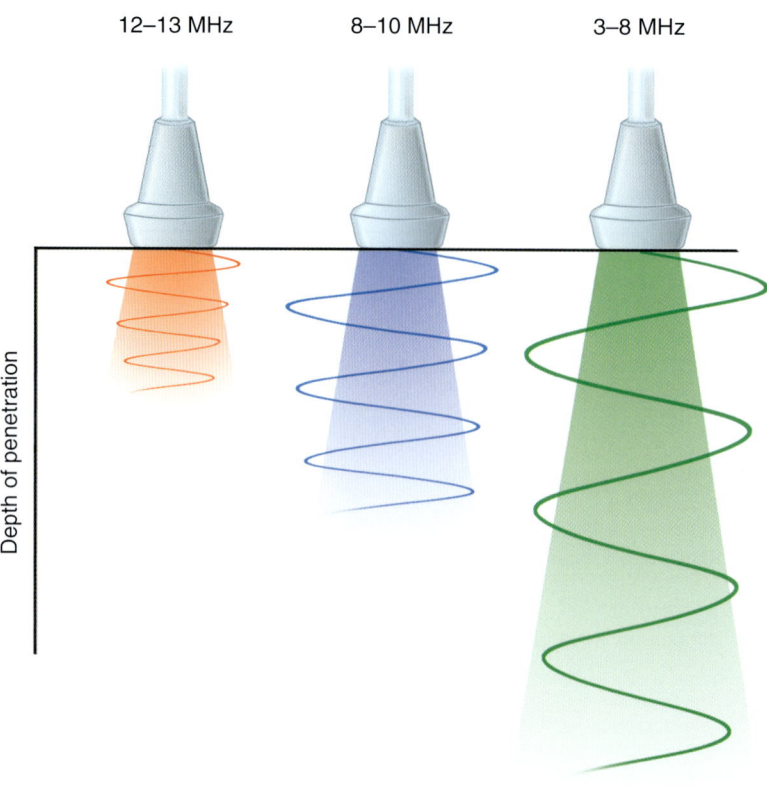

Fig. 3.8 Probe frequency and depth of tissue penetration. Higher-frequency ultrasound attenuates to a larger degree at more superficial depths, although it provides more image detail.

Although there are several different types of resolution, anesthesiologists are mostly concerned with lateral resolution (left–right distinction) and axial resolution (front–back distinction). Ultrasonography systems with higher frequencies have better resolution and can effectively discriminate closely spaced peripheral neural structures. However, because of a process known as *attenuation*, high-frequency ultrasound cannot penetrate into deep tissue (Fig. 3.8). Attenuation is the loss of ultrasound energy into the surrounding tissue, primarily as heat. For superficial blocks between 1 and 4 cm in depth, frequencies greater than 10 MHz are preferred. For blocks at depths greater than 4 cm, frequencies less than 8 MHz should result in adequate tissue penetration, with a predictable degradation in resolution.

Focus. Although axial resolution is related simply to the frequency of ultrasound, lateral resolution also depends on beam thickness. Any maneuver that generates a narrow beam will increase the lateral resolution. Most ultrasonography machines have an electronic focus that generates a focal point (narrowest part of the beam) that can be placed directly over the target of interest. However, this increases the divergence of the beam beyond the region of the focus point (far field), resulting in image degradation of structures beyond this focal point. Thus the beam focus should be placed at the level of the object that is being assessed to provide the clearest possible picture of the object (Fig. 3.9).

Gain. The overall gain controls allow the operator to increase or decrease the signal intensity for a darker or a brighter image. The time gain compensation (TGC) adjusts gain at specific depths of the image. The goal of TGC is to compensate for the attenuation in the signal as result of depth. Accordingly, appropriate TGC adjustment allows structures with similar reflecting characters to be seen with similar brightness regardless of depth. Inappropriately low gain settings may result in the apparent absence of an existing structure (i.e., "missing structure" artifact), whereas inappropriately high gain settings can easily obscure existing structures.

Reflection. The sound waves bounce back to the transducer at the interface of tissues with different acoustic impedance (*reflection*). The quantity of energy reflected determines the amplitude (brightness) of the image processed and mainly depends on the nature of the tissue, with bone having the highest impedance and air having the lowest impedance. A smooth large surface can reflect the beam more effectively than the surrounding tissue, which is called *specular reflection*. When two specular reflectors are close to each other, reverberation of the beam between those surfaces can occur. Clinically it shows as parallel, equally spaced lines, deep to and parallel to the reflecting surfaces (*reverberation artifact*). The comet tail artifact is an example of this reverberation when scanning the two layers of pleura, when in proximity with no fluids or air in-between. Hyperechoic reverberation is another example of this artifact caused by the two walls of the hollow block needles.

COLOR DOPPLER

Color-flow Doppler ultrasonography relies on the fact that if an ultrasound pulse is sent out and strikes moving red blood cells, the ultrasound that is reflected back to the

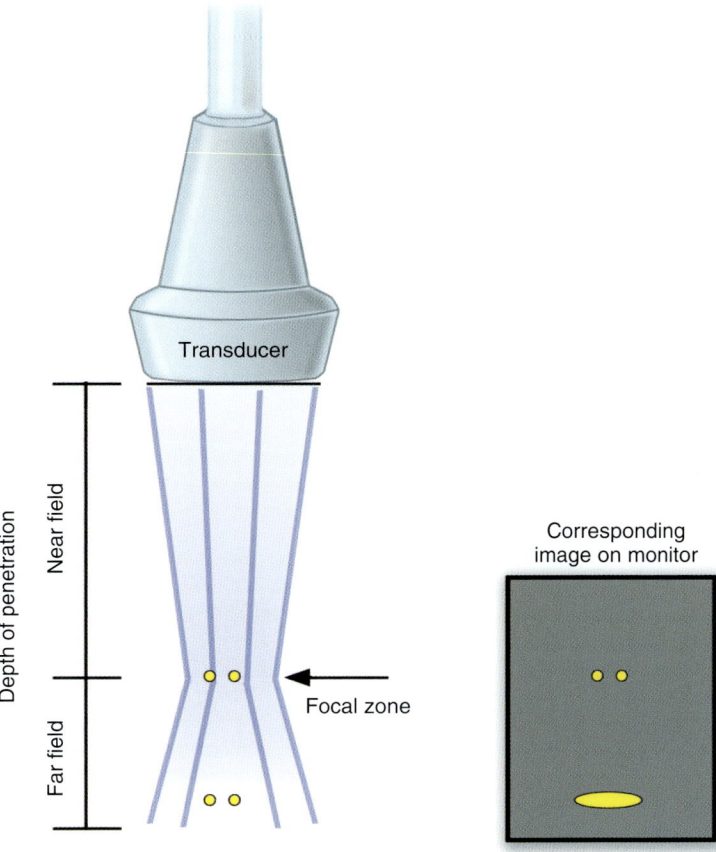

Fig. 3.9 Basics of ultrasonographic probe focusing.

transducer will have a frequency that is different from the original emitted frequency. This change in frequency is known as the *Doppler shift*. It is this frequency change that can be used in cardiac and vascular applications to calculate both blood flow velocity and blood flow direction. The Doppler equation states that

$$\text{Frequency shift} = 2 \times V \times Ft \times \text{cosine } \Phi / c$$

where V is velocity of the moving object, Ft is the transmitted frequency, Φ is the angle of incidence of the ultrasound beam and the direction of blood flow, and c is the speed of ultrasound in the medium. The direction of blood flow is not as crucial for regional anesthesia as it is for cardiovascular anesthesia. What is most important is being able to positively identify blood vessels by visualizing color flow. This is especially important when interrogating a projected trajectory of the needle when placing a block. By placing color-flow Doppler over the expected needle path, the clinician should be able to screen for and avoid any unanticipated vasculature.

GENERAL PRINCIPLES OF AN ULTRASONOGRAPHY-GUIDED NERVE BLOCK

During ultrasonographic needle guidance, most nerves are imaged in cross section (short axis). Alternatively, if the transducer is moved 90 degrees from the short-axis view, the long-axis view is generated. The short-axis view is generally preferred because it allows the operator to assess the lateromedial perspective of the target nerve, which is lost in the long-axis view (Fig. 3.10).

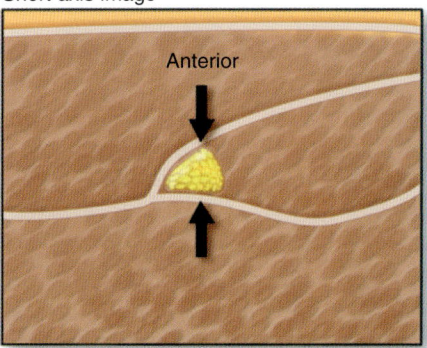
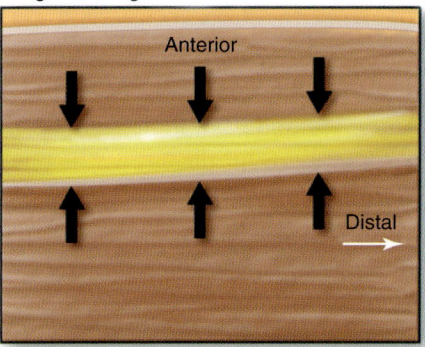

Fig. 3.10 Short-axis *(top)* and long-axis *(bottom)* imaging of the median nerve.

Two techniques have emerged regarding the orientation of the needle with respect to the ultrasound beam (Fig. 3.11). The in-plane approach generates a long-axis view of the needle, allowing full visualization of the shaft and tip of the needle. The out-of-plane view generates a

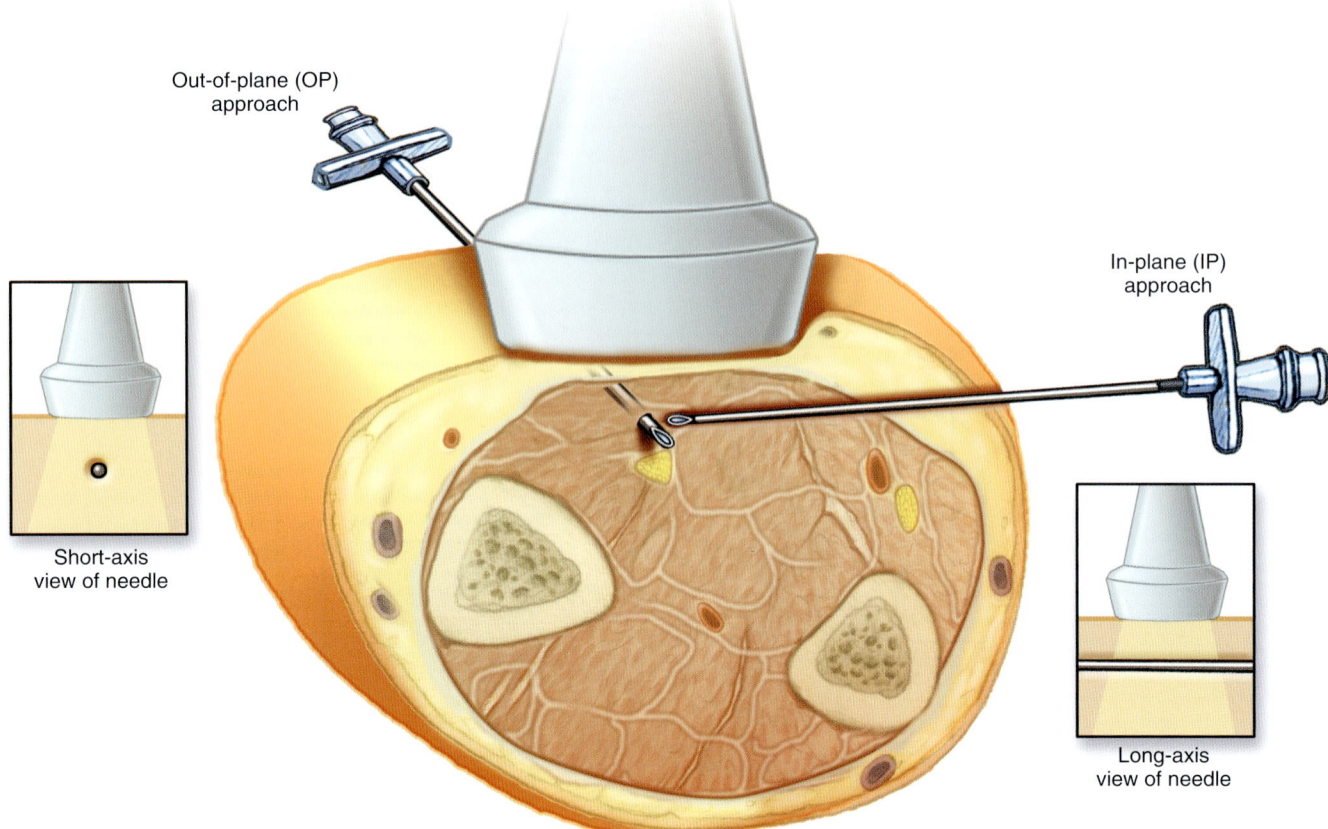

Fig. 3.11 The in-plane *(right)* and out-of-plane *(left)* needle approaches for needle insertion and ultrasonographic visualization.

short-axis view of the needle. One disadvantage of the in-plane approach is the challenge of maintaining needle imaging with a very thin ultrasound beam. A limitation of the out-of-plane view is that it generates a short-axis view of the block needle, which may be very hard to visualize. With the out-of-plane view, the operator cannot confirm that the needle tip (rather than part of the shaft) is being imaged, and therefore the needle location is often inferred from tissue movement or small injections of solution.

Two main types of ultrasound probes are used for regional anesthesia:

1. Linear probe (usually higher frequency probe) that allows better resolution and more accurate identification of the margins for the target structure, with narrower ultrasonographic window.
2. Curvilinear probe (generally with lower frequency), which makes it more suitable for deeper structures, providing a wider view to detect important structures adjacent to the target nerve. The caveat with the curvilinear probe is a lower degree of resolution (Figs. 3.12, 3.13A, and 3.13B).

Regardless of the machine or transducer selected, there are four basic transducer manipulation techniques, which can be described as the "PART" of scanning:

Pressure (P): Various degrees of pressure are applied to the transducer that are translated onto the skin.

Alignment (A): Sliding the transducer defines the lengthwise course of the nerve and reference structures.

Rotation (R): The transducer is turned in either a clockwise or counterclockwise direction to optimize the image (either long or short axis) of the nerve and needle.

Tilting (T): The transducer is tilted in both directions to maximize the angle of incidence of the ultrasound beam to the target nerve, thereby maximizing reflection and optimizing image quality.

The primary objective of PART maneuvers is to optimize the amount of ultrasound that reflects off an object and returns to the transducer (Fig. 3.14).

Constant and frequent manipulations of the probe, mainly rotation and tilting, allow better appreciation of the anatomical structures, particularly nerves and tendons, due to **anisotropy**.

This characteristic mainly indicates the change in amplitude of the reflected signal based on the angle of incidence of the beam. Small changes in the angle of the beam striking the object can result in significantly unequal amplitude of the reflected image (anisotropic), with the largest amplitude when this angle is perpendicular to the long axis of the structure in short axis view. Clear visualization of the targeted structure versus no visualization at all can be a function of change in this angle of incidence, highlighting the importance of acquiring this hand skill.

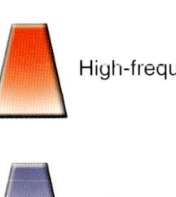 High-frequency setting (12–13 MHz)

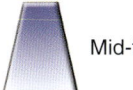 Mid-frequency setting (8–10 MHz)

IP = In-plane technique
OP = Out-of-plane technique

 Low-frequency setting (3–8 MHz)

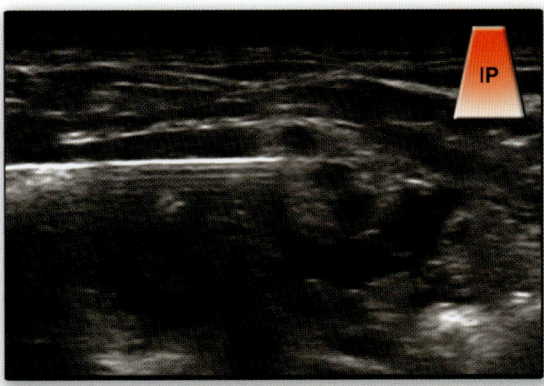

Fig. 3.12 Our system for ultrasonographic needle guidance recommendations. For a block for which we would recommend a high-frequency setting with the in-plane (IP) technique of needle visualization, a red scan plane with an "IP" inside the plane is shown. For a low-frequency setting with the out-of-plane (OP) technique for needle visualization, we show a green scan plane with an "OP" in the plane. The midfrequency setting is indicated by a blue scan plane. An example is shown in the upper right of the figure. In this case, we recommend starting with a high-frequency probe setting and an in-plane technique for needle visualization.

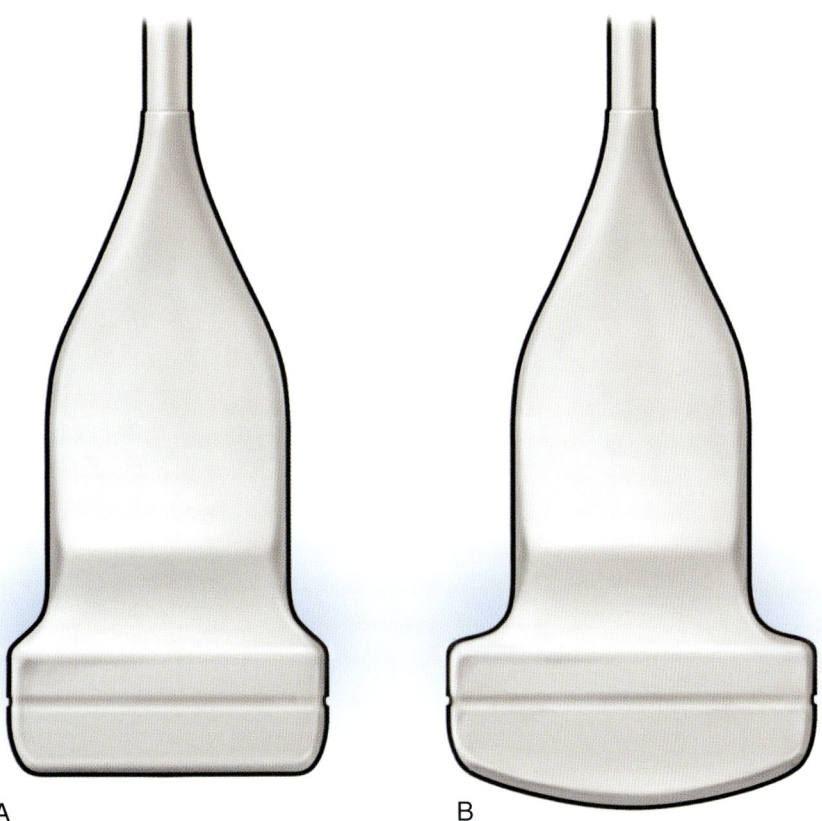

Fig. 3.13 (A) Linear probe; (B) Curvilinear probe.

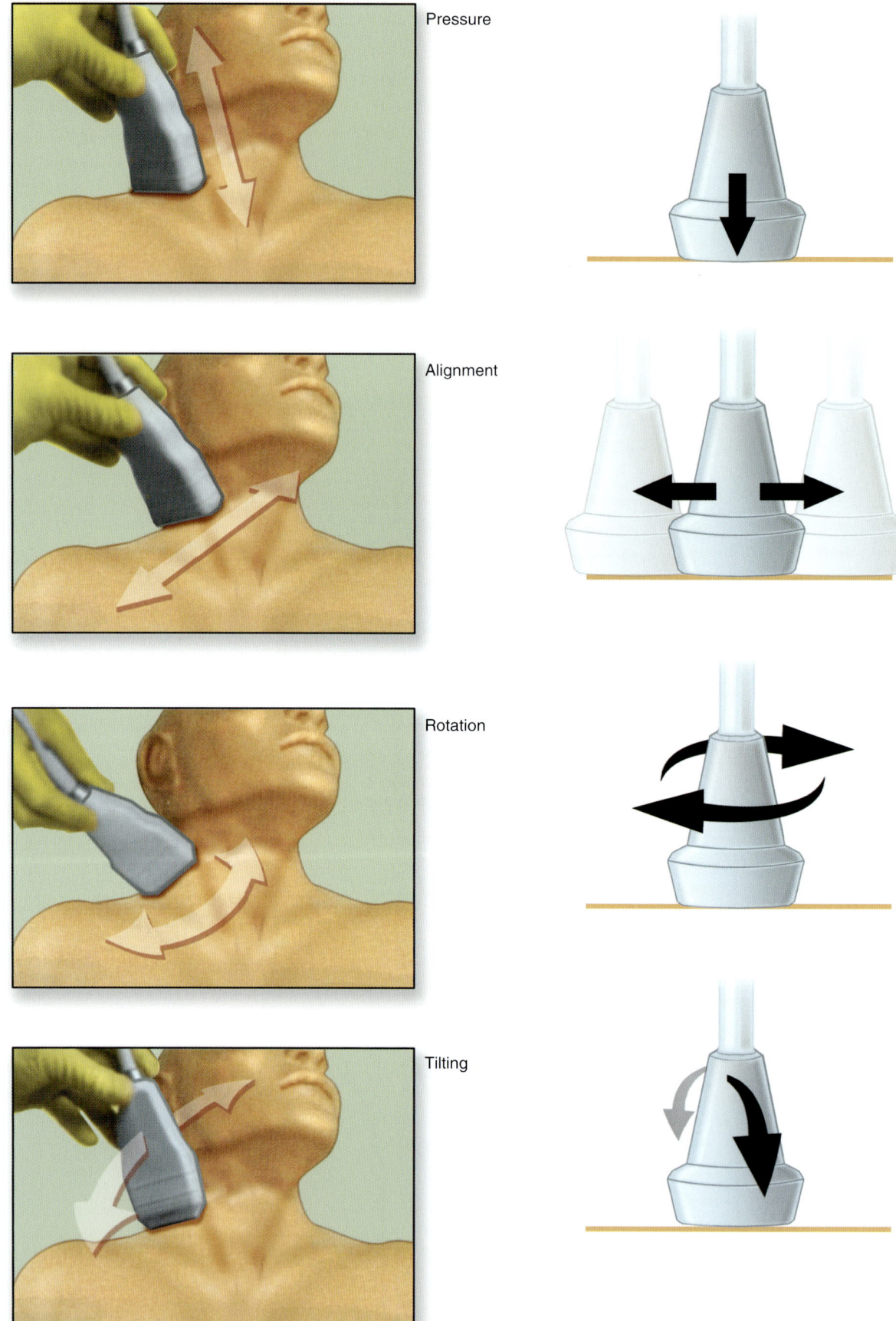

Fig. 3.14 PART maneuvers: pressure, alignment, rotation, and tilting.

SECTION 2
Upper Extremity Blocks

Upper Extremity Block Anatomy

4

David L. Brown

Key Points

- Along its course above the clavicle, the brachial plexus is bounded by the anterior and middle scalene muscles. The two muscles constitute the scalene triangle with its apex at the transverse processes of cervical vertebrae and its base formed by the first rib.
- The phrenic nerve runs anterior to the brachial plexus, separated by the anterior scalene muscle. The distance between the phrenic nerve and the brachial plexus is a few millimeters at the apex of the scalene triangle and reaches a few centimeters towards the base of the triangle.
- The vertebral artery lies anterior to the roots of the brachial plexus as they leave the cervical vertebrae.
- Nerves supplying the ventral part of the upper extremity originate from the anterior divisions of the trunks of the brachial plexus forming the medial and lateral cords.
- Nerves supplying the dorsal part of the upper extremity originate from the posterior divisions of the trunks of the brachial plexus forming the posterior cord.
- The cords of the brachial plexus get their names according to their relationship to the second part of the axillary artery in the standard anatomical position (arm adducted, extended parallel to the trunk).

Man uses his arms and hands constantly … as a result he exposes his arms and hands to injury constantly. … Man also eats constantly. … Man's stomach is never really empty. … The combination of man's prehensibility and his unflagging appetite keeps a steady flow of patients with injured upper extremities and full stomachs streaming into hospital emergency rooms. This is why the brachial plexus is so frequently the anesthesiologist's favorite group of nerves.

Classical Anesthesia Files, David Little, 1963.

The late David Little's appropriate observations do not always lead anesthesiologists to choose a regional anesthetic for upper extremity surgery. However, those selecting regional anesthesia recognize that there are multiple sites at which the brachial plexus block can be induced.

If anesthesiologists are to deliver comprehensive anesthesia care, they should be familiar with brachial plexus blocks. Familiarity with these techniques demands an understanding of brachial plexus anatomy. One problem with understanding this anatomy is that the traditional wiring diagram for the brachial plexus is unnecessarily complex and intimidating.

Fig. 4.1 illustrates that the plexus is formed by the ventral rami of the fifth to eighth cervical nerves and the greater part of the ramus of the first thoracic nerve. In addition, small contributions may be made by the fourth cervical and the second thoracic nerves. The intimidating part of this anatomy is what happens from the time these ventral rami emerge from between the middle and anterior scalene muscles until they end in the four terminal branches to the upper extremity: the musculocutaneous, median, ulnar, and radial nerves. Most of what happens to the roots on their way to becoming peripheral nerves is not clinically essential information for an anesthesiologist. There are some broad concepts that may help clinicians understand the brachial plexus anatomy; throughout this chapter, my goal is to simplify this anatomy.

After the roots pass between the scalene muscles, they reorganize into trunks—superior, middle, and inferior. The trunks continue toward the first rib. At the lateral edge of the first rib, these trunks undergo a primary anatomic division into ventral and dorsal divisions. This is also the point at which understanding of brachial plexus anatomy gives way to frustration and often unnecessary complexity. This anatomic division is significant, because nerves destined to supply the originally ventral part of the upper extremity separate from those that supply the dorsal part. As these divisions enter the axilla, the divisions give way to cords. The posterior divisions of all three trunks unite to form the posterior cord; the anterior divisions of the superior and middle trunks form the lateral cord; the un-united anterior division of the inferior trunk forms the medial cord. These cords are named according to their relationship to the second part of the axillary artery.

At the lateral border of the pectoralis minor muscle (which inserts onto the coracoid process), the three cords reorganize to give rise to the peripheral nerves of the upper extremity. Simplified, the branches of the lateral and medial cords are all "ventral" nerves to the upper extremity. The posterior cord, in contrast, provides all "dorsal" innervation to the upper extremity. Thus the radial nerve supplies all the dorsal musculature in the upper extremity below the shoulder. The musculocutaneous nerve supplies muscular

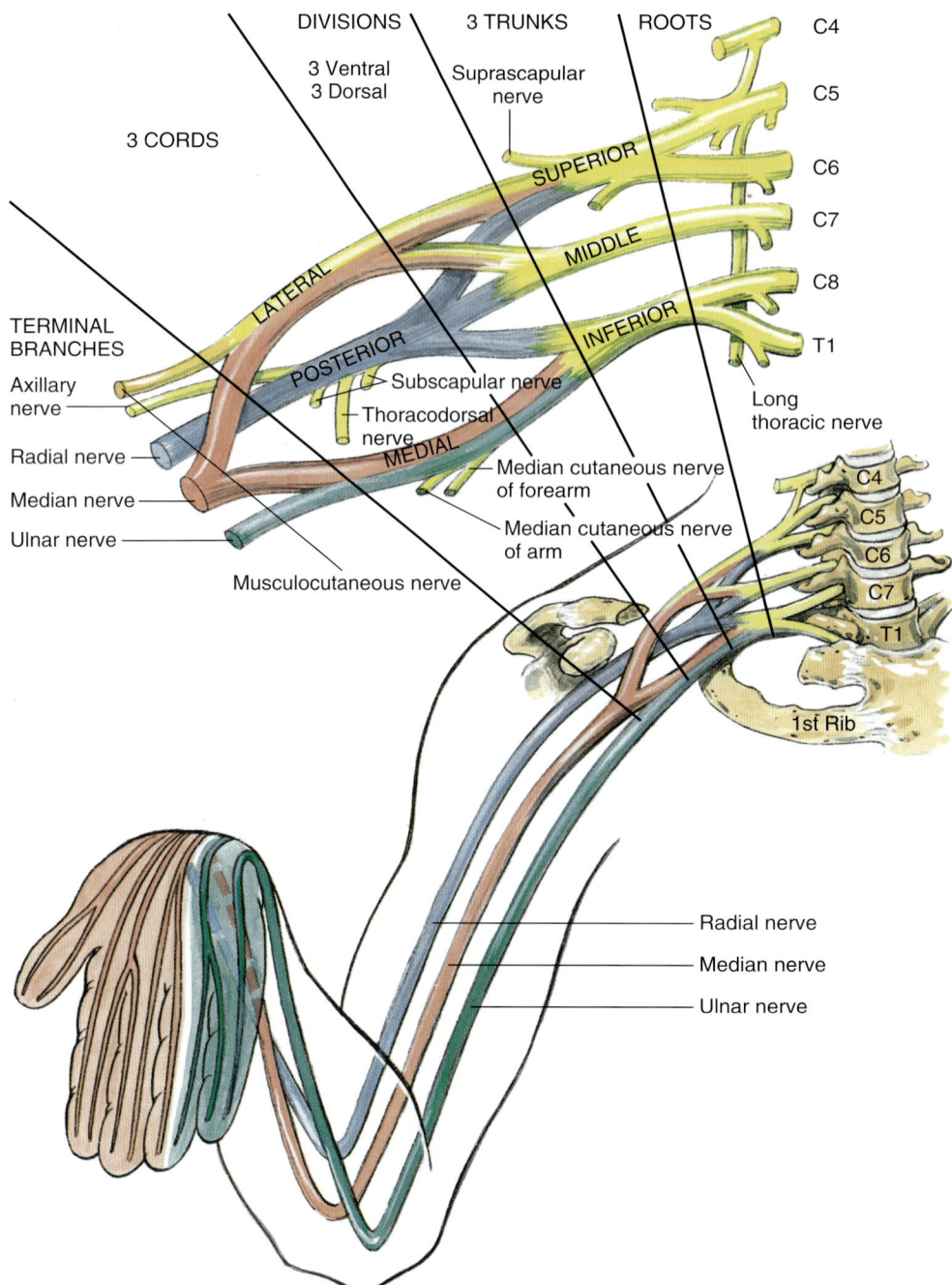

Fig. 4.1 Brachial plexus anatomy.

innervation in the arm while providing cutaneous innervation to the forearm. In contrast, the median and ulnar nerves are nerves of passage in the arm, but in the forearm and hand they provide the ventral musculature with motor innervation. These nerves can be further categorized: the median nerve innervates more heavily in the forearm, whereas the ulnar nerve innervates more heavily in the hand.

Some writers have focused anesthesiologists' attention on the fascial investment of the brachial plexus. As the brachial plexus nerve roots leave the transverse processes, they do so between the prevertebral fascia, which divides to invest both the anterior and the middle scalene muscles. Many suggest that this prevertebral fascia surrounding the brachial plexus is tubular throughout its course, thus allowing needle placement within the "sheath" to produce brachial plexus block easily. There is no question that the brachial plexus is invested with prevertebral fascia; however, the fascial covering is discontinuous, with septa subdividing portions of the sheath into compartments that clinically may prevent adequate spread of local anesthetics. Ultrasonographic observation of injections near the brachial plexus confirms our earlier clinical impressions of fascial discontinuity. My clinical impression is that the discontinuity of the "sheath" increases as one moves from transverse process to axilla.

Most upper extremity surgery is performed with the patient resting supine on an operating table with the arm extended on an arm board. Thus anesthesiologists must understand and clearly visualize the innervation of the upper extremity while the patient is in this position. Figs. 4.2 through 4.7 illustrate these features with the arm in the supinated and pronated positions for the cutaneous nerves, and dermatomal and osteotomal patterns, respectively.

Upper Extremity Block Anatomy

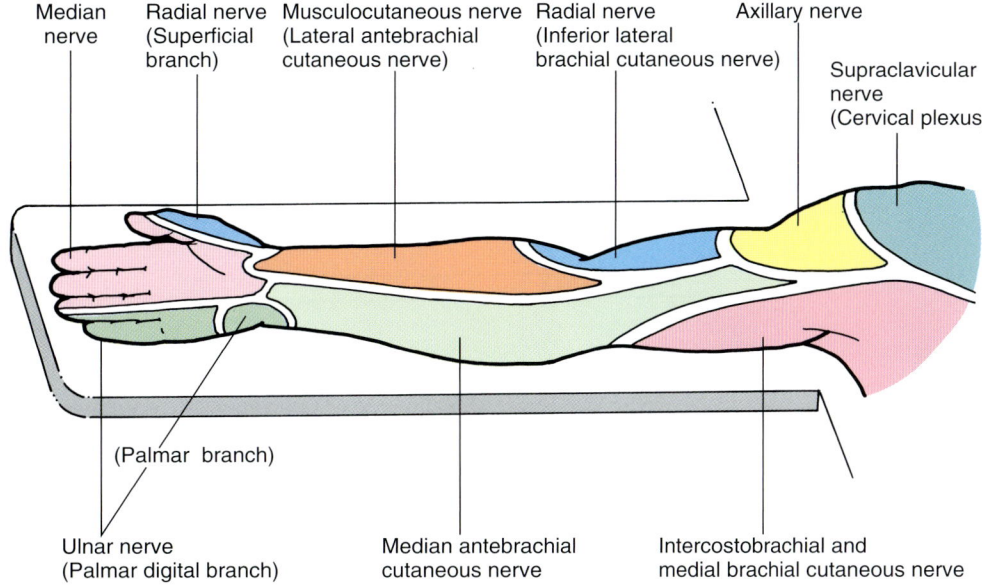

Fig. 4.2 Upper extremity peripheral nerve innervation with arm supinated on arm board.

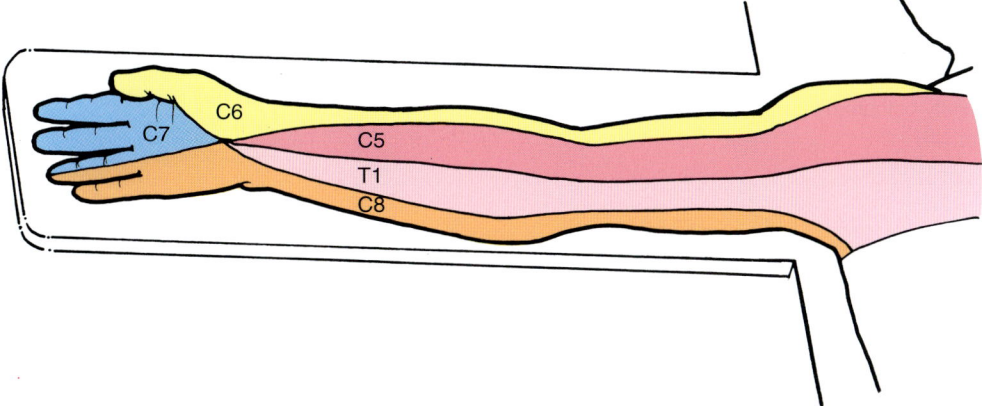

Fig. 4.3 Upper extremity dermatome innervation with arm supinated on arm board.

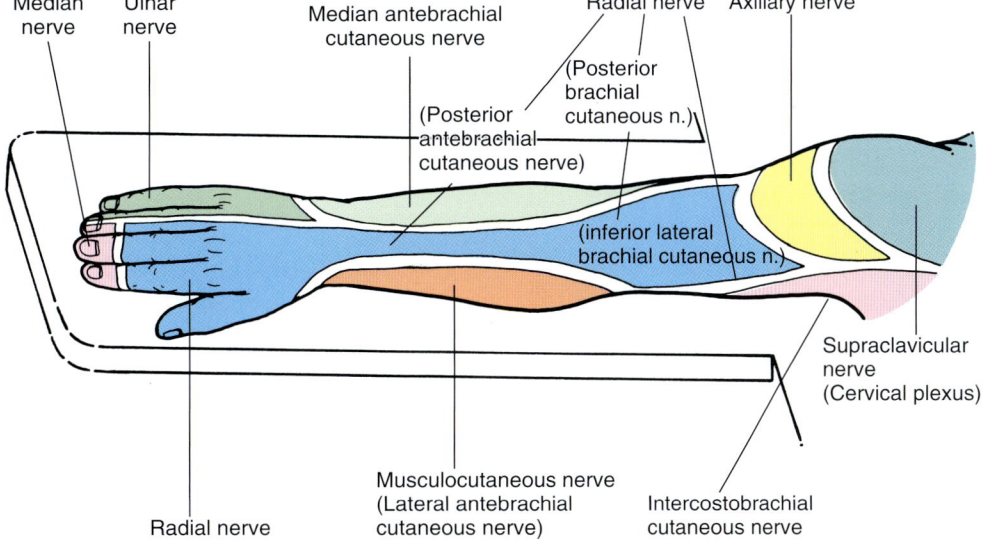

Fig. 4.4 Upper extremity peripheral nerve innervation with arm pronated on arm board.

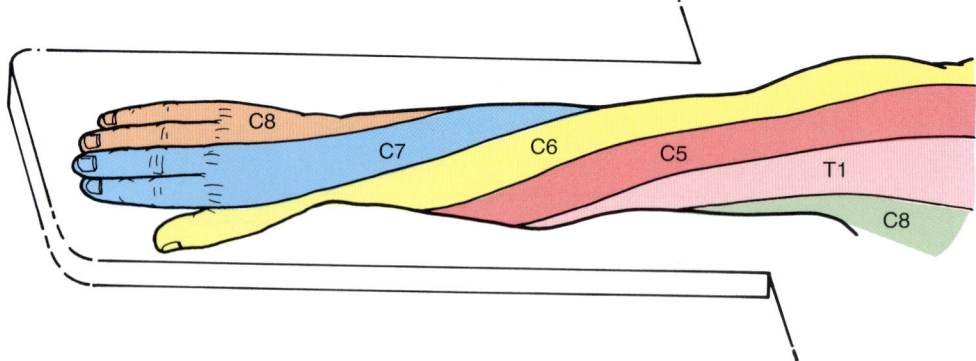

Fig. 4.5 Upper extremity dermatome innervation with arm pronated on arm board.

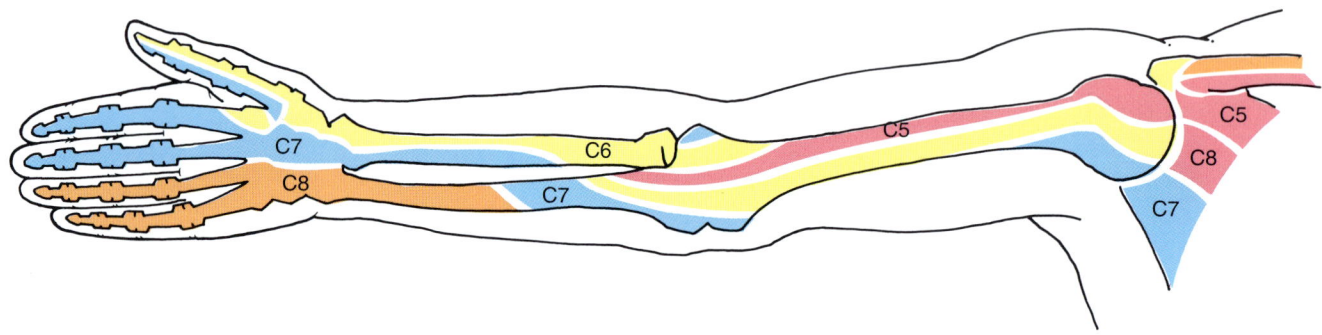

Fig. 4.6 Upper extremity osteotomes with arm supinated.

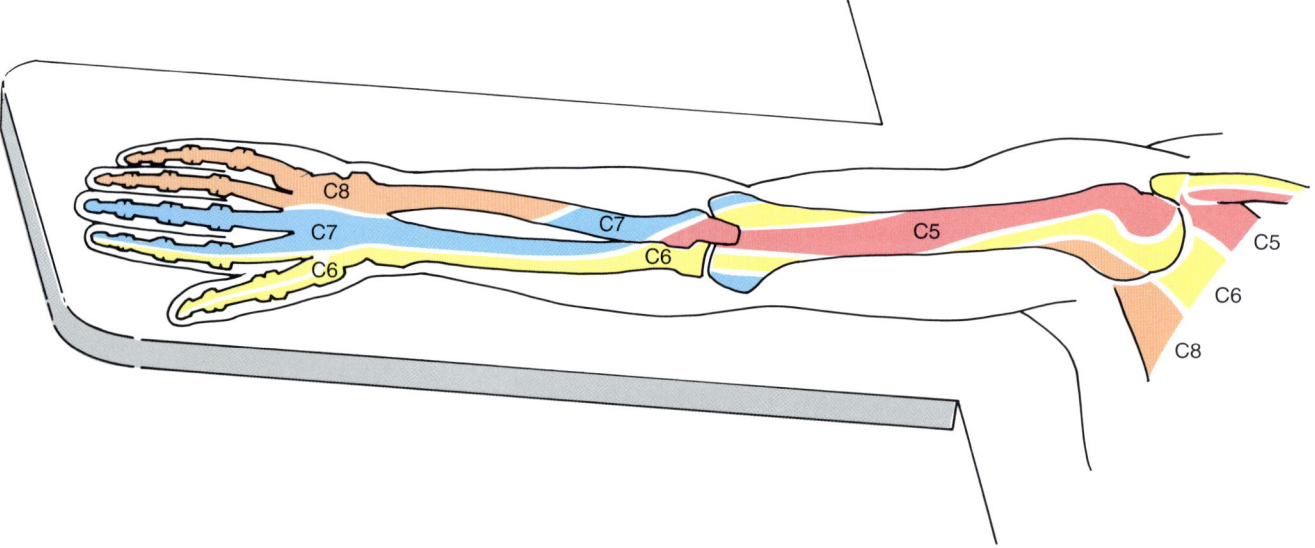

Fig. 4.7 Upper extremity osteotomes with arm pronated on arm board.

An additional clinical "pearl" that will help anesthesiologists check brachial plexus block before initiation of the surgical procedure is the "four Ps." Fig. 4.8 shows how the mnemonic "push, pull, pinch, pinch" can help an anesthesiologist remember how to check the four peripheral nerves of interest in the brachial plexus block. By having the patient resist the anesthesiologist's pulling the forearm away from the upper arm, motor innervation to the biceps muscle is assessed. If this muscle has been weakened, one can be certain that local anesthetic has reached the musculocutaneous nerve. Likewise, by asking the patient to attempt to extend the forearm by contracting the triceps muscle, one assesses the radial nerve. Finally, pinching the fingers in the distribution of the ulnar or median nerve—that is, at the base of the fifth or second digit, respectively—helps the anesthesiologist develop a sense of the adequacy of block of both the ulnar and median nerves. Typically, if these maneuvers are performed shortly after brachial plexus block, motor weakness will be evident before sensory block. As a historical highlight, this technique for checking the upper extremity was developed during World War II to allow medics a method of quick analysis of injuries to the brachial plexus.

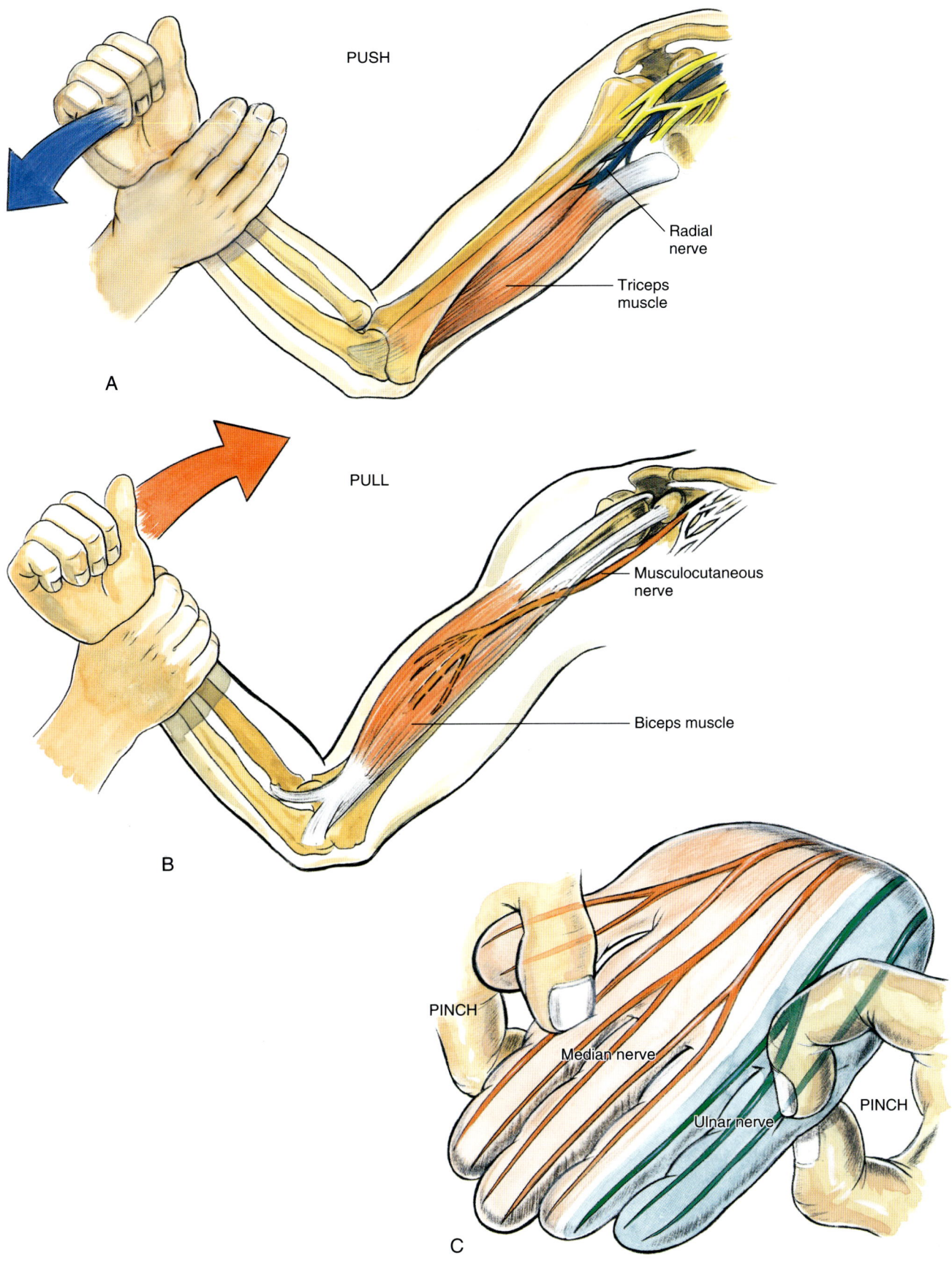

Fig. 4.8 Upper extremity peripheral nerve function mnemonic: "push (A), pull (B), pinch, pinch (C)."

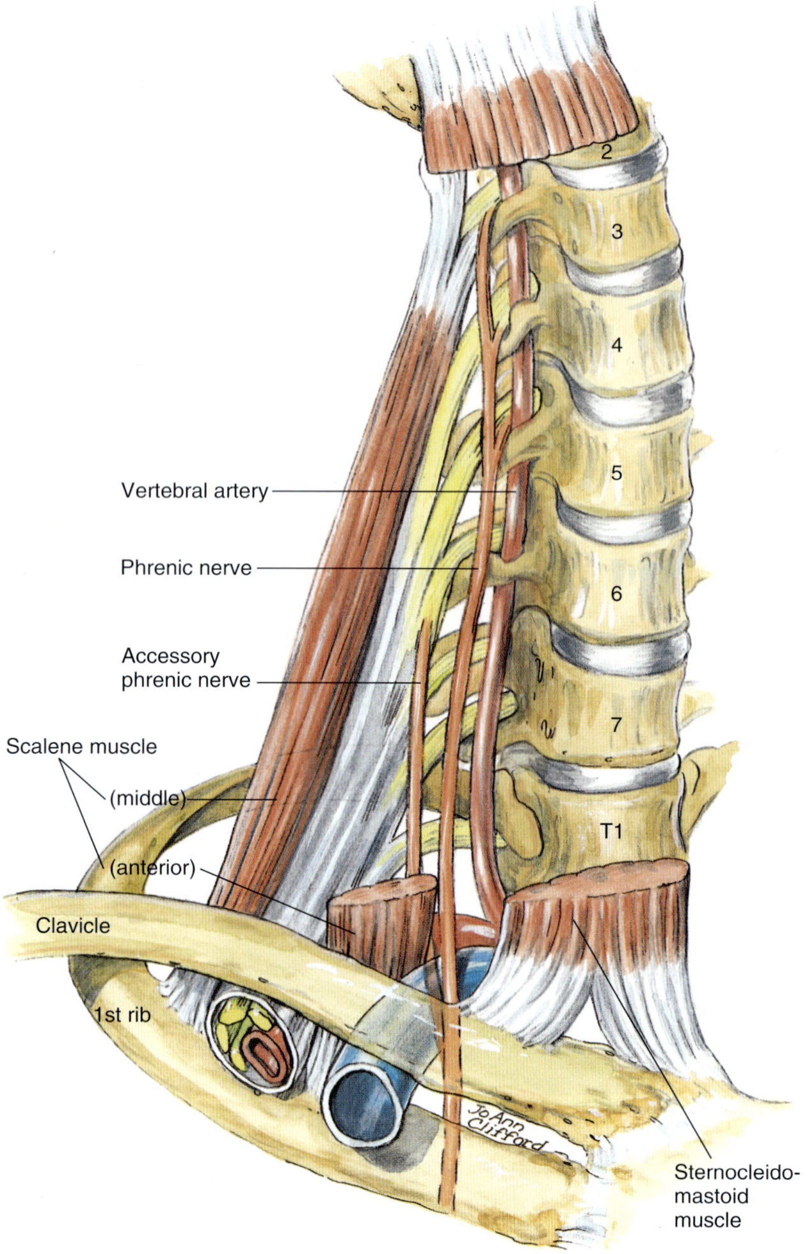

Fig. 4.9 Supraclavicular regional block: functional anatomy.

Although some of the brachial plexus neural anatomy of interest to anesthesiologists has been outlined, there are some anatomic details that should be highlighted (Fig. 4.9). As the cervical roots leave the transverse processes on their way to the brachial plexus, they exit in the gutter of the transverse process immediately posterior to the vertebral artery. The vertebral arteries leave the brachiocephalic and subclavian arteries on the right and left, respectively, and travel cephalad, normally entering a bony canal in the transverse process at the level of C6 and above. Thus one must be constantly aware of needle tip location in relationship to the vertebral artery. It should be remembered that the vertebral artery lies anterior to the roots of the brachial plexus as they leave the cervical vertebrae.

Another structure of interest in the brachial plexus anatomy is the phrenic nerve. It is formed from branches of the third, fourth, and fifth cervical nerves and passes through the neck on its way to the thorax on the ventral surface of the anterior scalene muscle. It is almost always blocked during interscalene block and less frequently with supraclavicular techniques or with cervical paravertebral block. Avoidance of phrenic blockade is important in only a small percentage of patients, although phrenic nerve location should be kept in mind for those with significantly decreased pulmonary function—that is, those whose day-to-day activities are limited by their pulmonary impairment.

Another detail of the brachial plexus anatomy that needs amplification is the organization of the brachial plexus nerves (divisions) as they cross the first rib. Textbooks often depict the nerves in a stacked arrangement at this point. However, radiologic, clinical, ultrasonographic, and anatomic investigations demonstrate that the nerves are not discretely "stacked" at this point, but rather assume a posterior and cranial relationship to the subclavian artery (Fig. 4.10). This is important when one is carrying out

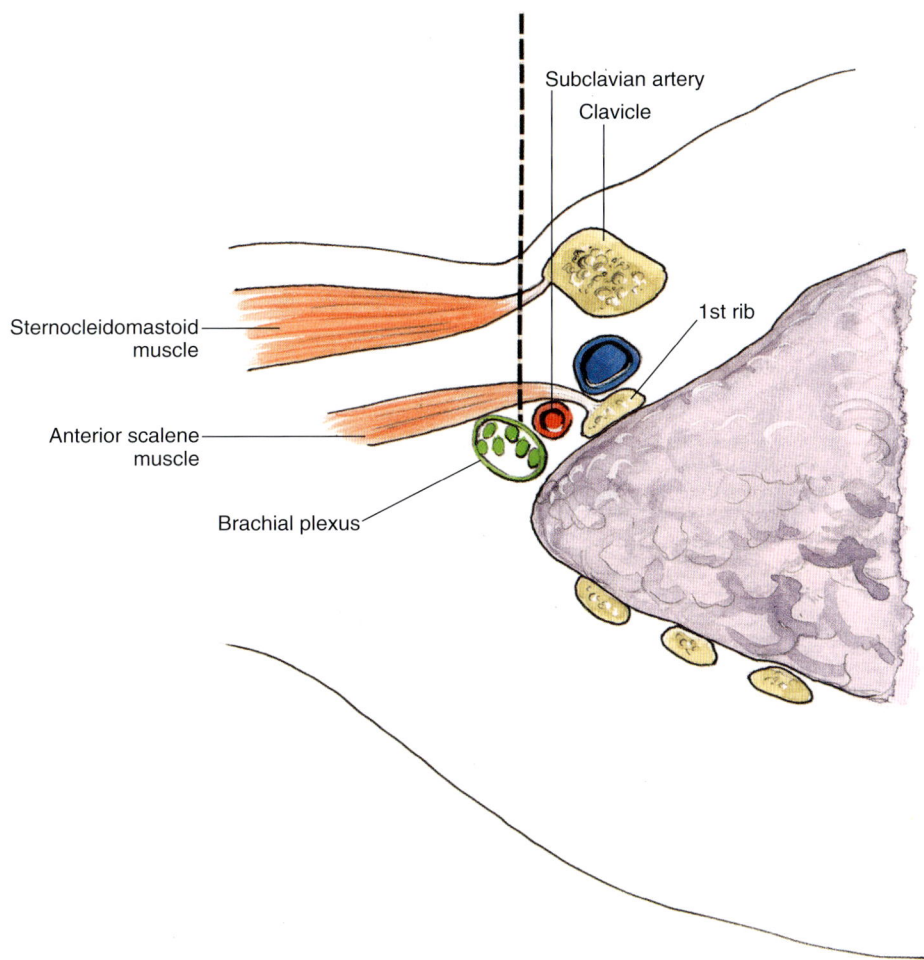

Fig. 4.10 Supraclavicular block anatomy: functional anatomy of brachial plexus, subclavian artery, and first rib.

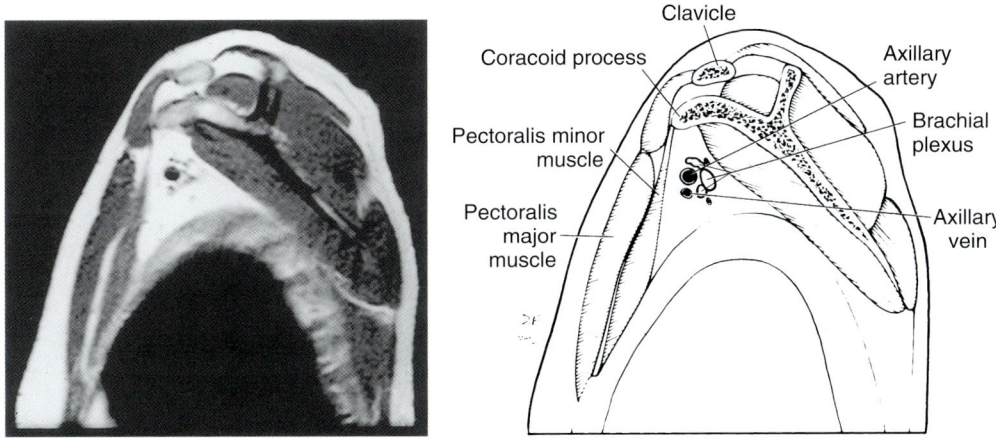

Fig. 4.11 Parasagittal magnetic resonance image and line drawing of the important anatomy in the infraclavicular block. *(From Brown DL: Regional Anesthesia and Analgesia. Philadelphia, WB Saunders, 1996. "Used with permission of Mayo Foundation for Medical Education and Research. All rights reserved.")*

supraclavicular nerve block and is using the rib as an anatomic landmark. The relationship of the nerves to the artery means that if one simply walks the needle tip closely along the first rib, one may not elicit paresthesias as easily, because the nerves are more cranial in relationship to the first rib.

Another anatomic detail that needs highlighting is the proximal axillary anatomy at a parasagittal section through the coracoid process. At this transition site, the brachial plexus is changing from the brachial plexus cords to the peripheral nerves as it surrounds the subclavian and axillary arteries (Fig. 4.11). At the site of this parasagittal section, the borders of the proximal axilla are formed by the following anatomic structures:

Anterior: posterior border of the pectoralis minor muscle and brachial head of the biceps

Posterior: scapula and subscapularis, latissimus dorsi, and teres major muscles

Medial: lateral aspect of chest wall, including the ribs and intercostal and serratus anterior muscles

Lateral: medial aspect of upper arm

These anatomic relationships are important during continuous techniques of infraclavicular block.

Interscalene Block

5

Ehab Farag with David L. Brown

PERSPECTIVE

Interscalene block (classic anterior approach) is especially effective for surgery of the shoulder or upper arm because the roots of the brachial plexus are most easily blocked with this technique. Frequently the ulnar nerve and its more peripheral distribution in the hand can be spared, unless one makes a special effort to inject local anesthetic caudad to the site of the initial paresthesia. This block is ideal for reduction of a dislocated shoulder and often can be achieved with as little as 10–15 mL of local anesthetic. This block also can be performed with the arm in almost any position and thus can be useful when brachial plexus block needs to be repeated during a prolonged upper extremity procedure.

Patient Selection. Interscalene block is applicable to nearly all patients because even obese patients usually have identifiable scalene and vertebral body anatomy. However, interscalene block should be avoided in patients with significantly impaired pulmonary function. This point may be moot if one is planning to use a combined regional and general anesthetic technique, which allows intraoperative control of ventilation. Even when a long-acting local anesthetic is chosen for the interscalene technique, usually phrenic nerve, and thus pulmonary function will return to a level that patients can tolerate by the time the average-length surgical procedure is completed.

Pharmacologic Choice. Useful agents for interscalene block are primarily the amino amides. Lidocaine and mepivacaine provide surgical anesthesia for 2–3 hours without epinephrine and for 3–5 hours when epinephrine is added. These drugs can be useful for less complex or outpatient surgical procedures. For more extensive surgical procedures requiring hospital admission, longer-acting agents such as bupivacaine or ropivacaine can be chosen. The more complex surgical procedures on the shoulder often require muscle relaxation; thus bupivacaine concentrations of at least 0.5% are needed. Plain bupivacaine produces surgical anesthesia lasting from 4–6 hours; the addition of epinephrine may prolong this to 8–12 hours. Ropivacaine's effects are slightly shorter in duration.

TRADITIONAL BLOCK TECHNIQUE

PLACEMENT

Anatomy. Surface anatomy of importance to anesthesiologists includes the larynx, sternocleidomastoid muscle, and external jugular vein. Interscalene block is most often performed at the level of the C6 vertebral body, which is at the level of the cricoid cartilage. Thus by projecting a line laterally from the cricoid cartilage, one can identify the level at which one should roll the fingers off the sternocleidomastoid muscle onto the belly of the anterior scalene and then into the interscalene groove. When firm pressure is applied, in most individuals it is possible to feel the transverse process of C6, and in some people it is possible to elicit a paresthesia by deep palpation. The external jugular vein often overlies the interscalene groove at the level of C6, although this should not be relied on (Fig. 5.1).

It is important to visualize what lies under the palpating fingers; again, the key to carrying out successful interscalene block is the identification of the interscalene groove. Fig. 5.2 allows us to look beneath surface anatomy and develop a sense of how closely the lateral border of the anterior scalene muscle deviates from the border of the sternocleidomastoid muscle. This feature should be constantly kept in mind. The anterior scalene muscle and the interscalene groove are oriented at an oblique angle to the long axis of the sternocleidomastoid muscle. Fig. 5.3 removes the anterior scalene and highlights the fact that at the level of C6, the vertebral artery begins its route to the base of the brain by traveling through the root of the transverse process in each of the more cephalad cervical vertebrae.

Position. The patient lies supine with the neck in the neutral position and the head turned slightly opposite the site to be blocked. The anesthesiologist then asks the patient to lift the head off the table to tense the sternocleidomastoid muscle and allow identification of its lateral border. The fingers then roll onto the belly of the anterior scalene and subsequently into the interscalene groove. This maneuver should be carried out in the horizontal plane through the cricoid cartilage—thus at the level of C6. To roll the

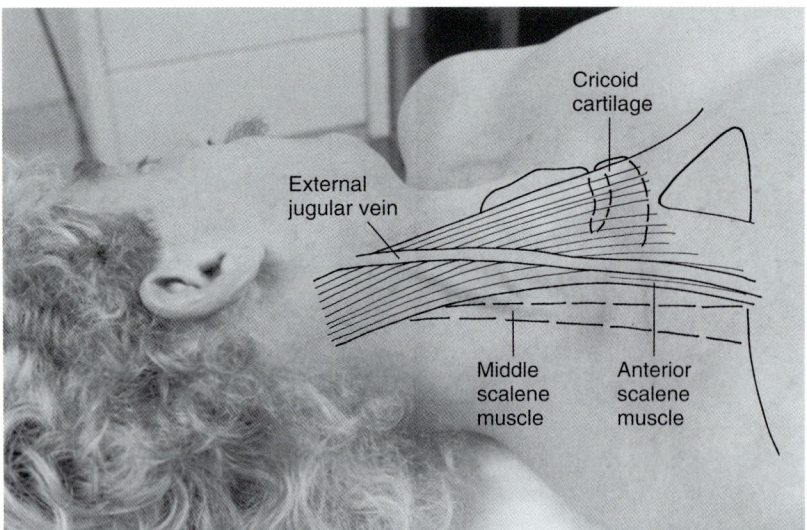

Fig. 5.1 Interscalene block: surface anatomy.

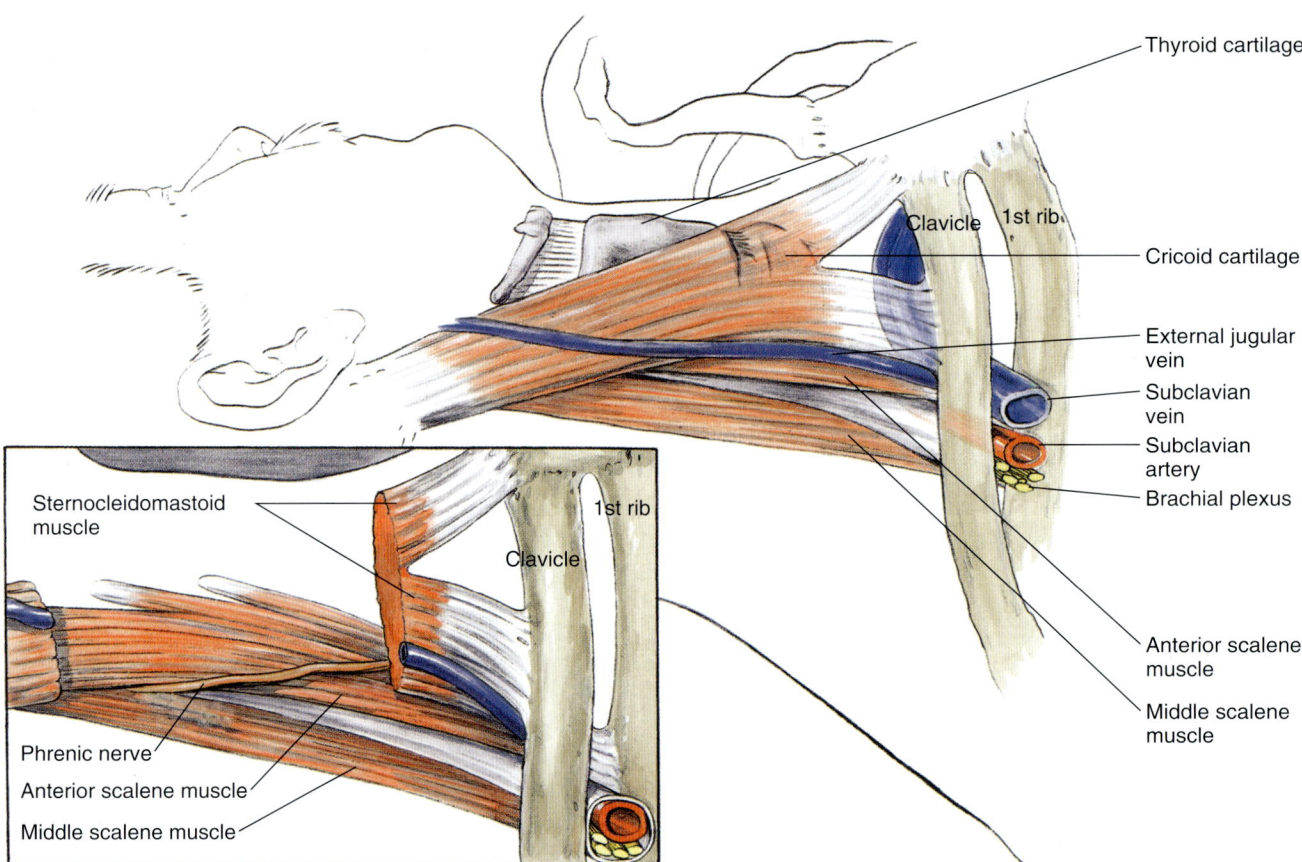

Fig. 5.2 Interscalene block: functional anatomy of scalene muscles.

fingers effectively the operator should stand at the patient's side (Fig. 5.4).

Needle Puncture. When the interscalene groove has been identified and the operator's fingers are firmly pressing in it, the needle is inserted, as shown in Fig. 5.5, in a slightly caudal and slightly posterior direction. As a further directional help, if the needle for this block is imagined to be long and inserted deeply enough, it would exit the neck posteriorly in approximately the midline at the level of the C7 or T1 spinous process. If a paresthesia or motor response is not elicited on insertion, the needle is "walked" while maintaining the same needle angulation as shown in Fig. 5.4 in a plane joining the cricoid cartilage to the C6 transverse process. Because the brachial plexus traverses the neck at virtually a right angle to this plane, a paresthesia or motor response is almost guaranteed if small enough steps of needle reinsertion are carried out. When undertaking the block for shoulder surgery, this is probably the one brachial plexus block in which a large volume of local anesthetic coupled with a single needle position allows effective anesthesia. For shoulder surgery 25–35 mL of lidocaine, mepivacaine, bupivacaine, or ropivacaine can be used. If the interscalene block is being carried out for forearm or hand surgery, a second, more caudal needle position is desirable, in which 10–15 mL of additional local anesthetic is injected to allow spread along more caudal roots.

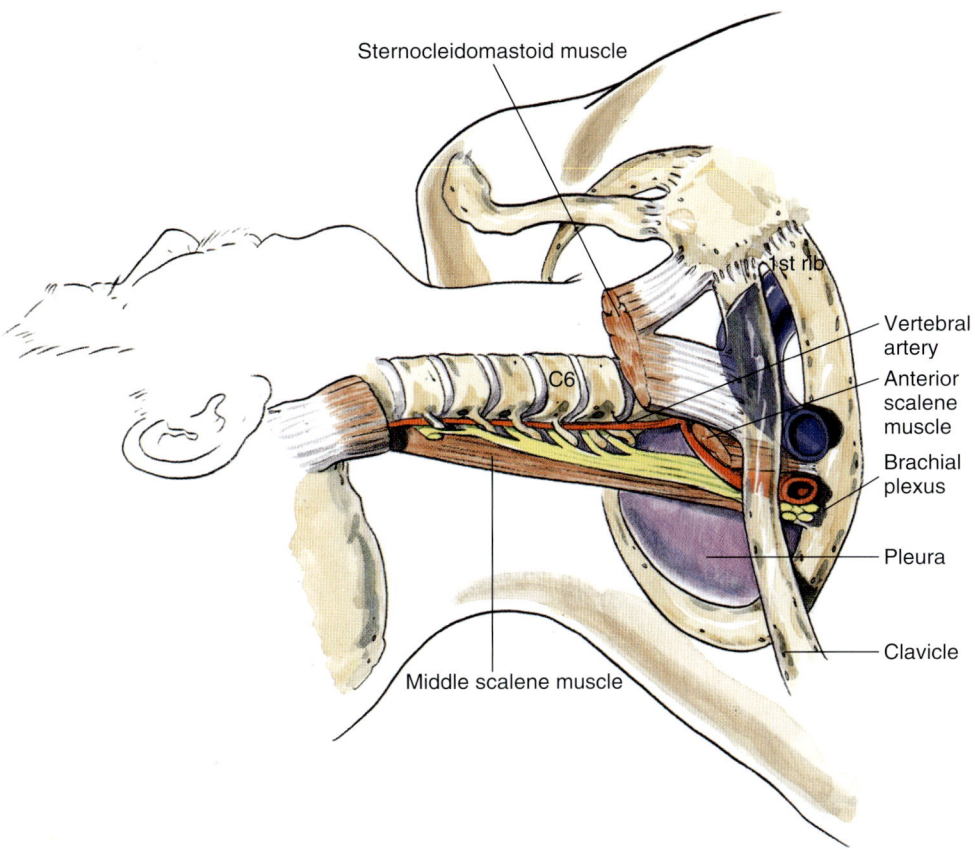

Fig. 5.3 Interscalene block: functional anatomy of vertebral artery.

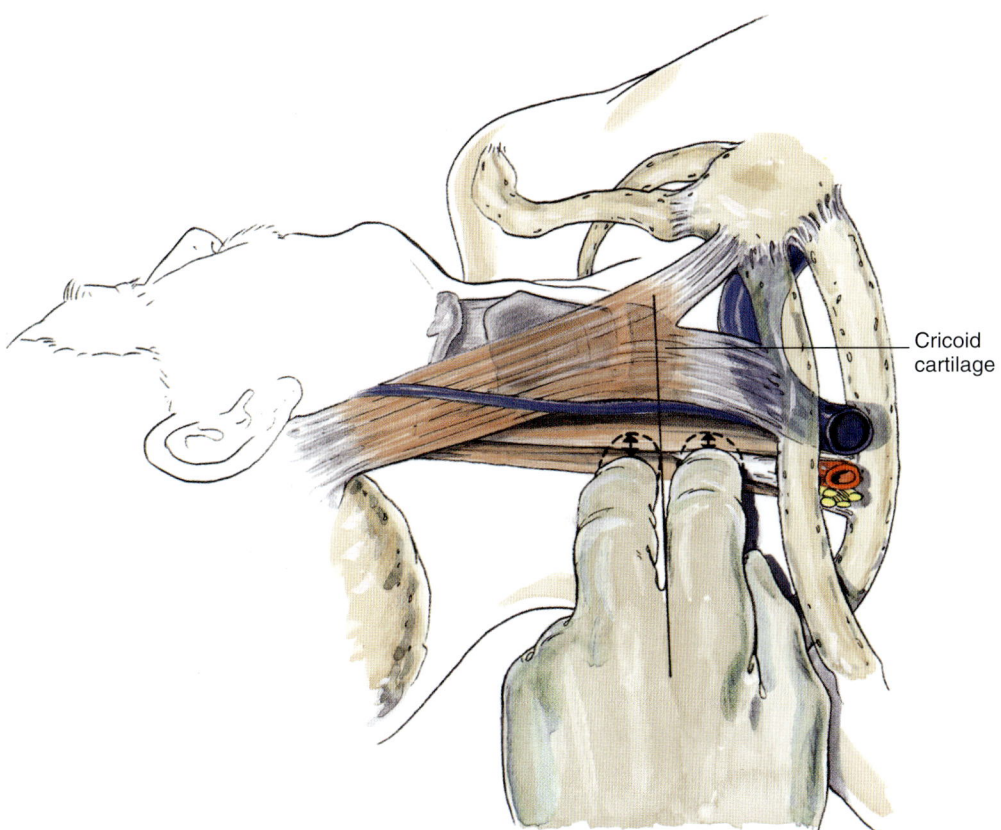

Fig. 5.4 Interscalene block technique: palpation.

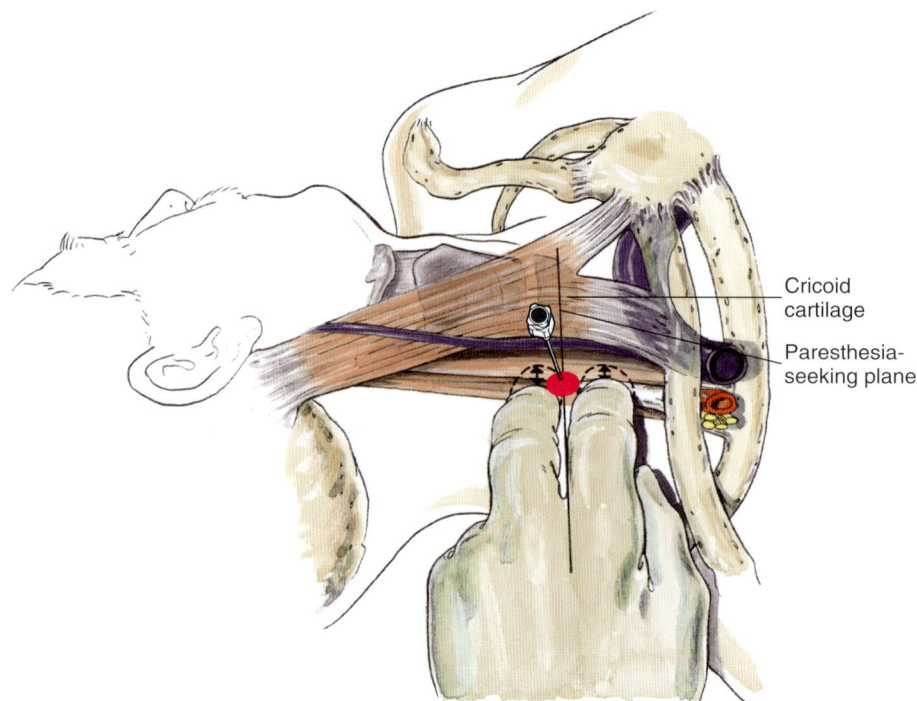

Fig. 5.5 Interscalene block technique: "paresthesia-seeking" plane.

POTENTIAL PROBLEMS

Problems that can arise from interscalene block include subarachnoid injection, epidural block, intravascular injection (especially in the vertebral artery), pneumothorax, and phrenic block.

PEARLS

This block is most applicable to shoulder procedures, as opposed to forearm and hand surgical procedures, although some practitioners combine interscalene and axillary blocks to produce an approximation of a supraclavicular block. For shoulder surgery block that requires muscle relaxation, a local anesthetic concentration that provides adequate motor block should be chosen (i.e., mepivacaine and lidocaine at 1.5%, bupivacaine at 0.5%, and ropivacaine at 0.75% concentrations). Because this block is most often carried out through a single injection site and the operator relies on the spread of local anesthetic solution, one must allow sufficient "soak time" after the injection. This often means from 20–35 minutes.

If there is difficulty in identifying the anterior scalene muscle, one maneuver is to have the patient maximally inhale while the anesthesiologist palpates the neck. During this maneuver the scalene muscles should contract before the sternocleidomastoid muscle contracts, and this may allow clarification of the anterior scalene muscle in the difficult-to-palpate neck. Further, if the operator is finding it difficult to elicit a paresthesia or produce a motor response during nerve stimulation with this block, it is almost always because the needle entry site has been placed too far posteriorly. For example, Fig. 5.6 shows that if the right side of the neck is divided into a 180-degree arc, the needle entry site should be approximately at 60 degrees from the sagittal plane to optimize production of the block.

Most of the injection difficulties that result in complications can be avoided if one remembers that this should be a very "superficial" block; if the palpating fingers apply sufficient pressure, no more than 1–1.5 cm of the needle should be necessary to reach the plexus. It is when the needle is inserted deeply that one must be cautious about subarachnoid, epidural, and intravascular injection. For an operation that requires ulnar nerve block, I would not choose the interscalene block. The ulnar nerve is difficult to block with the interscalene approach because it is derived from the eighth cervical nerve (this nerve is difficult to block after injection at a more cephalic injection site). Finally, one should be cautious about using this block in a patient with significant pulmonary impairment because phrenic block is almost guaranteed with the interscalene block.

ULTRASOUND FOR INTERSCALENE BLOCK

KEY POINTS

- A small linear (20- to 25-mm) footprint is preferred for this block.
- The most successful way to perform this block is to visualize the brachial plexus in the supraclavicular region and then scan cephalad to identify the roots that are sandwiched between the anterior scalene and middle scalene muscles.
- Insertion of the needle and the catheter between C5 and C6 or C6 and C7 will help to properly anchor the catheter and ensure good analgesia after shoulder surgery.

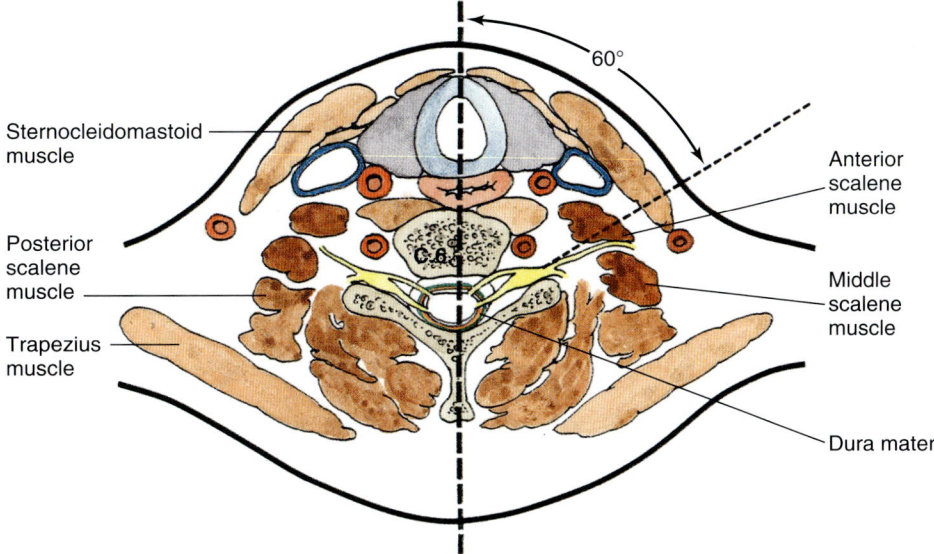

Fig. 5.6 Interscalene block anatomy: an angle of approximately 60 degrees from the sagittal plane is the optimal needle angle for the block.

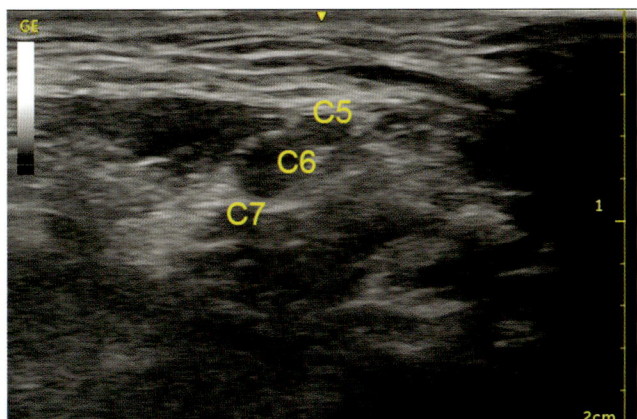

Fig. 5.7 Interscalene ultrasound.

SONOANATOMY

The interscalene block is performed in the posterior triangle (Figs. 5.7 through 5.9), which lies between the posterior border of the sternocleidomastoid muscle and the trapezius muscle, next to the sixth and seventh cervical vertebra. In the interscalene block, the brachial plexus is made of nerve roots (C5, C6, C7) or trunks. The brachial plexus in the interscalene block appears as hypoechogenic nodules (due to the high ratio of neural/nonneural tissue in this region) located between the anterior and middle scalene muscles under the prevertebral fascia. The dorsal scapular and long thoracic nerves of the brachial plexus are frequently located in the middle scalene muscle at less than 1 cm posterior to the plexus. The nerves appear as hyperechoic structures containing a hypoechoic center.

INDICATIONS

- The principal indication for interscalene block is surgery of the shoulder. Local anesthetic spread after the block includes the supraclavicular (nonbrachial plexus) nerve (C3 to C4), which supplies sensory innervation to the cape of the shoulder.
- The interscalene block can be used for surgery on the humerus neck; however, it is not sufficient for hand surgeries, as it misses the lower roots and the trunk of the plexus.

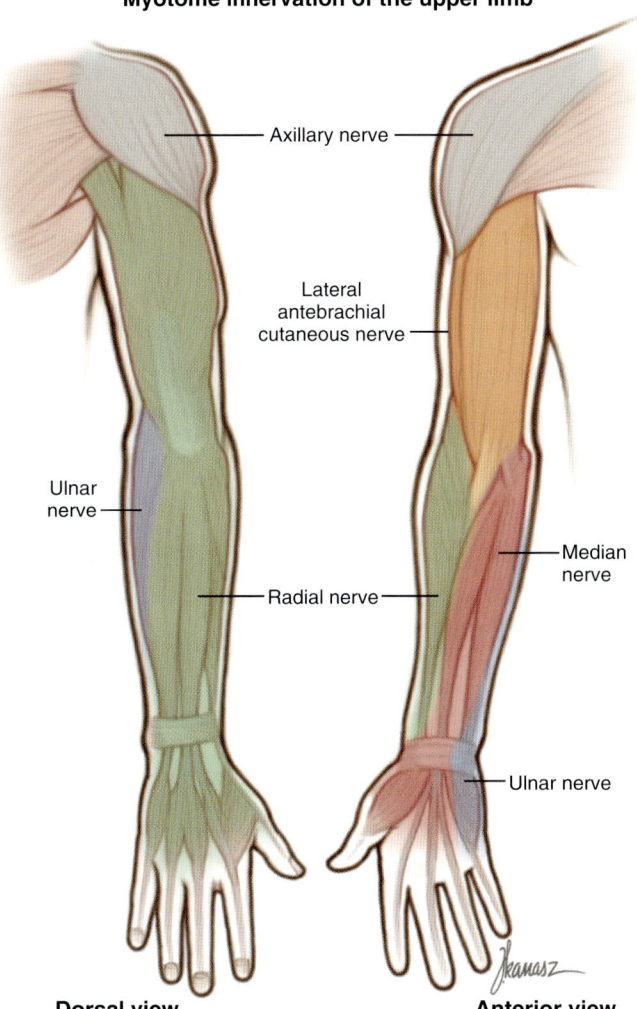

Fig. 5.8 The myotome innervation of the upper limb.

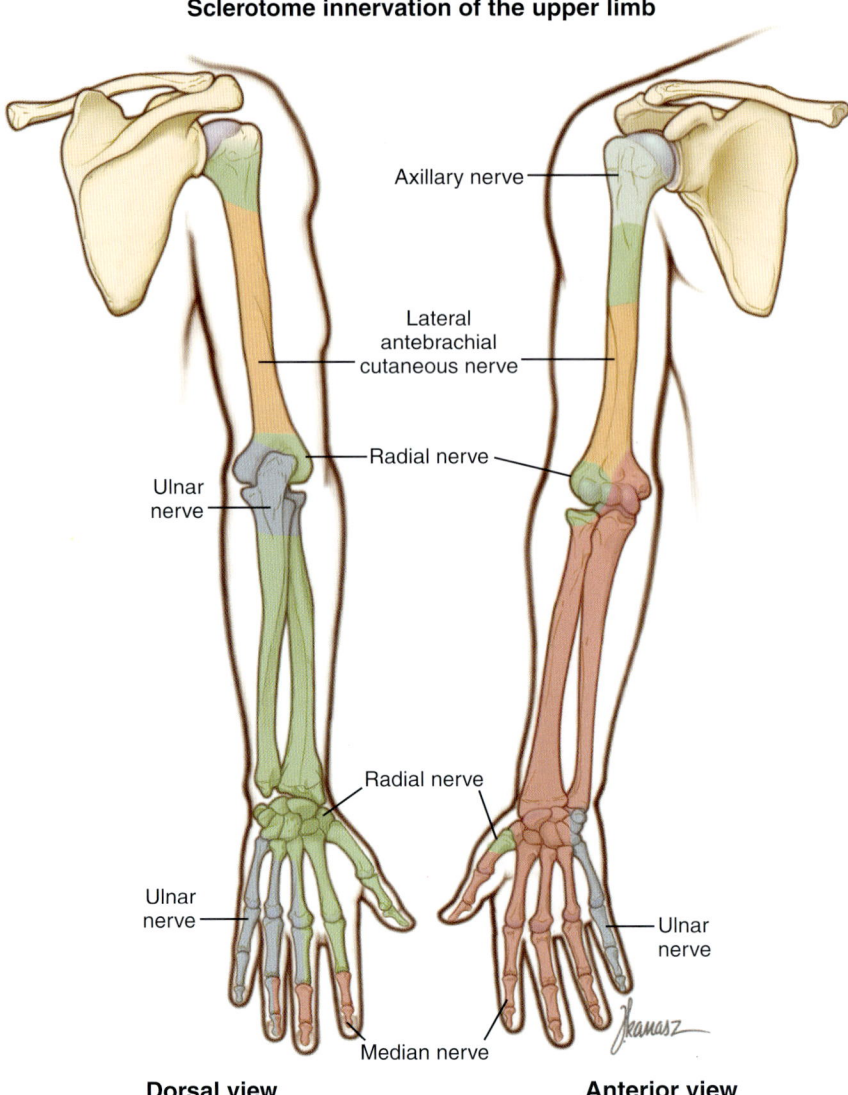

Fig. 5.9 Sclerotome innervation of the upper limb.

TECHNIQUE

The patient position is usually either supine with the head turned to the opposite side to be blocked or in the lateral decubitus position. We prefer to insert the block in the lateral decubitus position, especially during the catheter insertion. The supraclavicular region is usually scanned to identify the brachial plexus superficial and lateral to the subclavian artery. The brachial plexus is then followed cephalad to identify the roots of the brachial plexus in the interscalene region sandwiched between the anterior scalene and middle scalene muscles. In the transverse short-axis view of the plexus, the in-plane needle passes from the lateral into the medial direction in the supine position or from the posterior into the anterior direction in the lateral decubitus direction. The needle should be positioned between C5 and C6 or C6 and C7 in order to achieve a proper block for the shoulder surgery. In the case of catheter insertion, we prefer to pass the Tuohy needle through the middle scalene muscle below the dorsal scapular and long thoracic nerves to give the catheter better anchoring into the plexus. A fascial click is often felt when the needle penetrates the middle scalene fascia in order to reach the interscalene space (Figs. 5.10 through 5.17).

PEARLS

- The phrenic nerve and brachial plexus are within 2 mm of each other at the cricoid cartilage level, with additional 3 mm separation for every cm more caudal in the neck. Therefore puncture localization 1–2 cm caudal to the cricoid cartilage can be helpful in reducing phrenic nerve palsy after interscalene block.
- The transverse cervical artery or dorsal scapular artery is sometimes visible at the targeted site of injection. Therefore color Doppler can be useful to identify those vessels, as they might be misidentified as nerve structures.
- The needle insertion in the middle scalene muscle should be at a lower level to the dorsal scapular and long thoracic nerves. Injury to the dorsal scapular nerve is characterized by a dull ache along the medial border of the scapula and weakness and hypotrophy of the rhomboid and/or the levator scapulae muscles. Injury to the long thoracic nerve will result in chronic pain syndrome of the shoulder and different degree of serratus muscle weakness.

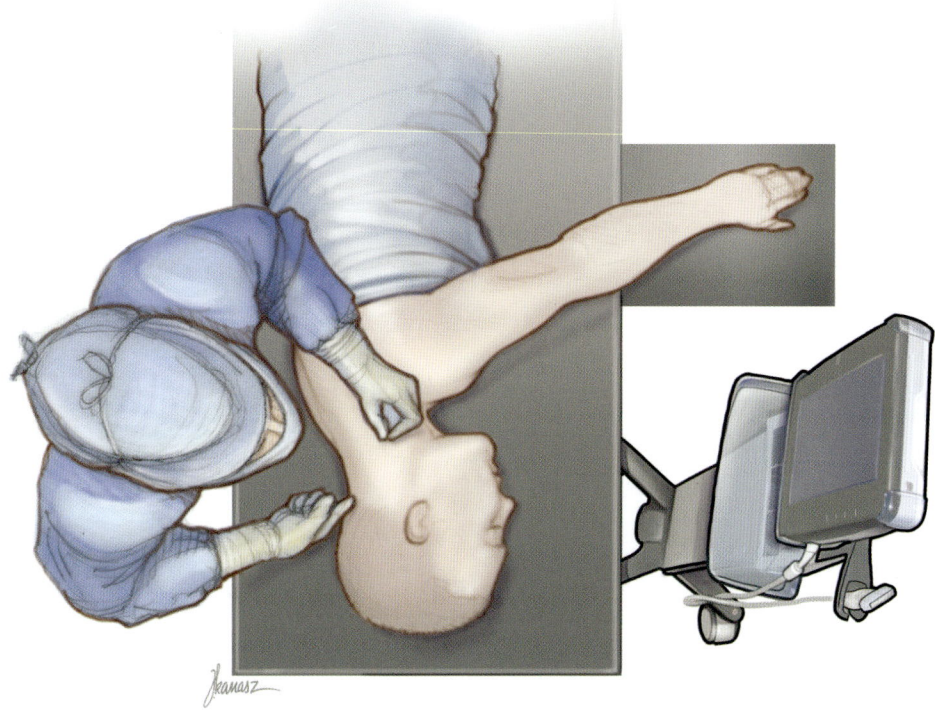

Fig. 5.10 Lateral decubitus position (posterior approach) for the interscalene block.

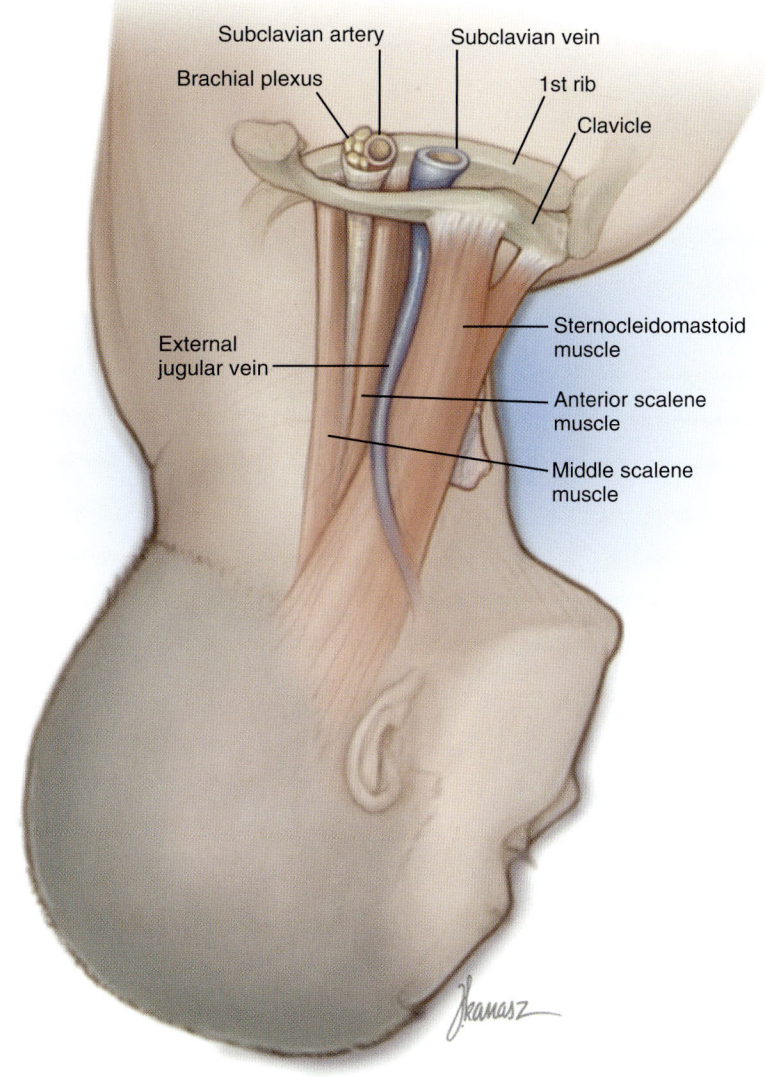

Fig. 5.11 Anatomy of the interscalene block and the lateral decubitus position.

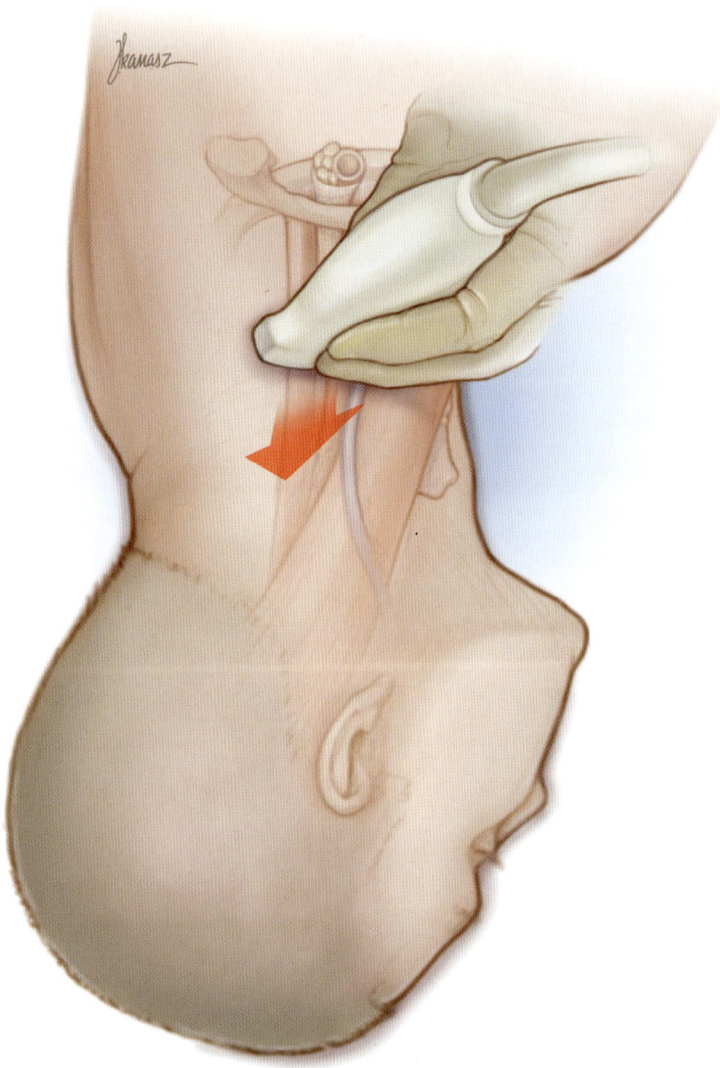

Fig. 5.12 The brachial plexus is scanned in the cephalad direction from supraclavicular region to identify the roots of brachial plexus in the interscalene region between anterior and middle scalene muscle.

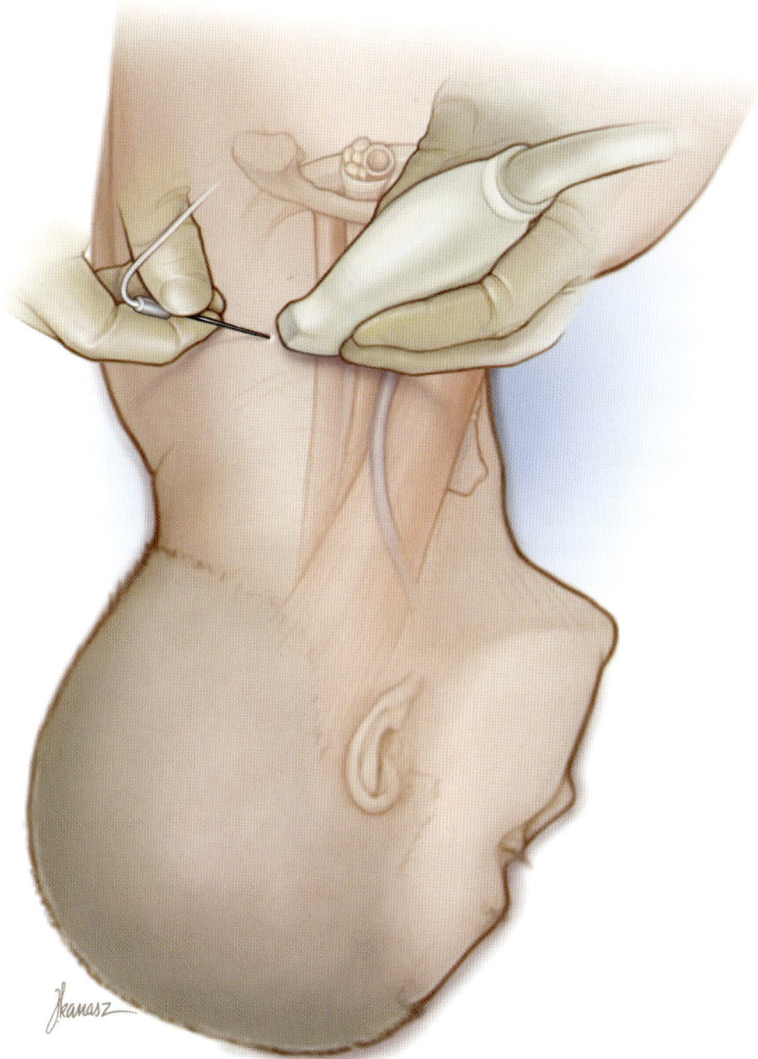

Fig. 5.13 In-plane technique for interscalene block with the needle direction from posterior to anterior in the lateral decubitus position.

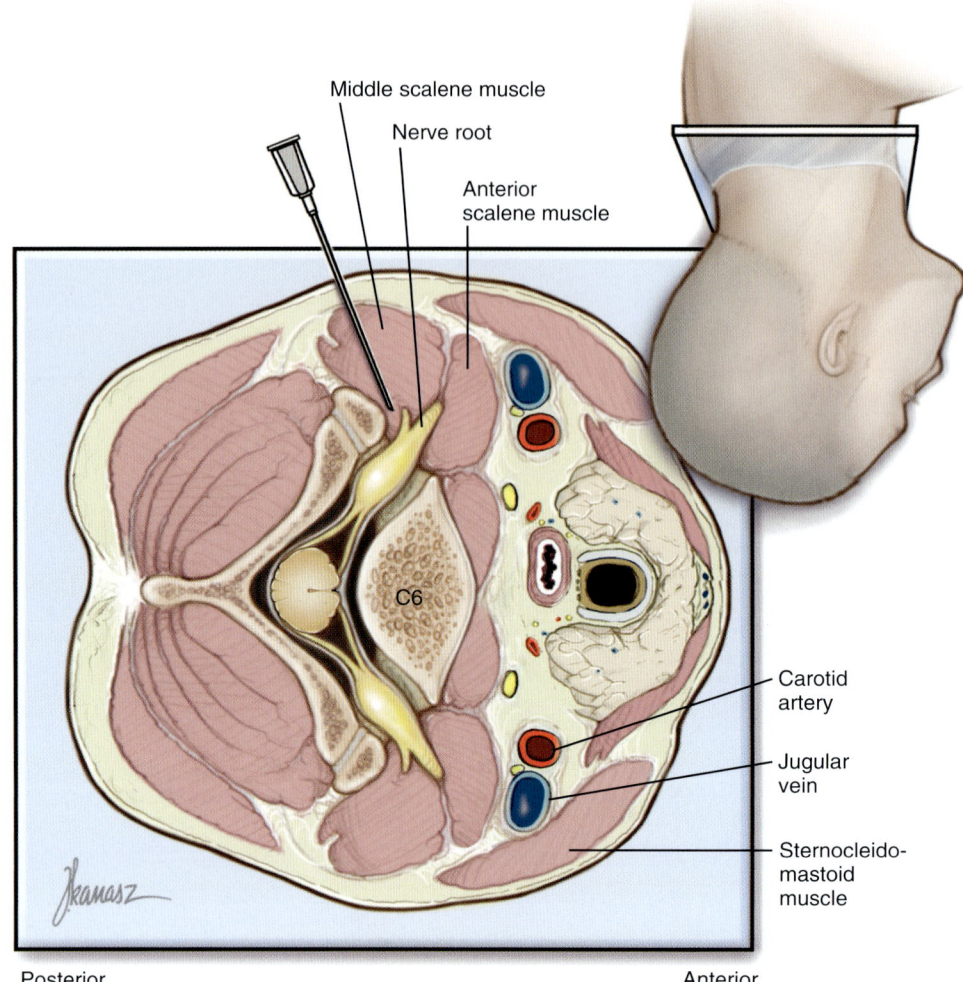

Fig. 5.14 Interscalene block. Notice the needle has to pass through middle scalene muscle to reach the roots of the brachial plexus in the interscalene groove.

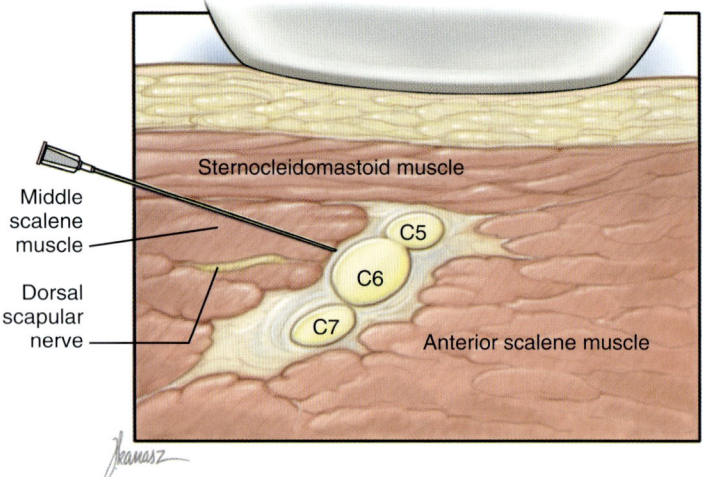

Fig. 5.15 The needle position between C5 and C6 roots of the brachial plexus.

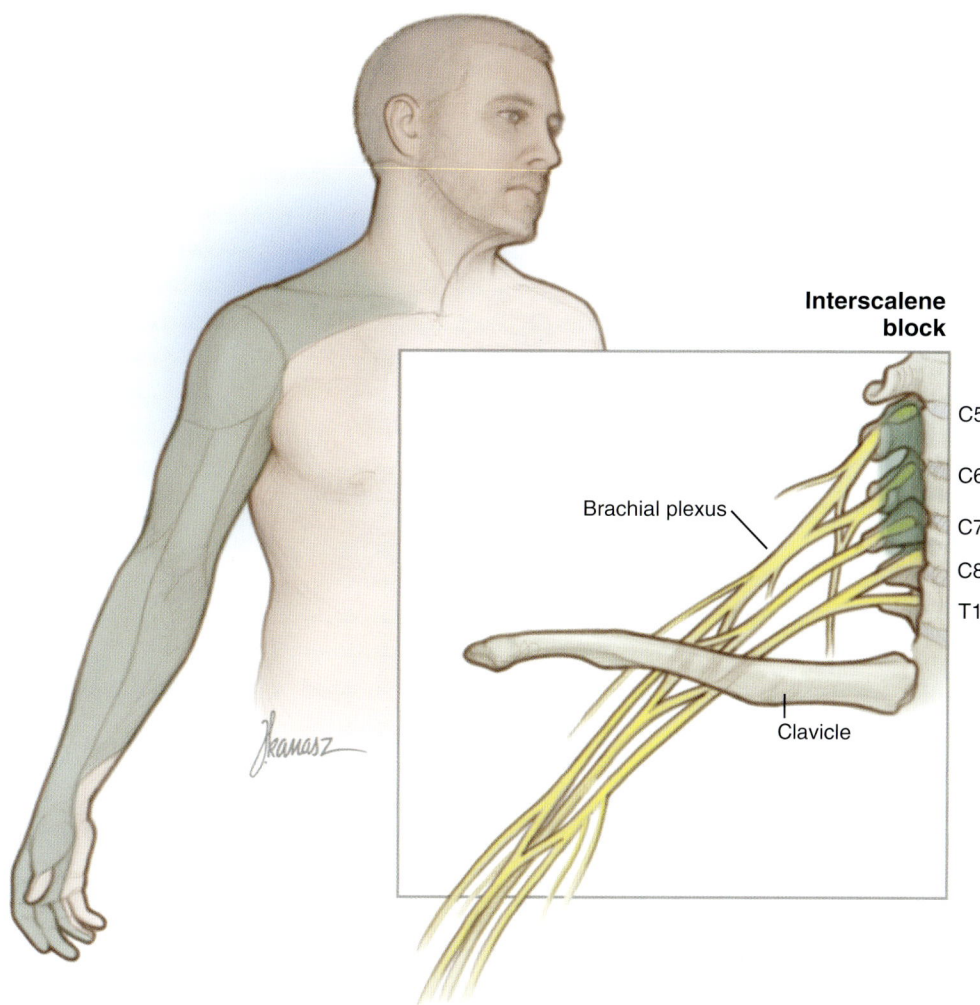

Fig. 5.16 The anatomy of the interscalene block. Notice the roots are blocked in this technique.

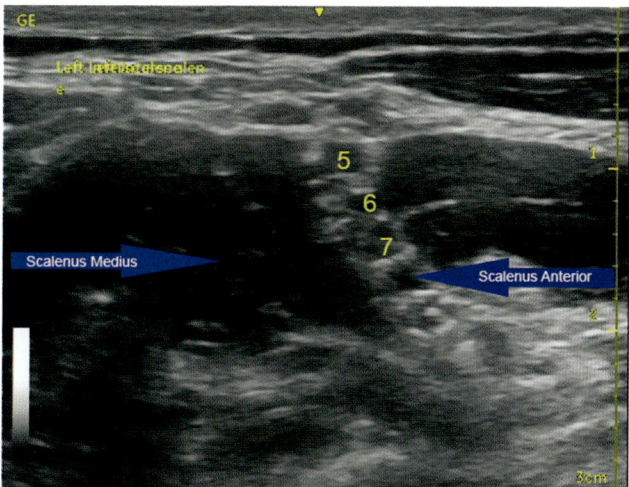

Fig. 5.17 Ultrasound of interscalene. Note the roots of the brachial plexus are sandwiched between the scalenus anterior and the scalenus medius.

Supraclavicular Block 6

Ehab Farag and David L. Brown

PERSPECTIVE

Supraclavicular block provides anesthesia of the entire upper extremity in the most consistent, efficient manner of any brachial plexus technique. It is the most effective block for all portions of the upper extremity and is carried out at the division level of the brachial plexus; perhaps this is why there is often little or no sparing of peripheral nerves if an adequate paresthesia is obtained. If this block is to be used for shoulder surgery, it should be supplemented with a superficial cervical plexus block to anesthetize the skin overlying the shoulder.

Patient Selection. Almost all patients are candidates for this block, with the exception of those who are uncooperative. In addition, in less experienced hands it may be inappropriate for outpatients. Although pneumothorax is an infrequent complication of the block, such an event often becomes apparent only after a delay of several hours, when an outpatient may already be at home. Also, because the supraclavicular block relies principally on bony and muscular landmarks, very obese patients are not good candidates because they often have supraclavicular fat pads that interfere with easy application of this technique.

Pharmacologic Choice. As with other brachial plexus blocks, the prime consideration in drug selection should be the length of the procedure and the degree of motor blockade desired. Mepivacaine (1%–1.5%), lidocaine (1%–1.5%), bupivacaine (0.5%), and ropivacaine (0.5%– 0.75%) are all applicable to brachial plexus block. Lidocaine and mepivacaine will produce 2–3 hours of surgical anesthesia without epinephrine and 3–5 hours when epinephrine is added. These drugs can be useful for less involved or outpatient surgical procedures. For extensive surgical procedures requiring hospital admission, a longer-acting agent like bupivacaine can be chosen. Plain bupivacaine produces surgical anesthesia lasting from 4–6 hours, and the addition of epinephrine may prolong this time to 8–12 hours, whereas ropivacaine is slightly shorter acting.

TRADITIONAL BLOCK TECHNIQUE

PLACEMENT

Anatomy. The anatomy of interest for this block is the relationship between the brachial plexus and the first rib, the subclavian artery, and the cupola of the lung (Fig. 6.1). Our experience suggests that this block is more difficult to teach than many of the other regional blocks, and for that reason two approaches to the supraclavicular block are illustrated: the classic Kulenkampff approach and the vertical ("plumb bob") approach. The vertical approach has been developed in an attempt to overcome the difficulty and time necessary to become skilled in the classic supraclavicular block approach. Both techniques are clinically useful once mastered. As the subclavian artery and brachial plexus pass over the first rib, they do so between the insertion of the anterior and middle scalene muscles onto the first rib (Fig. 6.2). The nerves lie in a cephaloposterior relationship to the artery; thus a paresthesia may be elicited before the needle contacts the first rib. At the point where the artery and plexus cross the first rib, the rib is broad and flat, sloping caudad as it moves from posterior to anterior, and although the rib is a curved structure, there is a distance of 1–2 cm on which a needle can be "walked" in a parasagittal anteroposterior direction. Remember that immediately medial to the first rib is the cupola of the lung; when the needle angle is too medial, pneumothorax may result.

Position: Classic Supraclavicular Block. The patient lies supine without a pillow, with the head turned opposite the side to be blocked. The arms are at the sides, and the anesthesiologist can stand either at the head of the table or at the side of the patient, near the arm to be blocked.

Needle Puncture: Classic Supraclavicular Block. In the classic approach, the needle insertion site is approximately 1 cm superior to the clavicle at the clavicular midpoint (Fig. 6.3). This entry site is closer to the middle of the clavicle than to the junction of the middle and medial thirds (as often described in other regional anesthesia texts). In addition, if the artery is palpable in the supraclavicular fossa, it can be used as a landmark. From this point, the needle and syringe are inserted in a plane approximately parallel to the patient's neck and head, taking care that the axis of the syringe and needle does not aim medially toward the cupola of the lung. A 22-gauge, 5-cm needle typically will contact the rib at a depth of 3 to 4 cm, although in a very large patient it is sometimes necessary to insert it to a depth of 6 cm. The initial needle insertion should not be carried out past 3–4 cm until a careful search in an anteroposterior plane does not identify the first rib. During the insertion of the needle and syringe, the assembly should be controlled with the hand, as illustrated in Fig. 6.4.

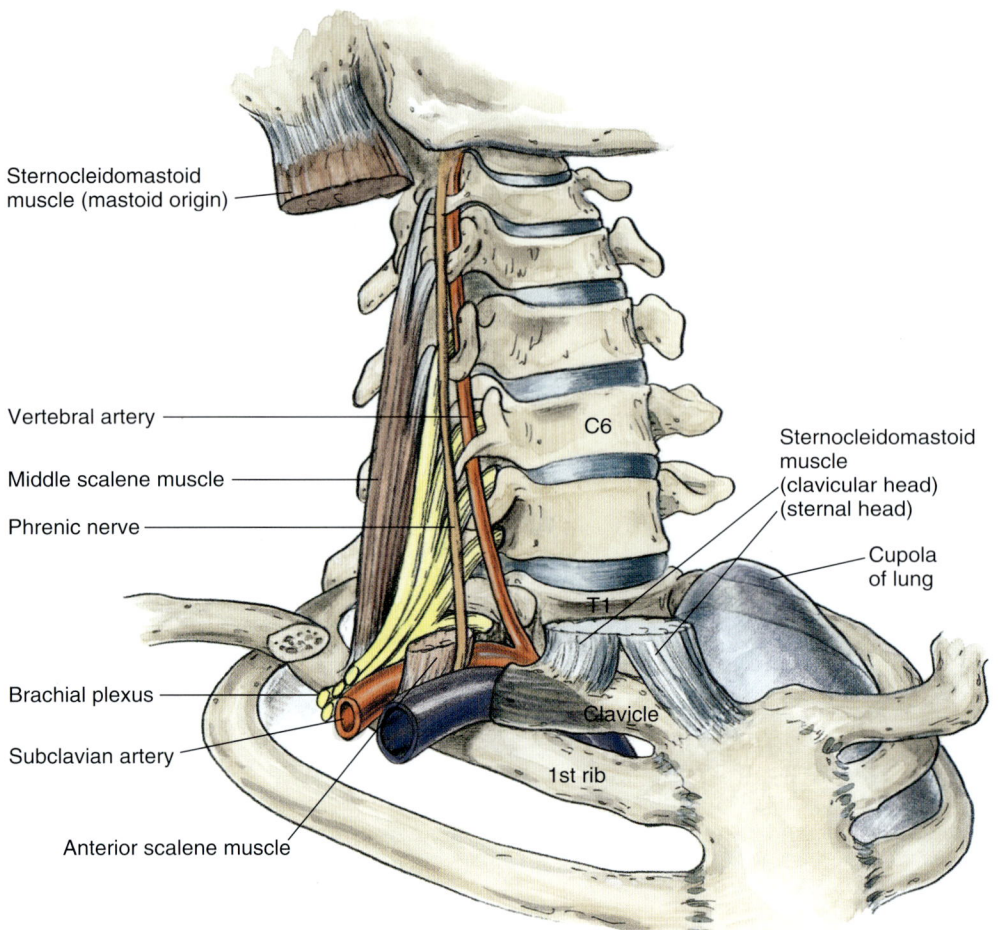

Fig. 6.1 Supraclavicular block: anatomy.

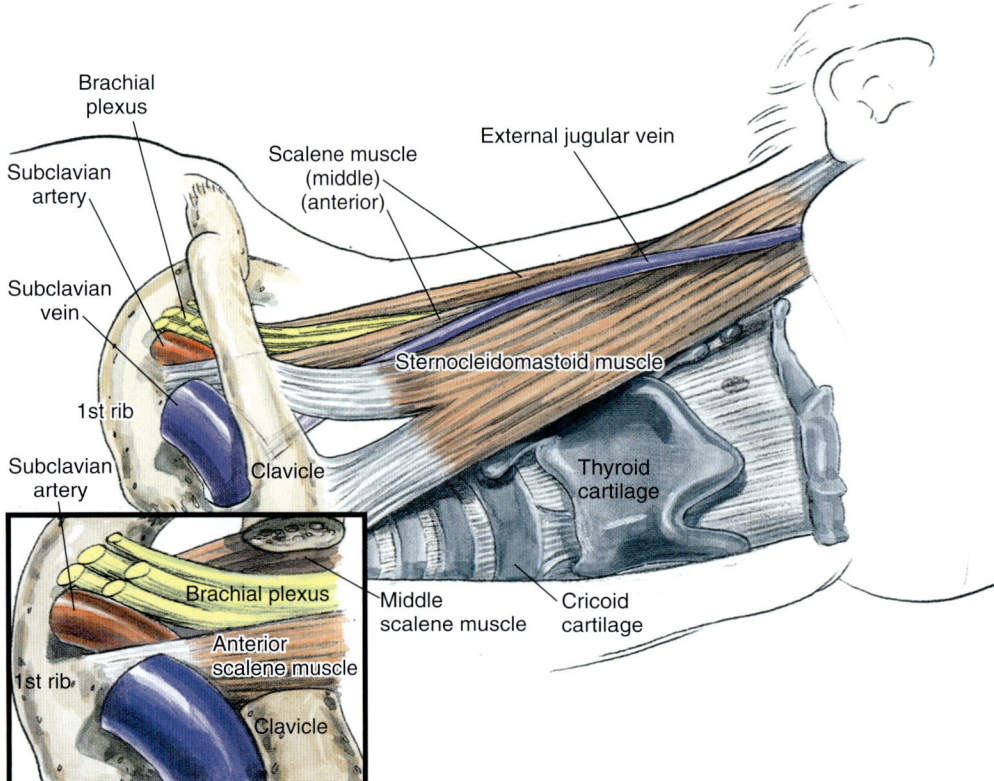

Fig. 6.2 Supraclavicular block: functional anatomy (with detail).

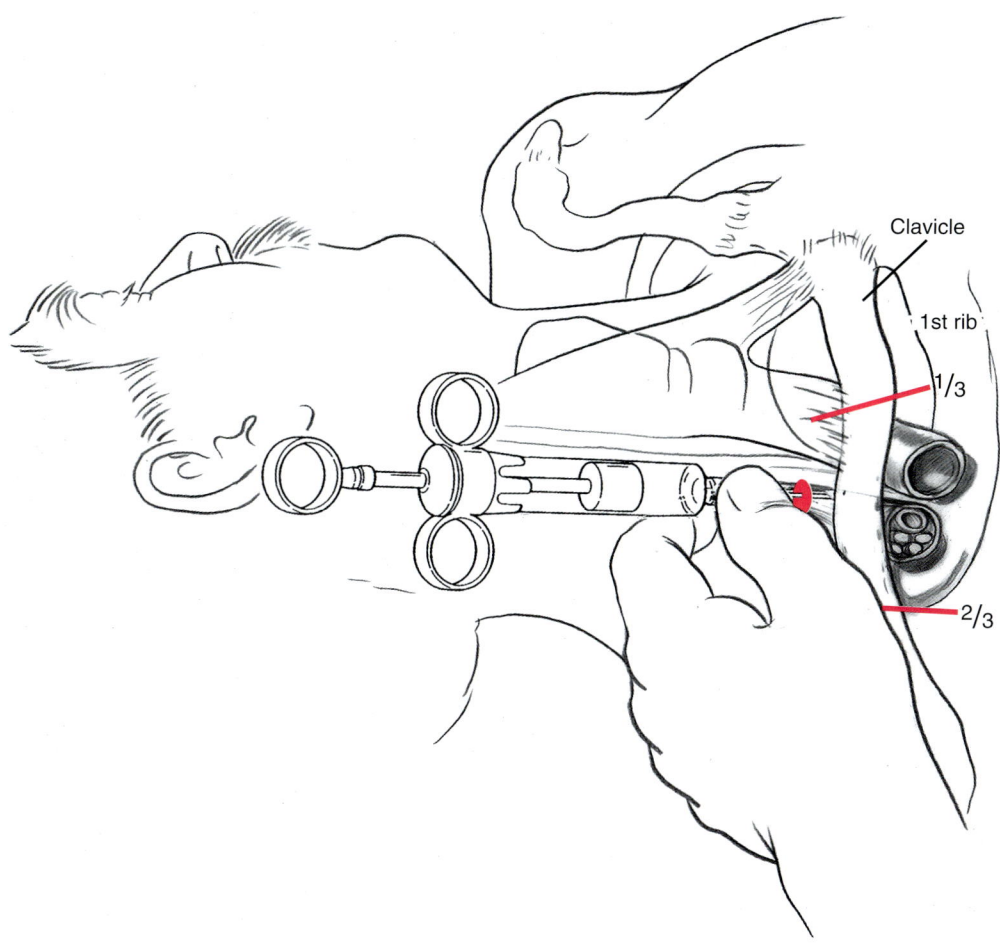

Fig. 6.3 Supraclavicular block (classic approach): insertion site.

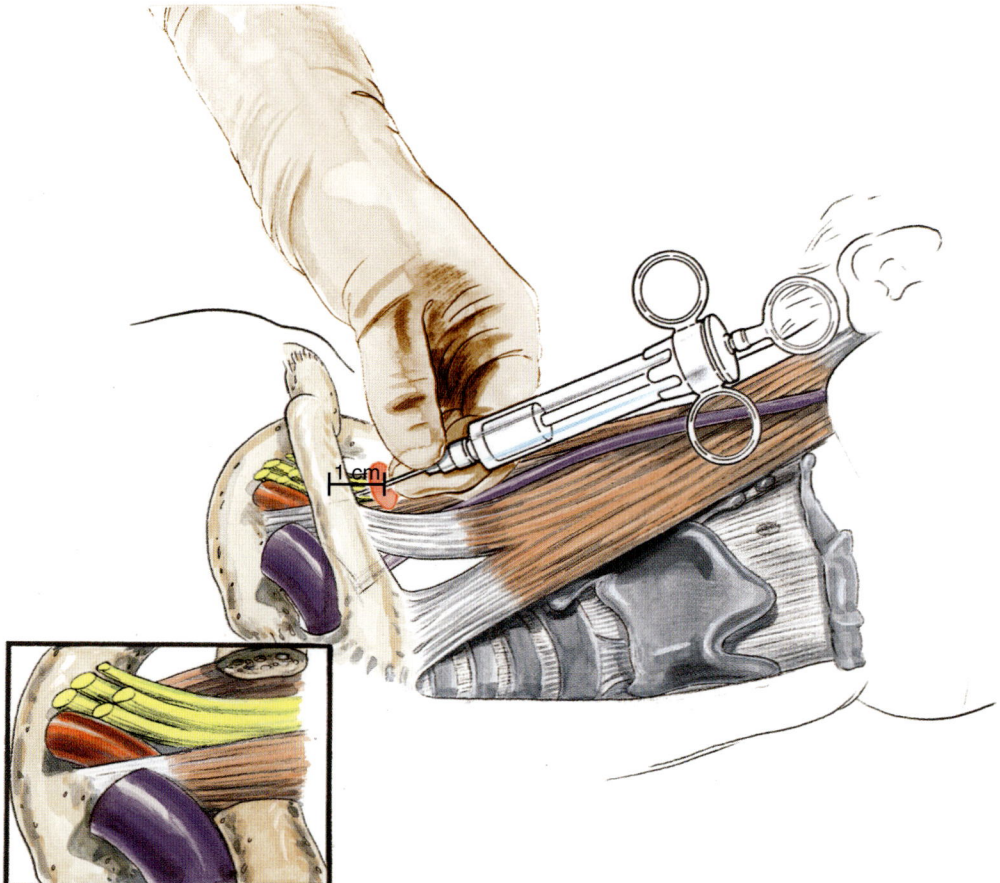

Fig. 6.4 Supraclavicular block (classic approach): hand and syringe assembly positioning.

The hand can rest lightly against the patient's supraclavicular fossa because patients often move the shoulder with elicitation of a paresthesia.

Position: Vertical (Plumb Bob) Supraclavicular Block. The vertical approach to the supraclavicular block was developed to simplify the anatomic projection necessary for the block. The patient should be positioned in a manner similar to that used for the classic approach, lying supine without a pillow, with the head turned slightly away from the side to be blocked. The anesthesiologist should stand lateral to the patient at the level of the patient's upper arm. This block involves inserting the needle and syringe assembly at approximately a 90-degree angle to that used in the classic approach.

Needle Puncture: Vertical (Plumb Bob) Supraclavicular Block. Patients are asked to raise the head slightly off the block table so that the lateral border of the sternocleidomastoid muscle can be marked as it inserts onto the clavicle. From that point, a plane is visualized running parasagittally through that site (Fig. 6.5). The name "plumb bob" was chosen for this block concept because if one were to suspend a plumb bob vertically over the entry site (Fig. 6.6), needle insertion through that point, along the continuation of the vertical line defined by the plumb bob, would result in contact with the brachial plexus in most patients. Fig. 6.6 also illustrates a parasagittal section obtained by magnetic resonance imaging in the sagittal plane necessary to carry out this block. As illustrated, the brachial plexus at the level of the first rib lies posterior and cephalad to the subclavian artery. Once this skin mark has been placed immediately superior to the clavicle at the lateral border of the sternocleidomastoid muscle as it inserts into the clavicle, the needle is inserted in the parasagittal plane at a 90-degree angle to the tabletop. If a paresthesia is not elicited on the first pass, the needle and syringe are redirected cephalad in small steps through an arc of approximately 20 degrees. If a paresthesia still has not been obtained, needle and syringe are reinserted at the starting position and then moved in small steps through an arc of approximately 20 degrees caudad (Fig. 6.7).

Because the brachial plexus lies cephaloposterior to the artery as it crosses the first rib, often a paresthesia can be elicited before either the artery or the first rib is contacted. If that occurs, approximately 30 mL of local anesthetic is inserted at this single site.

If a paresthesia is not elicited with the maneuvers described, but the first rib is contacted, the block is carried out just as it is in the classic approach—by "walking" along the first rib until a paresthesia is elicited. As in the classic

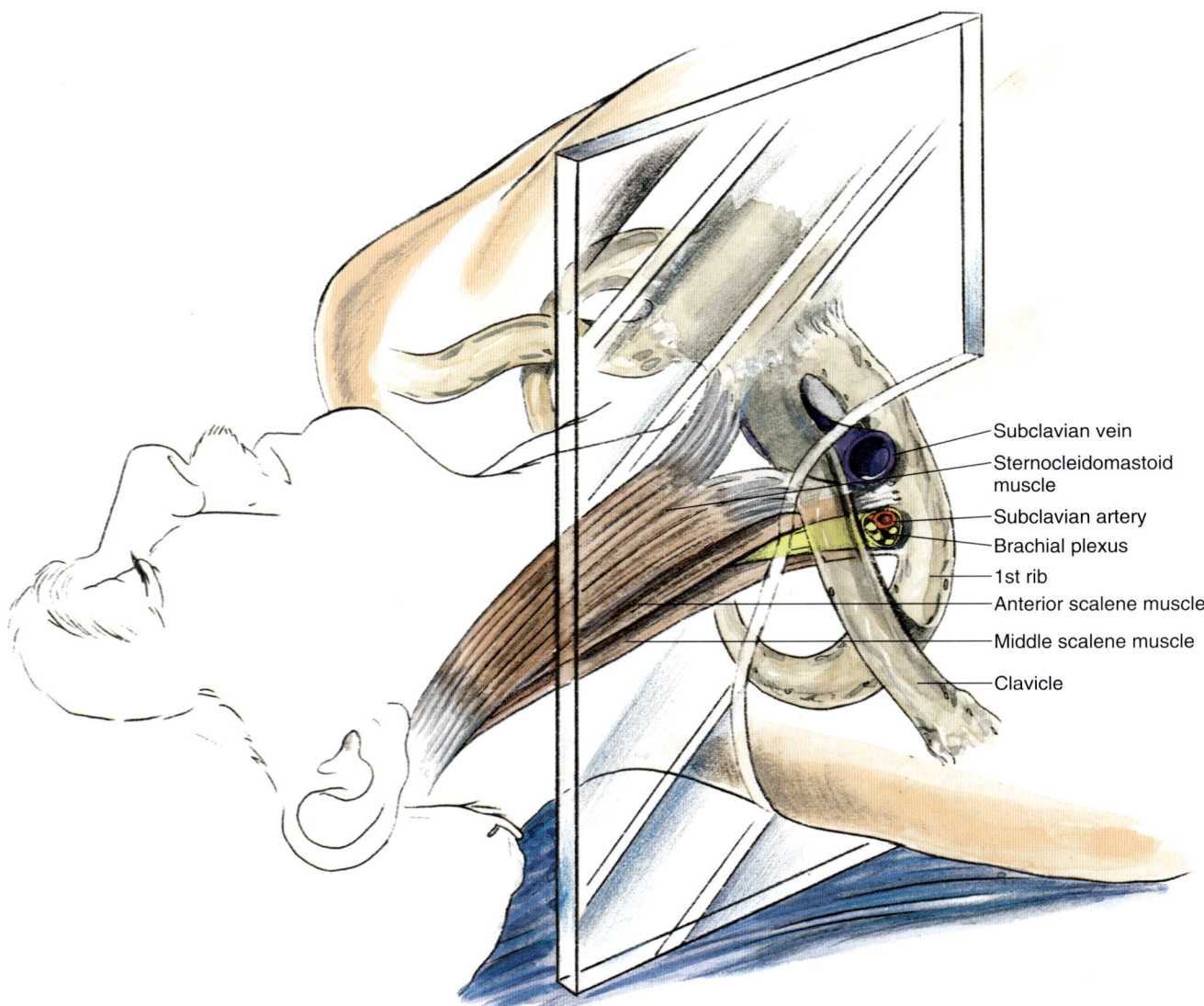

Fig. 6.5 Supraclavicular block (plumb bob): functional anatomy.

Supraclavicular Block

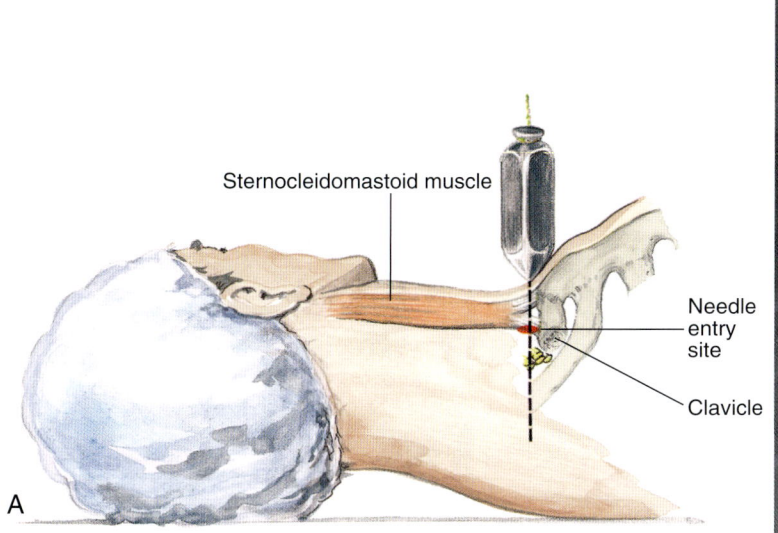
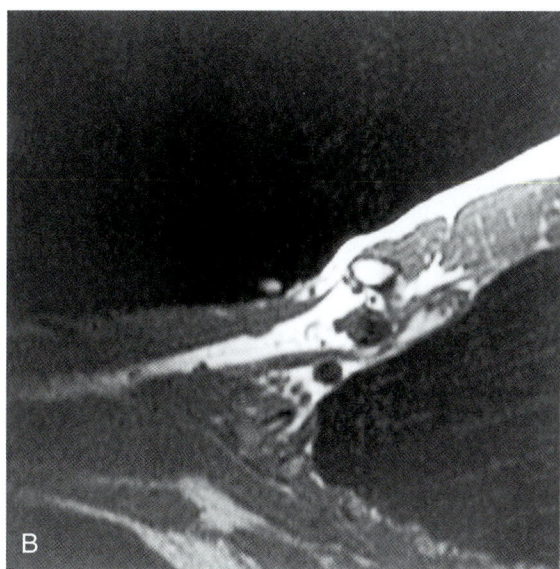
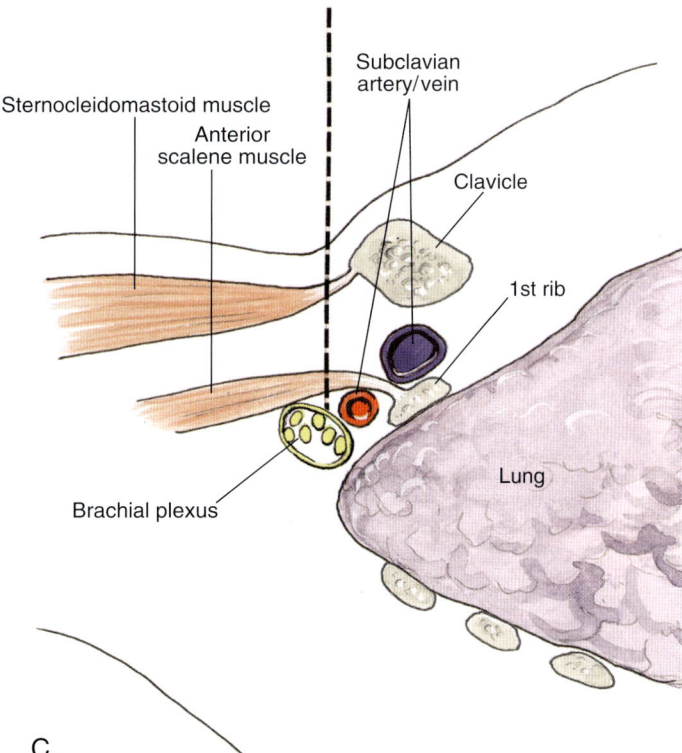

Fig. 6.6 Supraclavicular block (plumb bob): parasagittal anatomy. (A) Schematic, showing plumb bob and needle path. (B) Magnetic resonance image. (C) Needle path.

approach, care should be taken not to allow the syringe and needle assembly to aim medially toward the cupola of the lung.

POTENTIAL PROBLEMS

The most feared complication of this block is pneumothorax, the principal cause of which is a needle/syringe angle that aims toward the cupola of the lung. Special attention should be directed to "walking" the needle in a strict anteroposterior direction. Pneumothorax incidence is between 0.5% and 5% and becomes less frequent as an anesthesiologist becomes skilled. The cupola of the lung rises proportionally higher in the neck in thin, asthenic individuals, and perhaps in these individuals the incidence of pneumothorax is higher. Pneumothorax most often develops over a number of hours as the result of impingement of the needle on the lung, rather than due to immediate entrance of air into the pleural space as the needle is inserted. Phrenic nerve block occurs probably in the range of 30%–50% of patients, and the block's use in patients with significantly impaired pulmonary function must be weighed. The development of hematoma after supraclavicular block as a result of puncture of the subclavian artery usually simply requires observation.

PEARLS

The predictability and rapid onset of this block allow the anesthesiologist to keep up with a fast orthopedic surgeon.

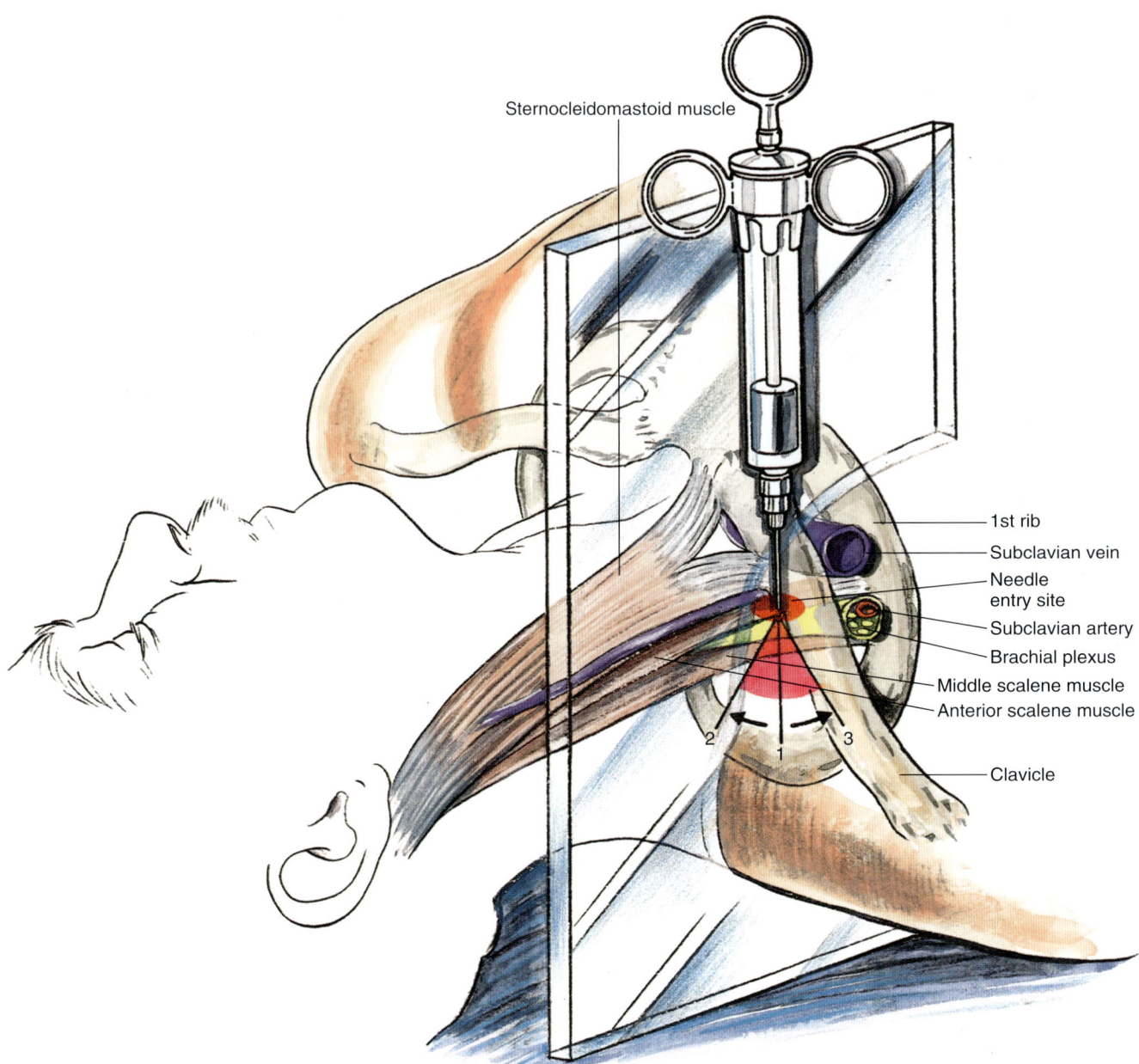

Fig. 6.7 Supraclavicular block (plumb bob): paresthesia-seeking approach.

Use of this block allows regional anesthesia to be used for hand surgery, even in a busy practice. Because this block requires a longer time for the anesthesiologist to attain proficiency than most other regional blocks, the anesthesiologist should develop a system for its use. "Wishful" probing at the root of the neck without a system is not the way to approach this block. Likewise, one should choose either the classic or the vertical approach and give each a fair trial before abandoning either.

If a pneumothorax occurs after supraclavicular block, it most often can be observed while the patient is reassured. If the pneumothorax is large enough to cause dyspnea or patient discomfort, aspiration of the pneumothorax through a small-gauge catheter is often all that is necessary for treatment. The patient should be admitted for observation; however, it is the exceptional patient who needs formal, large-bore chest tube placement for reexpansion of the lung. Obviously, difficult patients should not be chosen as subjects while the anesthesiologist is developing expertise with this block.

Some anesthesiologists combine the axillary and interscalene blocks (in the so-called AXIS block) to approximate the results achieved from a more typical supraclavicular block. An AXIS block requires that the total doses of local anesthetic be increased; one must be willing to use almost 60 mL of whichever drug is injected. Time will tell whether this combined approach offers any advantages over the supraclavicular block. In the AXIS block, the axillary portion should be blocked first, with the interscalene block performed second to minimize the risk of injecting into an area already blocked by local anesthetic.

ULTRASONOGRAPHY-GUIDED TECHNIQUE

SONOANATOMY

The brachial plexus in the supraclavicular region is composed mainly of three trunks: superior, middle, and inferior.

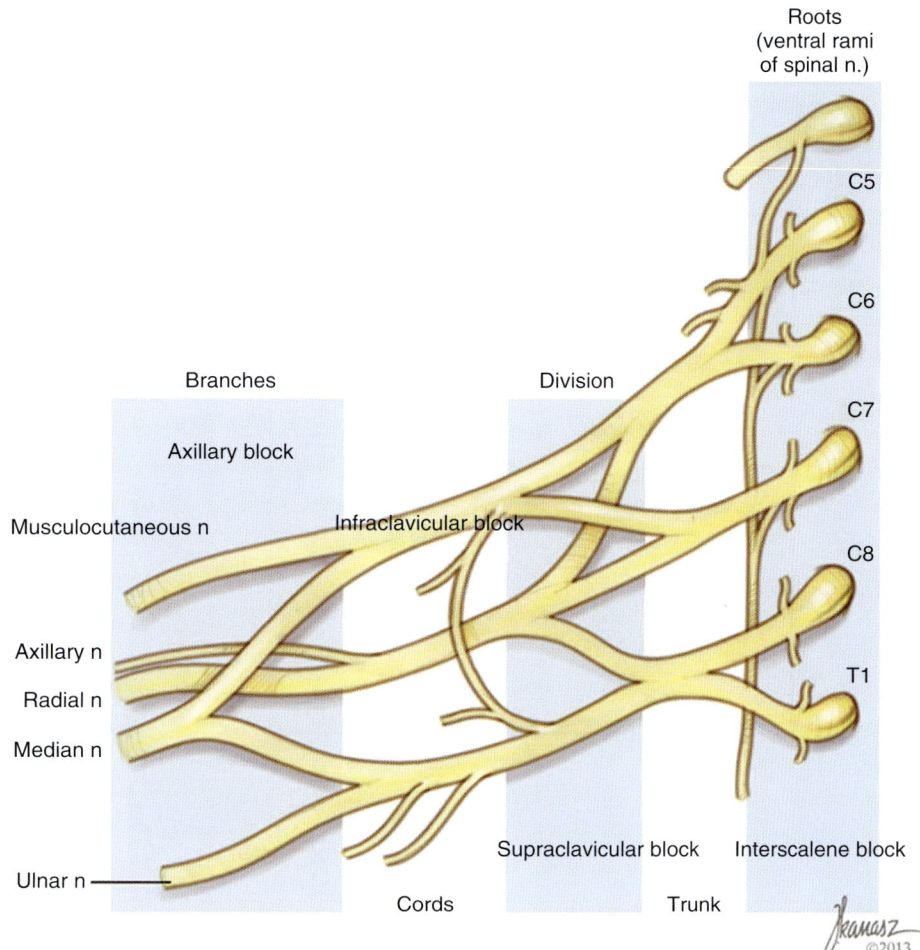

Fig. 6.8 Comparing the different block positions for the different techniques of brachial plexus block.

These trunks pass across the upper surface of the first rib, where they lie posterior and superior to the subclavian artery. The trunks then divide into anterior and posterior divisions behind the clavicle. With ultrasonography, the six divisions can be seen compactly arranged and located superior and posterior to the subclavian artery as the artery passes over the first rib. Practically, in the supraclavicular approach for the brachial plexus, the trunks and the divisions appear as a compact group of nerves (like a bunch of grapes) lying superior and posterior to the artery (Figs. 6.8 through 6.10).

INDICATIONS

- The supraclavicular block is very efficient for upper limb and hand surgeries.
- This block can be used for shoulder surgery; however, it can miss the suprascapular nerve, which supplies the sensory innervation to the glenohumeral joint. Therefore the block could fail to provide appropriate analgesia after shoulder surgery.

TECHNIQUE

The patient could be in either a semisitting position (beach-chair position) by elevating the head of the bed 45 degrees or a supine position with the patient's head turned to the opposite side to be blocked. The first position is preferable in obese patients. The usual probe position is in the coronal oblique plane behind the midpoint of the clavicle to obtain the short-axis view. Scan the supraclavicular fossa to identify the subclavian artery and brachial plexus in the short-axis view. The first rib and the cervical pleura should be identified in this view as well. We prefer to use the in-plane approach for this technique, and the needle will be inserted from the posterior to anterior direction (Figs. 6.11 through 6.14).

KEY POINTS

- A small linear (20- to 25-mm footprint) transducer is preferred for this block.
- Try to identify the cervical pleura and keep the needle direction in a parallel position to the first rib to avoid injuring the pleura and prevent the development of pneumothorax.
- For catheter insertion, the Tuohy needle is usually used. The catheter is typically inserted superior to the subclavian artery in the case of shoulder surgery or in the corner pocket between the artery and the first rib in the case of hand surgery. The correct position of the catheter can be confirmed under ultrasound by either injecting local anesthetic or 1 mL of air via the catheter and observing its distribution in relation to the plexus.

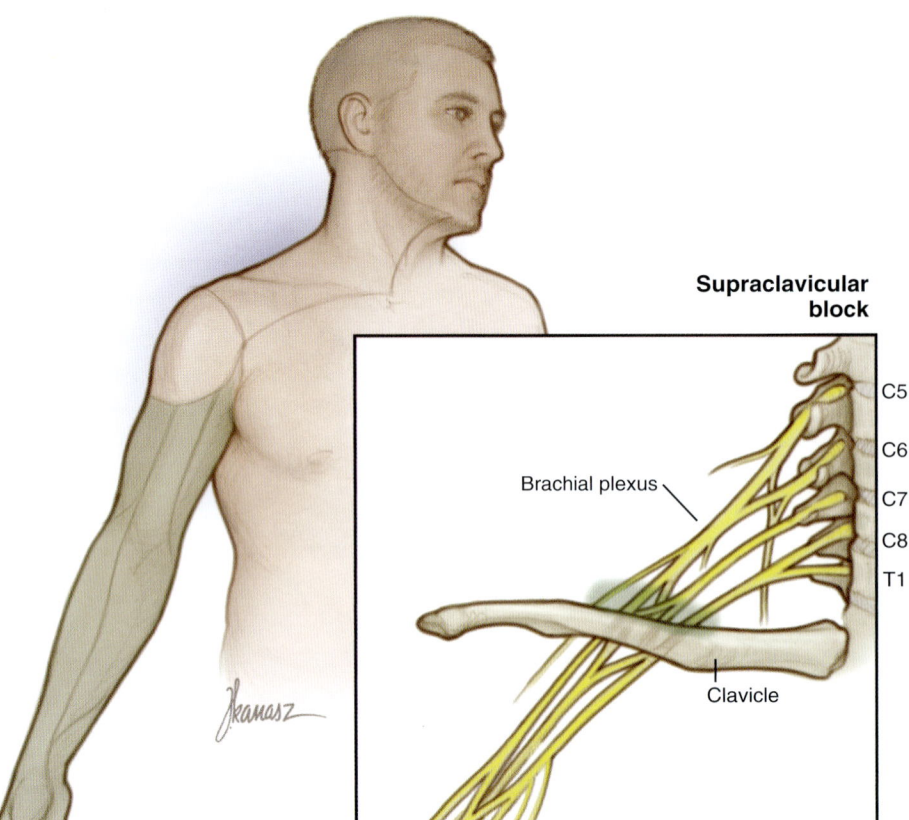

Fig. 6.9 Anatomy of supraclavicular block. Note the block is performed at the level of trunks and divisions of brachial plexus.

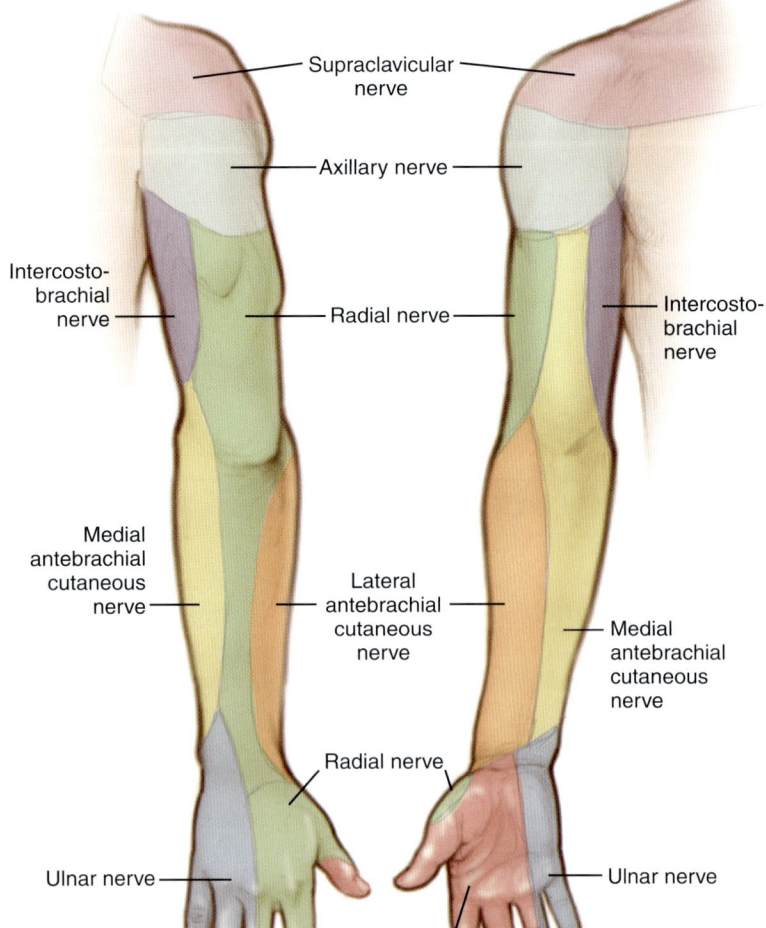

Fig. 6.10 Anatomy for Supraclavicular Block.

Supraclavicular Block

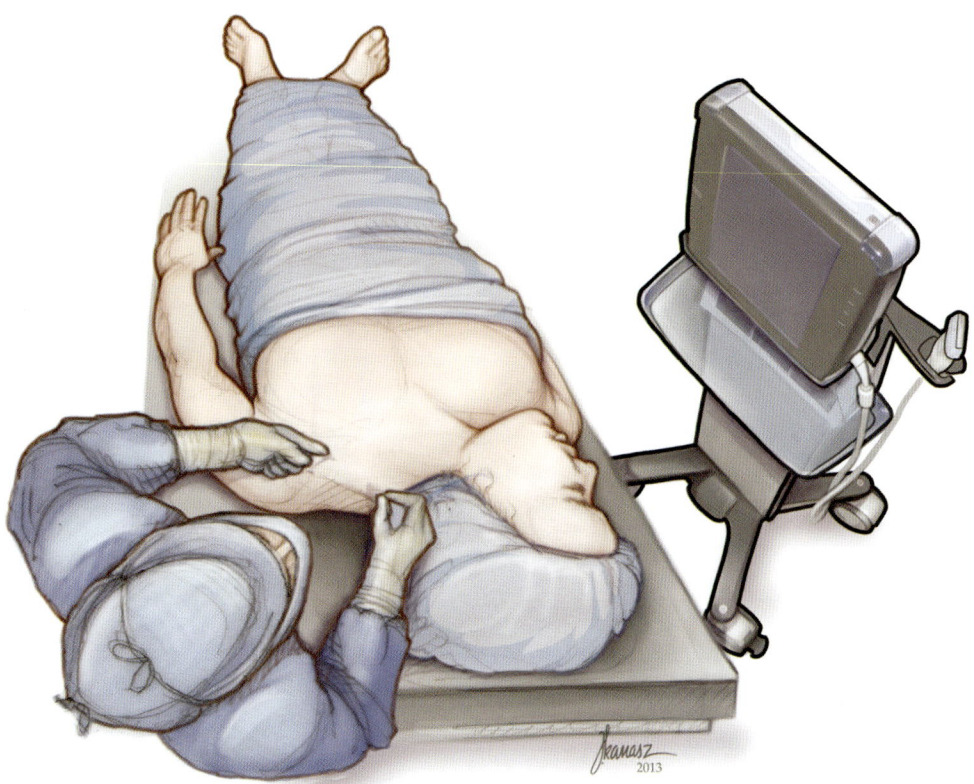

Fig. 6.11 Patient position with the ultrasound machine for the supraclavicular block.

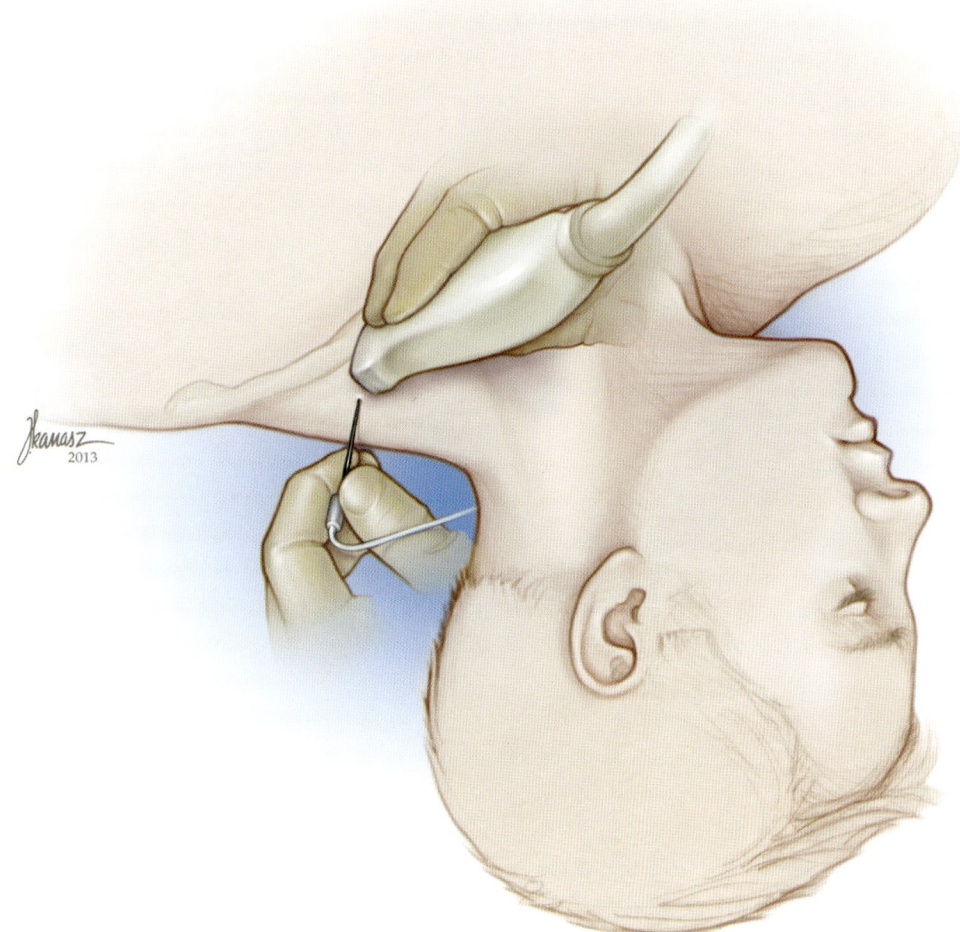

Fig. 6.12 The probe is in the coronal oblique plane. Note the in-plane position of the needle with the direction of the needle from posterior to anterior.

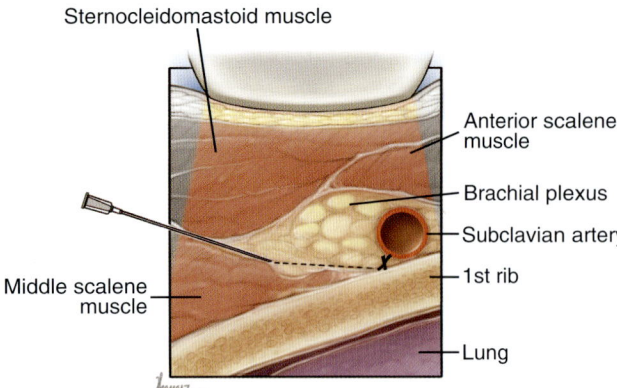

Fig. 6.13 The needle position beneath the brachial plexus parallel to the first rib.

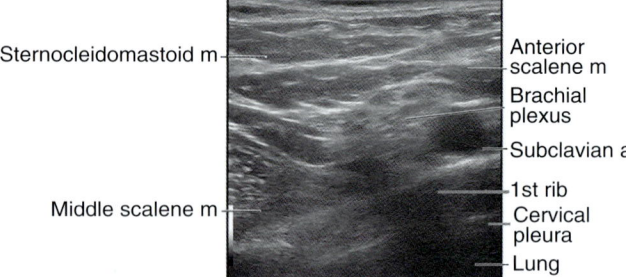

Fig. 6.14 Ultrasound image of Fig. 6.13.

PEARLS

- For hand surgery, the local anesthetic should be inserted in the corner pocket between the subclavian artery and the first rib to avoid missing the lower trunk/divisions and therefore the ulnar nerve.
- For shoulder surgeries, try to visualize the suprascapular nerve by scanning more proximal away from the artery.
- If the patient developed chest pain and cough during the procedure, they might have developed pneumothorax. The procedure should be abandoned and chest x-ray should be ordered to confirm the diagnosis.
- Try to examine the anterior chest wall by ultrasound after every supraclavicular block to confirm the absence of pneumothorax by visualizing the intact pleura (sliding sign).
- Injury to the suprascapular nerve following supraclavicular block is usually presented by severe shoulder pain followed by weakness in the supraspinatus and infraspinatus muscles. To prevent this complication, try not to inject above the plexus to avoid exposing the nerve to toxic high concentrations of local anesthetics. In addition, avoiding injection above the plexus might decrease the incidence of phrenic nerve palsy after the block.
- Parsonage-Turner syndrome has the same physical presentations as suprascapular nerve injury. However, Parsonage-Turner syndrome is often idiopathic in its etiology, although its onset has been associated with physical stressors, including surgery.

Suprascapular Block

Wael Ali Sakr Esa

Key Points

- High-frequency, 38-mm broadband linear array transducer is preferred for this block.
- For catheter insertion, the Tuohy needle is usually used. The catheter is placed beneath the transverse scapular ligament around the suprascapular nerve (SSN). The correct position of the catheter can be confirmed under ultrasound by injecting either local anesthetic or 1 mL of air via the catheter and observing its distribution in relation to the SSN and the transverse scapular ligament.
- The incidence of pneumothorax associated with SSN block is reported as less than 1%. The use of ultrasound and the in-plane approach will decrease this risk markedly.

SONOANATOMY

The SSN arises from the C5 and C6 nerve roots, emerges from the superior trunk of the brachial plexus, and then enters the supraspinatus fossa via the suprascapular notch underneath the superior transverse scapular ligament. With application of color Doppler, the SSN can be visualized medial to the pulsation of the suprascapular artery as an oval or round, slightly hyperechoic structure. In the supraspinous fossa, the nerve is in direct contact with bone and exits the suprascapular fossa lateral to the infrascapular fossa and lateral to the spinoglenoid notch (Fig. 7.1).

INDICATIONS

- Shoulder arthroscopic surgeries that approach the joint from its posterior aspect. The SSN innervates up to 70% of the superior and posterior part of the shoulder. The superior articular branch from the SSN supplies the coracohumeral ligament, subacromial bursa, and posterior aspect of the acromioclavicular joint capsule, whereas the inferior articular branch from the SSN supplies the posterior joint capsule. The SSN has no innervation to the anterior and inferior shoulder regions.
- Frozen shoulder, dislocated shoulder, rotator cuff syndrome, and scapular fracture.
- Supplementation to the supraclavicular block for shoulder replacement surgeries if the patient has pain on the posterior part of the shoulder joint postoperatively.

TECHNIQUE

The patient ideally should be placed in a sitting position, and the operator should be behind the patient with the ultrasound machine in front of the patient and facing the operator. This will allow an uninterrupted field of view of the ultrasound screen. The ultrasound transducer should be placed parallel to the scapular spine. A transverse plane of imaging is optimum for the ultrasound-guided SSN block. By moving the transducer cephalad, the suprascapular fossa can be identified. While imaging the supraspinatus muscle and the bony fossa underneath, the ultrasound transducer should be slowly moved laterally to locate the suprascapular notch. The SSN should be seen as a round, hyperechoic structure beneath the transverse scapular ligament in the scapular notch. Also, with application of color Doppler, the SSN can be visualized medial to the pulsation of the suprascapular artery as an oval or round, slightly hyperechoic structure. We prefer to use the in-plane approach for this technique. The echoic needle should be advanced using the in-plane approach medial to lateral to visualize the whole length of the needle (Fig. 7.2). The endpoint for injection is an ultrasound image demonstrating the needle tip in proximity to the SSN in the suprascapular notch below the transverse scapular ligament and the spread of the local anesthetic confirmed as a separation between the supraspinatus muscle and the spine of the scapula (Figs. 7.3 and 7.4).

PEARLS

- Adjust the focal point to the suprascapular notch to get a better image.
- If possible, ask the patient to adduct the arm and move it forward, thus bringing the nerve more superficially.
- Using color Doppler can be very helpful, as the SSN usually lies medial to the suprascapular artery.
- The block is painful, as the needle will pass through muscles, so prepare your patient with local anesthesia, midazolam, and fentanyl.

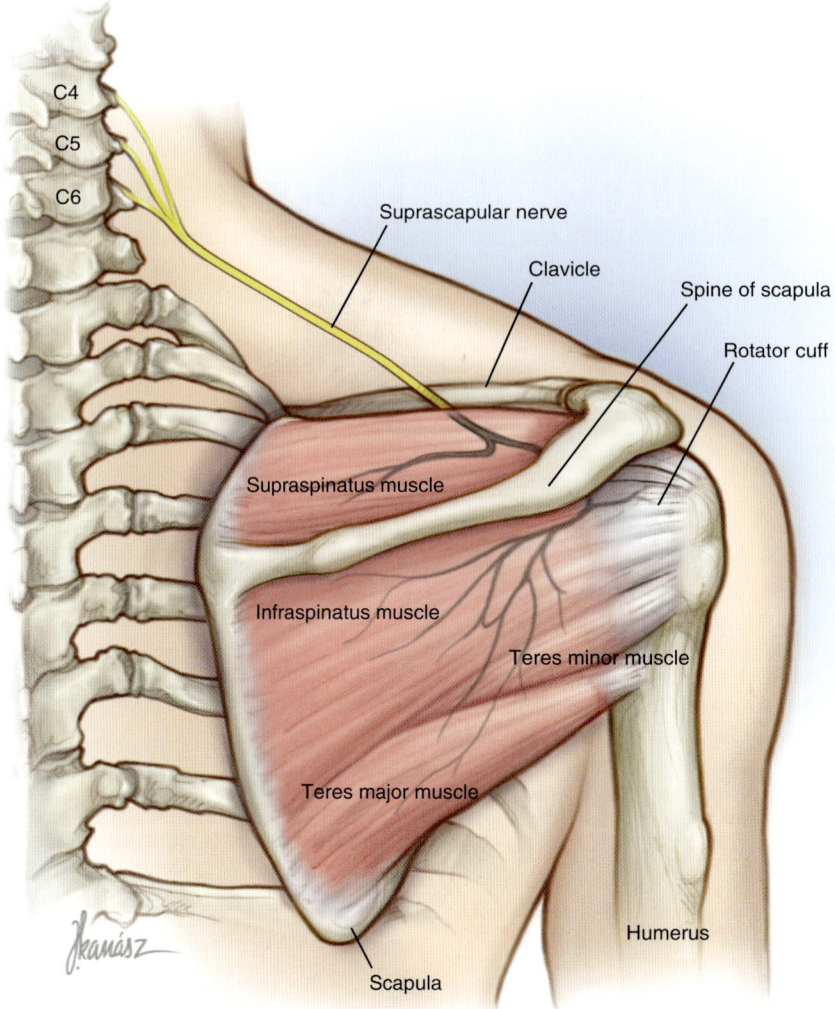

Fig. 7.1 Anatomy of the suprascapular nerve.

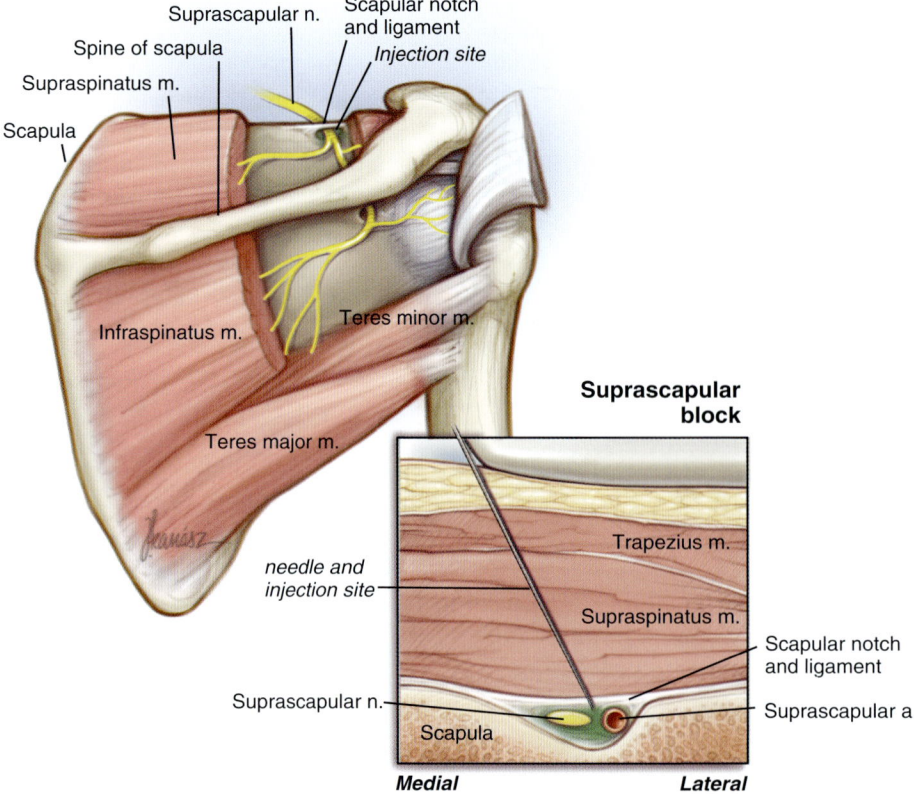

Fig. 7.2 In-plane technique for suprascapular block. The needle direction is from medial to lateral.

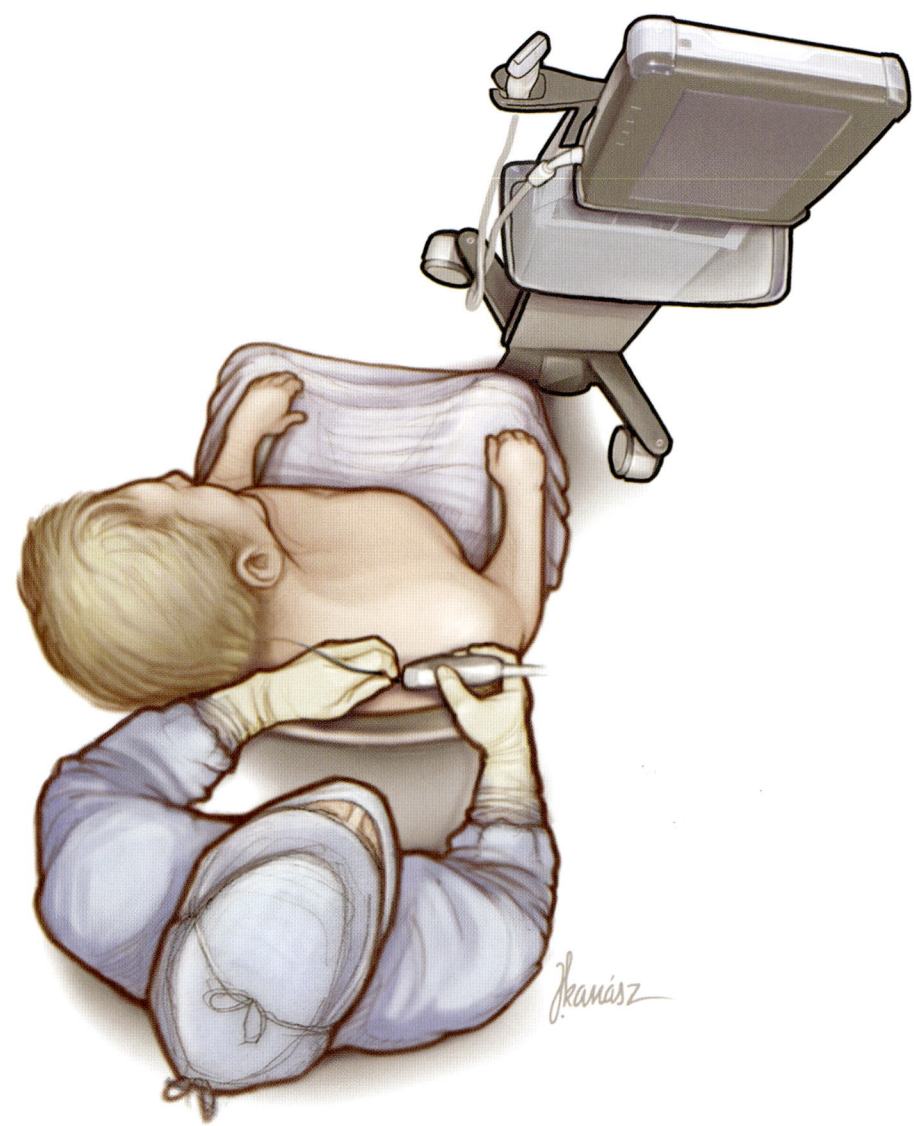

Fig. 7.3 Position of the patient and ultrasound machine.

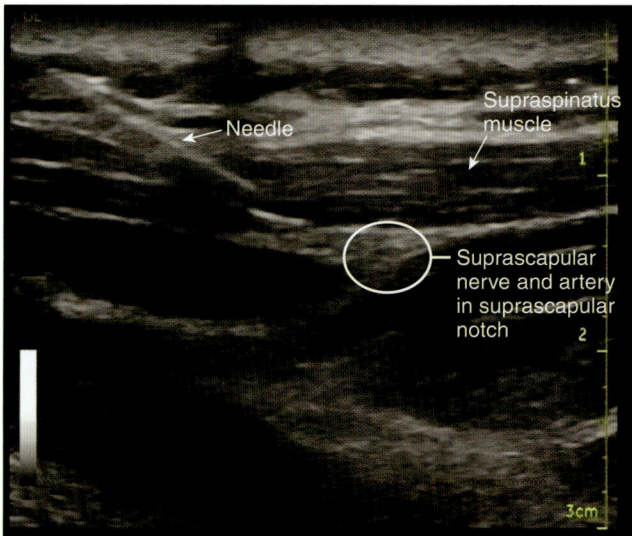

Fig. 7.4 Ultrasound image of a 22-gauge needle directed toward the suprascapular nerve.

- Always use echogenic needles, as visualization of the needle is difficult due to the steep angle used in performing this block. Also, you can reduce the needle angle by using an insertion point as far as possible from the ultrasound probe while still maintaining an in-line approach and visualization of the entire needle during the block.

SUPRASCAPULAR BLOCK ANTERIOR APPROACH

This technique was described by Siegenthaler, et al. The SSN originates from the superior trunk of the brachial plexus, runs in a dorsocaudal direction, crosses deep to the inferior belly of the omohyoid muscle, and reaches the suprascapular fossa.

The patient is placed in slightly lateral position and using a high frequency linear ultrasound probe a 17 gauge Tuohy needle is advanced using in-plane technique deep to the inferior belly of the omohyoid muscle and superficial (anterior) to the prevertebral fascia. Five to 10 mL of a local anesthetic is then injected and spread around the SSN. A 19 gauge catheter is threaded through the 17 gauge Tuohy needle and left around the SSN. If the SSN is not well visualized, the local anesthetic is injected deep into the inferior belly of the omohyoid and superficial to the prevertebral fascia, lateral to the main bulk of brachial plexus. Care should be taken when advancing the needle to avoid puncturing the omohyoid muscle. Tracing the SSN from its origin (nerve root C5) can facilitate its identification. After placing the SSN catheter, a ropivacaine 0.2% infusion should be started at a basal rate of 5 mL/h and a demand dose of 5mL/h using an automated infusion pump, which the patient can take home for 5 days after surgery.

Advantages of SSN block over interscalene block are a marked decrease in the incidence of Horner syndrome and phrenic nerve blockade.

Infraclavicular Block

Kenneth C. Cummings III and Ehab Farag

PERSPECTIVE

Infraclavicular brachial plexus block is useful for both single-injection and continuous infusion techniques. This technique results in a sensory and motor block similar to a traditional axillary approach, albeit with certain advantages. Thus it is most useful for patients undergoing procedures on the elbow, forearm, or hand. Like the axillary block, this technique is carried out distant from both the neuraxial structures and the lung, thus minimizing complications associated with those areas.

Patient Selection. To undergo an infraclavicular block the patient need not abduct the arm at the shoulder, as is required for the axillary block, and thus the technique can substitute for an axillary block in patients who cannot abduct their arms due to pain or other limitation. However, abduction of the arm at the shoulder elevates the clavicle and pulls the plexus anteriorly, usually improving the ease of the procedure.

Pharmacologic Choice. Because prolonged brachial plexus analgesia requires less motor block than is needed for surgical anesthesia, the concentration of local anesthetic can be decreased during postoperative analgesia regimens. Appropriate drugs for infusion are bupivacaine 0.1%–0.15% or ropivacaine 0.2%, both administered at initial rates of 8–12 mL/hr. If a single-injection technique is used, appropriate drugs are lidocaine (1%–1.5%), mepivacaine (1%–1.5%), bupivacaine (0.5%), or ropivacaine (0.5%–0.75%). Lidocaine and mepivacaine produce 2–3 hours of surgical anesthesia without epinephrine and 3–5 hours with the addition of epinephrine. These drugs are useful for less involved procedures or outpatient surgical procedures. For more extensive surgical procedures (or where a longer block is desired), longer-acting agents such as bupivacaine or ropivacaine are appropriate. Plain bupivacaine and ropivacaine produce surgical anesthesia lasting 4 to 6 hours; the addition of epinephrine may prolong this period to 8–12 hours. With the addition of adjuvants such as dexamethasone, blocks lasting as long as 18–24 hours are possible with higher concentrations of ropivacaine or bupivacaine.

TRADITIONAL BLOCK TECHNIQUE

PLACEMENT

Anatomy. At the level of the proximal axilla, where the infraclavicular block is performed, the axilla is a pyramid-shaped space with an apex, a base, and four sides (Fig. 8.1A). The base is the concave armpit, and the anterior wall is composed of the pectoralis major and minor muscles and their accompanying fasciae. The posterior wall of the axilla is formed by the scapula and the scapular musculature, the subscapularis, and the teres major. The latissimus dorsi muscle abuts the teres major muscle to form the inferior aspect of the posterior wall of the axilla (Fig. 8.1B). The medial wall of the axilla is composed of the serratus anterior muscle and its fascia, and the lateral wall is formed by the converging muscle and tendons of the anterior and posterior walls as they insert into the humerus (see Fig. 8.1B). The apex of the axilla is triangular and is formed by the convergence of the clavicle, the scapula, and the first rib. The neurovascular structures of the limb pass into the pyramid-shaped axilla through its apex (Fig. 8.2A).

The contents of the axilla are blood vessels and nerves—the axillary artery and vein and the brachial plexus, respectively—in addition to lymph nodes and loose areolar tissue. The neurovascular elements are enclosed within the anatomically variable, multipartitioned axillary sheath, a fascial extension of the prevertebral layer of cervical fascia covering the scalene muscles. The axillary sheath adheres to the clavipectoral fascia behind the pectoralis minor muscle and continues along the neurovascular structures until it enters the medial intramuscular septum of the arm (Fig. 8.2B).

The brachial plexus divisions become cords as they enter the axilla. The posterior divisions of all three trunks unite to form the posterior cord; the anterior divisions of the superior and middle trunks join to form the lateral cord; and the anterior division of the inferior trunk forms the medial cord. These cords are named according to their relationship to the second part of the axillary artery (Fig. 8.3). From these cords nerves to the subscapularis, pectoralis major and minor, and latissimus dorsi muscles leave the brachial plexus. The medial brachial cutaneous,

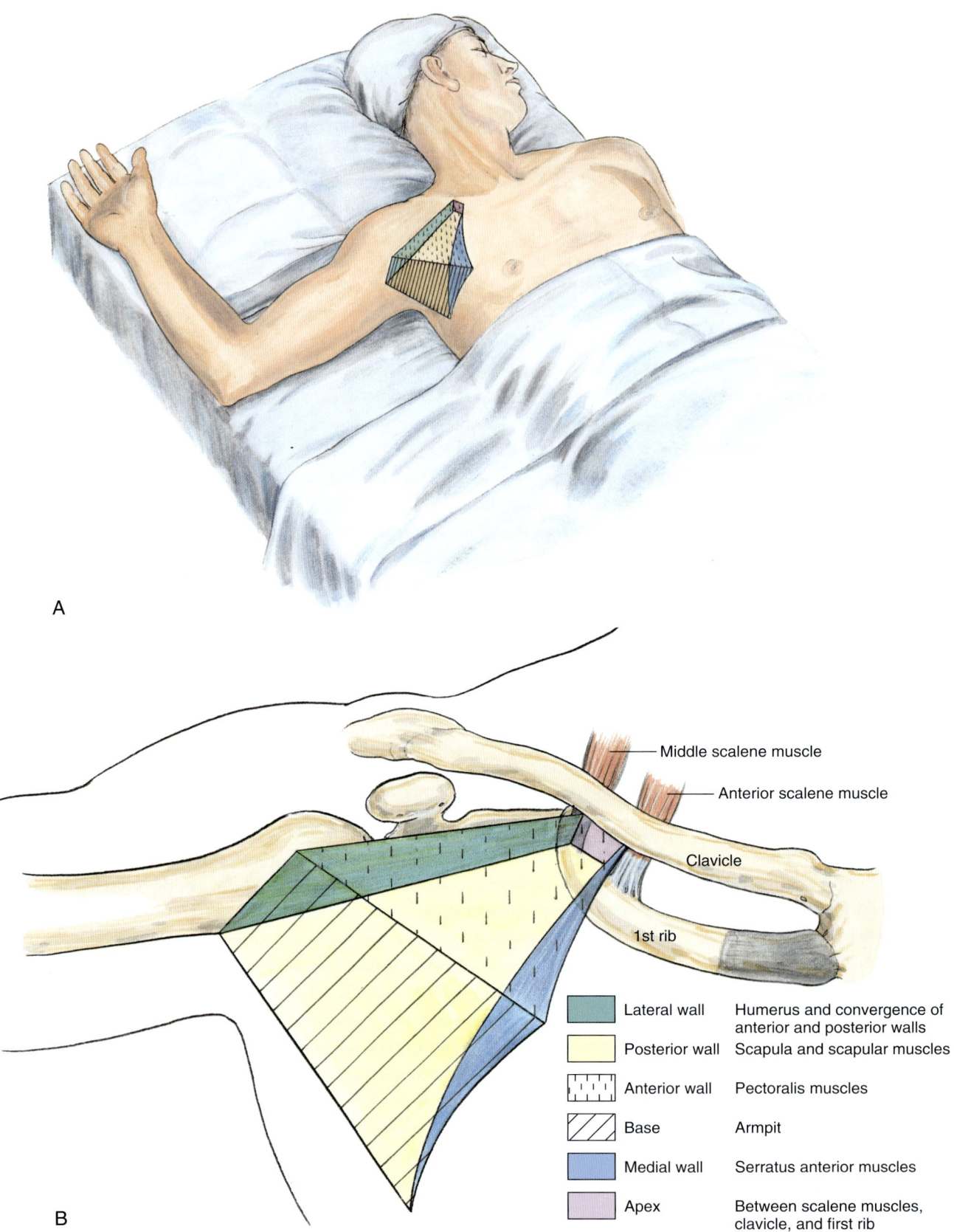

Fig. 8.1 (A) Surface anatomy of infraclavicular block. (B) The concept of the pyramid-shaped axilla is important for infraclavicular block.

medial antebrachial cutaneous, and axillary nerves also leave the brachial plexus at the level of the cords.

At the lateral border of the pectoralis minor muscle (which inserts onto the coracoid process), the three cords reorganize to give rise to the peripheral nerves of the upper extremity. In a simplified scheme, the branches of the lateral and medial cords are all "ventral" nerves to the upper extremity. The posterior cord, in contrast, provides all "dorsal" innervation to the upper extremity. Thus the radial nerve supplies all the dorsal muscles in the upper extremity below the shoulder. The musculocutaneous nerve supplies muscular innervation in the arm and provides cutaneous innervation to the forearm. In contrast, the median and ulnar nerves are nerves of passage in the

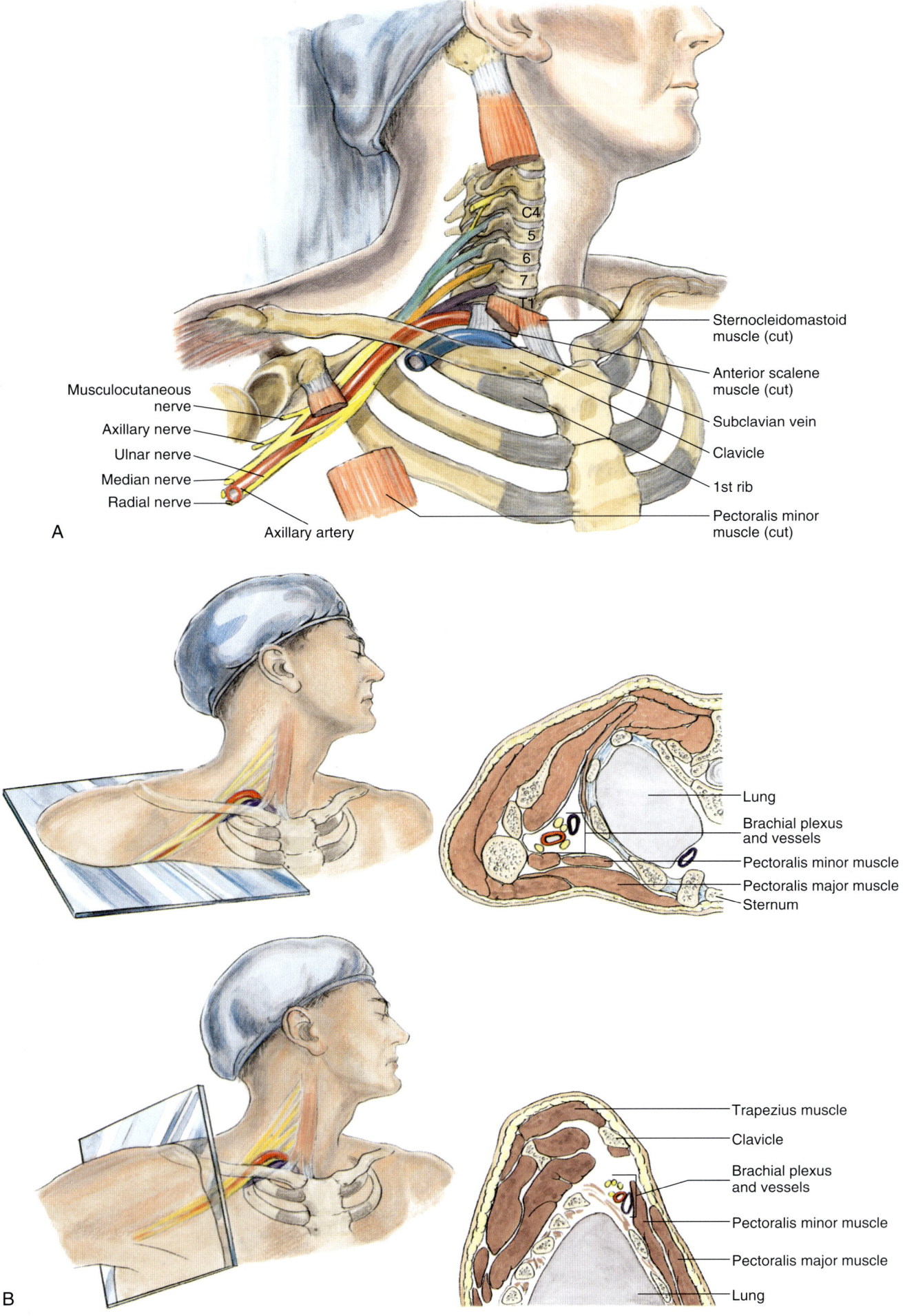

Fig. 8.2 Anatomy important for infraclavicular block. (A) Muscles, bones, and neurovascular structures. (B) Cross-sectional *(top)* and parasagittal *(bottom)* anatomy.

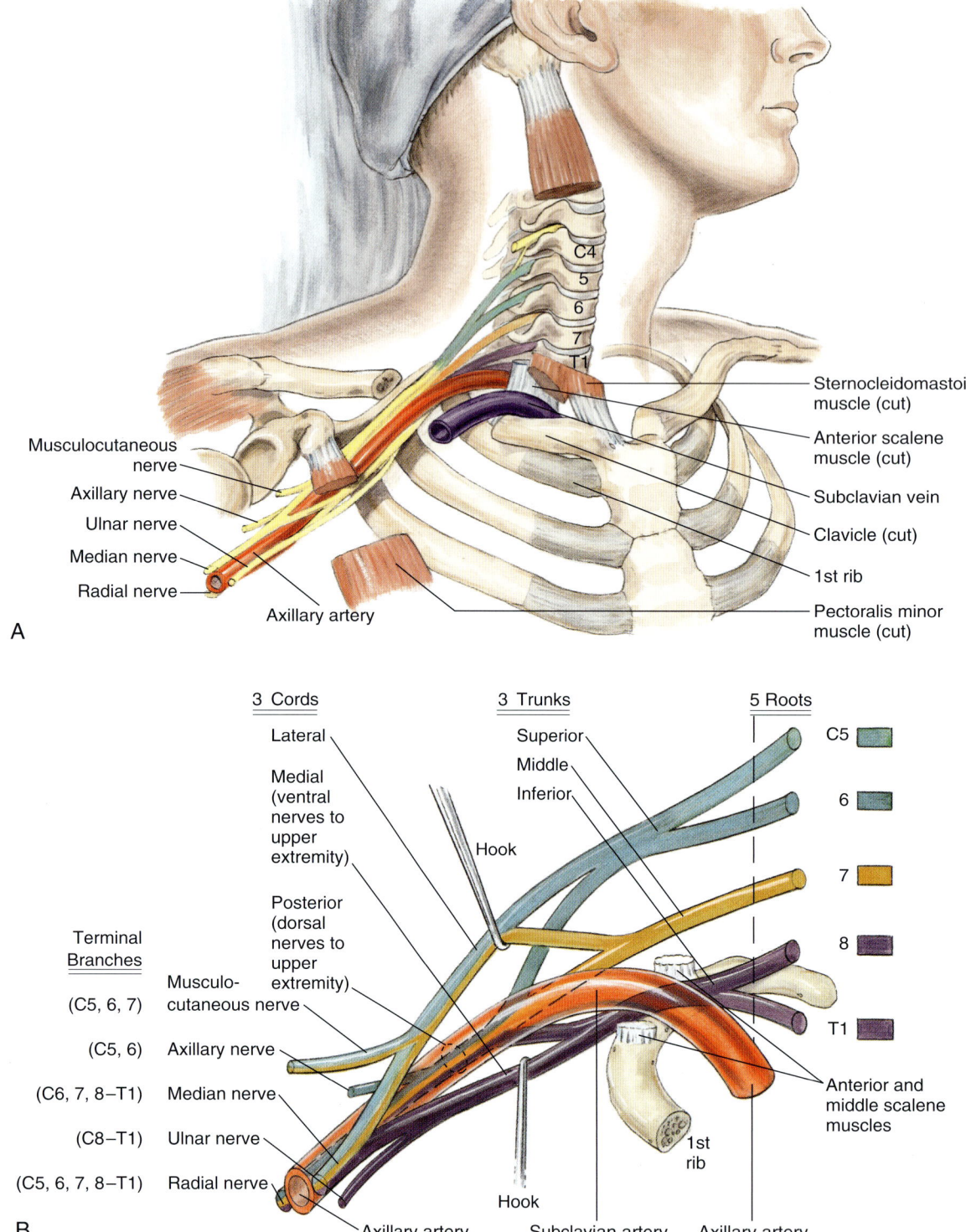

Fig. 8.3 Brachial plexus anatomy important for infraclavicular block. (A) Regional anatomy. (B) Detailed infraclavicular anatomy.

arm, but in the forearm and hand they provide the ventral musculature with motor innervation. These nerves can be further categorized: the median nerve innervates more heavily in the forearm, whereas the ulnar nerve innervates more heavily in the hand.

Position. The patient is placed supine, with the arm to be blocked abducted at the shoulder at a 90-degree angle if possible. If pain prevents this, the arm can be left at the patient's side and adjustments can be made with skin markings. The anesthesiologist can stand on the ipsilateral or the contralateral side of the patient, depending on his or her preference and the patient's body habitus. We prefer to stand on the ipsilateral side of the patient.

Traditional Approach. The coracoid process is identified by palpation and a skin mark placed at its most prominent portion. The skin entry mark is then made at a point 2 cm medial and 2 cm caudad to the previously marked coracoid process (Fig. 8.4A). Deeper infiltration is then performed with a 25-gauge, 5-cm needle while the needle is directed from the insertion site in a vertical parasagittal plane. Then a 7- to 9.5-cm, 20- to 22-gauge needle is inserted in a direction similar to that taken by the infiltration needle. If a

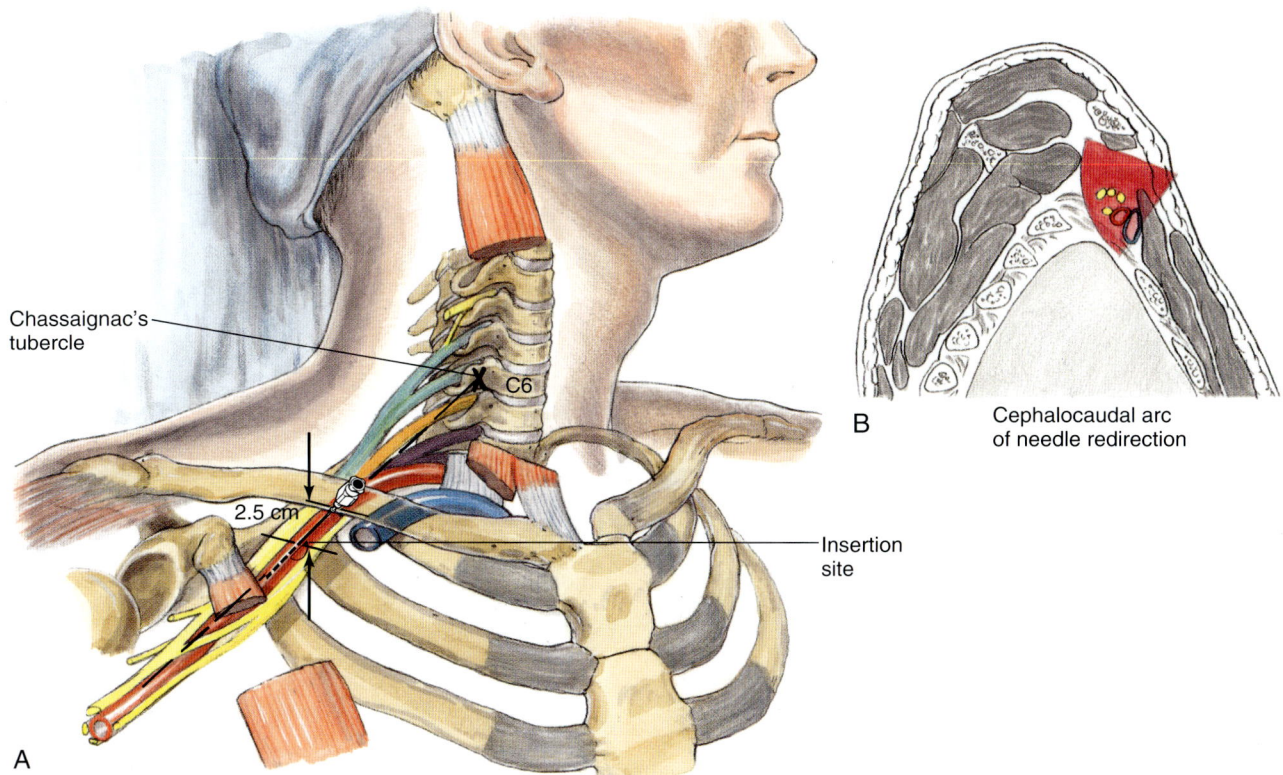

Fig. 8.4 Technique of infraclavicular block. (A) Surface markings for block. (B) Parasagittal view showing arc of needle redirection.

paresthesia technique is used, a distal upper extremity paresthesia is sought; if a nerve stimulator technique is used, a distal upper extremity motor response is sought. If needle redirection is needed to achieve either a paresthesia or a motor response, the needle should be redirected only in a cephalocaudal arc (Fig. 8.4B). To avoid inadvertent entry into the thorax, it is important not to direct the needle path medially. The depth of contact with the brachial plexus depends on body habitus and needle angulation; it ranges from 2.5–3 cm in slender patients and from 8–10 cm in larger individuals.

Once adequate needle position has been achieved, either the single-injection dose of local anesthetic is administered incrementally, or 20 mL of preservative-free normal saline solution (5% dextrose if a stimulating catheter is used) is injected before threading the continuous brachial plexus catheter. For a single-injection technique, the block can be administered in a manner similar to that used in either a supraclavicular or an axillary block. For a continuous technique, we currently use a stimulating catheter device to optimize catheter placement.

POTENTIAL PROBLEMS

An infraclavicular block should not cause neuraxial or pulmonary complications. Although vascular compromise (puncture of the axillary artery or vein) is theoretically possible, in our experience this occurs infrequently. If a continuous catheter technique is chosen, there is the possibility that despite adequate initial needle position, the catheter may be threaded too far away from the plexus to result in an effective block. However, the use of stimulating catheters has decreased this concern.

ULTRASONOGRAPHY-GUIDED TECHNIQUE

SONOANATOMY

The brachial plexus in the infraclavicular region consists of three cords, each named for its classical position relative to the second portion of the axillary artery: medial, lateral, and posterior. There is, however, significant anatomic variation. The cords and axillary vessels lie deep to the pectoralis major and minor muscles, just below the fascia of the pectoralis minor. The ultrasound transducer should be placed in a parasagittal orientation caudal to the coracoid process, roughly perpendicular to the clavicle, so that the plane of the ultrasound beam cuts the brachial plexus cords and axillary vessels in the short-axis view. The axillary artery is seen in cross section as a hypoechoic, noncompressible pulsatile structure, whereas the axillary vein usually lies inferior and/or superficial to the artery. With the left side of the screen oriented cephalad, the lateral, posterior, and medial cords are often found at 9 to 10 o'clock, 6 to 7 o'clock, and 4 to 5 o'clock relative to the artery, respectively. The cords are often difficult to distinctly identify, emphasizing the importance of placing the local anesthetic deep to the pectoral fascia (Fig. 8.5). Depending on how medially the transducer is placed, ribs and/or pleura may be identified in the inferior part of the image.

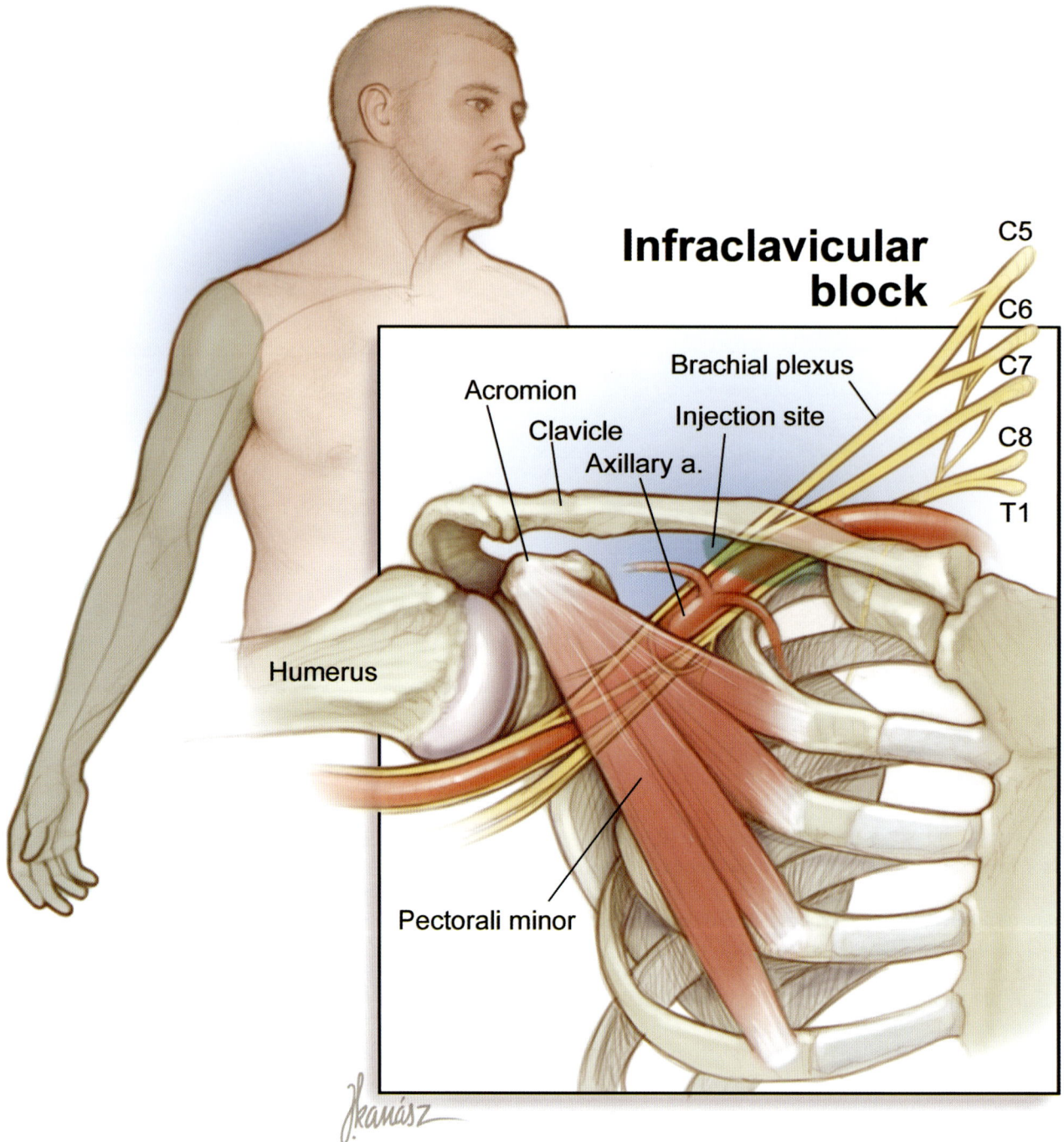

Fig. 8.5 Anatomy of infraclavicular block.

INDICATIONS

- Infraclavicular blocks are very effective for arm, elbow, forearm, and hand surgeries.
- Both single-shot and continuous techniques are possible. Continuous infraclavicular nerve blocks may provide superior analgesia compared with other techniques.[1]

TECHNIQUE

The patient may be placed either supine or semisitting. The patient's head should be turned away from the side to be blocked. In the classic technique for the infraclavicular block, the arm is adducted to the side; therefore it is called the lateral infraclavicular technique. However, to improve visualization of the cords, we prefer to use the medial infraclavicular approach in which the arm is abducted 110 degrees, externally rotated, and the elbow is flexed 90 degrees. This will bring the cords closer together, superior to the axillary artery, and they may lie closer to the skin. The puncture site is made at the apex of the deltopectoral groove in the parasagittal plane. An in-plane approach is recommended from the cephalad end of the probe along its long axis. In the case of catheter insertion, we prefer using a 22-gauge needle to inject the local anesthetics around the three cords separately first; then we use a Touhy needle to place the catheter beneath the posterior cord (Figs. 8.6 through 8.8).

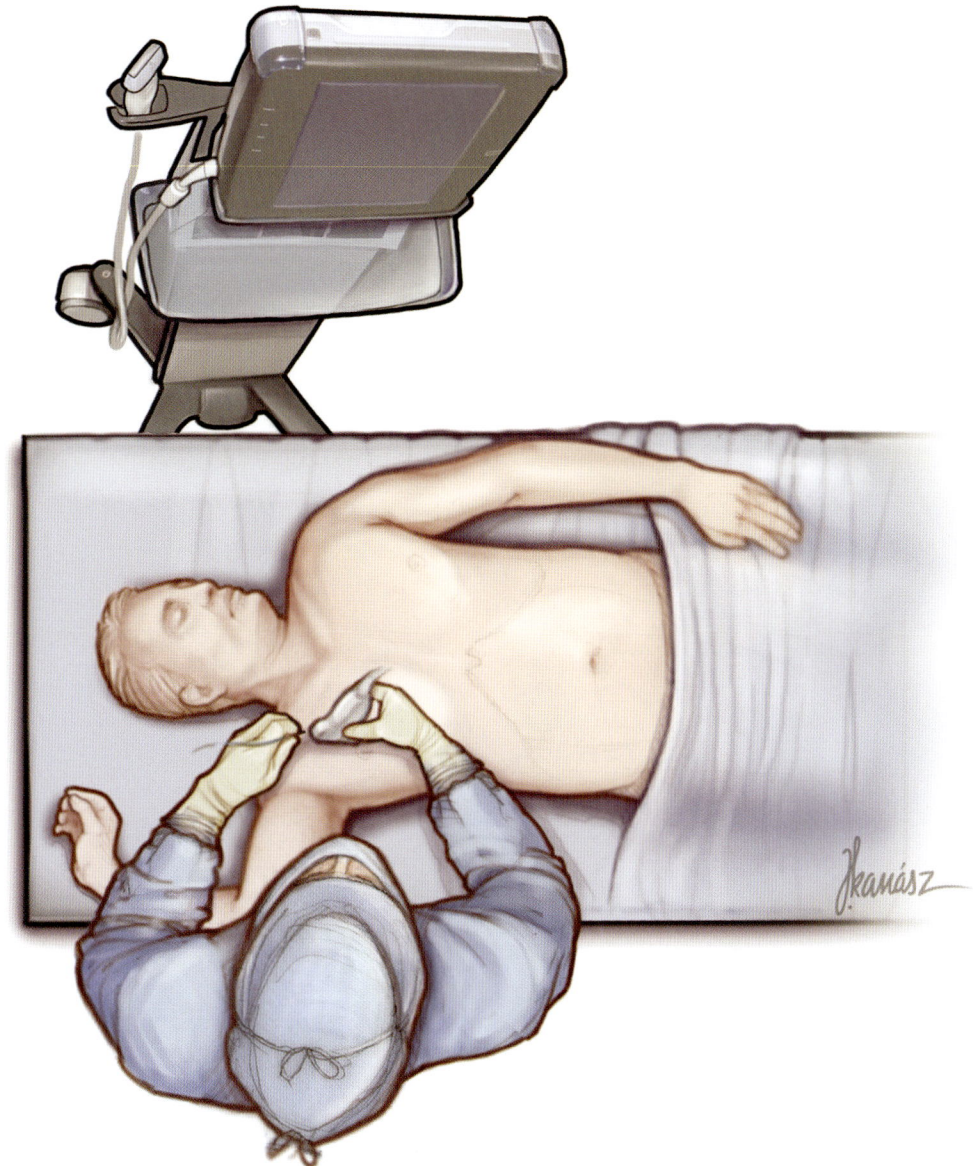

Fig. 8.6 Medial approach for infraclavicular block. Note the arm is abducted.

Alternative Approaches

Costoclavicular Block

The costoclavicular space lies deep to the clavicle and superficial to the second rib. In this space, the cords of the brachial plexus are more closely positioned and are typically all lateral to the axillary artery. This allows the use of lower doses of local anesthetic (20 mL has been reported as an effective volume). The patient is placed supine with the arm abducted at the shoulder with the head turned slightly away. The transducer is placed immediately caudad to and parallel with the clavicle in the midclavicular line (Fig. 8.9). The transducer is angled caudally slightly, to direct the plane of the ultrasound beam cranially underneath the clavicle. Using an in-plane technique, the needle path is lateral to medial, with the target location between the three cords just lateral to the axillary artery (Fig. 8.10). In principle, this should show the neurovascular structures in short axis. However, the transducer may be rotated relative to the clavicle to optimize the short axis view. As with any block closer to the thorax, this block carries the risk of pneumothorax.

Retroclavicular Block

An alternative approach has been proposed in which the needle entry point is superior to the clavicle rather than between the clavicle and transducer. This allows easier visualization of the needle as it approaches the plexus due to a more perpendicular orientation relative to the ultrasound beam. We do not endorse this approach due to the inability to visualize the needle as it passes posterior to the clavicle and the close proximity of the suprascapular nerve to the needle path.[2]

KEY POINTS

- A linear or small curved transducer is preferred for this block to minimize the transducer footprint.
- The axillary artery is usually 4–5 cm below the skin in a typical patient.
- Because of the steep angle of needle insertion relative to the ultrasound beam, direct visualization of the needle may be difficult.

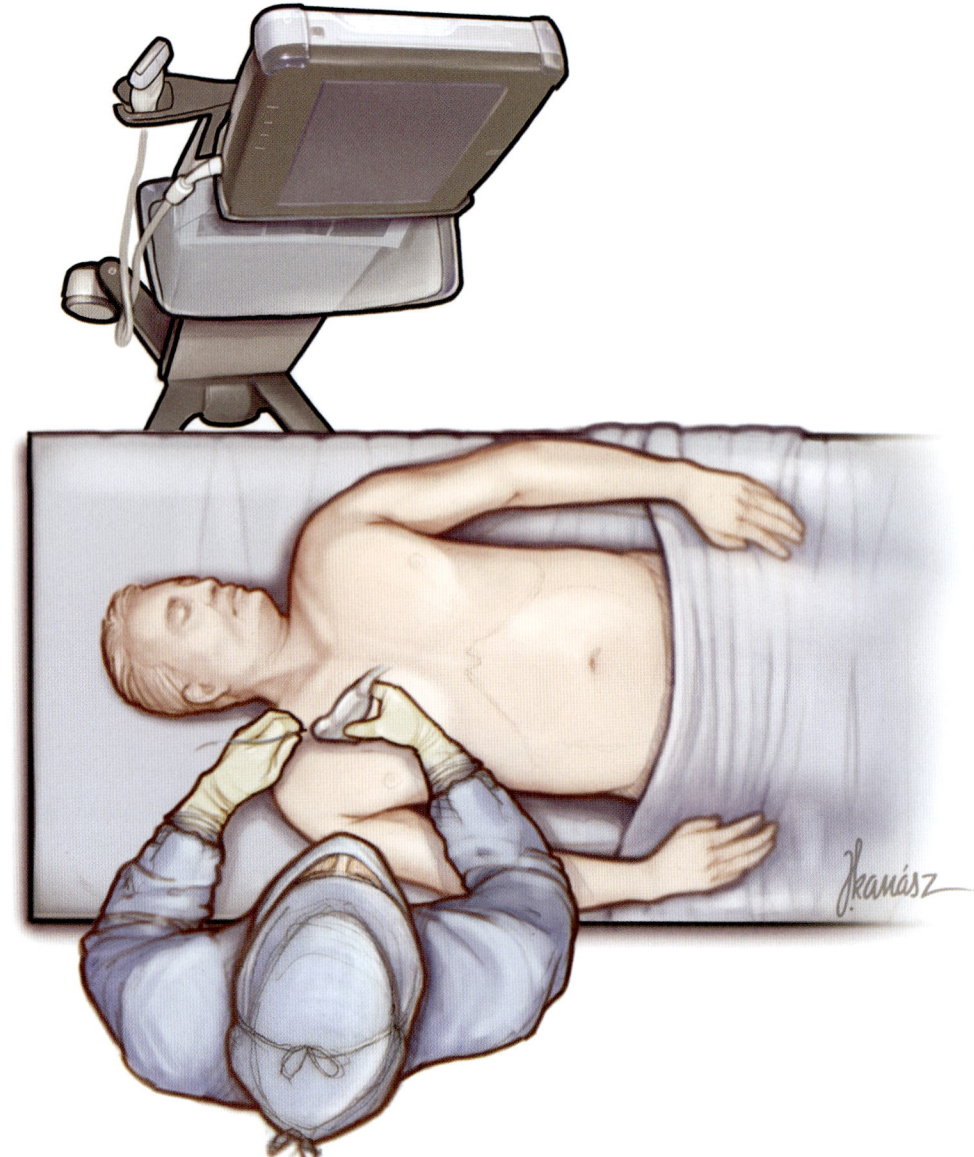

Fig. 8.7 Lateral approach for infraclavicular block. Note the arm is adducted. In both, the in-plane technique is used with the needle direction from proximal to distal.

- Approximately 15–30 mL of local anesthetic is typically sufficient to provide complete block of the plexus. A single injection at the 6 o'clock position commonly suffices, but multiple injections may be required to ensure spread around the three cords.
- Unlike an axillary block, the medial brachial and antebrachial cutaneous nerves are blocked with this technique. The intercostobrachial nerve (arising from T2) may be separately blocked under the arm if desired.
- For catheter insertion, a Tuohy needle is usually used. The catheter is usually inserted posterior to the axillary artery and advanced 2–3 cm past the needle tip. The correct position of the catheter can be confirmed under ultrasound by injecting either local anesthetic or 1 mL of air via the catheter and observing its distribution relative to the plexus.
- Catheters are typically coiled on the skin over the insertion site and covered with a transparent sterile dressing.

PEARLS

- If visualization of all three cords is not possible, it is typically sufficient to ensure that local anesthetic spreads in a "U" shape surrounding the axillary artery. The contrast provided by the local anesthetic commonly improves visualization of the cords during the block.
- A reverberation artifact from the axillary artery may lead to the incorrect impression of a nerve structure deep to the artery.
- Because of the acute needle-to-transducer angle, it may be necessary to rely on indirect signs of needle location such as hydrodissection with normal saline or tissue movement while jiggling the needle. Textured ("echogenic") needles may be easier to visualize with this approach.
- Excessive transducer pressure may occlude veins and increase the chance of inadvertent intravenous injection or hematoma formation

Infraclavicular Block 67

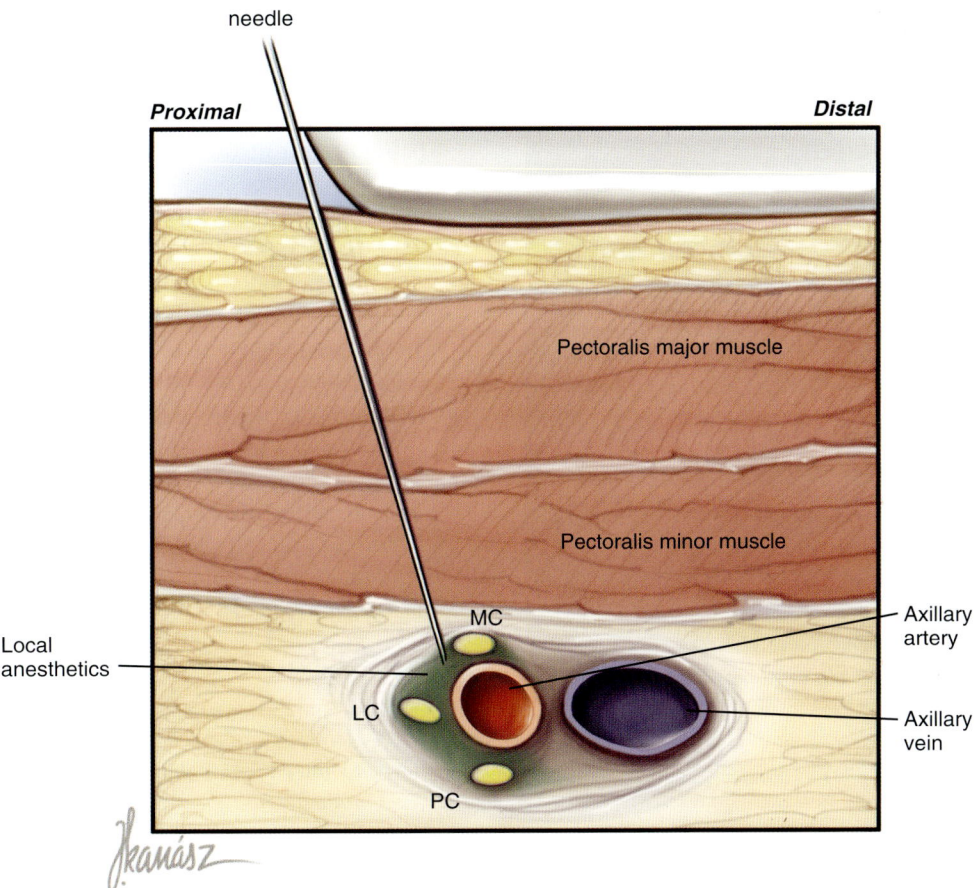

Fig. 8.8 In-plane technique of infraclavicular block. The needle direction is from proximal to distal. *LC*, Lateral cord; *MC*, medial cord; *PC*, posterior cord.

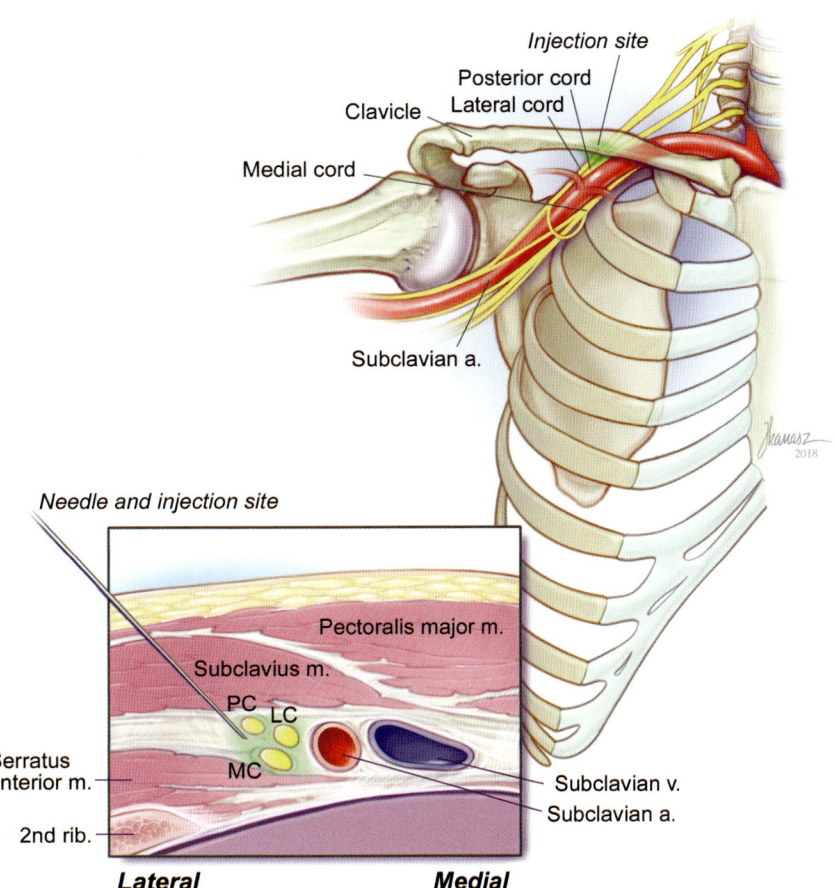

Fig. 8.9 Transducer position and needle approach for costoclavicular block. The inset demonstrates the transducer angulation and relative position of the neurovascular structures.

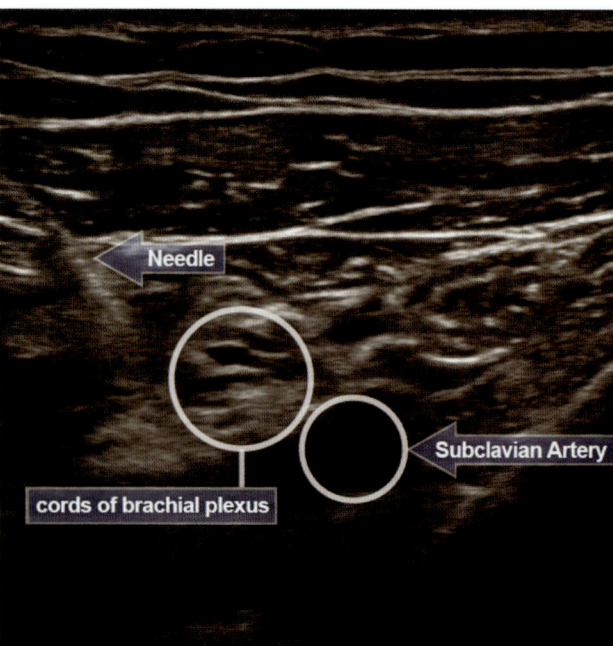

Fig. 8.10 Ultrasound image of the brachial plexus and needle path using the costoclavicular approach. *(Image courtesy Ehab Farag MD, FRCA.)*

- Placing the transducer as laterally as possible (but still medial to the coracoid process) increases the distance to the pleura and provides a larger margin of safety.

- Because of the greater distance between the plexus structures at this level, a larger volume of local anesthetic is commonly needed compared with more proximal brachial plexus blocks. Larger patient-controlled or programmed boluses (8 – 12 mL once per hour in our practice) via an indwelling catheter are also often needed to provide adequate analgesia.

- The infraclavicular location is particularly appealing for continuous blocks because the insertion site is away from the patient's head and neck, and passing through the pectoral muscles stabilizes the catheter.

- In contrast to the interscalene or supraclavicular approaches to the brachial plexus, the infraclavicular approach does not produce phrenic nerve paralysis. This characteristic makes infraclavicular blocks an appealing option in patients with compromised pulmonary function.

References

1. Mariano ER, Sandhu NS, Loland VJ, et al. A randomized comparison of infraclavicular and supraclavicular continuous peripheral nerve blocks for postoperative analgesia. *Region Anesth Pain M*. 2011;36:26–31.
2. Sancheti SF, Uppal V, Sandeski R, Kwofie MK, Szerb JJ. A cadaver study investigating structures encountered by the needle during a retroclavicular approach to infraclavicular brachial plexus block. *Region Anesth Pain M*. 2018;3:752–755.

Axillary Block

Wael Ali Sakr Esa and David L. Brown

PERSPECTIVE

Axillary brachial plexus block is most effective for surgical procedures distal to the elbow. Some patients can undergo procedures on the elbow or lower humerus with an axillary technique, but strong consideration should be given to a supraclavicular block for those requiring more proximal procedures. It is discouraging to carry out a "successful" axillary block only to find that the surgical procedure extends outside the area of the block. This block is appropriate for hand and forearm surgery; thus it is often the most appropriate technique for outpatients in a busy hand surgery practice. Some anesthesiologists find the axillary block suitable for elbow surgical procedures, and continuous axillary catheter techniques may be indicated for postoperative analgesia in these patients. Because this block is carried out distant from both the neuraxial structures and the lung, complications associated with those areas are avoided.

Patient Selection. To undergo an axillary block, patients must be able to abduct the arm at the shoulder. As the experience of the operator increases the need for abduction decreases, but this block cannot be carried out with the arm at the side. Because the block is most appropriate for forearm and hand surgery, it is a rare patient with a surgical condition at those sites who cannot abduct the arm as needed.

Pharmacologic Choice. Because hand and wrist procedures often require less motor blockade than procedures on the shoulder, the concentration of local anesthetic needed for axillary block can usually be slightly less than that needed for supraclavicular or interscalene block. Appropriate drugs are lidocaine (1% to 2%), mepivacaine (1% to 2%), bupivacaine (0.5%), and ropivacaine (0.5% to 0.75%). Lidocaine and mepivacaine produce 2 to 3 hours of surgical anesthesia without epinephrine and 3 to 5 hours with the addition of epinephrine. These drugs can be useful for less involved procedures or outpatient surgical procedures. For more extensive surgical procedures requiring hospital admission, a longer-acting agent such as bupivacaine can be chosen. Plain bupivacaine and ropivacaine produce surgical anesthesia that lasts from 4 to 6 hours; the addition of epinephrine may prolong this period to 8 to 12 hours. The local anesthetic timeline must be considered when prescribing a drug for outpatient axillary block because blocks lasting as long as 18 to 24 hours can result from higher concentrations of bupivacaine with added epinephrine. With continuous catheter techniques used for postoperative analgesia or chronic pain syndromes, 0.25% bupivacaine or 0.2% ropivacaine may be used, and even lower concentrations of these drugs may be used after a trial.

TRADITIONAL BLOCK TECHNIQUE

PLACEMENT

Anatomy. At the level of the distal axilla, where the axillary block is undertaken (Fig. 9.1), the axillary artery can be visualized as the center of a four-quadrant neurovascular bundle. We conceptualize these nerves in quadrants like a clock face because multiple injections during axillary block result in more acceptable clinical anesthesia than does injection at a single site. The musculocutaneous nerve is found in the 9 to 12 o'clock quadrant in the substance of the coracobrachialis muscle. The median nerve is most often found in the 9 to 12 o'clock quadrant; the ulnar nerve is "inferior" to the median nerve in the 2 to 3 o'clock quadrant; and the radial nerve is located in the 5 to 6 o'clock quadrant. The block does not need to be performed in the axilla; in fact, needle insertion in the middle to lower portion of the axillary hair patch or even more distal to this is effective. It is clear from radiographic and anatomic study of the brachial plexus and the axilla that separate and distinct sheaths are associated with the plexus at this point. Keeping this concept in mind will help decrease the number of unacceptable blocks performed. This more distal approach to axillary block is similar to the midhumeral brachial plexus block.

Position. The patient is placed supine, with the arm forming a 90-degree angle with the trunk, and the forearm forming a 90-degree angle with the upper arm (Fig. 9.2). This position allows the anesthesiologist to stand at the level of the patient's upper arm and palpate the axillary artery, as illustrated in Fig. 9.2. A line should be drawn tracing the course of the artery from the midaxilla to the lower axilla; overlying this line, the index and third fingers of the anesthesiologist's left hand are used to identify the artery and minimize the amount of subcutaneous tissue overlying the neurovascular bundle. In this manner, the

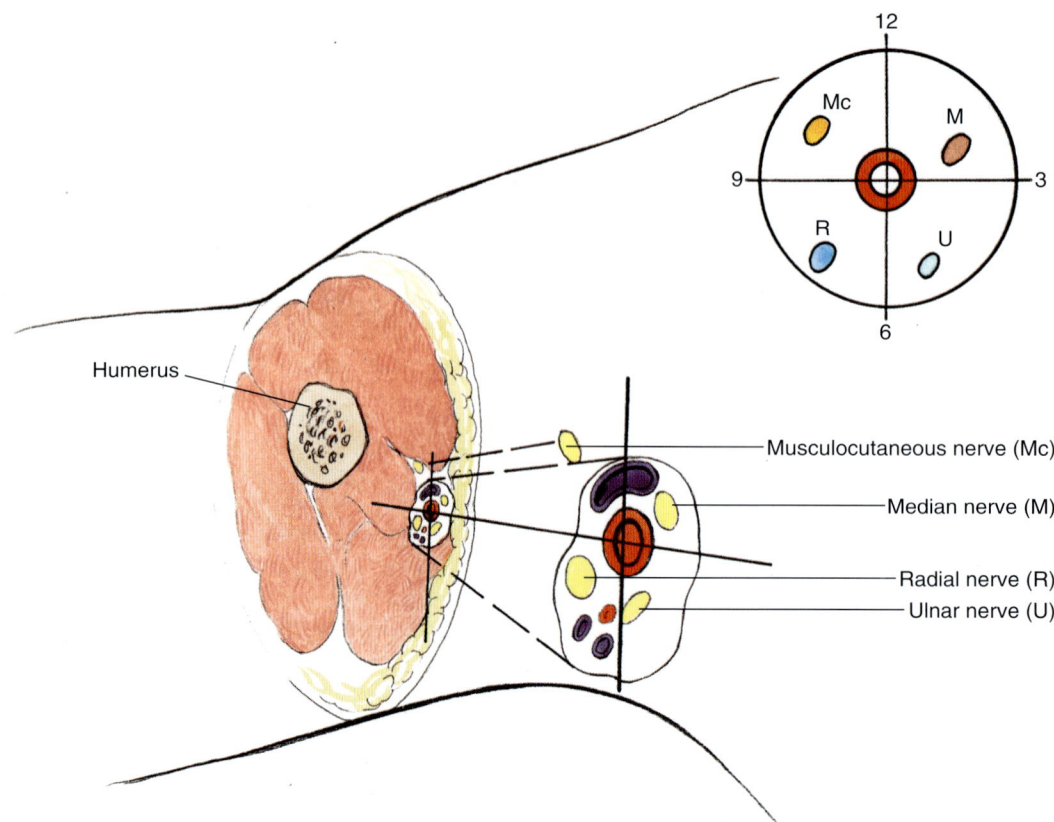

Fig. 9.1 Axillary block: functional quadrant anatomy of distal axilla.

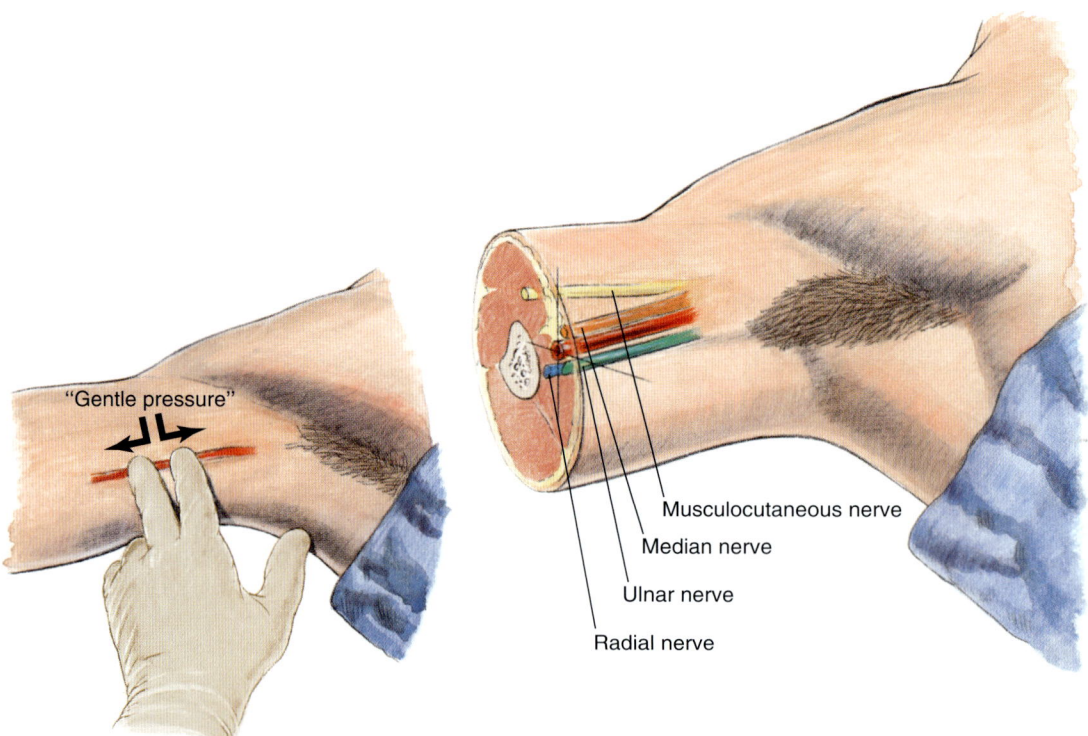

Fig. 9.2 Axillary block: position of patient arm and clinician's fingers for palpation of axillary artery.

anesthesiologist can develop a sense of the longitudinal course of the artery, which is essential for performing an axillary block.

Needle Puncture. While the axillary artery is identified with two fingers, the needle and syringe are inserted as shown in Fig. 9.3. Some local anesthetic should be deposited in each of the quadrants surrounding the axillary artery. If paresthesia is obtained, it is beneficial, although undue time should not be expended or patient discomfort incurred from an attempt to elicit a paresthesia. As

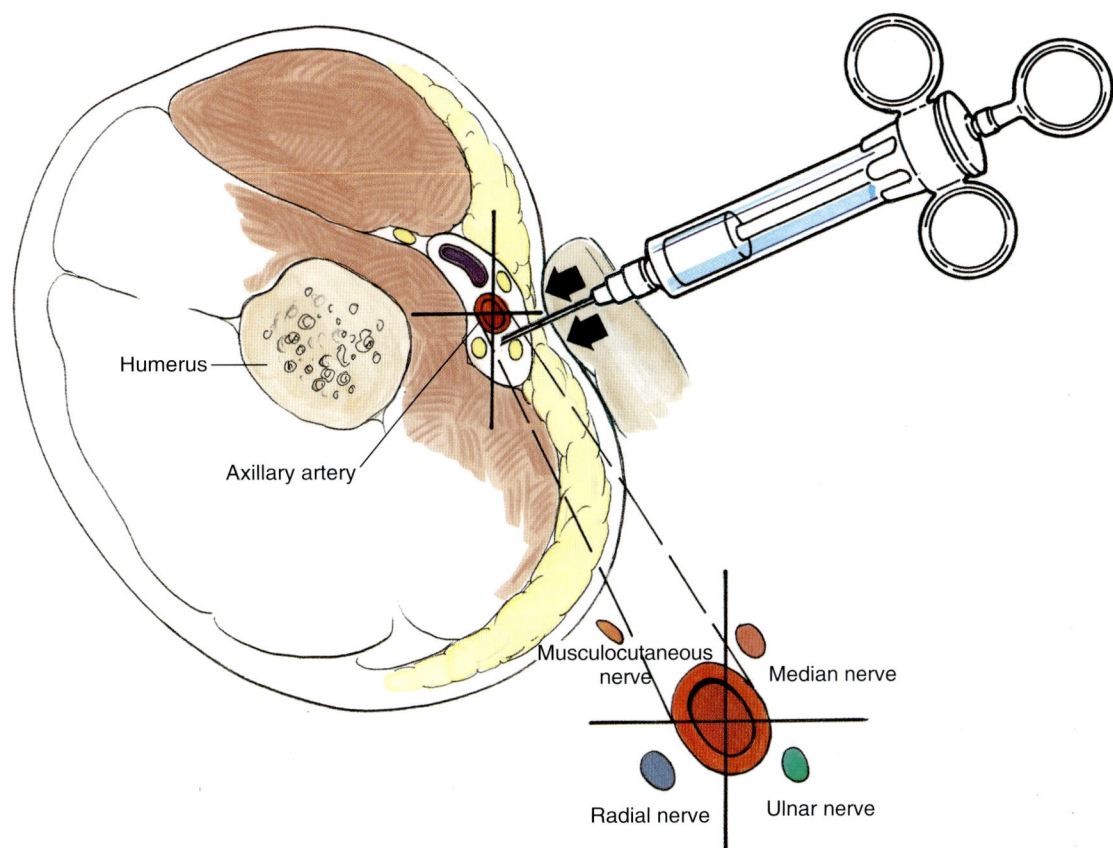

Fig. 9.3 Axillary block: needle and syringe insertion.

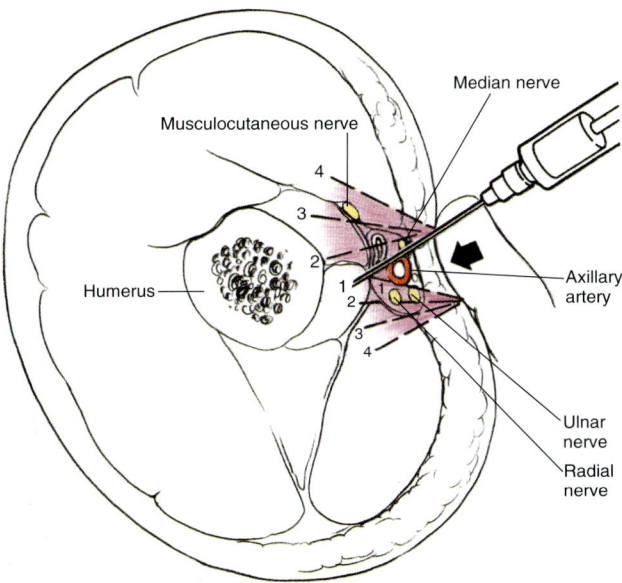

Fig. 9.4 Axillary block: fanlike injection pattern using axillary artery as guide.

illustrated in Fig. 9.4, effective axillary block is produced by using the axillary artery as an anatomic landmark and infiltrating in a fanlike manner around the artery. Anesthesia of the musculocutaneous nerve is best achieved by infiltrating into the mass of the coracobrachialis muscle. This maneuver can be carried out by identifying the coracobrachialis and injecting anesthetic into its substance, or by inserting a longer needle until it contacts the humerus and injecting in a fanlike manner near the humerus (see Fig. 9.4).

When using a continuous catheter technique for an axillary block, stimulating or nonstimulating catheter kits may be used; we prefer the stimulating catheter (Fig. 9.5). With the nonstimulating catheter, the epidural needle is positioned either with the assistance of a nerve stimulator or with elicitation of paresthesia as an endpoint. After the needle is positioned, 20 mL of preservative-free normal saline solution is injected through the needle, and then the appropriate-size catheter is inserted approximately 10 cm past the needle tip. Once the catheter has been secured with a plastic occlusive dressing, the initial bolus of drug is injected and the infusion is started.

POTENTIAL PROBLEMS

Problems with axillary block are infrequent because of the distance of this block from neuraxial structures and the lung. One occasional complication, which can be minimized by using multiple injections rather than a fixed needle, is systemic toxicity. Use of a single immobile needle to inject large volumes of a local anesthetic increases the potential for systemic toxicity relative to the use of smaller volumes of local anesthetic injected at multiple sites. Another potential problem with axillary block is the development of postoperative neuropathy, but one should not assume that axillary block is the cause of all neuropathy after upper extremity surgery. One must follow a logical and systematic approach when seeking the cause

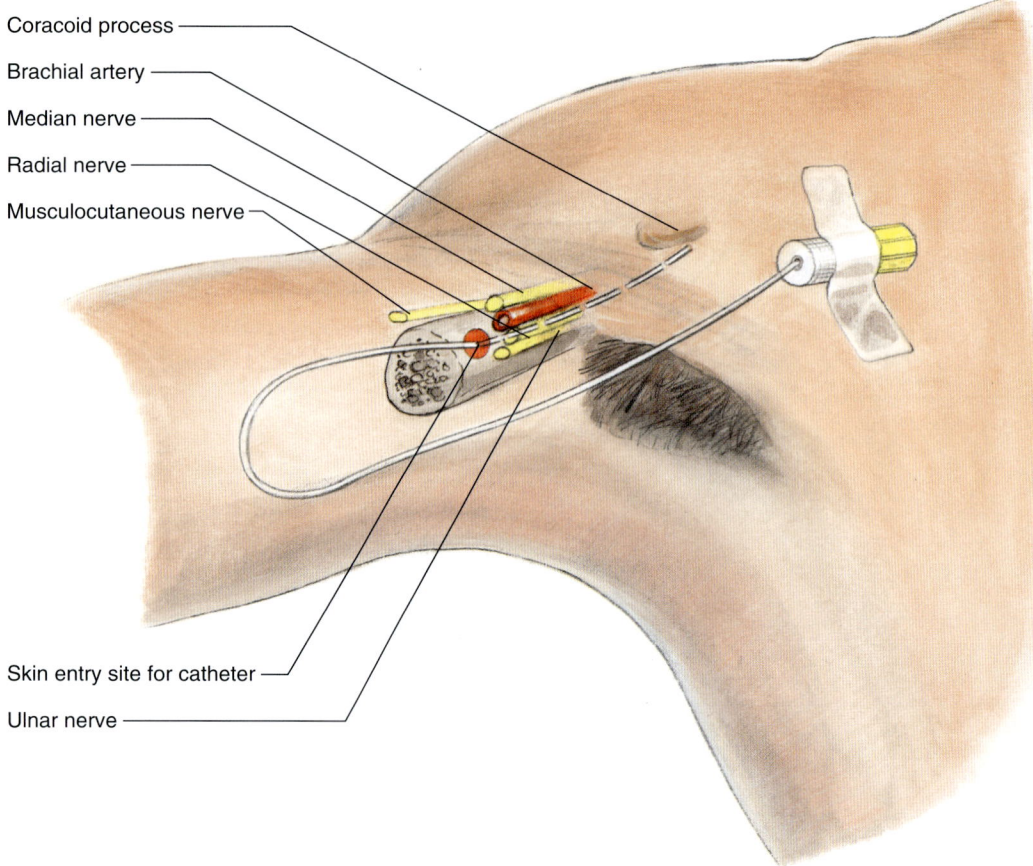

Fig. 9.5 Axillary block: continuous catheter technique after threading 10 cm of catheter proximally.

of a neuropathy if we are to understand the true incidence and causes of this condition after brachial plexus block and upper extremity surgery.

SONOANATOMY

The lateral cord of the brachial plexus divides into the musculocutaneous nerve and the lateral portion of the median nerve, the medial cord divides into the ulnar nerve and medial portion of the median nerve, and the posterior cord divides into the radial nerve and the axillary nerve. In the axilla, the median, ulnar, and radial nerves travel in a neurovascular bundle with the axillary artery medial to the humerus. The musculocutaneous nerve travels separately and usually lies in the plane between the biceps and coracobrachialis muscles or in the body of the coracobrachialis.

The target nerves for the axillary block are the radial, median, ulnar, and musculocutaneous nerves. The structures of interest, including the axillary artery and surrounding nerves, are superficial (1 to 3 cm) from the skin surface of the anteromedial aspect of the proximal arm. The median nerve is located superficial and lateral to the artery, whereas the ulnar nerve is superficial and medial to the artery, and the radial nerve is posterior and lateral or medial to the artery.

Under ultrasound, the median, ulnar, and radial nerves have a honeycomb appearance or can be seen as round hyperechoic structures. The musculocutaneous nerve is usually seen under ultrasound as a hypoechoic, flattened oval, with a bright hyperechoic border (Figs. 9.6, 9.7B, 9.8A-B).

INDICATIONS

- Surgeries from midarm down to elbow (brachiobasilic fistula, elbow fixation).
- Surgeries on the hand and wrist.

TECHNIQUE

The patient ideally should be placed in the supine position, with the arm abducted 90 degrees and externally rotated so the dorsum of the hand rests on the bed, and preferably the operator should be positioned behind the patient, with the ultrasound machine in front of the patient and facing the operator. Injured extremities should be well supported during positioning. The ultrasound probe is placed transversely on the proximal medial upper aspect of the arm in order to view the axillary artery and surrounding nerves in short-axis view. This starting point should place the ultrasound transducer over both the biceps and triceps muscles. Then slide the ultrasound transducer across the axilla until the thick-walled pulsatile axillary artery and the hyperechoic surrounding nerves are visualized. Relative to the axillary artery, the median nerve usually lies around the 9 to 12 o'clock position, the ulnar nerve around 2 to 3 o'clock, and the radial nerve around 5 to 6 o'clock. We prefer to use the in-plane approach and a 2-inch, 22-gauge

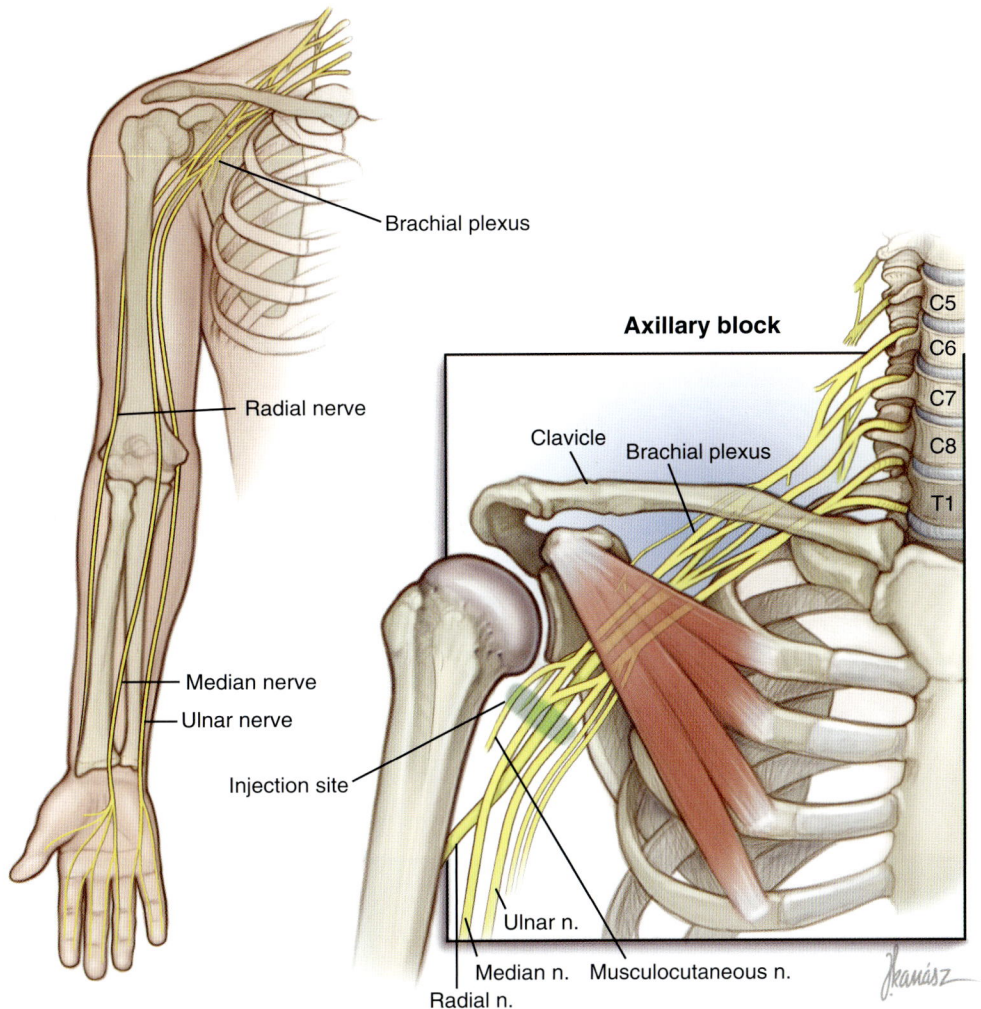

Fig. 9.6 Anatomy of axillary approach of brachial plexus block.

echogenic needle. The needle is inserted in plane from the cephalad aspect and directed to the location of the median, ulnar, and radial nerves using careful hydrodissection with a small amount of local anesthetic. Finally, the needle is withdrawn to the biceps muscle and redirected toward the hypoechoic flattened oval with a bright hyperechoic border musculocutaneous nerve (see Figs. 9.7A-B and 9.8A-B).

KEY POINTS

- High-frequency, 38-mm broadband linear array transducer is preferred for this block.
- Use between 20 and 25 mL of 0.5% ropivacaine or bupivacaine to inject the four nerves.
- We usually block the nerves around the axillary artery first—which are the median, ulnar, and radial nerves—and then the needle is withdrawn to the biceps muscle and redirected toward the hypoechoic, flattened oval musculocutaneous nerve.

PEARLS

- A reverberation artifact deep to the artery is often misinterpreted for the radial nerve. When you are in doubt, you can use nerve stimulation to confirm the location of the nerve.
- The axillary nerve is not blocked because it departs from the posterior cord high up in the axilla; that's why the deltoid muscle is not anesthetized by the axillary block.
- Always aspirate before injection, and watch for the spread and the dose of the local anesthetic to avoid toxicity.
- When scanning, use minimal pressure with the ultrasound transducer to avoid obliteration of the veins, rendering the veins invisible and easily prone to being punctured with the needle if care is not taken.
- Unintentional multiple punctures of the veins surrounding the axillary artery can predispose the patient to local anesthetic toxicity.

AXILLARY CATHETER TECHNIQUE

Axillary block is performed first targeting the median, ulnar, radial, and musculocutaneous nerves using a 22-gauge needle 4 inches in length, to speed the onset of the block and to avoid vascular punctures with a Tuohy needle. From the same entry point the 19-gauge axillary catheter is then

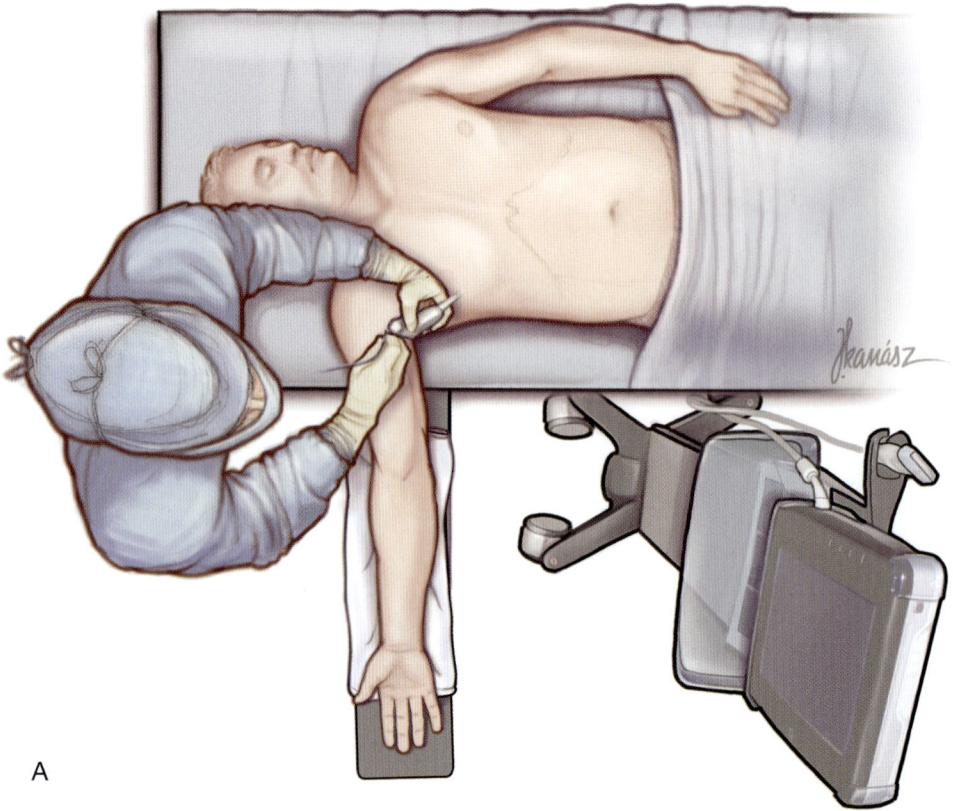

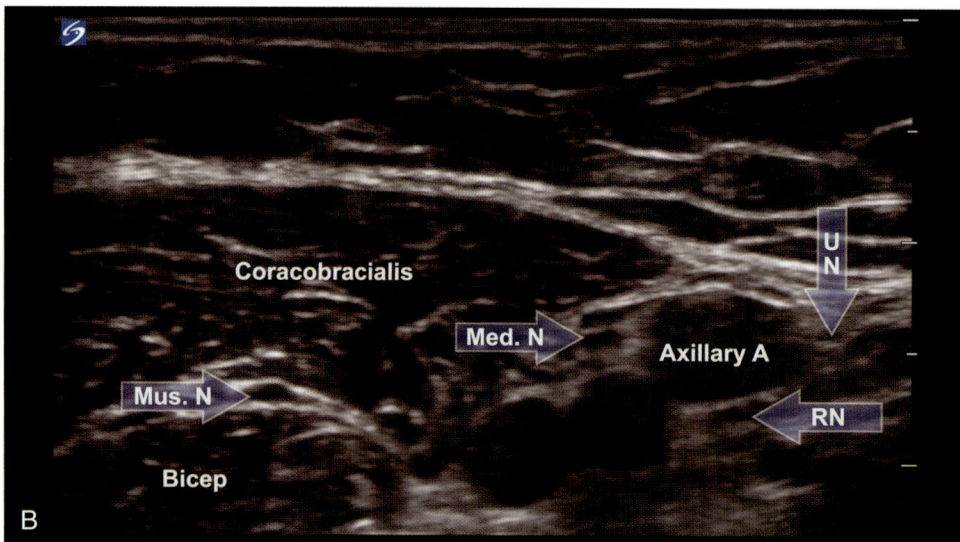

Fig. 9.7 (A) Patient position with the arm abducted 90 degrees and externally rotated. (B) Ultrasound for the brachial plexus. *RN,* Radial nerve; *UN,* ulnar nerve.

placed using a 17-gauge Tuohy needle, 3 inches in length, and the catheter is threaded around the targeted nerves for the surgical procedure. For example, if the surgery involves the little finger, then we thread the catheter around the ulnar nerve. If the surgery involves the whole hand, then we thread the catheter between the median and ulnar nerve, and usually the local anesthetic spreads to the radial nerve. Then we tunnel the catheter for 2 to 3 inches under the skin away from the axilla to decrease catheter migration and we use an adhesive dressing with built-in slow releasing chlorhexidine to prevent infection. We use a ropivacaine 0.2% infusion at 5mL basal rate in the hospital, and 5mL per hour demand rate using an automated programmed pump to deliver the medication when the patient is at home. The axillary catheter is usually kept in place for 5 days after surgery. The catheter is then removed either by the patient or a family member, or by the surgeon at his office during the patient's postoperative visit.

If there are multiple vessels around the axillary artery and between the nerves, infraclavicular block or supraclavicular block may be a better option to block surgeries for the hand, forearm, and elbow.

INDICATIONS FOR AXILLARY CATHETER

- Surgeries for hand, forearm, and elbow.
- Patients with morbid obesity (cannot have a good image to perform an infraclavicular block and

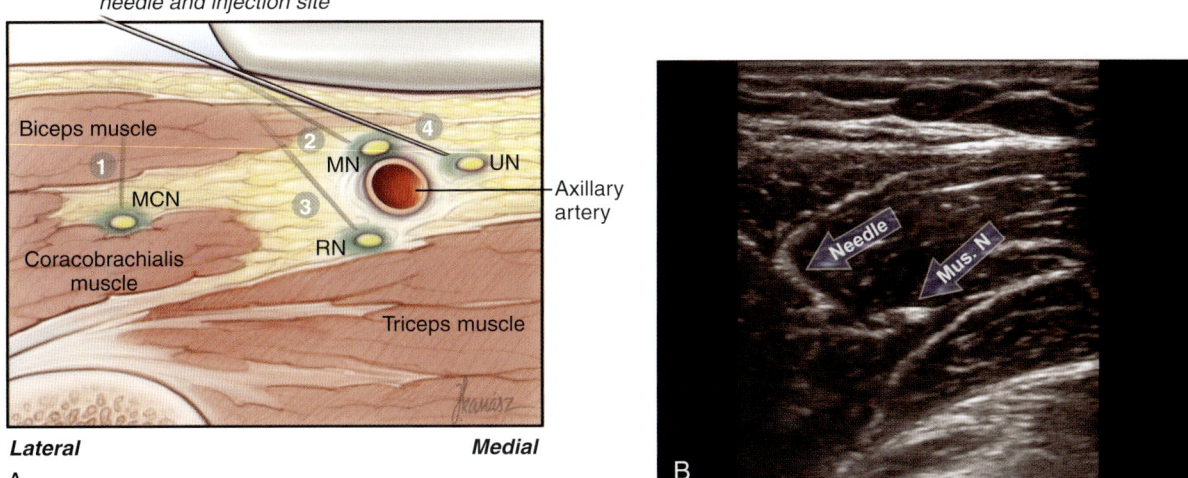

Fig. 9.8 (A) In-plane technique for axillary block. Note the multiple injections of local anesthetics around the musculocutaneous nerve (MCN), median nerve (MN), radial nerve (RN), and ulnar nerve (UN). (B) Ultrasound image for musculocutaneous nerve injection. Notice the needle in close proximity to the nerve.

concerned about phrenic block when using a supraclavicular block).
- Patients with severe COPD (chronic obstructive pulmonary disease), sleep apnea, asthma, on home oxygen, phrenic nerve palsy on the contralateral side of surgery, and refusal to have an infraclavicular block.

COMPLICATIONS FOR AXILLARY CATHETER

- Infections.
- Partially working block.
- Catheter migration and dislodgement.

Distal Upper Extremity Blocks

10

Sree Kolli and Sanchit Ahuja

Key Points

- Blockade of peripheral nerves of the upper extremity is often accomplished by brachial plexus approaches. However, conditions such as infections to brachial plexus sites, coagulopathy, single nerve distribution, minor procedures (not requiring a tourniquet), and rescue supplementations of brachial plexus block may require individual nerve blockade.
- Distal peripheral nerve blocks are associated with a slightly higher likelihood of nerve injury, possibly because of the anatomical location of these sites where the nerve is contained within bony and ligamentous surroundings.
- As most distal forearm and hand surgery procedures are performed using a tourniquet, the patients may require deeper sedation to tolerate the high tourniquet inflation pressures.
- A high-frequency linear array transducer is preferred for these peripheral nerves; also it is easier to locate a nerve in short axis at a determined landmark and then follow in a cranial to caudal direction.
- Continuous nerve catheters are not recommended, perhaps because these nerves are confined in a tight space and carry the risk of compartment syndrome. Nevertheless, if prolonged analgesia is needed, axillary continuous catheters may be considered.

SONOANATOMY

The three major peripheral nerves of the upper extremity, namely median, radial, and ulnar, may be blocked at various levels as follows: arm, elbow, forearm, and wrist.

The *median nerve* is composed of both motor and sensory components derived from the medial and lateral cords of the brachial plexus. It is bounded in a neurovascular bundle in the upper arm where it accompanies the brachial artery. At the elbow, the median nerve courses medial to the brachial artery, and lies between the humeral and ulnar heads of the pronator teres muscle (Fig. 10.1). At mid-forearm, the median nerve separates from ulnar artery and is sandwiched between the muscle of the flexor digitorium superficialis (FDS) and flexor digitorum profundus (FDP) before entering through the carpal tunnel at the wrist. Motor branches (anterior interosseous nerve) supply the deep volar muscles in the forearm and thenar eminence of the hand, whereas sensory distribution is limited to the radial aspect of the hand. Notably, the median nerve does not provide any sensory distribution to the forearm; however, it innervates all muscles of the forearm except flexor carpi ulnaris and the ulnar aspect of flexor carpi radialis.

The *ulnar nerve* originates from the C8 and T1 nerve roots as the terminal branch of the medial cord of the brachial plexus and has mixed motor-sensory components. At the upper level of the arm, the ulnar nerve is medial to the axillary artery, and posterior to the brachial artery and median nerve. It does not provide any motor or sensory innervation at this level. However, in midarm, it descends along the posteromedial aspect and passes between the olecranon process and medial epicondyle to enter the forearm, where it lies superficial to the FDP and medial to the ulnar artery. At the forearm, the ulnar nerve can be located medial to the ulnar artery in close proximity, and hence facilitates sonographic determination. At the level of wrist, the nerve runs lateral to flexor carpi ulnaris and enters the hand superficial to the flexor retinaculum.

The *radial nerve* is a mixed motor-sensory nerve originating from the posterior cord of the brachial plexus via C5 to T1 nerve roots. It travels from medial to lateral within the spiral groove of the humerus and further descends along the medial and lateral heads of the triceps muscle to lie anterior to the lateral epicondyle in the elbow (see Fig. 10.1). At this level, the nerve divides into superficial and deep branches.

TECHNIQUE

MEDIAN NERVE

Landmark technique. At the level of elbow—antecubital crease, the median nerve is located 1 cm medial to pulsation of the brachial artery approximately 1–2 cm deep (Fig. 10.2). The needle is inserted at 45 degrees cephalad, and a resistance click of the bicipital aponeurosis may be felt 1–2 cm deep to the skin. At this point, paresthesia may be achieved, and after

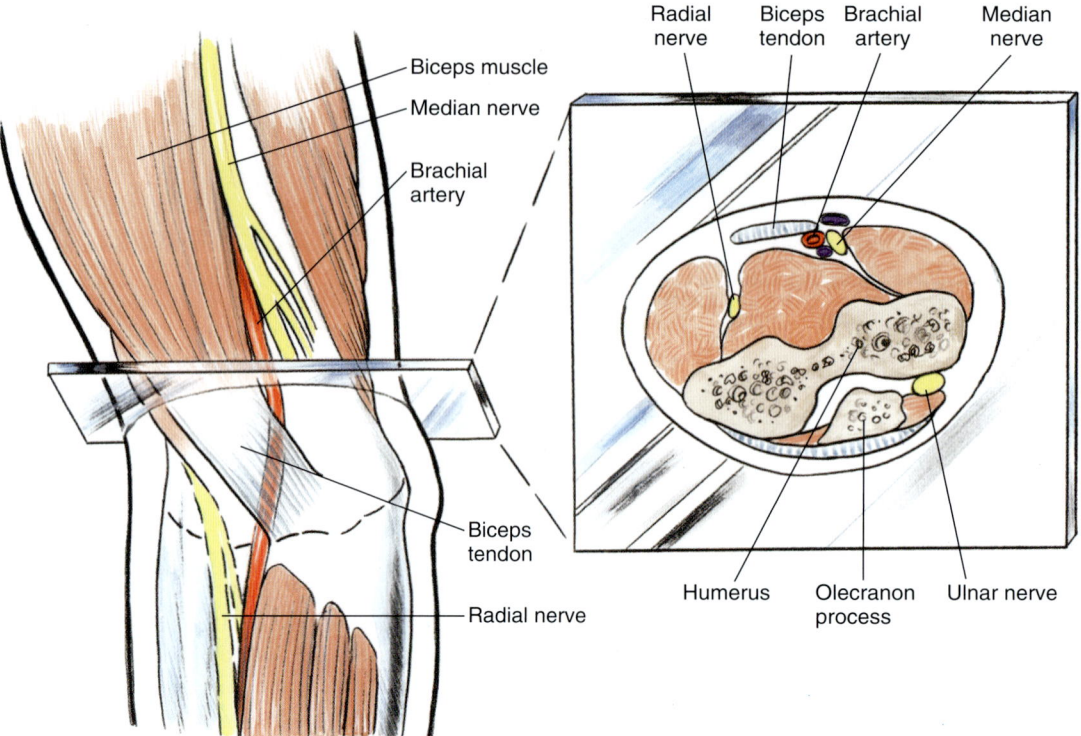

Fig. 10.1 Elbow nerve blocks: functional anatomy.

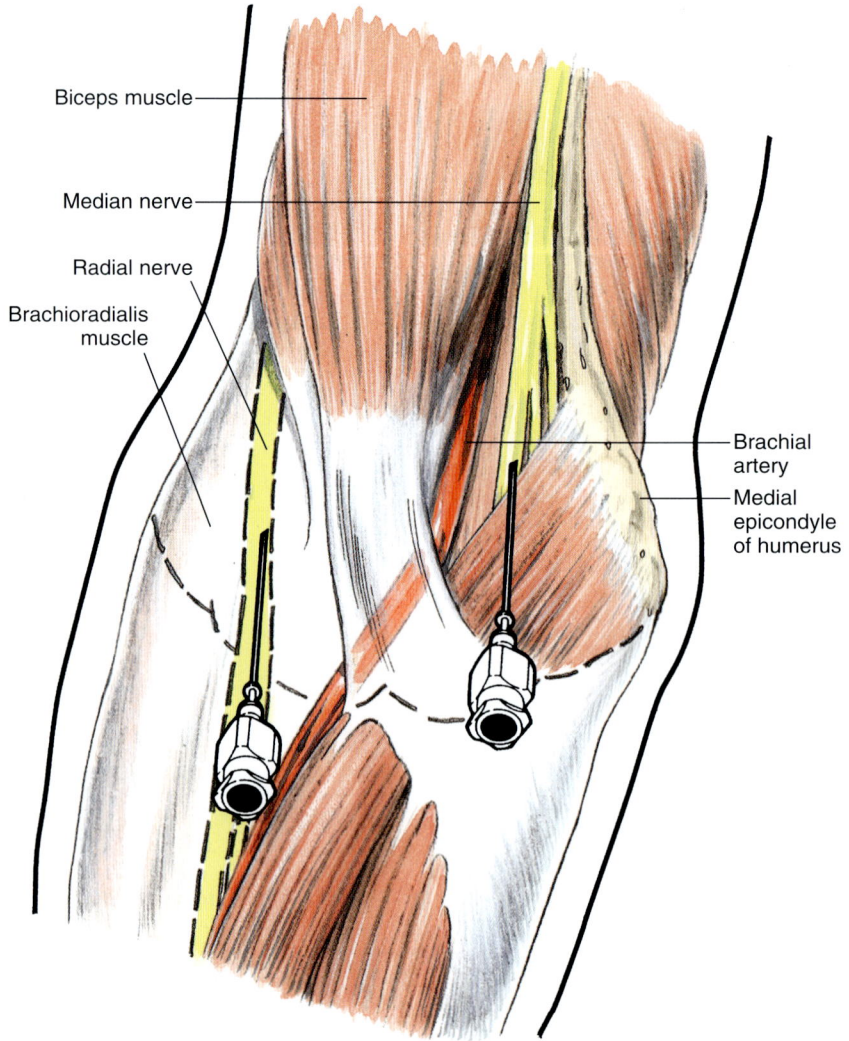

Fig. 10.2 Elbow nerve blocks: median and radial nerves.

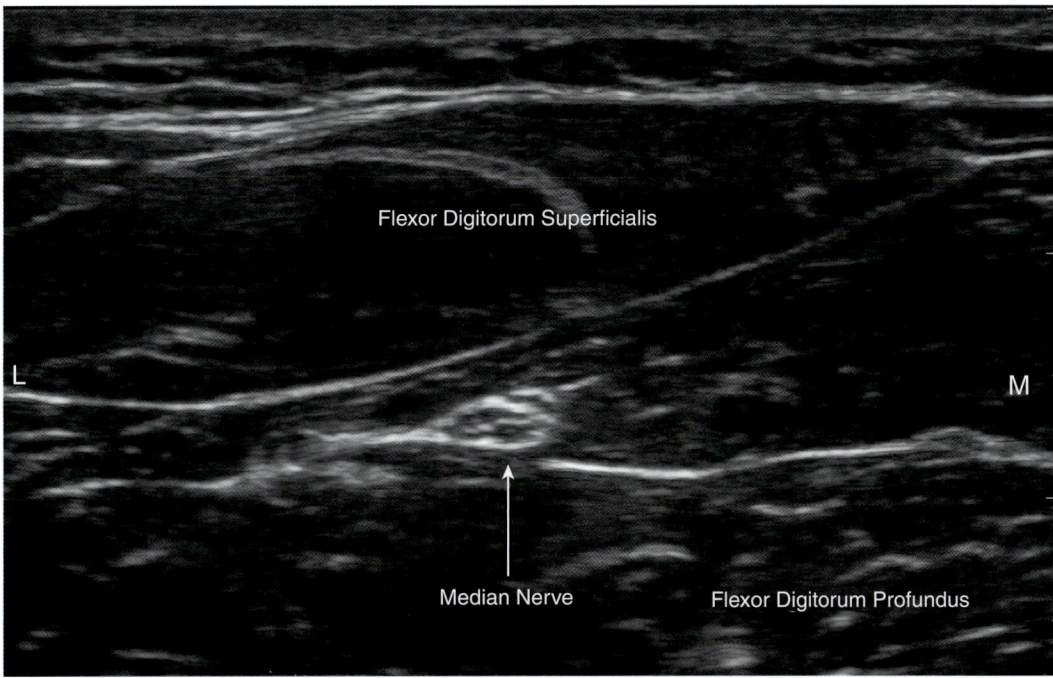

Fig. 10.3 Ultrasound of mid-forearm showing median nerve.

confirming, 5–10 mL of local anesthetic (LA) can be injected.

Ultrasound technique. Distal to the elbow, at the level of the mid-forearm, the median nerve is found as a hyperechoic structure embedded in hypoechoic FDS and FDP (Fig. 10.3). The nerve should be confirmed by fanning the probe along its course. Using an *in-plane* view, with a high frequency linear probe, the needle tip is advanced towards the base of the median nerve and 2–3 mL of LA is injected. The needle is then readjusted to the superior border of the nerve in order to effectively surround the nerve completely with LA. The total volume should be limited to 5–7 mL.

ULNAR NERVE

Landmark technique. At the level of elbow, the ulnar nerve can be accessed by mid-range flexion and abduction. Identification of ulnar groove and medial epicondyle landmarks are made, followed by insertion of a needle 1–2 cm deep and proximal to the medial epicondyle at 45 degrees cephalad to the skin (Fig. 10.4). After appropriate paresthesia is achieved, 3–5 mL of LA can be injected. Within the ulnar groove the nerve is immobile and care must be taken with regard to restricting the total volume (preferably less than 5 mL) injected to avoid causing pressure neurapraxia.

Ultrasound technique. We suggest an ulnar nerve block at the level of the mid-forearm for the following reasons: 1) the nerve is easily found at the ulnar artery landmark; 2) the nerve starts to separate and risk of arterial puncture may be avoided at a somewhat distal location; 3) there is a low risk of compartment syndrome; and 4) the ability to cover the dorsal and volar terminal branches of the ulnar nerve, which divides distal to this location. After the nerve is located (Fig. 10.5), the confirmation is done by fanning the probe along in a proximal to distal direction. Using an *in-plane view* with a low frequency probe, the needle is inserted along the ulnar side of the transducer and no more than 3–5 mL of LA is used to surround the nerve. The ulnar nerve can also be blocked at the elbow, where it can be easily identified medial to the pulsatile brachial artery, appearing as a bright hyperechoic oval structure.

RADIAL NERVE

Landmark technique. At the level of elbow, the antecubital crease, medial epicondyle, lateral epicondyle, biceps and brachioradialis tendons are identified. The median nerve is located within the groove of brachioradialis and biceps tendon (see Fig. 10.2). An imaginary line can be drawn connecting the medial and lateral epicondyle and the needle is inserted between the brachioradialis muscle and the biceps tendon, 2–4 cm deep to the skin. After appropriate paraesthesia (wrist extension) is achieved, 5–10 mL of LA can be injected.

Ultrasound technique. We recommend blocking the nerve at the upper arm level, which theoretically assures broader coverage. This technique involves placing a low frequency probe in an *out-of-plane* view and a transverse direction, approximately between the upper and middle third of the arm, over the triceps muscle as it crosses the humerus shaft. At this level, the radial nerve and deep brachial artery are visible. Color Doppler may be helpful in visualization. Scanning more distally, just

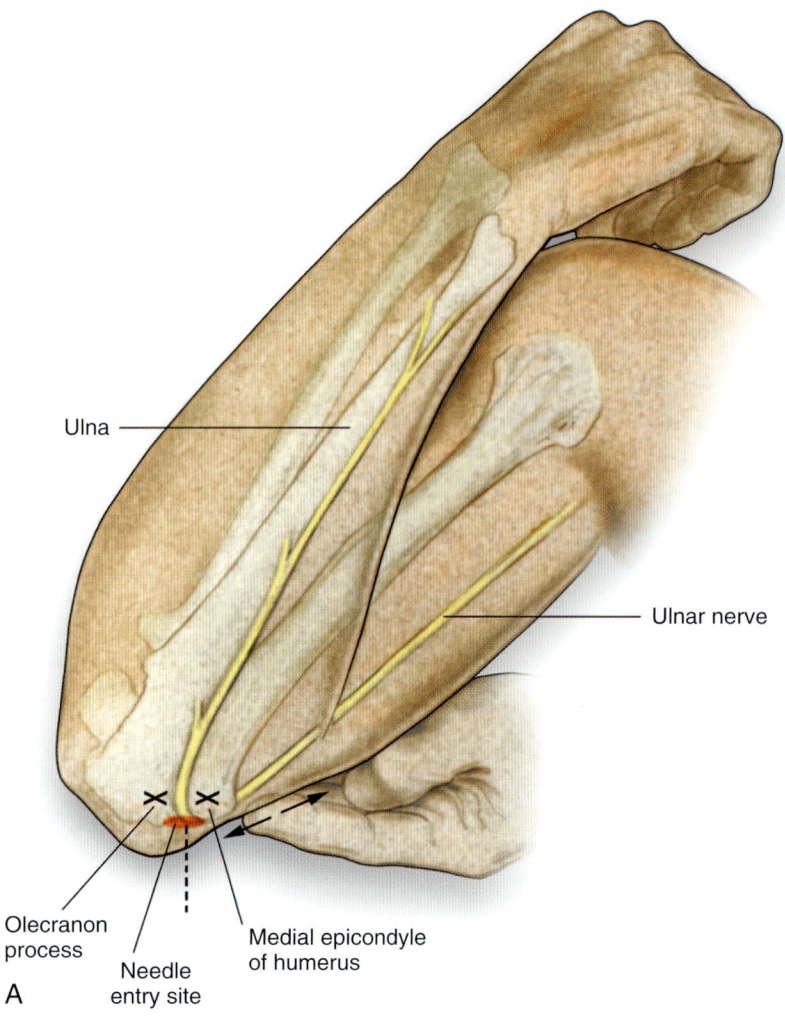

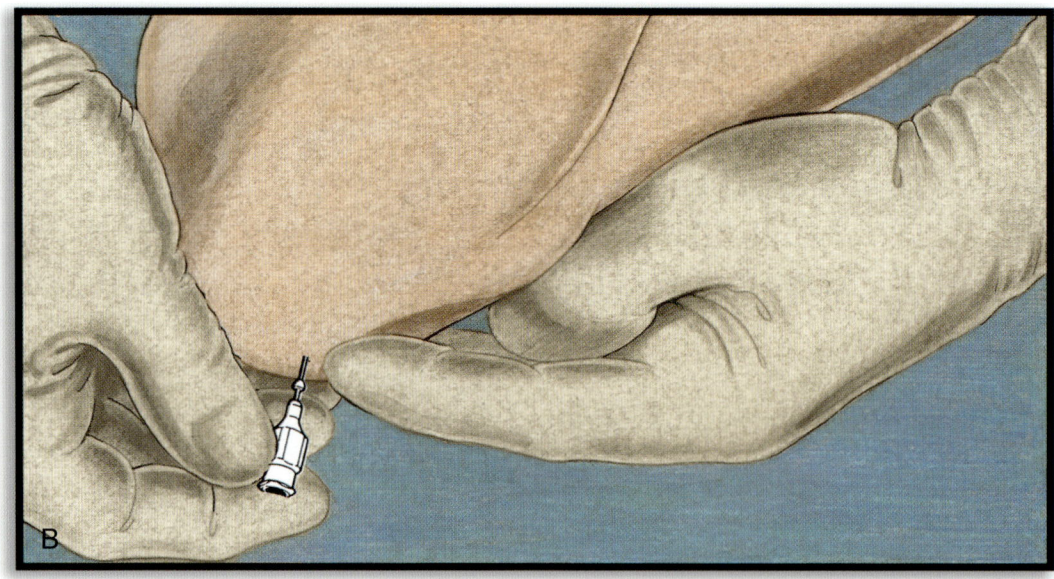

Fig. 10.4 Ulnar nerve block: (A) positioning and (B) palpation of the ulnar groove and needle position.

above the elbow, the nerve may be seen sandwiched between the brachioradialis and brachialis muscle and more distal to this point it divides into superficial and deep branches. The radial nerve may also be traced from the cubital fossa more proximally to the mid-humeral level. However, the nerve is more superficial proximally, and the chance of vascular injury may be decreased when the injection is done at the cubital fossa. It can also be blocked at the mid-forearm level (Fig. 10.6), but does not get the benefit of blocking higher up in the mid-humeral or at the level of elbow.

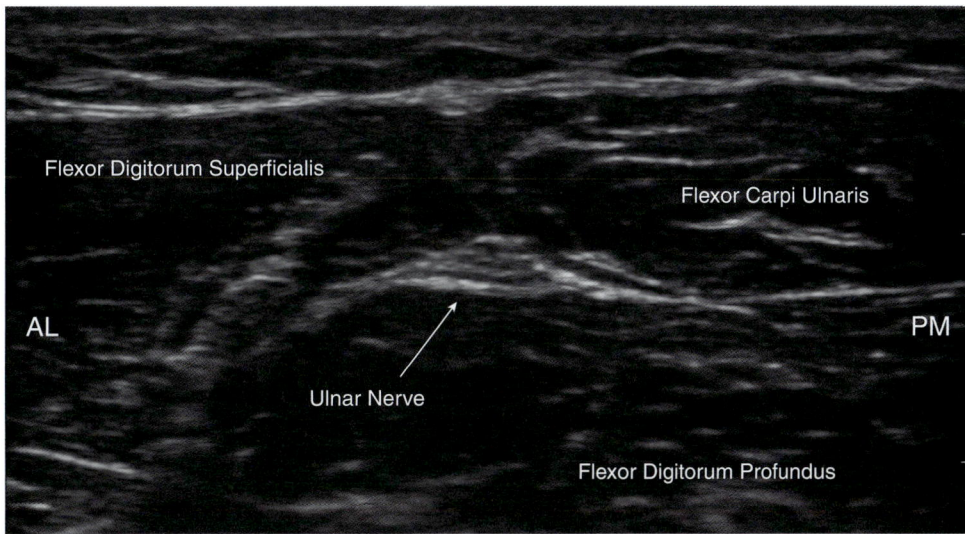

Fig. 10.5 Ultrasound of mid-forearm showing ulnar nerve.

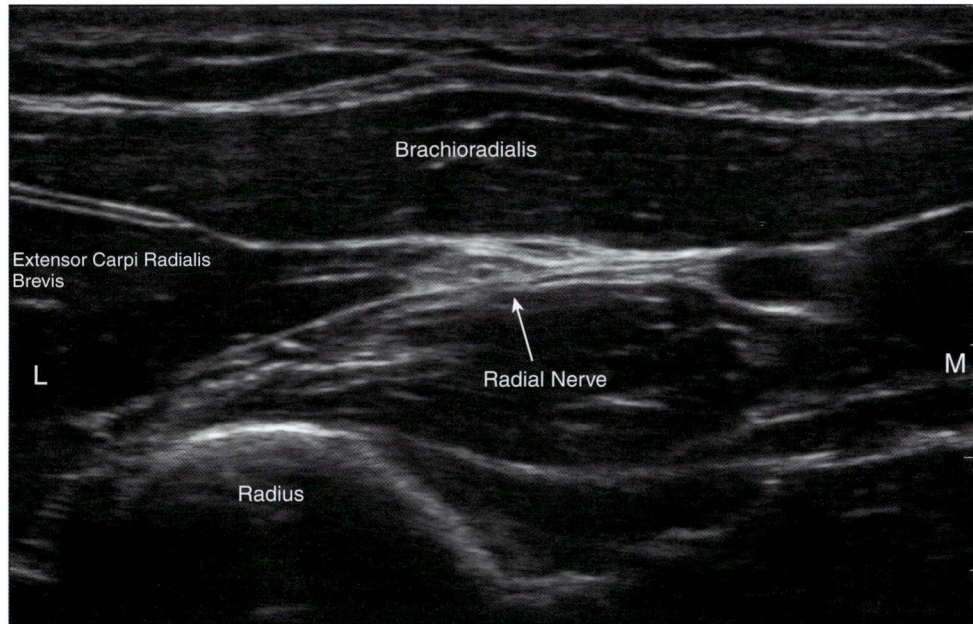

Fig. 10.6 Ultrasound of mid-forearm showing radial nerve.

WRIST BLOCK

At the level of wrist (See Fig. 10.7)	Median nerve	Ulnar nerve	Radial nerve
Landmark technique *Position of wrist*: Supine	Located between tendons of palmaris longus and flexor carpi radialis. Palmaris longus is the more prominent of these two and presents in 85% of the population. Median nerve is blocked by inserting a needle at 45 degrees to skin, 1 to 1.5 cm deep until a fascial click is felt. At this level paresthesia (thumb or index finger) can be achieved and 3 to 5 mL of LA is injected.	Located between flexor carpi ulnaris and ulnar artery. Blocked by inserting the needle to a depth of 1–1.5 cm, 5–10 mm past the flexor carpi ulnaris tendon towards the radial border of wrist, close to the ulnar styloid. 3–5 mL of LA is injected after achieving appropriate paresthesia.	LA is injected subcutaneously between the radial styloid and the dorsal midpoint of the wrist.
Ultrasound technique *Probe position*: Transverse at level of wrist	Nerve appears as an oval hypoechoic structure beneath the flexor retinaculum, confirmed by scanning proximally 5–10 cm. Needle is inserted in-plane and 3–5 mL of LA injected in a circumferential pattern.	Nerve appears as a triangular hyperechoic structure medial to the ulnar artery. Hyperechoic ulnar bone shadow is also seen posteriorly. Following negative aspiration 3–5 mL of LA is injected around the nerve.	A subcutaneous field block around radial styloid process can be used at this level. The radial styloid process is lateral to radial artery.

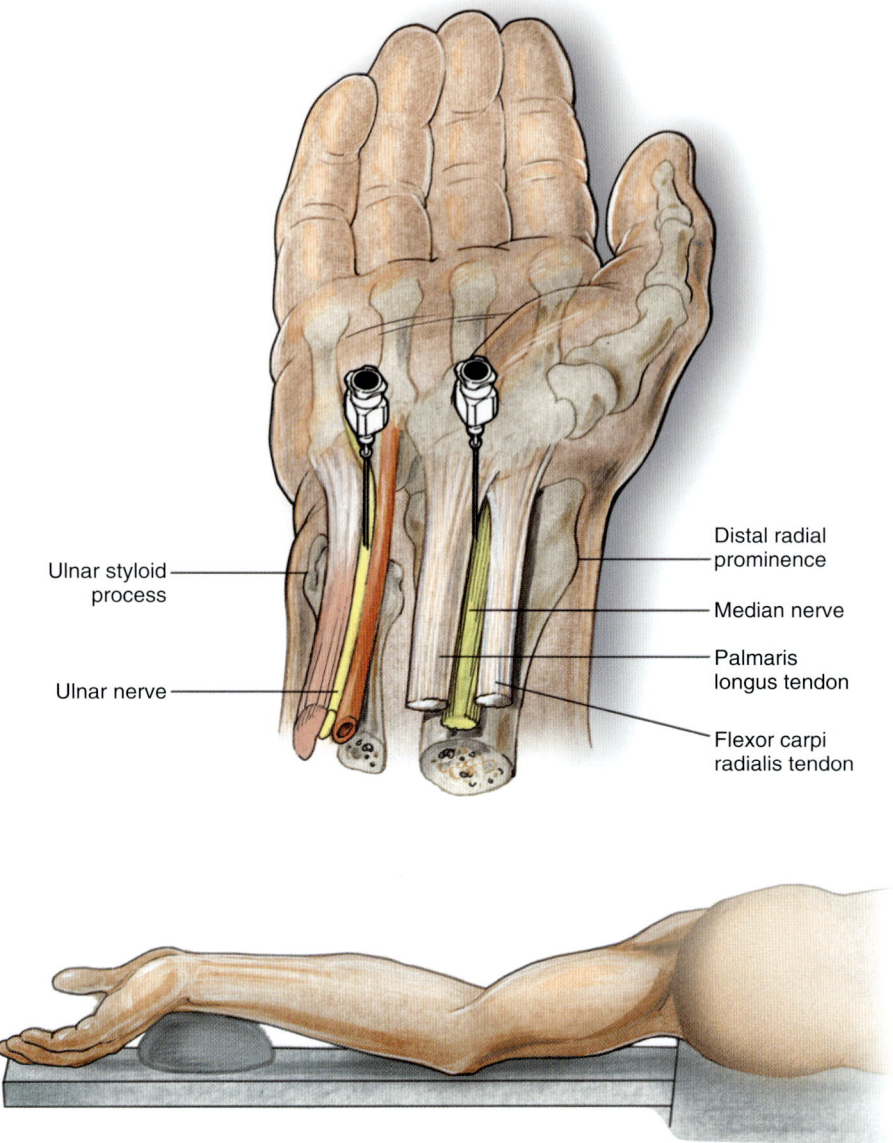

Fig. 10.7 Wrist nerve blocks: functional anatomy, needle insertion and arm positioning.

DIGITAL BLOCK

The most common use of the digital block in the emergency room is for the repair of lacerations and drainage of digital abscesses. It can also be used in certain elective digital surgeries.

The nerves appear to traverse laterally on a cross section of a digit. The digital nerves are the distal continuations of both the median and ulnar nerves (Fig. 10.8). They provide anesthesia distal to the distal interphalangeal joint.

Many techniques for performing a digital nerve block have been described. With the hand pronated the block is performed using a 27-gauge needle and injecting slowly and laterally into the base of a digit—1cm distal to the web space, along the side of periosteum. Angle the needle towards the palmar and dorsal surface and inject 1.5–2 mL of LA. A small subcutaneous swelling can be observed. Repeat on the opposite side.

PEARLS

- Caution should be observed when injecting LA into the olecranon fossa. The ulnar nerve is located in a confined tight space at this location. To prevent intraneural injection it is preferable to use less than 5 mL of anesthetic, ensure that injection pressure is not high, and avoid overflexing the elbow.
- Color Doppler may be helpful in identifying and distinguishing the brachial artery and radial nerve in the proximal third of the upper arm, and also the forearm.
- In morbidly obese patients, it can be difficult to identify individual nerves. Therefore we recommend determining arterial location first and following its course, and finally confirming the location of the nerve with a peripheral nerve stimulator.

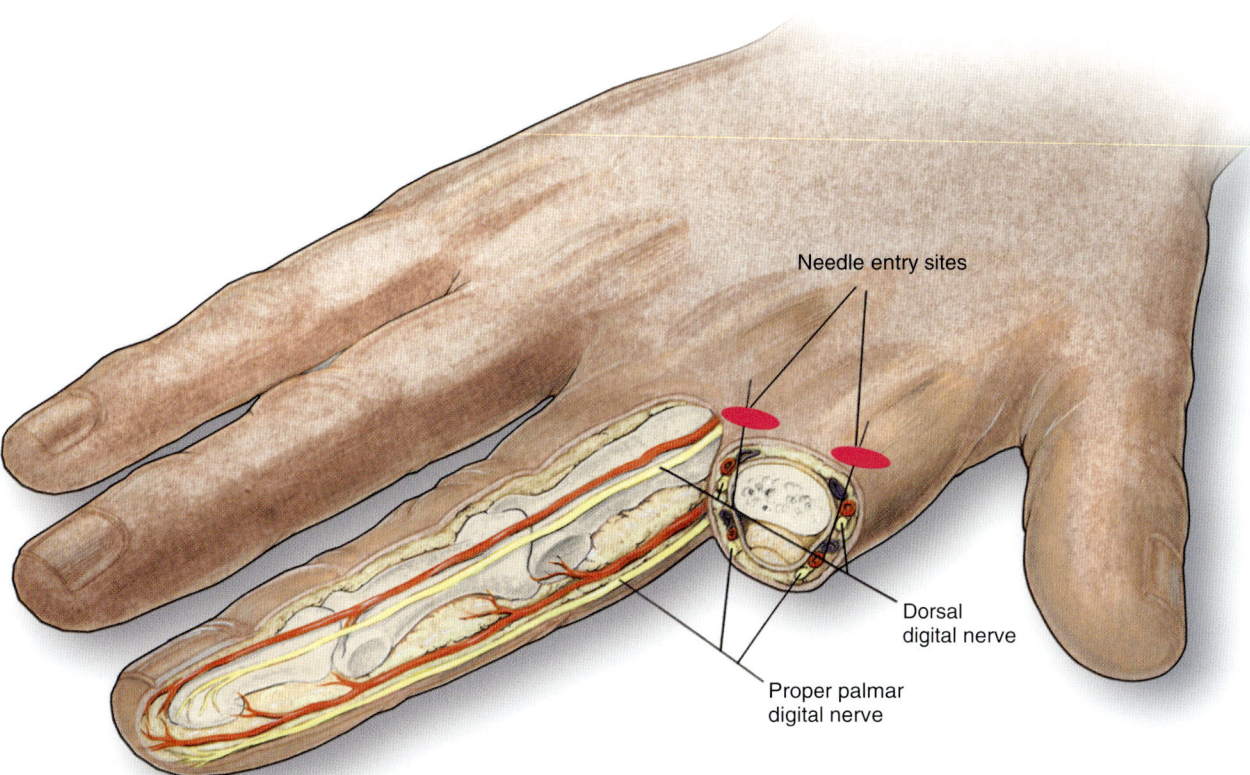

Fig. 10.8 Digital nerve block: anatomy and needle insertion.

- Inadvertent vascular injection can be avoided by applying firm pressure to the vascular structure via a transducer.
- When using an out-of-plane technique, injecting a small amount of normal saline may be helpful in determining the location of the tip of the needle.
- At times the median nerve can be confused with a muscle tendon; asking the patient to flex fingers and wrist may be helpful in distinguishing.
- Advantages of blocking terminal nerves 5–10 cm proximal to the wrist—more room for maneuverability, wider coverage can be ensured by additional blockage of palmar branches of median and ulnar nerves, risk of neurapraxia may be reduced by avoiding injection in tight structures at the wrist.
- Never use LA with epinephrine for digital nerve block. Digital arteries are end arteries and epinephrine may cause ischemia and potentially necrosis.

Intravenous Regional Block

11

David L. Brown

Key Points

- Intravenous (IV) regional anesthesia is usually achieved using dilute lidocaine 0.5%; 50 mL of prilocaine has also been used successfully.
- The IV regional block is useful for procedures lasting 90–120 minutes. This time limit is due to tourniquet time constraints rather than to diminution of the local anesthetic effect.

PERSPECTIVE

IV regional anesthesia was introduced by Bier in 1908. As illustrated in Fig. 11.1, in the initial description, a surgical procedure was required to cannulate a vein, and both proximal and distal tourniquets were used to contain the local anesthetic in the venous system. After its introduction, the technique fell into disuse until the less toxic amino amides became available in the mid-20th century. This technique can be used for a variety of upper extremity operations, including both soft tissue and orthopedic procedures, primarily in the hand and forearm. The technique has also been used for foot procedures with a calf tourniquet.

Patient Selection. The technique is best suited for patients in whom there is no disruption of the venous system of the involved upper extremity, because the technique relies on an intact venous system. It can be used for distal orthopedic fractures and soft tissue operations. Intravenous regional block may not be appropriate for patients in whom movement of the upper extremity causes significant pain, because movement of the upper extremity is required to exsanguinate blood from the venous system adequately.

Pharmacologic Choice. The most commonly used agent for IV regional anesthesia is a dilute concentration of lidocaine; however, prilocaine has also been used successfully. Lidocaine is used in a 0.5% concentration; approximately 50 mL is used for an upper extremity IV regional block.

PLACEMENT

Anatomy. The only anatomic detail necessary for clinical use of the IV regional block is identification of a peripheral vein; one must be cannulated in the involved extremity.

Position. The patient should be resting supine on the operating table with an IV tube already established in the nonsurgical arm. The involved arm should be extended on an armboard near available supplies (Fig. 11.2).

Needle Puncture. Before placement of the IV catheter in the operative extremity, a tourniquet, either double or single, should be placed around the upper arm of the patient. An IV cannula is then inserted in the operative extremity as distally as possible, most commonly in the dorsum of the hand (Fig. 11.3).

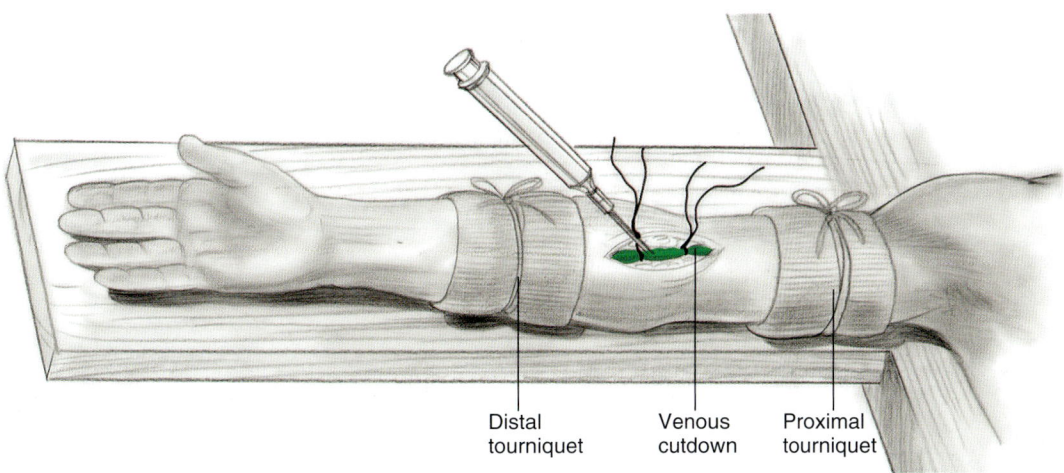

Fig. 11.1 Early Bier block: surgical technique.

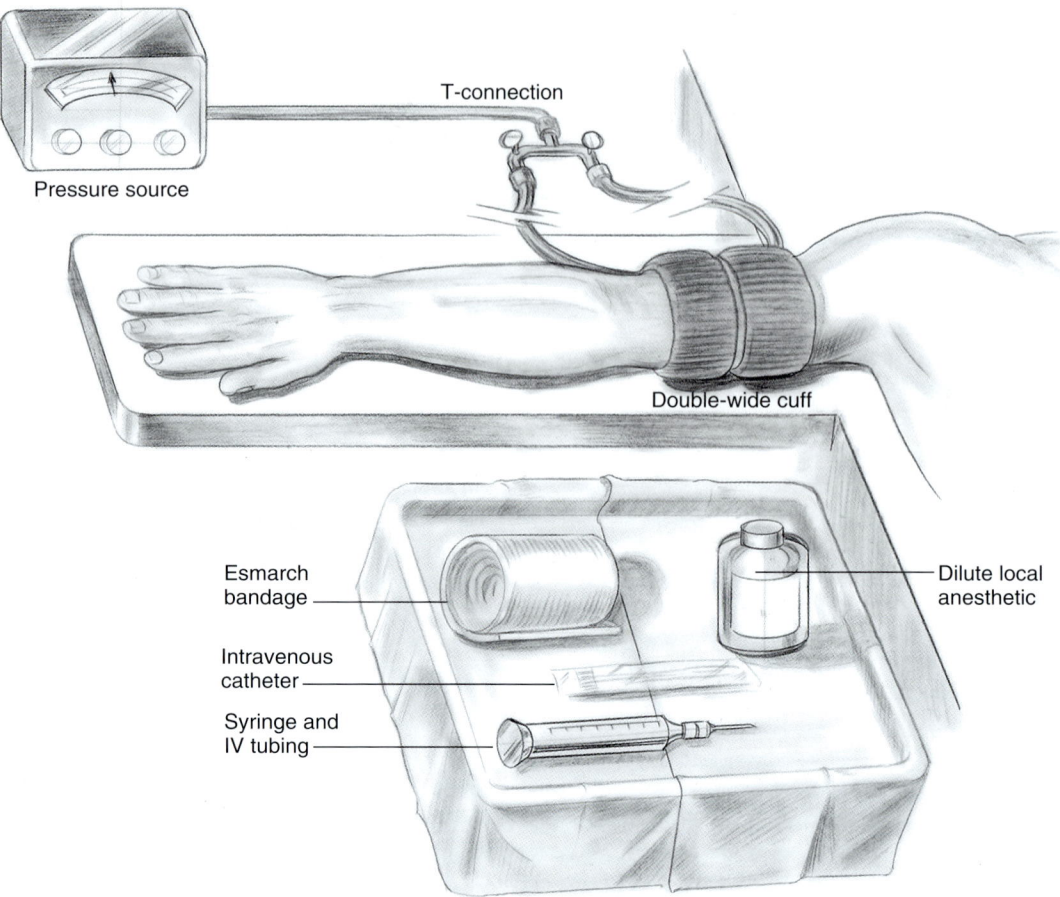

Fig. 11.2 Intravenous regional block: equipment.

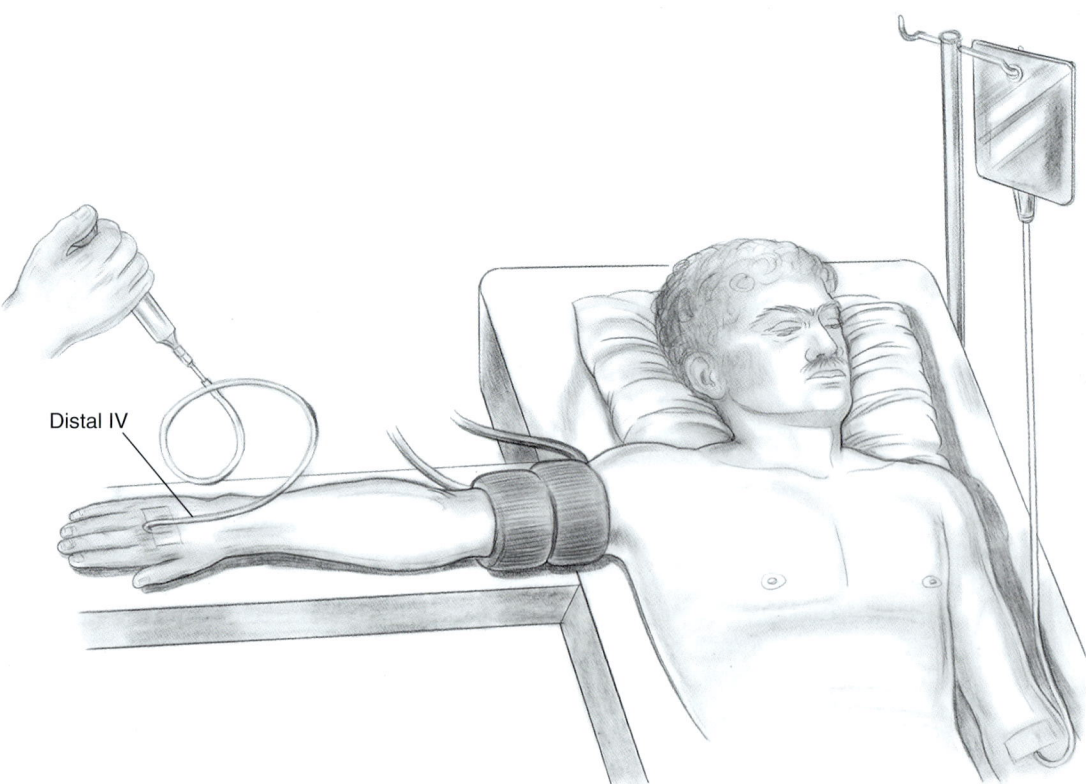

Fig. 11.3 Intravenous regional block: distal IV site.

There are two methods for exsanguinating the venous blood from the operative extremity. The traditional technique requires wrapping an Esmarch bandage from distal to proximal (Fig. 11.4). When the Esmarch bandage is not available or the patient is in too much pain to allow its placement, another method is to raise the arm for 3–4 minutes to allow gravity to exsanguinate the operative upper extremity (Fig. 11.5). After the blood has been exsanguinated from the upper extremity, the tourniquet is

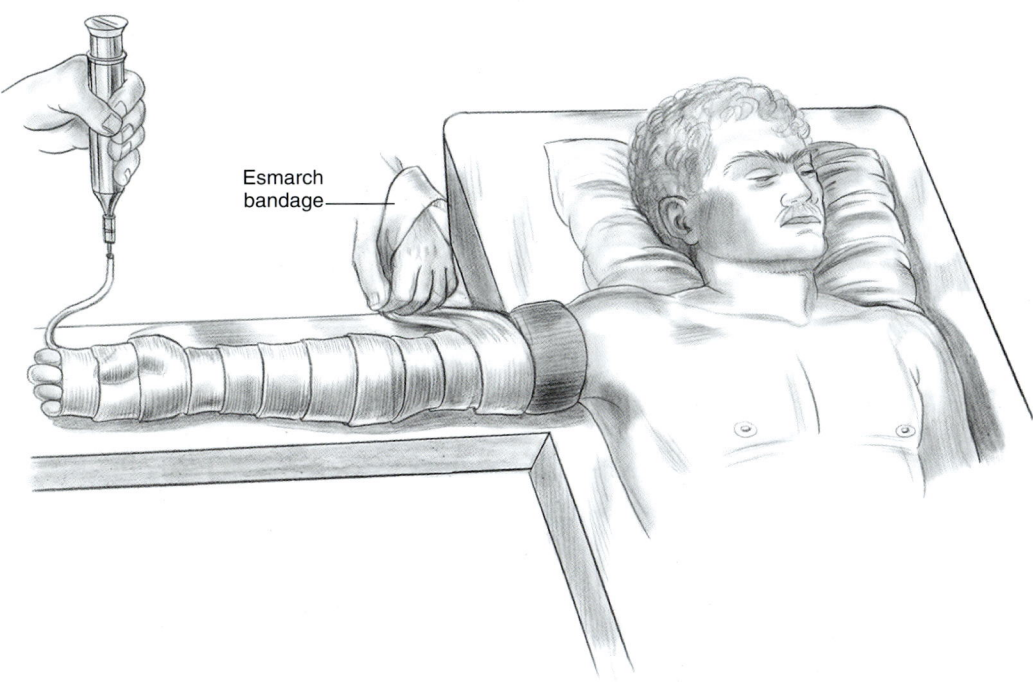

Fig. 11.4 Intravenous regional block: venous exsanguination with Esmarch bandage.

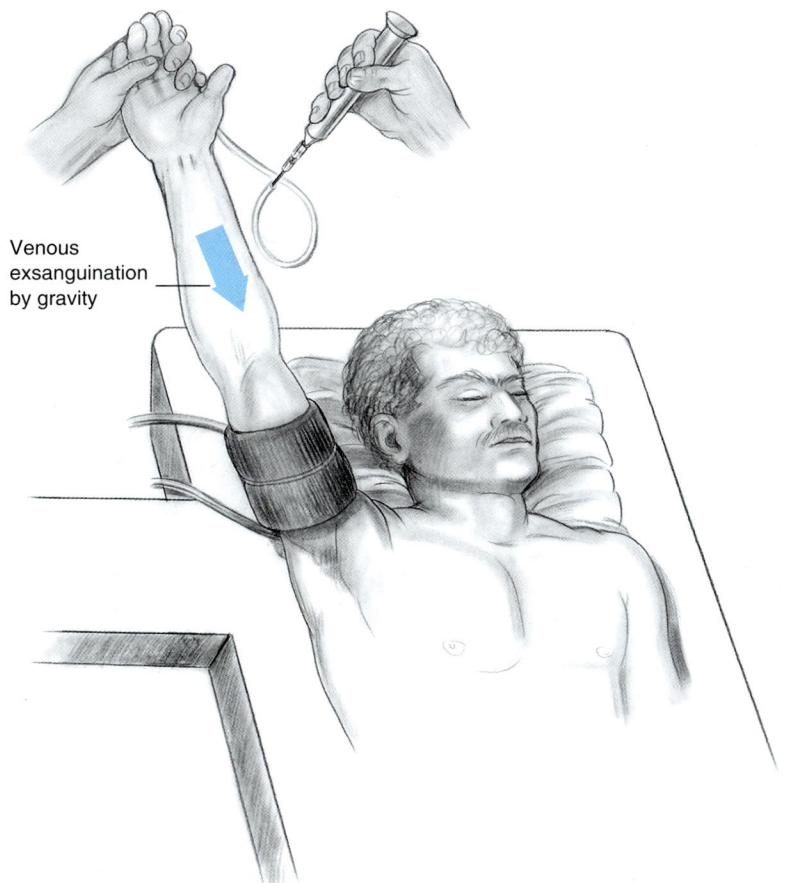

Fig. 11.5 Intravenous regional block: venous exsanguination by gravity.

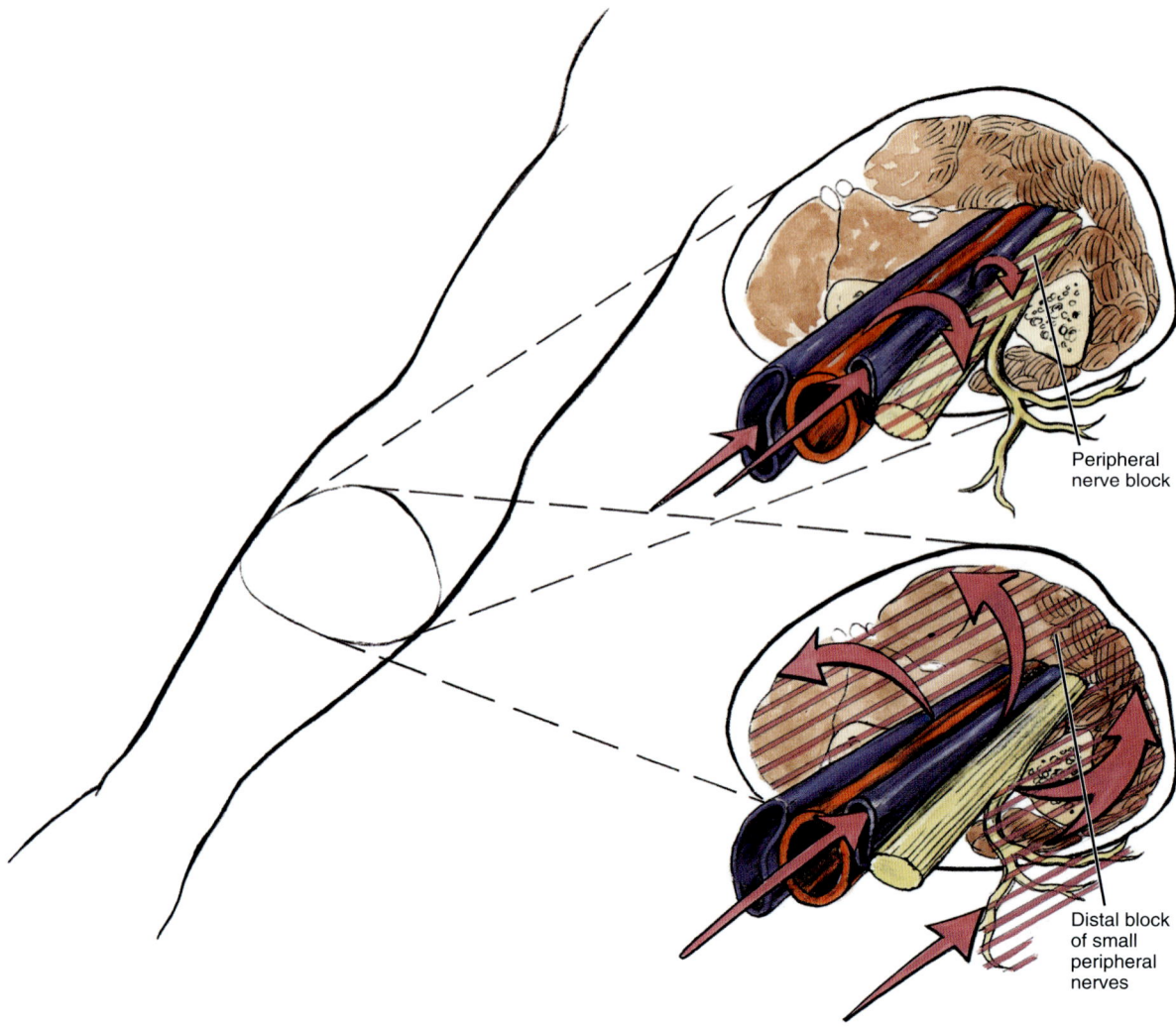

Fig. 11.6 Intravenous regional block: potential mechanism(s) of action.

inflated. If a double tourniquet is used, only the upper tourniquet is inflated. Recommendations for tourniquet inflation pressures range from 50 mm Hg above systolic blood pressure with a wide cuff, to a cuff pressure double the systolic blood pressure, to 300 mm Hg regardless of blood pressure. Until more information is available, I caution against using pressures greater than 300 mm Hg during upper extremity block.

If an Esmarch bandage has been used, the elastic bandage is then unwrapped, and in the average adult 50 mL of 0.5% lidocaine without a vasoconstrictor is injected. Onset of the block usually occurs within 5 minutes, and the block is effective for procedures lasting as long as 90–120 minutes. This time limit is due to tourniquet time constraints rather than to diminution of the local anesthetic effect. The IV cannula is removed before preparation for operation. The block persists as long as the cuff is inflated and disappears shortly after deflation.

POTENTIAL PROBLEMS

The principal disadvantage of IV regional anesthesia is that physicians unfamiliar with treating local anesthetic toxicity may use the technique when appropriate resuscitation measures are not available. Although some workers report successful use of IV regional anesthesia for lower extremity surgery, especially if a calf tourniquet is used for foot surgery, its use is not widespread. During upper extremity use, a considerable number of patients complain about tourniquet pressure even when a double tourniquet is used, and this is often the clinically limiting feature of this technique. Appropriate use of IV sedatives is important for patient comfort.

PEARLS

Fig. 11.6 illustrates the two complementary theories of how IV regional anesthesia produces block. The figure conceptualizes local anesthetic entering the venous system and producing block by blocking the peripheral nerves running with the venous structures. It also outlines a theory that may be complementary—that is, the local anesthetic leaves the veins and blocks small distal branches of peripheral nerves. It is likely that both of these theories are operative. If IV regional anesthesia is to be used successfully, all members of the operating team should understand the importance of tourniquet integrity because the most significant problems with the technique involve unintentional deflation of the tourniquet.

SECTION 3
Lower Extremity Blocks

Lower Extremity Block Anatomy

12

David L. Brown

Key Points

- Unlike the upper extremity, there are two nerve plexuses innervating the lower extremity; the lumbar plexus innervates the ventral aspect, whereas the lumbosacral plexus primarily innervates the dorsal aspect of the lower extremity.
- The three major branches of the lumbar plexus are the lateral femoral cutaneous, femoral, and obturator nerves. They exit from the pelvis anteriorly and innervate the ventral aspect of the lower extremity.
- The sciatic nerve is the combination of two major trunks: the tibial and common peroneal nerves.

Anesthesiologists are more comfortable carrying out lower extremity regional block than upper extremity regional block because of the ease and simplicity of blocking the lower extremities with neuraxial techniques. Also, in no anatomic site outside the neuraxis are the lower extremity plexuses as compactly packaged as are the nerves to the upper extremity in the brachial plexus. If one compares the path of lower extremity nerves over the pelvic brim with the path of the brachial plexus over the first rib, it is clear that the four major nerves to the lower extremity exit from four widely differing sites (Figs. 12.1 and 12.2). Thus regional block of the lower extremity focuses on block of individual peripheral nerves, and my approach to anatomy will follow that concept.

Two major nerve plexuses innervate the lower extremity: the lumbar plexus and the lumbosacral plexus. The lumbar plexus primarily innervates the ventral aspect, whereas the lumbosacral plexus primarily innervates the dorsal aspect of the lower extremity (see Fig. 12.2).

The lumbar plexus is formed from the ventral rami of the first three lumbar nerves and part of the fourth lumbar nerve. In approximately half of patients, a small branch from the twelfth thoracic nerve joins the first lumbar nerve. The lumbar plexus forms from the ventral rami of these nerves anterior to the transverse processes of the lumbar vertebrae deeply within the psoas muscle (Fig. 12.3). The cephalad portion of the lumbar plexus (i.e., the first lumbar nerve, and often a portion of the twelfth thoracic nerve) splits into superior and inferior branches. The superior branch redivides into the iliohypogastric and ilioinguinal nerves, and the smaller inferior branch unites with a small superior branch of the second lumbar nerve to form the genitofemoral nerve (see Fig. 12.1).

The iliohypogastric nerve penetrates the transversus abdominis muscle near the crest of the ilium and supplies motor fibers to the abdominal musculature. It ends in an anterior cutaneous branch to the skin of the suprapubic region and a lateral cutaneous branch in the hip region (Fig. 12.4).

The ilioinguinal nerve courses slightly inferior to the iliohypogastric nerve. It then traverses the inguinal canal and ends cutaneously in branches to the upper and medial parts of the thigh and near the anterior scrotal nerves, which supply the skin at the root of the penis and the anterior part of the scrotum in males (see Fig. 12.4). In females, the comparable anterior labial nerves supply the skin of the mons pubis and labia majora.

The genitofemoral nerve divides at a variable level into genital and femoral branches. The genital branch is small; it enters the inguinal canal at the deep inguinal ring and supplies the cremaster muscle, small branches to the skin and fascia of the scrotum, and adjacent parts of the thigh. The femoral branch is the more medial of the two branches and continues under the inguinal ligament on the anterior surface of the external iliac artery. Below the inguinal ligament, it pierces the femoral sheath and passes through the saphenous opening to supply the skin over the femoral triangle lateral to that supplied by the ilioinguinal nerve (see Fig. 12.4). These three nerves are clinically important during regional block for inguinal herniorrhaphy or other groin procedures carried out under regional block.

Caudal to these three nerves are three major nerves of the lumbar plexus that exit from the pelvis anteriorly and innervate the lower extremity. These are the lateral femoral cutaneous, femoral, and obturator nerves (see Figs. 12.1 and 12.2).

The lateral femoral cutaneous nerve passes under the lateral end of the inguinal ligament. It may be superficial or deep to the sartorius muscle, and it descends at first deep to the fascia lata. It provides cutaneous innervation to the lateral portion of the buttock distal to the greater trochanter and to the proximal two-thirds of the lateral aspect of the thigh.

The obturator nerve descends along the medial posterior aspect of the psoas muscle and through the pelvis to the

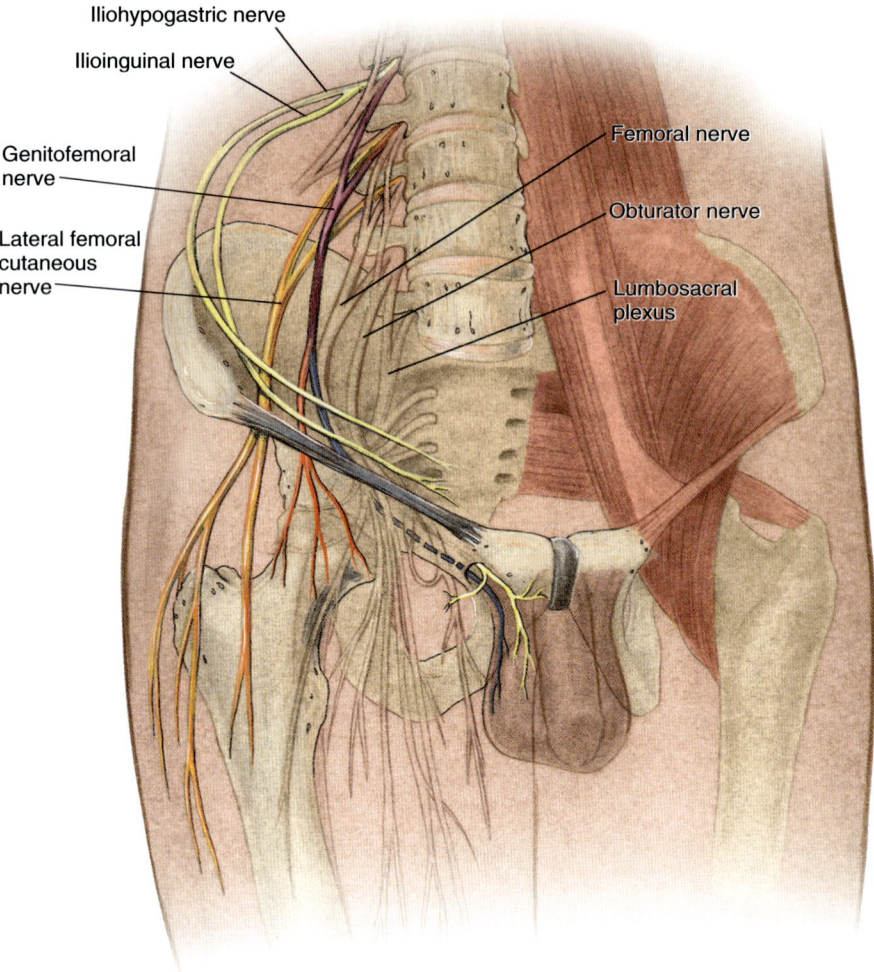

Fig. 12.1 Lower extremity anatomy: major nerves, anterior oblique view.

obturator canal into the thigh. This nerve supplies the adductor group of muscles, the hip and knee joints, and often the skin on the medial aspect of the thigh proximal to the knee.

The femoral nerve is the largest branch of the lumbar plexus. It emerges through the fibers of the psoas muscle at the muscle's lower lateral border and descends in the groove between the psoas and the iliacus muscles. It passes under the inguinal ligament within this groove. Slightly before or on entering the femoral triangle of the upper thigh, the femoral nerve breaks into numerous branches supplying the muscles and skin of the anterior thigh, knee, and hip joints.

The lumbosacral plexus is formed by the ventral rami of the lumbar fourth and fifth and the sacral first, second, and third nerves. Occasionally, a portion of the fourth sacral nerve contributes to the sacral plexus. The nerve from the plexus that is of primary interest to anesthesiologists during lower extremity block is the sciatic nerve. The posterior femoral cutaneous nerve is sometimes listed as an additional branch important to anesthesiologists. In reality, the sciatic nerve is the combination of two major nerve trunks: the first is the tibial nerve, derived from the anterior branches of the ventral rami of the fourth and fifth lumbar and the first, second, and third sacral nerves, whereas the second is the common peroneal nerve, derived from the dorsal branches of the ventral rami of the same five nerves. These two major nerve trunks pass as the sciatic nerve through the upper leg to the popliteal fossa, where they divide into their terminal branches: the tibial and common peroneal nerves.

Figs. 12.5 and 12.6 illustrate the cutaneous innervation of the peripheral nerves of the lower extremity. This subject is illustrated with the patient's lower extremity in both the anatomic and the lithotomy positions for greatest clinical utility. Fig. 12.7 illustrates the dermatomal innervation of the lower extremities in a similar manner. Fig. 12.8 illustrates the osteotome pattern of lower extremity innervation and will be most useful to anesthesiologists who are providing anesthesia for orthopedic procedures. Fig. 12.9 helps clarify the cross-sectional anatomy pertinent to regional block of the lower extremity.

Lower Extremity Block Anatomy

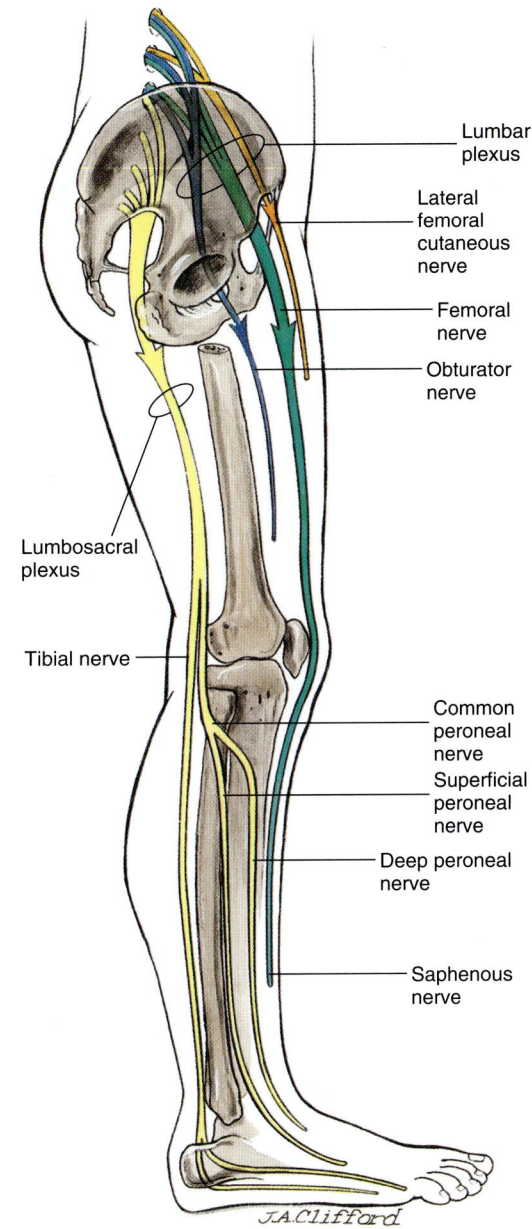

Fig. 12.2 Lower extremity anatomy: major nerves, lateral view.

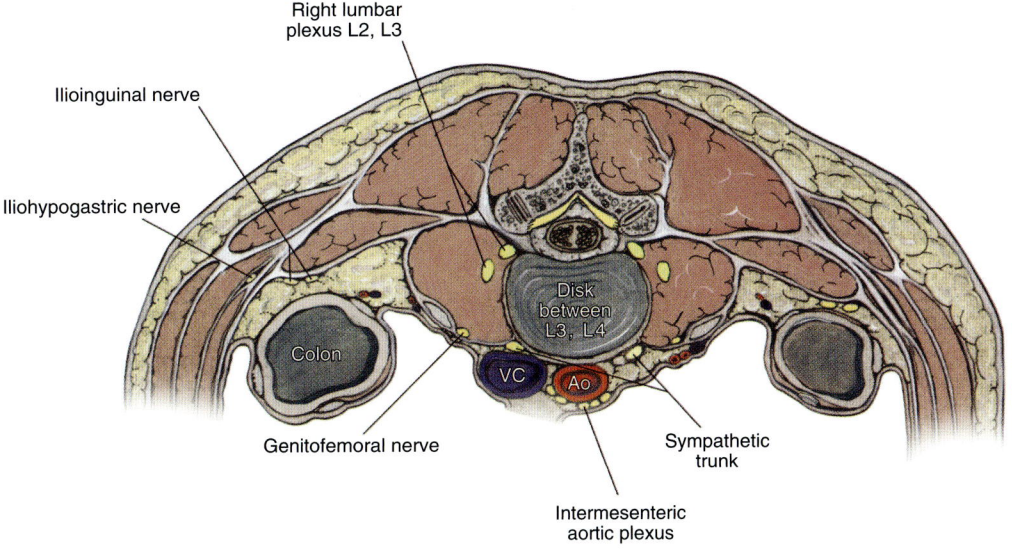

Fig. 12.3 Lumbar plexus anatomy: cross-sectional view. *Ao*, Aorta; *VC*, vena cava.

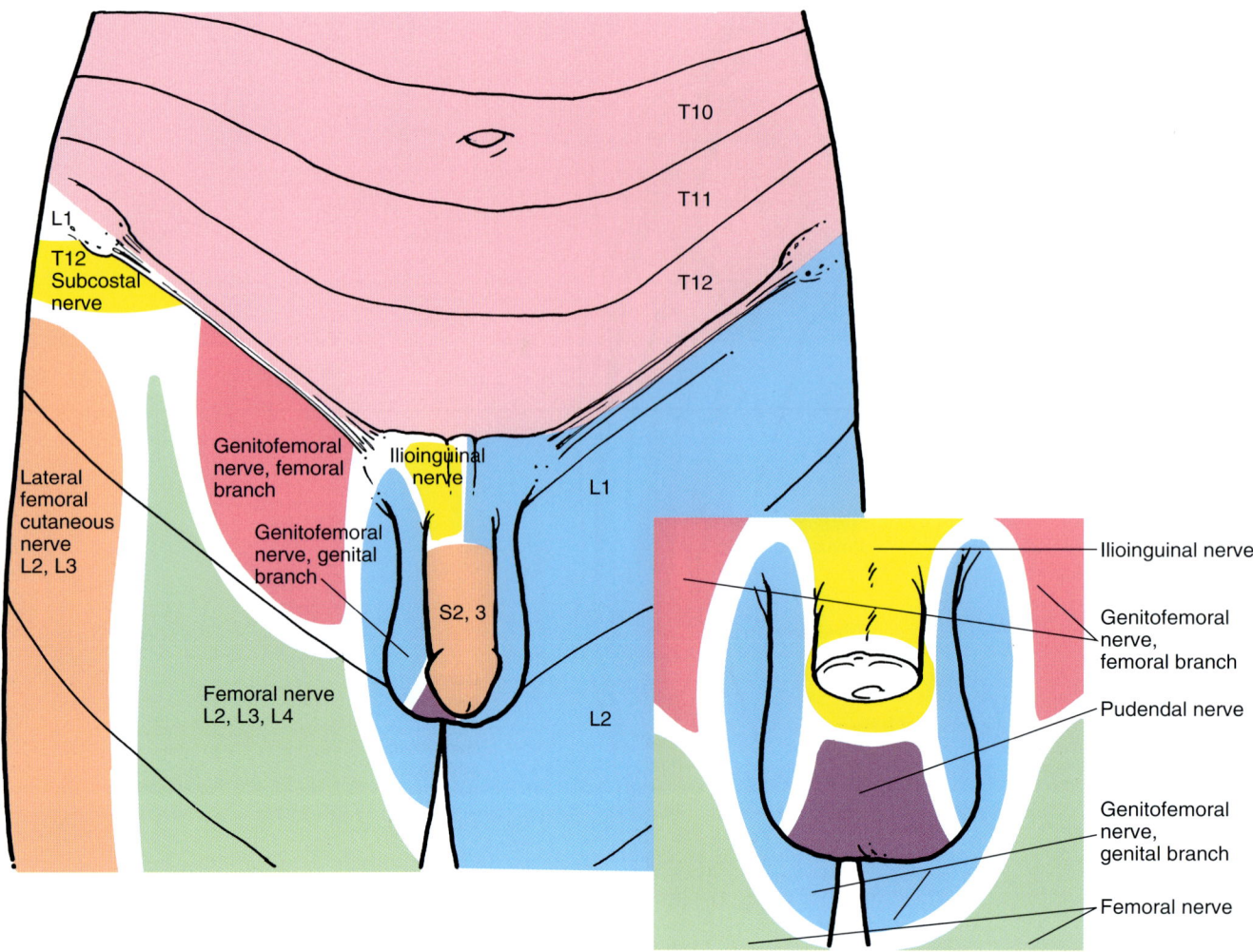

Fig. 12.4 Lower extremity anatomy: proximal innervation (peripheral nerves labeled on right side of the body, dermatomes on the left).

Lower Extremity Block Anatomy

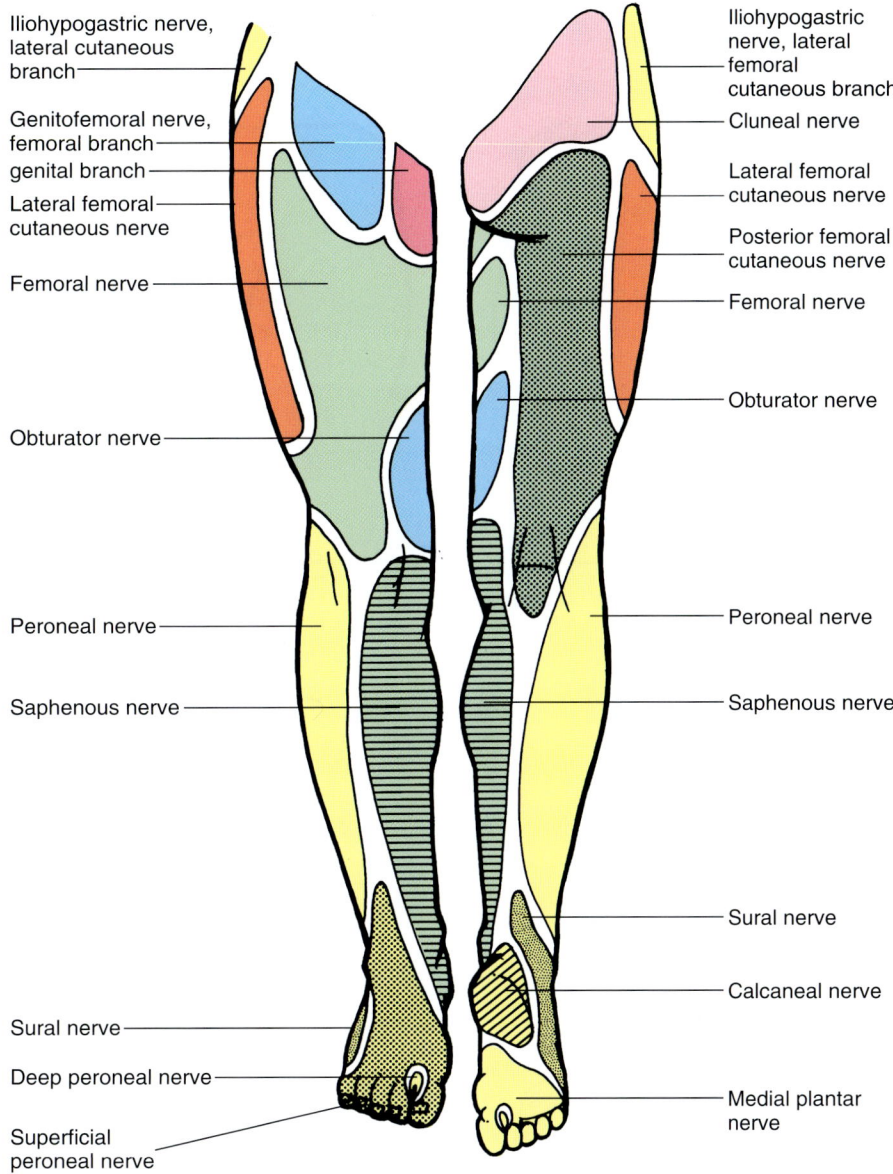

Fig. 12.5 Lower extremity anatomy: proximal and distal innervation.

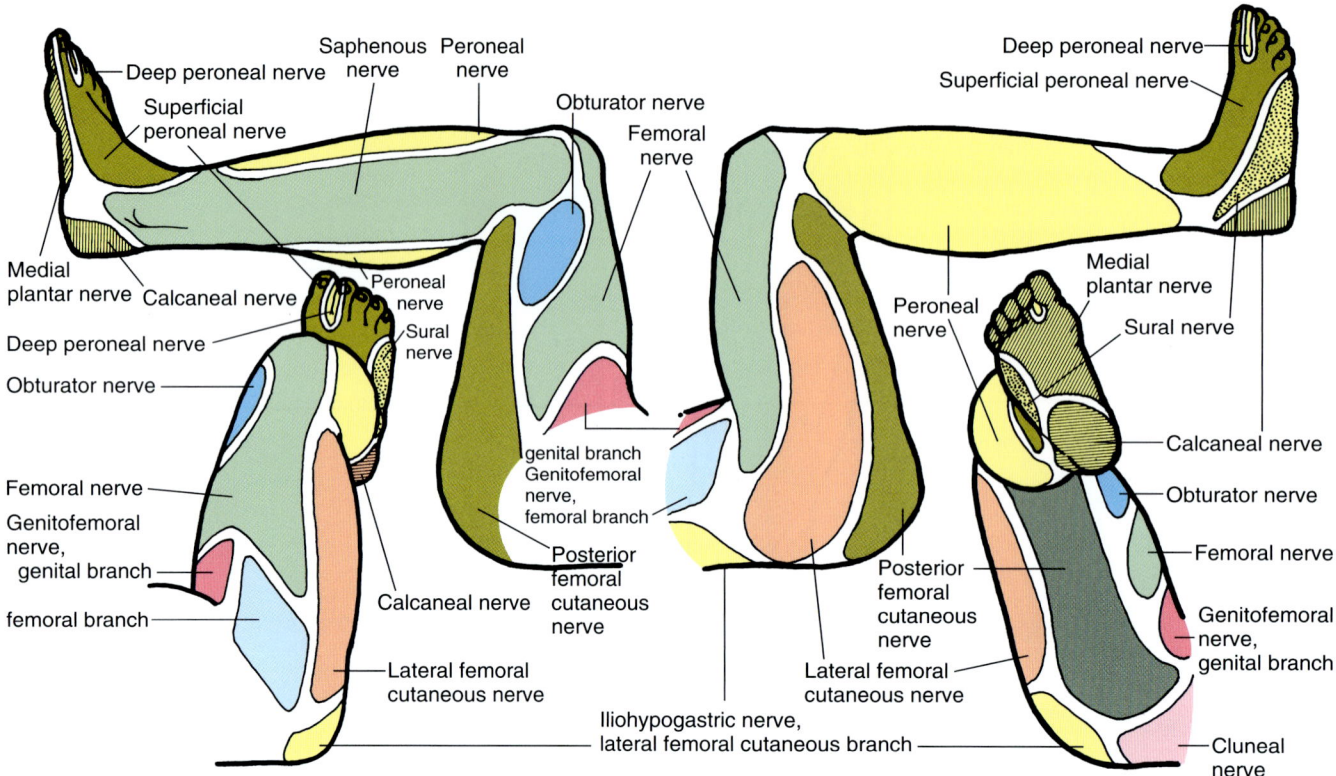

Fig. 12.6 Lower extremity anatomy in lithotomy position: proximal and distal peripheral nerves.

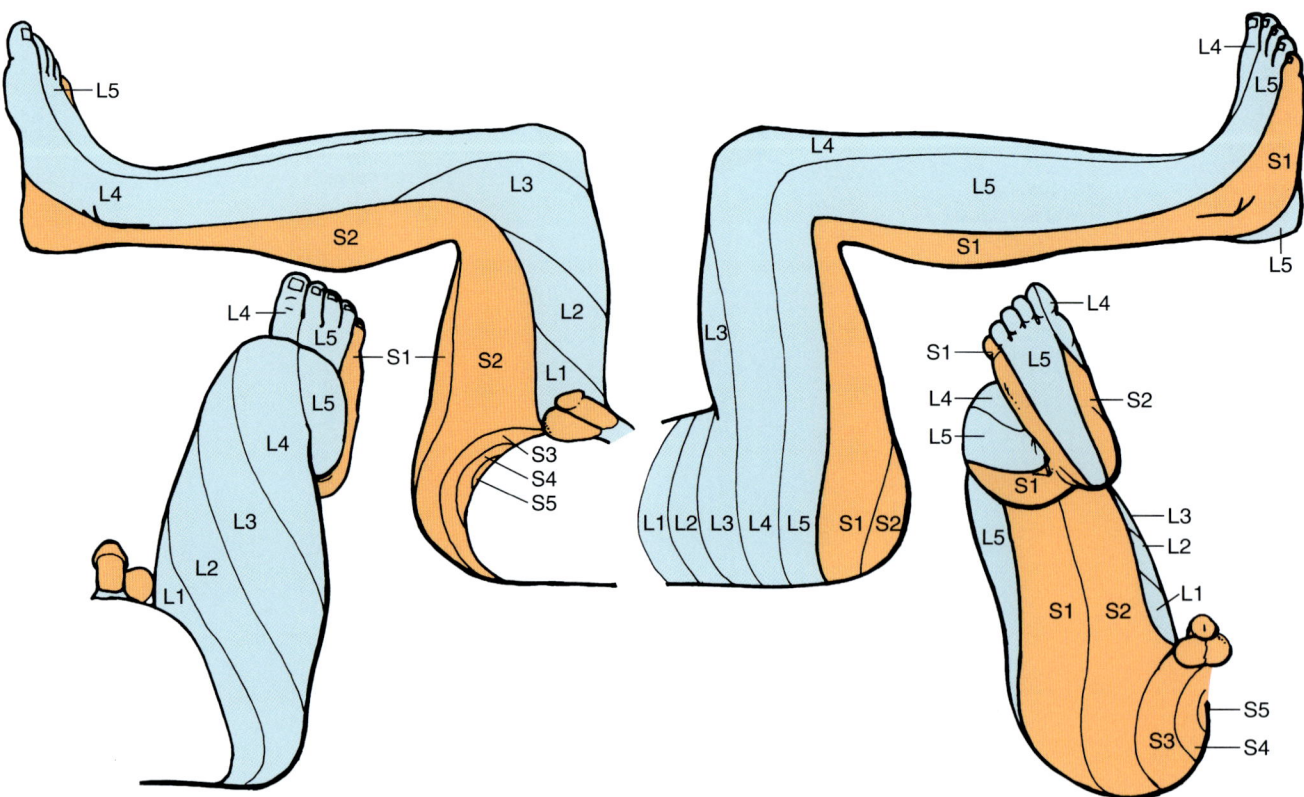

Fig. 12.7 Lower extremity anatomy in lithotomy position: dermatomes.

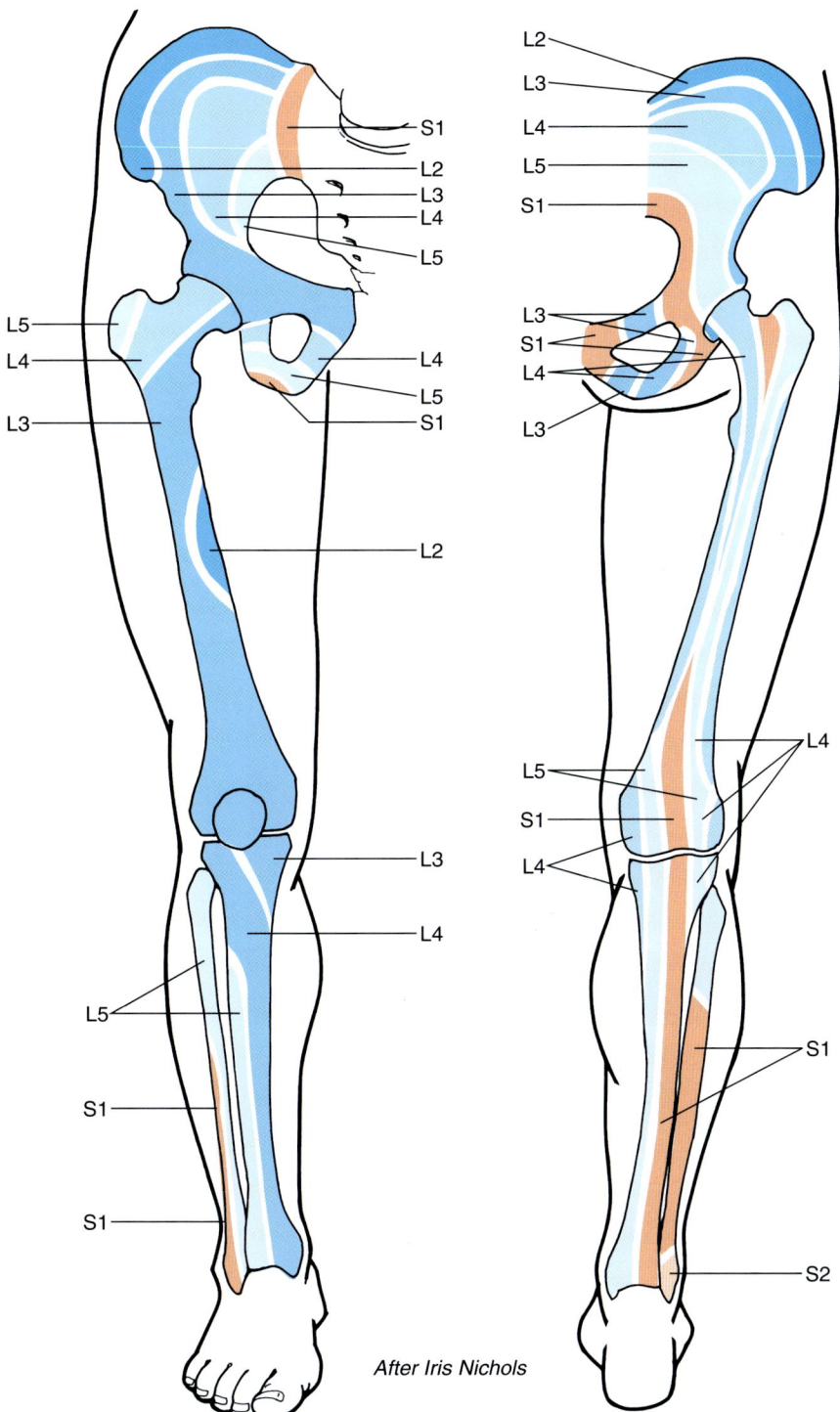

Fig. 12.8 Lower extremity anatomy: osteotomes.

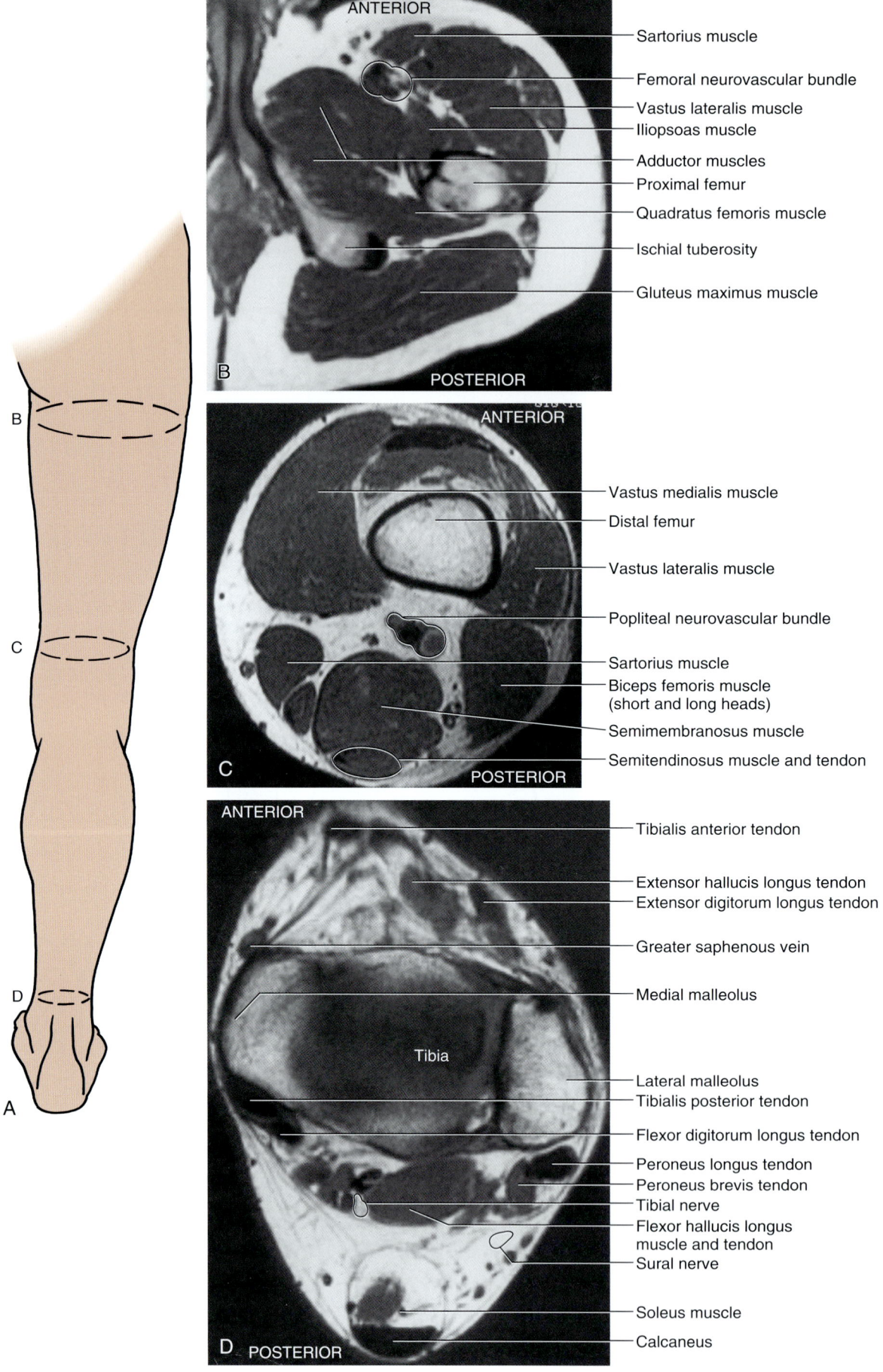

Fig. 12.9 Lower extremity anatomy: cross-sectional magnetic resonance images. (A) Location of sections. (B) Upper leg (below the hip). (C) Middle leg (above the knee). (D) Lower leg (above the ankle).

Lumbar Plexus Block

13

Loran Mounir-Soliman and David L. Brown

INGUINAL PERIVASCULAR BLOCK (THREE-IN-ONE BLOCK)

PERSPECTIVE

The inguinal perivascular block is based on the concept of injecting local anesthetic near the femoral nerve in an amount sufficient to track proximally along fascial planes to anesthetize the lumbar plexus. The three principal nerves of the lumbar plexus pass from the pelvis anteriorly: the lateral femoral cutaneous, the femoral, and the obturator nerves. As illustrated in Fig. 13.1, the theory behind this block presumes that the local anesthetic will track in the fascial plane between the iliacus and the psoas muscles to reach the region of the lumbar plexus roots.

Patient Selection. As outlined, lower extremity block is often most effectively and efficiently performed with neuraxial blocks. Nevertheless, in some patients avoidance of bilateral block or sympathectomy may make an alternative approach necessary.

Pharmacologic Choice. Local anesthetics should be selected by deciding whether a primarily sensory or a sensory and motor block is needed. Any of the amino amides can be used. It has been suggested that the volume of local anesthetic needed for adequate lumbar plexus block from this approach can be estimated by dividing the patient's height, in inches, by three. That number is the volume of local anesthetic in milliliters that theoretically will provide lumbar plexus block.

PLACEMENT

Anatomy. The concept behind this block is that the only anatomy one needs to visualize is the extension of sheath-like fascial planes that surround the femoral nerve.

Position. The patient should be placed supine on the operating table with the anesthesiologist standing at the patient's side in position to palpate the ipsilateral femoral artery.

Needle Puncture. A short-beveled, 22-gauge, 5-cm needle is inserted immediately lateral to the femoral artery, caudal to the inguinal ligament in the lower extremity to be blocked. It is advanced with cephalad angulation until femoral paresthesia occurs; alternatively, nerve stimulation or ultrasonographic guidance is used to identify the correct perineural location of the needle tip. At this point, the needle is firmly fixed, and while the distal femoral sheath is digitally compressed, the entire volume of local anesthetic is injected.

POTENTIAL PROBLEMS

Our clinical experience suggests that the principal problem with this technique is a lack of predictability. In addition, whenever a large volume of local anesthetic is injected through a fixed "immobile" needle, the risk of systemic toxicity is increased. If the technique is used, incremental injection of local anesthetic, accompanied by frequent aspiration for blood, should be carried out.

PEARLS

This block should be used when the goal is lower extremity analgesia, not anesthesia during an operation. We do not believe one needs to master this technique to provide comprehensive regional anesthesia care.

PSOAS COMPARTMENT BLOCK

PERSPECTIVE

In theory, the psoas compartment block produces block of all lumbar and some sacral nerves, thus providing anesthesia of the anterior thigh. Based on the anatomical site and the expected end result of this block, it is sometimes described as a *lumbar paravertebral block.*

LUMBAR PLEXUS BLOCK

RELEVANT ANATOMY OF THE LUMBAR PLEXUS

The lumbar plexus is formed by the ventral rami of the first three lumbar nerves and the greater part of the ventral ramus of the fourth nerve. The first lumbar nerve, frequently supplemented by the 12th thoracic nerve, splits into an upper branch that divides into the iliohypogastric

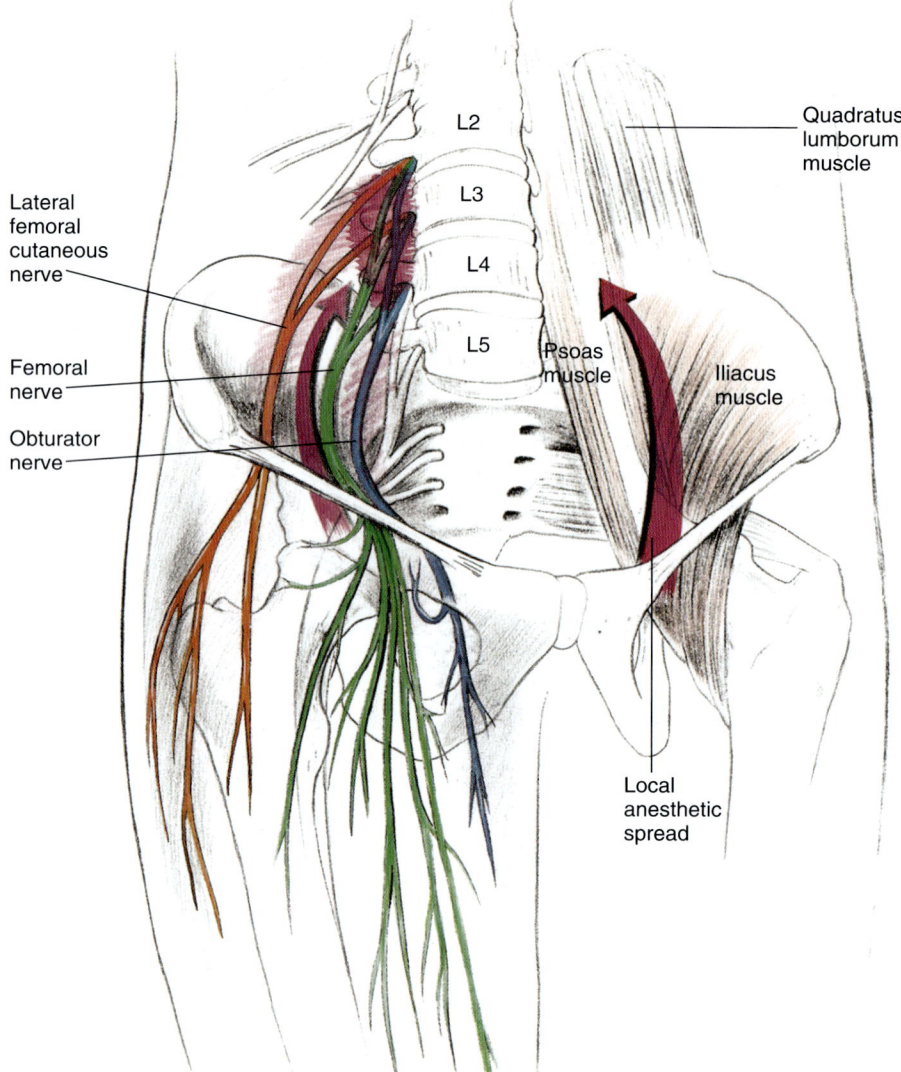

Fig. 13.1 Lumbar plexus anatomy: proposed mechanism of proximal local anesthetic spread.

and ilioinguinal nerves. The lower branch unites with a branch from the second lumbar to form the genitofemoral nerve.

From the remains of the second lumbar nerve, the third and fourth nerves divide into ventral and dorsal divisions. The anterior divisions unite to form the obturator nerves, and the dorsal divisions form the lateral femoral cutaneous nerve and the larger femoral nerve.

The lumbar plexus and its branches are formed within the psoas major muscle in front of the transverse processes of the lumbar vertebrae. The anterior two-thirds of the psoas muscle originate from the anterolateral aspect of the vertebral body, and the posterior one-third of the muscle originates from the anterior aspect of the transverse processes, creating a fascial plane between both compartments of the muscle that hosts the lumbar plexus.

It is important to appreciate that the lumbar plexus is located anterior to the transverse processes of the lumbar vertebrae and posterior (embedded in the post wall) of the psoas muscle. The erector spinae muscle covers the lumbar spine posteriorly medially and the quadratus lumborum muscle laterally.

Appreciation of the relations between the different muscles and spine anatomy, as well as the sonographic characteristics of these structures, is crucial to perform the block.

TECHNIQUE

The lumbar plexus block is a deep block that requires a lower-frequency (2-5 MHz), curvilinear ultrasound probe. A 4- to 6-inch needle is used, depending on the body habitus. Two techniques are described to perform the block.

Paramedian Longitudinal Scanning Technique
With the patient in the prone position (this can also be performed in the lateral position with the side blocked upwards), the ultrasound probe is placed parallel to the long axis of the sacrum to identify its flat surface. The probe is moved cephalad to identify the intervertebral space between L5 and S1 as an interruption of the sacral line continuity. The probe is moved 3-4 cm

laterally (keeping the same orientation) to identify the transverse process of L5. The transverse processes of the other lumbar vertebrae are identified by cephalad scan in ascending order. The acoustic shadow of the transverse processes has a characteristic appearance often referred to as a *trident sign*.

The psoas muscle is imaged through the acoustic windows between the hyperechoic shadows of the transverse processes. The lumbar plexus can be identified as hyperechoic striations in the posterior wall of the psoas muscle. However, appropriate identification of the plexus is confirmed by inducing quadriceps contraction or adduction when applying nerve stimulation to the insulated needle. The needle can be introduced using both the in-plane and out-of-plane techniques in the middle of the probe or using the in-plane technique from the lower edge of the probe (Fig. 13.2A-D).

Transverse Oblique Scanning Technique

This technique can be also used in the prone or lateral position with the side blocked up. The L3 to L4 transverse processes are identified by the same technique described earlier (scanning from the sacrum upwards). Once identified, the ultrasound probe is rotated horizontally parallel to the transverse processes. Next, it is directed slightly medially to scan the midline structures (transverse oblique orientation). The target structures of the ultrasound beam are:

- Quadratus lumborum (lateral) and erector spinae muscles (medial).
- Deeper to the muscles, the transverse processes of L3 to L4 and the anterolateral surface of the vertebral bodies can be scanned as hyperechoic structures with underlying drop-down shadows.
- The psoas muscle appears slightly hypoechoic with multiple hyperechoic striations deeper to the transverse processes.
- Slowly adjust the probe in the acoustic window between the transverse processes, allowing for visualization of the intervertebral foramen, and the articular process facet joint with the roots of the lumbar plexus as it emerges from the intervertebral foramen. The roots appear as hyperechoic structures adjacent to the posterior wall of the psoas muscle.

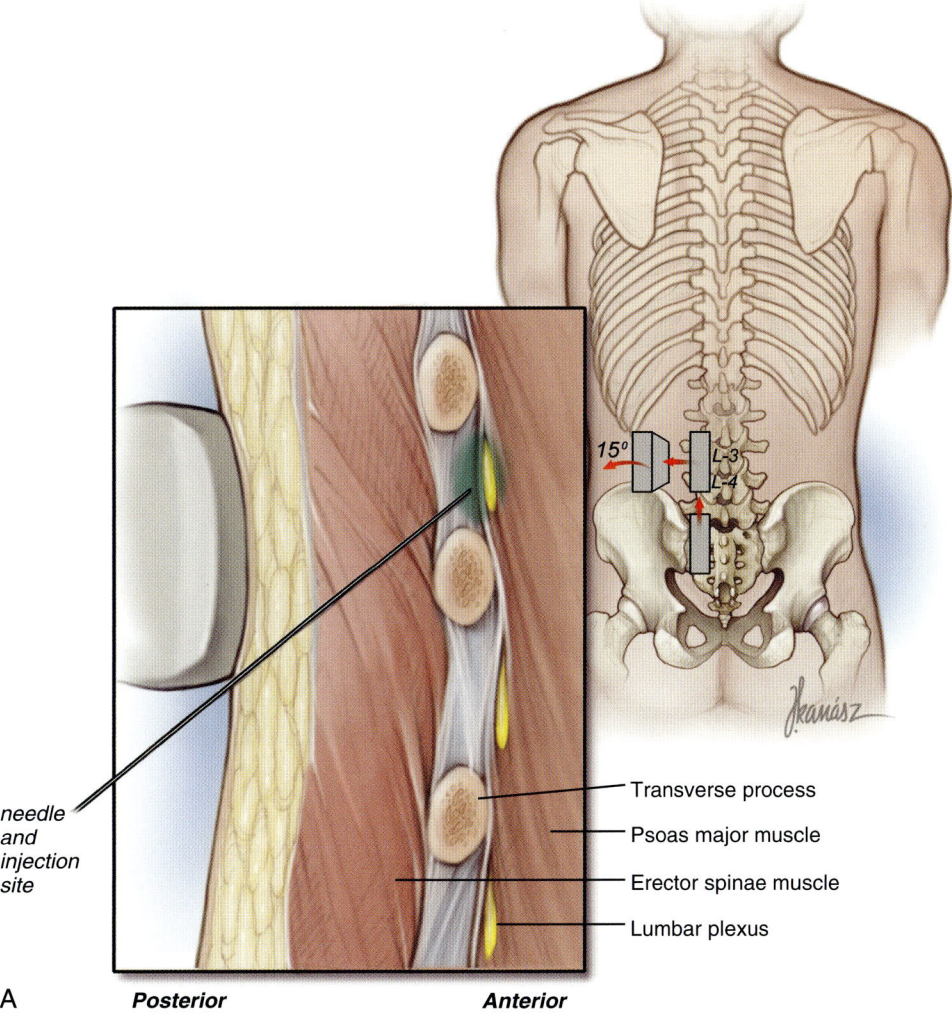

Fig. 13.2 (A) Anatomy of paramedian longitudinal technique for lumbar plexus block.

Continued

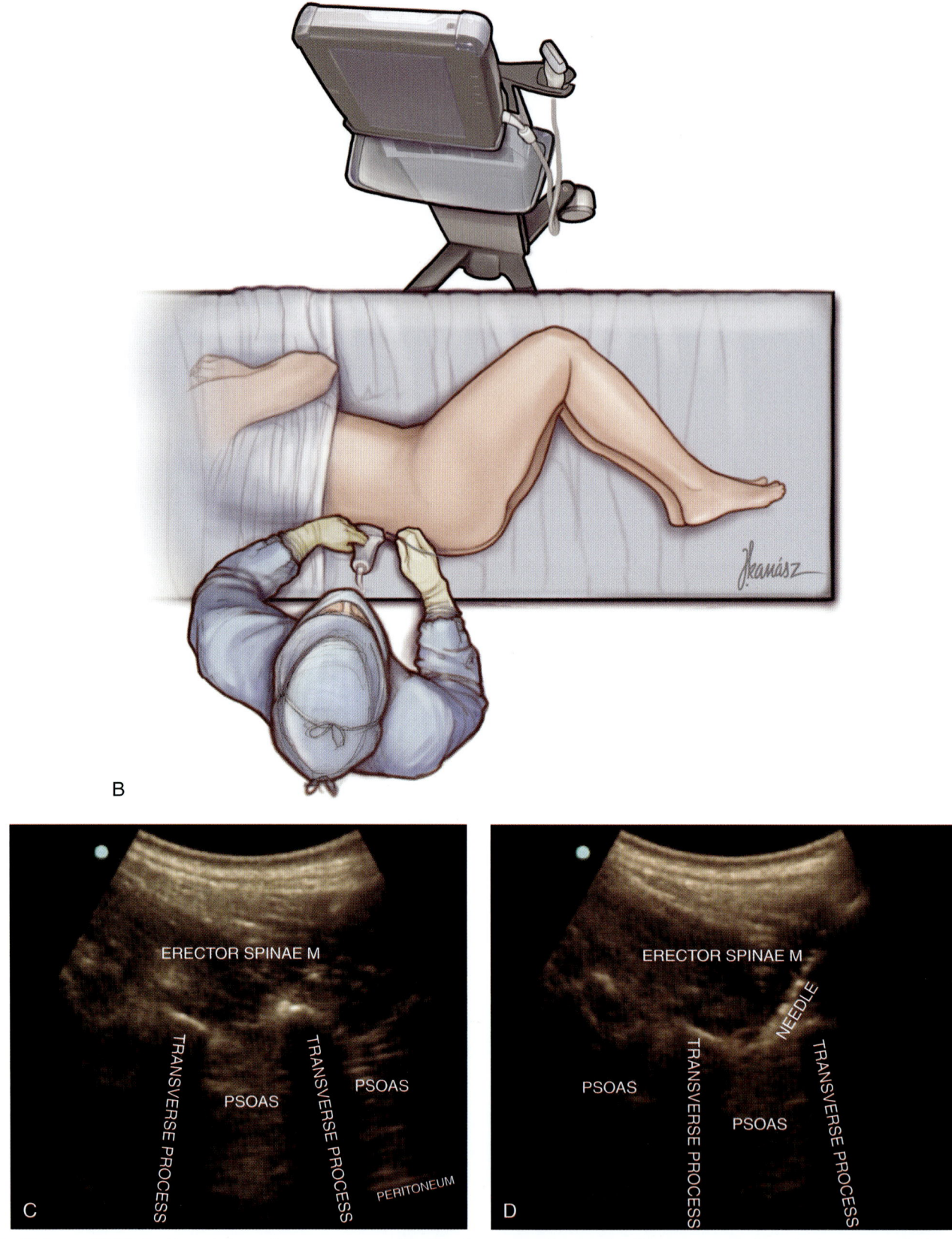

Fig. 13.2, cont'd **(B)** Position of the patient and probe orientation for paramedian longitudinal technique. Note the in-plane technique for the paramedian longitudinal approach. **(C)** and **(D)** Ultrasound images for the paramedian approach for lumbar plexus that show the transverse processes and psoas muscle, and the needle position.

The lumbar plexus is approached with the needle in the plane with the ultrasound beam from the lateral side of the probe (the approach from the medial side is also described), targeting the posterior border of the psoas muscle at the level of the intervertebral foramen. Using nerve stimulation is very helpful to confirm the proximity of the needle to the lumbar plexus and avoid intramuscular injection where local psoas contraction is induced. Care should be taken to avoid advancing the needle too medially, to reduce the risk of injury of the lumbar artery or its branches, and to avoid spread of local anesthetic into the neuraxial space (Fig. 13.3A-D).

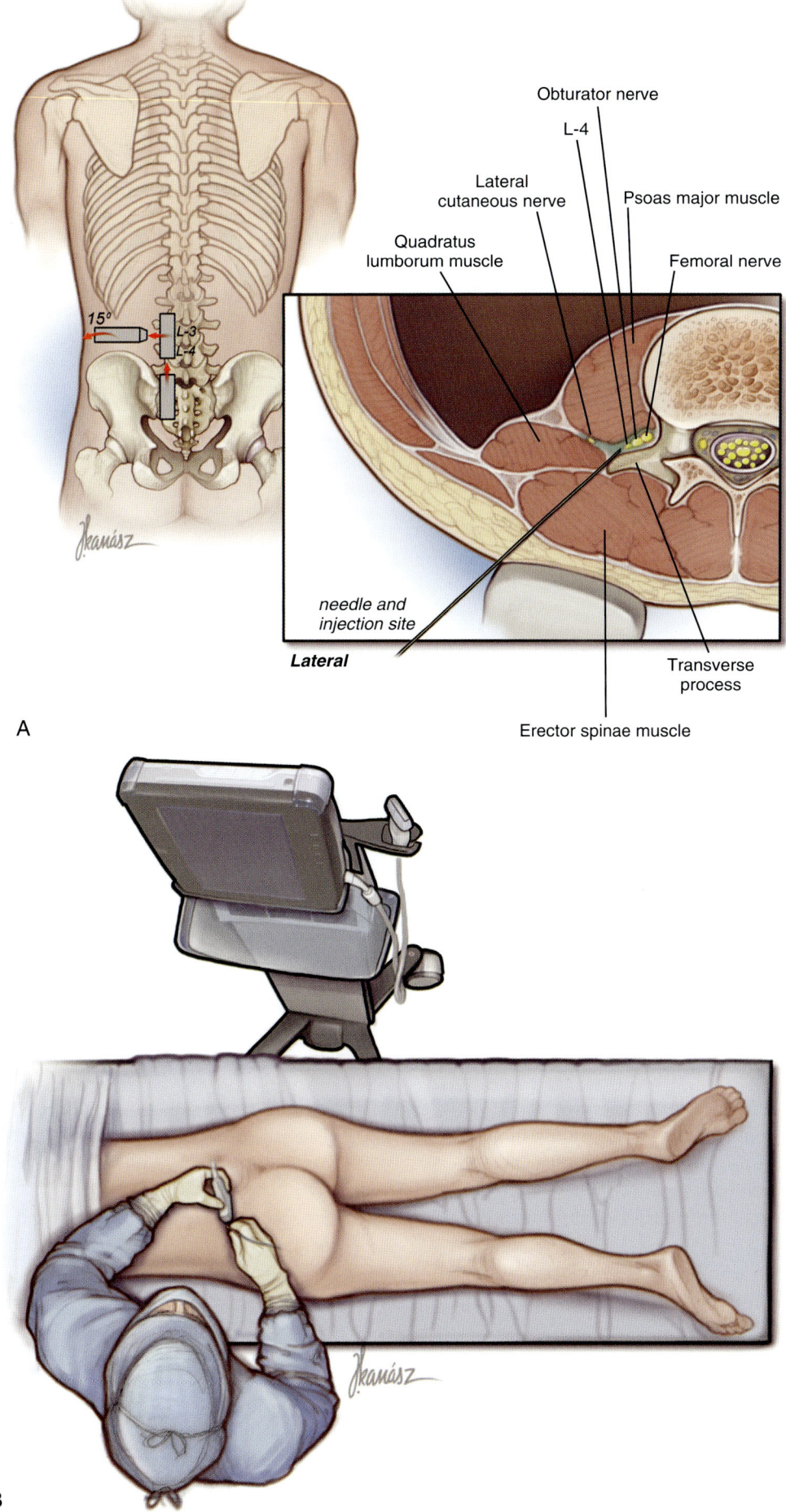

Fig. 13.3 (A) Anatomy of transverse oblique technique for lumbar plexus block. (B) Position of the patient for the transverse technique; note the in-plane technique used for the block.

Continued

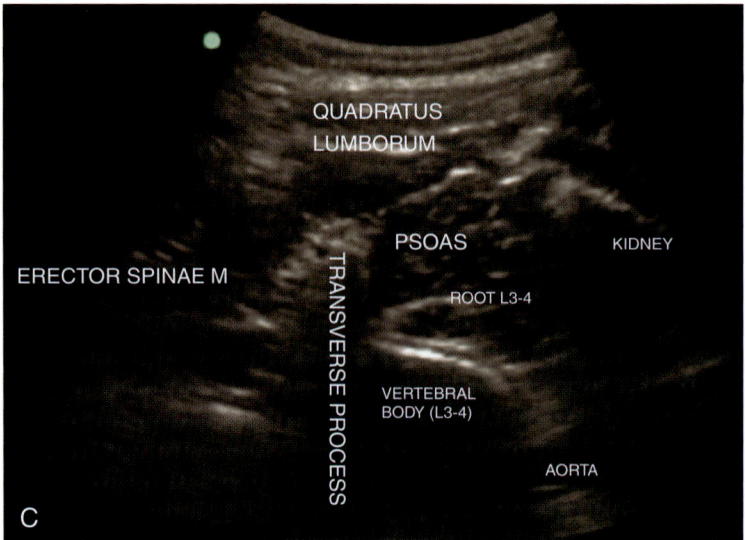

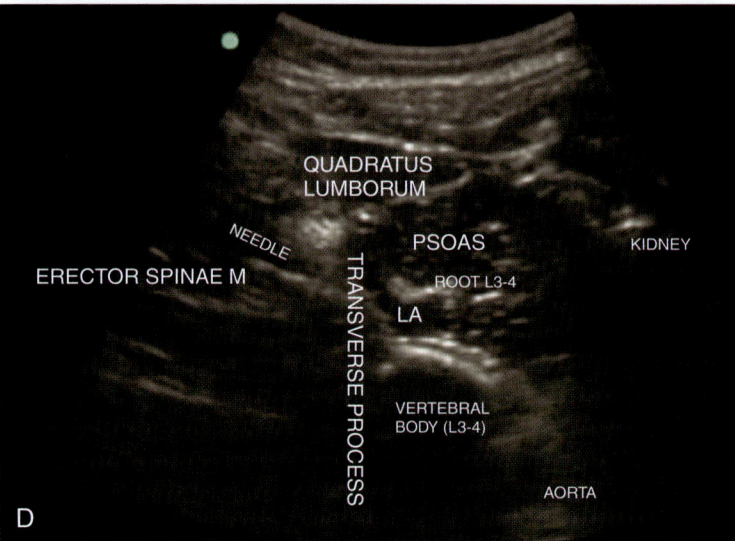

Fig. 13.3, cont'd (C) and (D) Ultrasound images for the transverse technique for lumbar plexus block; note the position of the needle in the psoas muscle deep to the quadratus lumborum muscle.

INDICATIONS

- The lumbar plexus block is the most proximal approach to the lumbar plexus, providing the most reliable block of its major branches (femoral, obturator, and lateral femoral cutaneous nerves).
- The block is ideal for hip surgeries and surgeries above the knee.
- When combined with sciatic nerve block, it provides complete unilateral lower limb anesthesia suitable for lower extremity surgeries.
- Continuous catheterization can be used for prolonged analgesia (Fig. 13.4).

KEY POINTS

- The lumbar plexus block is a deep block that makes it difficult to appreciate the difference in the echogenicity of the anatomic structures, especially in obese and elderly patients.
- The use of nerve stimulation is necessary to identify the lumbar plexus.
- Identification of small lumbar arteries is hard to visualize at deeper scan, and the block should be avoided in patients with coagulation disorders or at risk of bleeding.
- The spread of local anesthetic at the posterior surface of the psoas muscle is satisfactory.

PEARLS

- The lumbar plexus block is a technically advanced procedure with major potential for complications. Experience with ultrasound anatomy, scanning skills, and needle manipulations is necessary before attempting ultrasound-guided lumbar plexus block.
- The lumbar plexus is embedded within the body of the psoas muscle; hence the name *psoas block* is synonymous with lumbar plexus block.

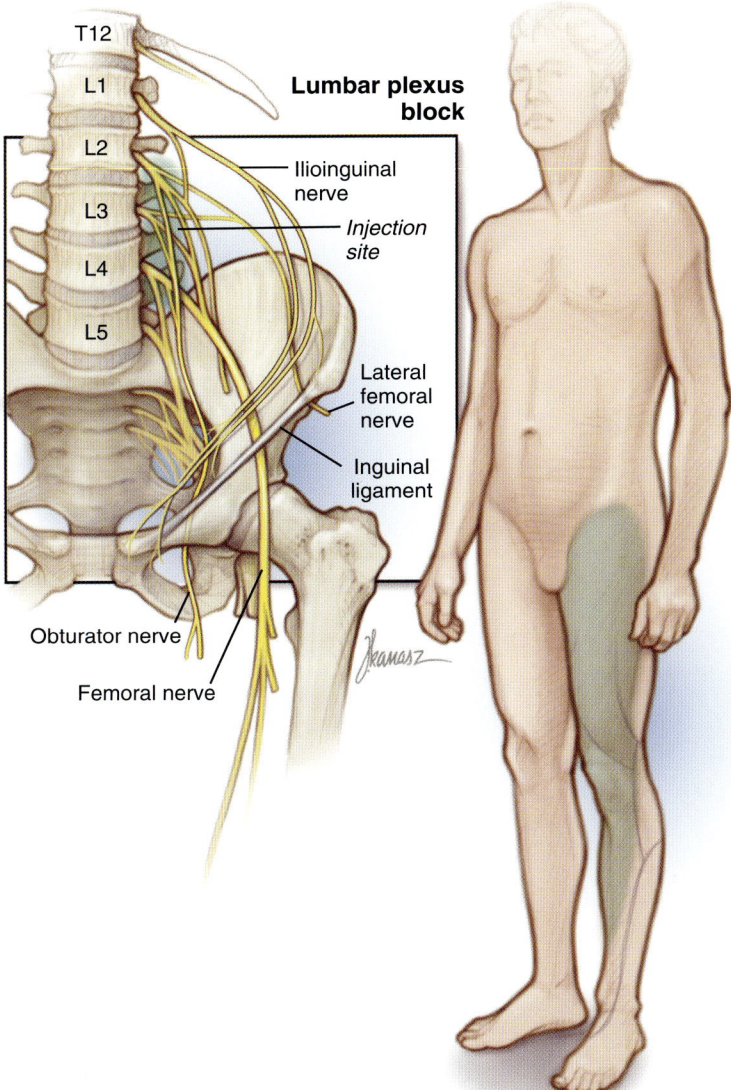

Fig. 13.4 Anatomical distribution of lumbar plexus block.

- The block can be performed in the prone and lateral positions. The advantage of the prone position is that it provides a more stable resting hand position, allowing more precise scanning and manipulations.
- At the level of L2 to L3, the kidney can be visualized as a hypoechoic structure that moves with respiration.
- Care should be taken to do frequent repeated aspiration and inject the local anesthetic in small increments to detect epidural or spinal spread early.
- The lumbar paravertebral space is a vascular and muscular space, which leads to significant systemic absorption of the local anesthetic and potentially high plasma levels.

Sciatic Block 14

Ehab Farag and David L. Brown

PERSPECTIVE

The sciatic nerve is one of the largest nerve trunks in the body, yet few surgical procedures can be performed with sciatic block alone. It is combined most often with femoral, lateral femoral cutaneous, or an obturator nerve block. The block is also effective for analgesia of the lower leg and may provide pain relief from ankle fractures or tibial fractures before operative intervention.

Patient Selection. This block may be indicated for patients needing analgesia before transport for definitive orthopedic surgical repair of lower leg or ankle fractures. For patients in whom it may be desirable to avoid the sympathectomy accompanying neuraxial block, sciatic block combined with femoral nerve block often allows ankle and foot procedures to be carried out. One group of patients in whom this block is often useful is those undergoing distal amputations of the lower extremity, who have vascular compromise based on diabetes or peripheral vascular disease.

Pharmacologic Choice. Sciatic nerve block requires from 20–25 mL of local anesthetic solution. When this volume is added to that required for other lower extremity peripheral blocks, the total may reach the upper end of an acceptable local anesthetic dose range. Conversely, uptake of local anesthetic from these lower extremity sites is not as rapid as with epidural or intercostal block; thus a larger mass of local anesthetic may be appropriate in this region. If motor blockade is desired with this block, 1.5% mepivacaine or lidocaine may be necessary, whereas 0.5% bupivacaine or 0.5%–0.75% ropivacaine will be effective.

TRADITIONAL BLOCK TECHNIQUE

PLACEMENT

Anatomy. The sciatic nerve is formed from the L4 through S3 roots. These roots of the sacral plexus form on the anterior surface of the lateral sacrum and are assembled into the sciatic nerve on the anterior surface of the piriformis muscle. The sciatic nerve results from the fusion of two major nerve trunks. The "medial" sciatic nerve is functionally the tibial nerve, which forms from the ventral branches of the ventral rami of L4 to L5 and S1 to S3; the posterior branches of the ventral rami of these same nerves form the "lateral" sciatic nerve, which is functionally the peroneal nerve. As the sciatic nerve exits the pelvis, it is anterior to the piriformis muscle and is joined by another nerve—the posterior cutaneous nerve of the thigh. At the inferior border of the piriformis, the sciatic and posterior cutaneous nerves of the thigh lie posterior to the obturator internus, the gemelli, and the quadratus femoris. At this point these nerves are anterior to the gluteus maximus. Here, the nerve is approximately equidistant from the ischial tuberosity and the greater trochanter (Figs. 14.1–14.3). The nerve continues downward through the thigh to lie along the posteromedial aspect of the femur. At the cephalad portion of the popliteal fossa, the sciatic nerve usually divides to form the tibial and common peroneal nerves. Occasionally this division occurs much higher, and sometimes the tibial and peroneal nerves are separate through their entire course. In the popliteal fossa, the tibial nerve continues downward into the lower leg, whereas the common peroneal nerve travels laterally along the medial aspect of the short head of the biceps femoris muscle.

CLASSIC APPROACH

Position. The patient is positioned laterally, with the side to be blocked nondependent. The nondependent leg is flexed and its heel placed against the knee of the dependent leg (Fig. 14.4). The anesthesiologist is positioned to allow insertion of the needle, as shown in Fig. 14.4.

Needle Puncture. A line is drawn from the posterior superior iliac spine to the midpoint of the greater trochanter. Perpendicular to the midpoint of this line, another line is extended caudomedially for 5 cm. The needle is inserted through this point (Fig. 14.5). As a cross-check for proper placement, an additional line may be drawn from the sacral hiatus to the previously marked point on the greater trochanter. The intersection of this line with the 5-cm perpendicular line should coincide with the needle insertion site.

At this site, a 22-gauge, 10- to 13-cm needle is inserted, as illustrated in Fig. 14.4. The needle should be directed through the entry site toward an imaginary point where the femoral vessels course under the inguinal ligament. The needle is inserted until paresthesia is elicited or until bone is contacted. If bone is encountered before paresthesia is elicited, the needle is redirected along the line joining the sacral hiatus and the greater trochanter until paresthesia or

108 ATLAS OF REGIONAL ANESTHESIA

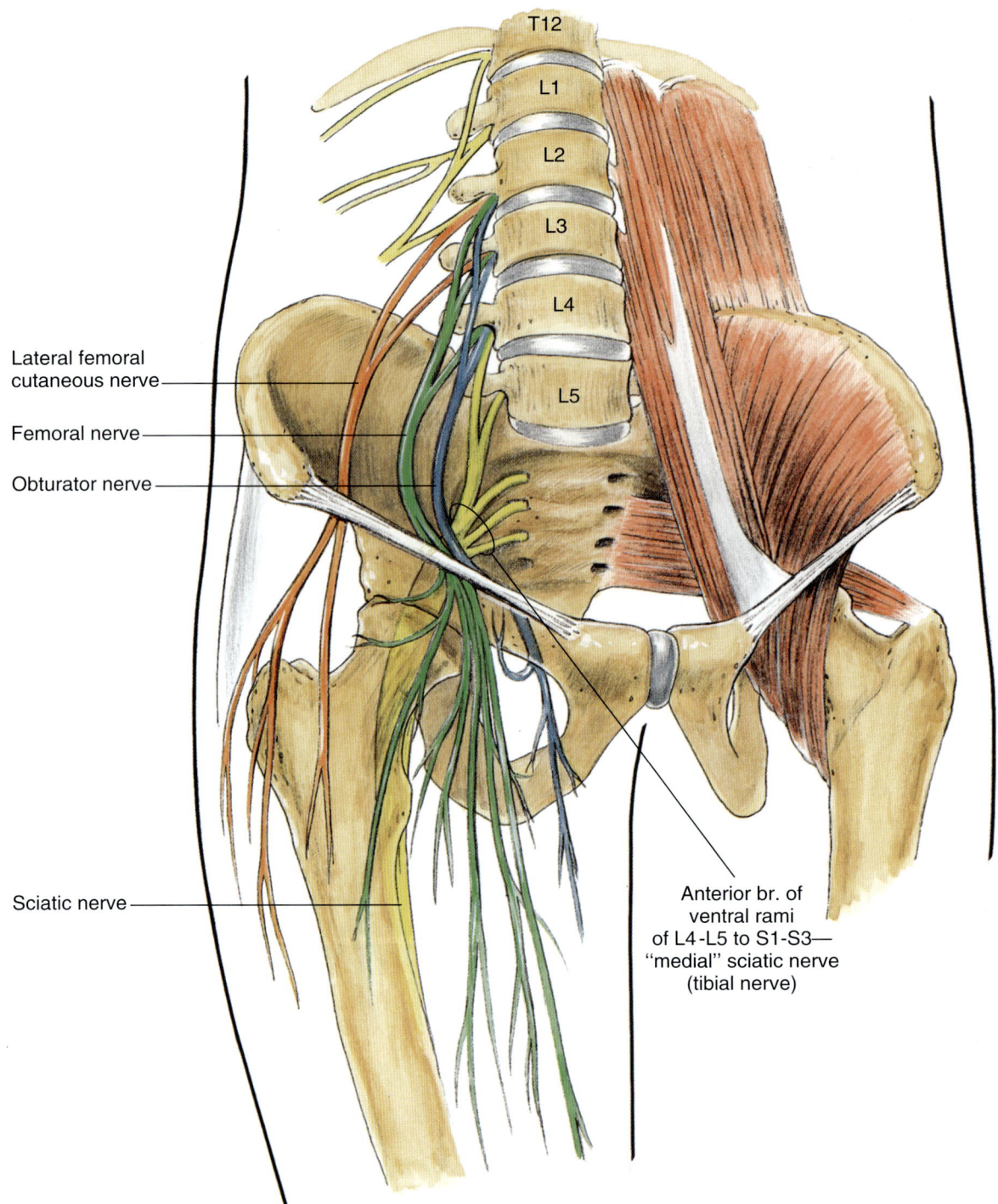

Fig. 14.1 Sciatic nerve anatomy: anterior oblique view.

a motor response is elicited. During this redirection the needle should not be inserted more than 2 cm past the depth at which bone was originally contacted, or the needle tip will be placed anterior to the site of the sciatic nerve. Once paresthesia or a motor response is elicited, 20–25 mL of local anesthetic is injected.

ANTERIOR APPROACH

Position. The anterior block of the sciatic nerve can be carried out in the supine patient whose leg is in the neutral position. The anesthesiologist should be at the patient's side, similar to positioning during femoral nerve block.

Needle Puncture. In the supine patient, a line should be drawn from the anterior superior iliac spine to the pubic tubercle. Another line should be drawn parallel to this line from the midpoint of the greater trochanter inferomedially, as illustrated in Fig. 14.6. The first line is trisected, and a perpendicular line is drawn caudolaterally from the juncture of the medial and middle thirds, as shown in Fig. 14.6. At the point where the perpendicular line crosses the more caudal line, a 22-gauge, 13-cm needle is inserted so that it contacts the femur at its medial border. Once the needle has contacted the femur, it is redirected slightly medially to

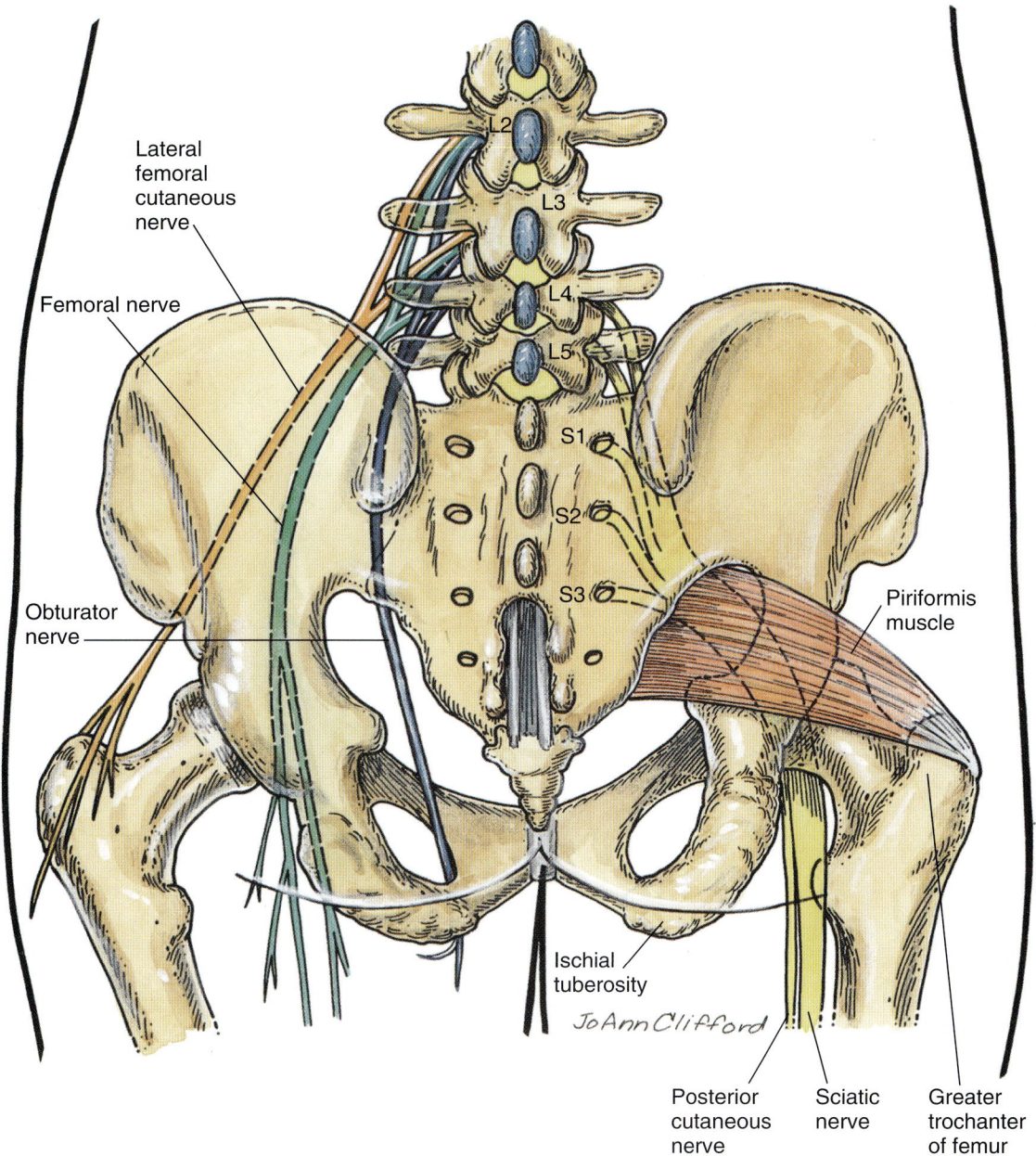

Fig. 14.2 Sciatic nerve anatomy: posterior view.

slide off the medial surface of the femur. At approximately 5 cm past the depth required to contact the femur, paresthesia or a motor response should be sought to ensure successful block (Fig. 14.7). Once paresthesia or a motor response is obtained, 20–25 mL of local anesthetic is injected.

POTENTIAL PROBLEMS

In patients in whom the block is being used for an injury to the lower extremity, the classic position is sometimes difficult to use. This block can also be of long duration, and patients should be warned of this before surgery. Although it is unsubstantiated, some consider that dysesthesia may be more common after this block than after other peripheral blocks. The same problems pertaining to the classic approach should be considered with the anterior approach.

PEARLS

CLASSIC APPROACH

The keys to making this block work are adequate positioning of the patient and a systematic redirection of the needle until paresthesia is obtained.

ANTERIOR APPROACH

Although the anterior approach is conceptually simple, we are able to produce anesthesia using it slightly less often than when using the classic approach. Perhaps with additional experience this difference would not be as apparent. One observation that may help to improve one's success rate with this block is to make sure that the lower extremity to be blocked is maintained in the neutral position and is not allowed to assume either a medially or a laterally rotated position. This block may be useful in supine patients who are in significant discomfort and cannot be positioned for the classic approach.

ULTRASONOGRAPHY-GUIDED TECHNIQUE

SONOANATOMY

The sciatic nerve in the subgluteal region lies in the middle between the greater trochanter laterally and the ischial tuberosity medially. Under ultrasound, the subgluteal sciatic nerve has a triangular shape defined by the long head of the biceps femoris (posterolateral), the semitendinosus (posteromedial), and the adductor magnus (anterior). If it is difficult to identify the sciatic nerve in the subgluteal region, it can be identified in the midthigh region by tracing the nerve from the popliteal region (Fig. 14.8).

TECHNIQUE

The prone position is the preferred one to provide better imaging for the in-plane technique from the lateral aspect of the thigh. If the patient is not able to lie in the prone position, the lateral position with the hips and the knees flexed will be utilized. The curved array ultrasound probe is placed at the level of the inferior border of the gluteus maximus to visualize the sciatic nerve in the short axis as a hyperechoic structure between the greater trochanter

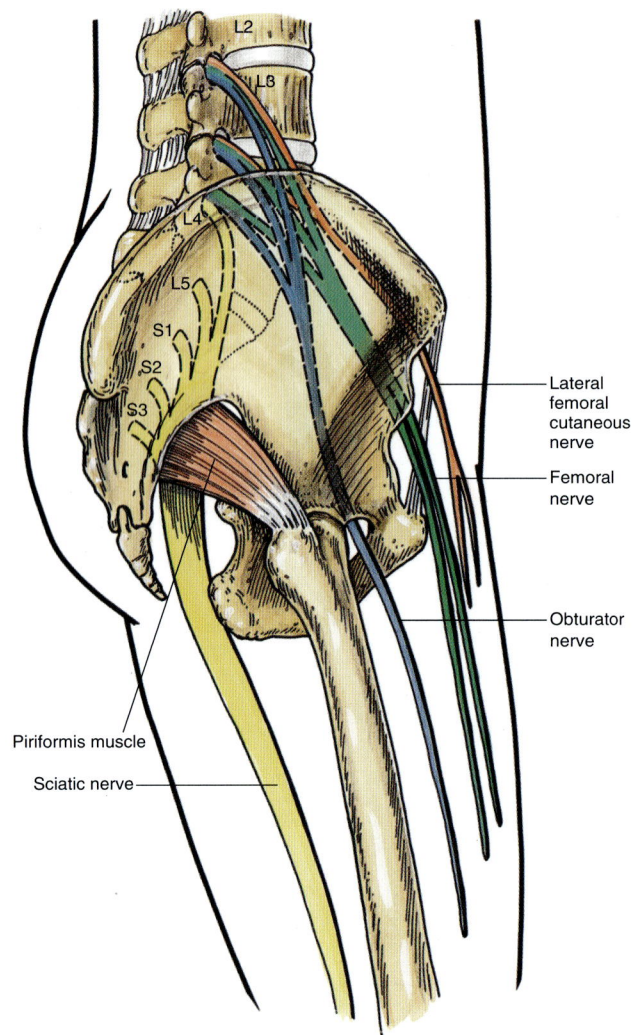

Fig. 14.3 Sciatic nerve anatomy: lateral view.

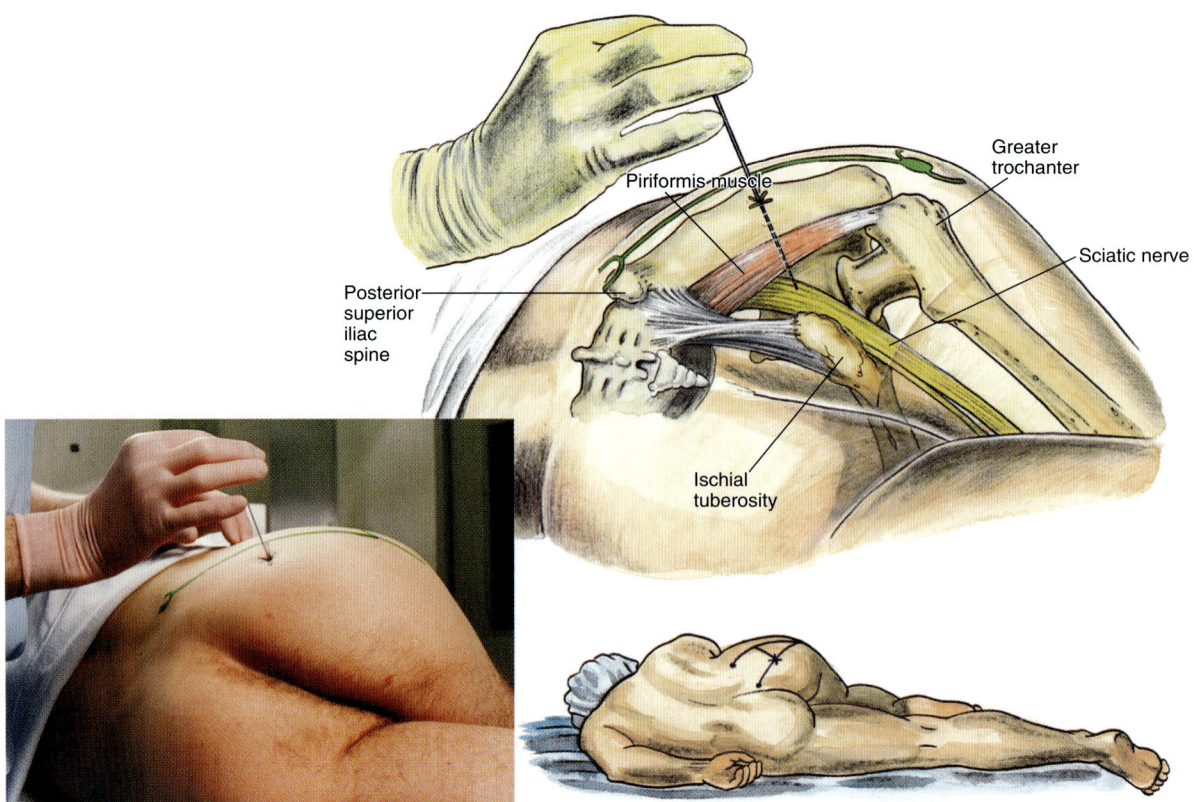

Fig. 14.4 Sciatic nerve block: classic technique and positioning.

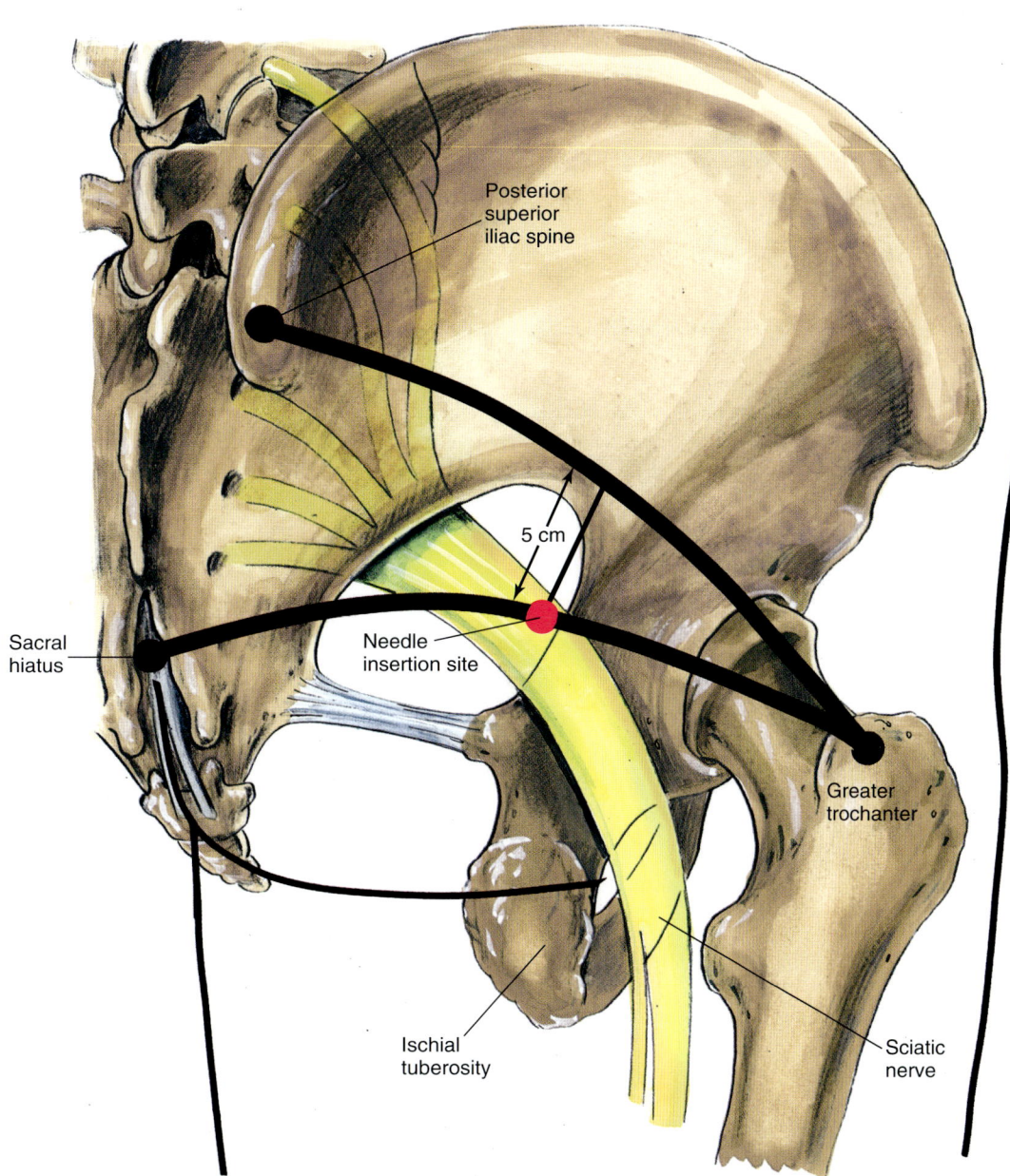

Fig. 14.5 Sciatic nerve block: surface marking technique.

and ischial tuberosity. The in-plane approach will be used with the needle direction from medial to lateral in the prone position; however, in the lateral position, the needle direction should preferably be from posterior to anterior. The use of nerve stimulation, in addition to the ultrasound, is preferred in this technique to confirm the nerve identification, especially in obese patients. The medium-frequency, linear, 50-mm footprint is used for the midthigh approach block for the sciatic nerve block. The continuous block can be performed using a catheter threaded through a Touhy needle. The catheter tip position can be identified by injecting local anesthetic and observing its distribution using ultrasound or by injecting 1 mL of air, which appears as a hyperechogenic artifact (Figs. 14.9–14.11).

CLINICAL PEARLS

- Continuous sciatic block is very helpful for managing phantom limb pain after either below-knee or above-knee amputations.
- Single-shot sciatic block using 0.1% ropivacaine is very helpful to manage posterior knee pain after total knee arthroplasty without affecting the motor power and/or neurological examination of the lower limb after total knee arthroplasty.
- Combined femoral and sciatic blocks are quite sufficient for lower limb procedures, especially in high-risk patients in whom general and/or neuraxial anesthesia can disturb their hemodynamic

112 ATLAS OF REGIONAL ANESTHESIA

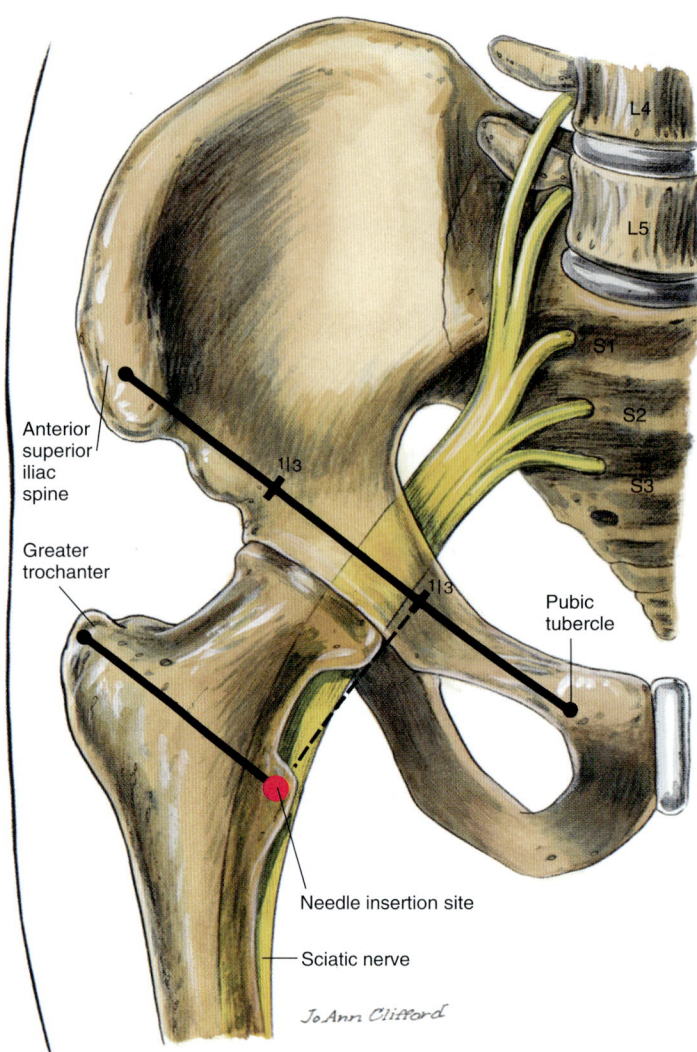

Fig. 14.6 Sciatic nerve block: anterior technique.

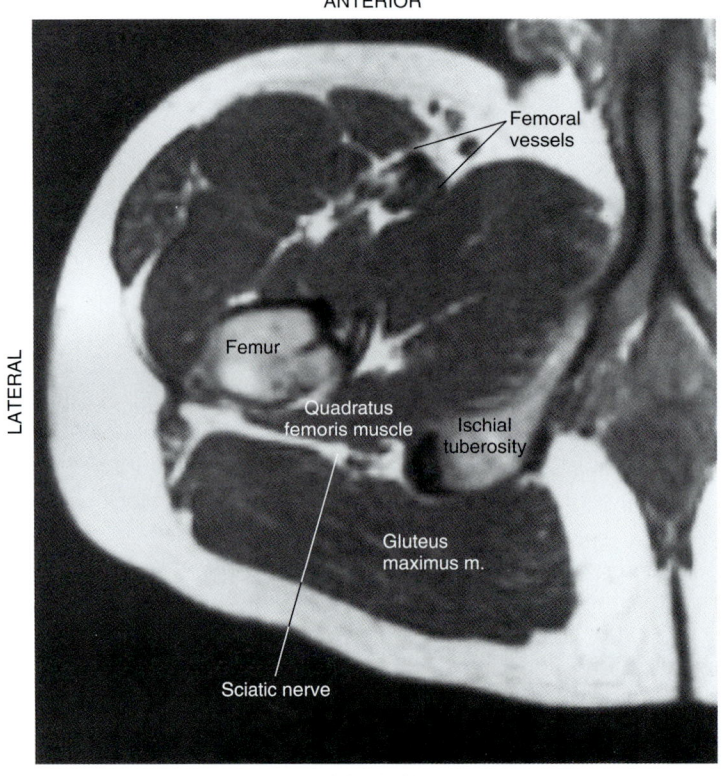

Fig. 14.7 Magnetic resonance image (cross-sectional) at level of anterior sciatic nerve.

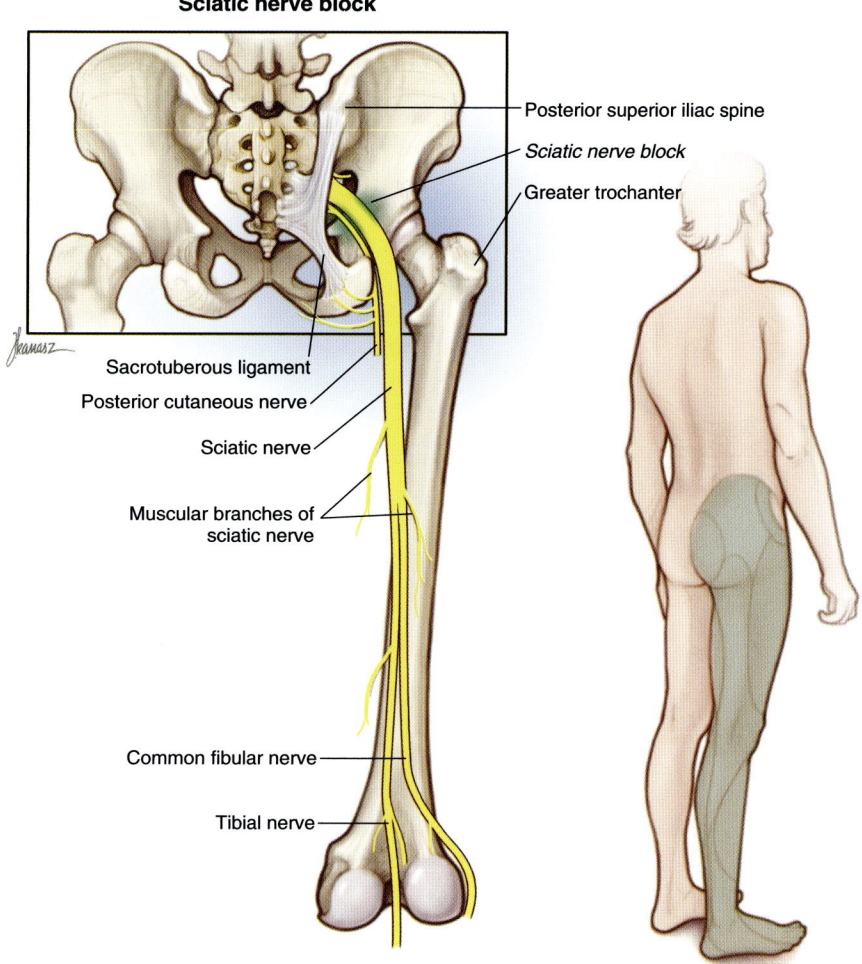

Fig. 14.8 Anatomy of the subgluteal sciatic nerve block.

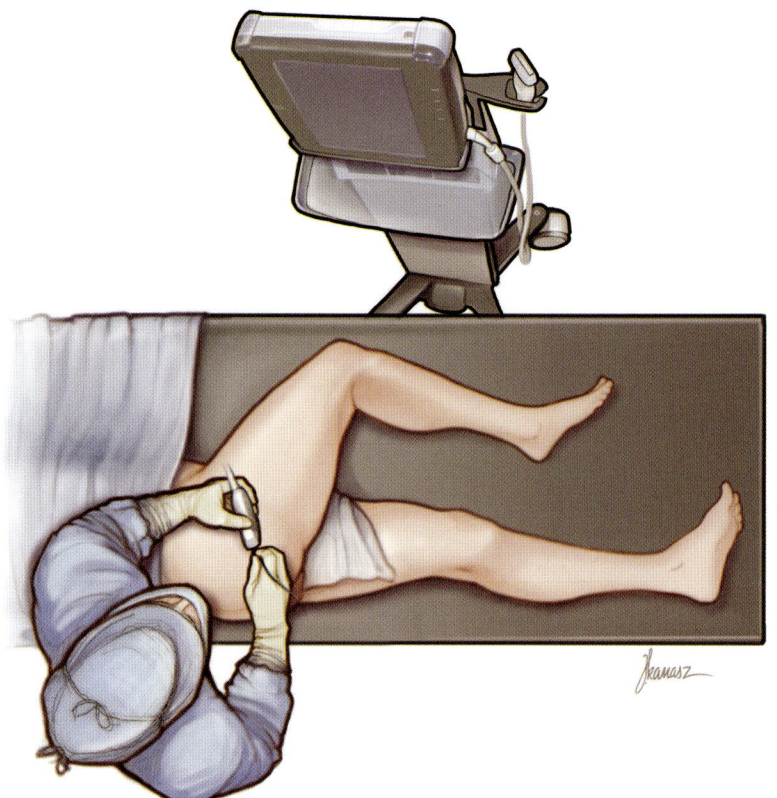

Fig. 14.9 Patient in lateral position. Note the in-plane approach with posterior to anterior needle direction.

114 ATLAS OF REGIONAL ANESTHESIA

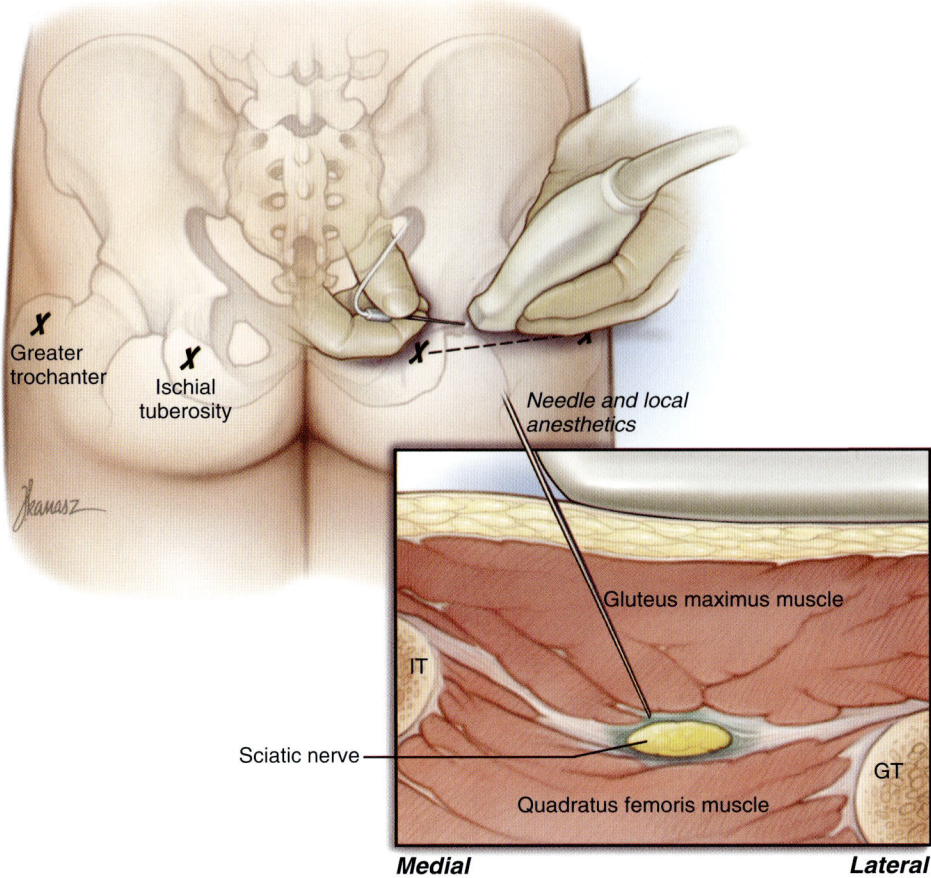

Fig. 14.10 In-plane technique for subgluteal sciatic nerve block in prone position. Note the medial to lateral needle direction.

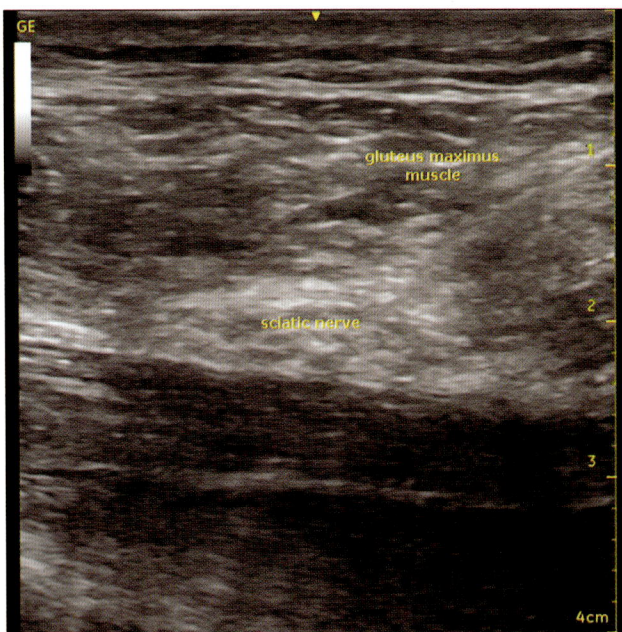

Fig. 14.11 Ultrasound still of sciatic nerve block.

stability, such as very tight aortic stenosis or heart failure.

KEY POINTS

- Subgluteal and midthigh approaches are the most commonly used techniques for sciatic nerve block using ultrasound.
- Short axis with in-plane approach with lateral to medial needle direction is the preferred ultrasound technique for both subgluteal and midthigh sciatic blocks.
- Using a nerve stimulator is very helpful to confirm the identification of the sciatic nerve in the subgluteal approach, especially in obese patients.

Femoral Block 15

Ehab Farag and David L. Brown

PERSPECTIVE

This block is useful for surgical procedures carried out on the anterior thigh, both superficial and deep. It is most frequently combined with other lower extremity peripheral blocks to provide anesthesia for operations on the lower leg and foot. As an analgesic technique, it is used for femoral fracture analgesia or for prolonged continuous catheter analgesia after surgery on the knee or femur.

Patient Selection. Because the patient is supine when this block is carried out, virtually any patient undergoing a surgical procedure of the lower extremity is a candidate. Because elicitation of paresthesia is not necessary to carry out femoral block, even anesthetized patients are candidates.

Pharmacologic Choice. As with all lower extremity blocks, a decision must be made about the extent of sensory and motor blockade desired. If motor blockade is necessary, higher concentrations of local anesthetic are needed. As with concerns about local anesthetic use in the sciatic block, the desire for motor blockade must be balanced against the volume of local anesthetic necessary if femoral, sciatic, lateral femoral cutaneous, and obturator blocks are combined. Approximately 20 mL of local anesthetic should be adequate to produce femoral block. With continuous catheter techniques used for postoperative analgesia, 0.25% bupivacaine or 0.2% ropivacaine may be used, and even lower concentrations of these drugs may be useful after a trial. With this technique, a rate of 8–10 mL per hour usually suffices.

TRADITIONAL BLOCK TECHNIQUE

PLACEMENT

Anatomy. The femoral nerve travels through the pelvis in the groove between the psoas and the iliacus muscles, as illustrated in Fig. 15.1. It emerges beneath the inguinal ligament, posterolateral to the femoral vessels, as illustrated in Fig. 15.2. It frequently divides into its branches at or above the level of the inguinal ligament.

Position. The patient is in a supine position, and the anesthesiologist should stand at the patient's side to allow easy palpation of the femoral artery.

Needle Puncture. A line is drawn connecting the anterosuperior iliac spine and the pubic tubercle, as illustrated in Fig. 15.3. The femoral artery is palpated on this line, and a 22-gauge, 4-cm needle is inserted, as illustrated in Fig. 15.4. The initial insertion should abut the femoral artery in a perpendicular fashion, as shown in Fig. 15.5 (*position 1*); a "wall" of local anesthetic is developed by redirecting the needle in a fanlike manner in progressive steps to *position 2*. (Ultrasonography highlights that the nerve is deep to the fascia iliaca, something difficult to appreciate without imaging guidance.) Approximately 20 mL of local anesthetic is injected incrementally in this fashion. It may also be useful to displace the needle entry site laterally 1 cm, direct the needle tip to lie immediately posterior to the femoral artery, and then inject an additional 2–5 mL of drug. This allows a block of those fibers that may be in a more posterior relationship to the femoral artery. Elicitation of paresthesia is variable with this block; however, if one does occur, the mediolateral injection should still be carried out because the nerve often divides into branches cephalad to the inguinal ligament.

When using a continuous catheter technique, either stimulating catheter block kits, or traditional epidural needles and matched catheters may be used in adults (Fig. 15.6). In the latter situation, the epidural needle is positioned either with the assistance of a nerve stimulator or with paresthesia elicitation as an endpoint. After the needle is positioned, 20 mL of preservative-free normal saline solution is injected through the needle, and then the appropriate-size catheter is inserted approximately 10 cm past the needle tip. Once the catheter has been secured with a plastic occlusive dressing, the initial bolus injection of the drug is carried out and the infusion is started.

POTENTIAL PROBLEMS

Patients with peripheral vascular disease often require unilateral lower extremity block; thus a number of patients with prosthetic femoral arteries may be suitable candidates for this block. If lower extremity peripheral regional block has been chosen in a patient who has recently undergone placement of a prosthetic femoral artery, efforts should be made to avoid the prosthesis.

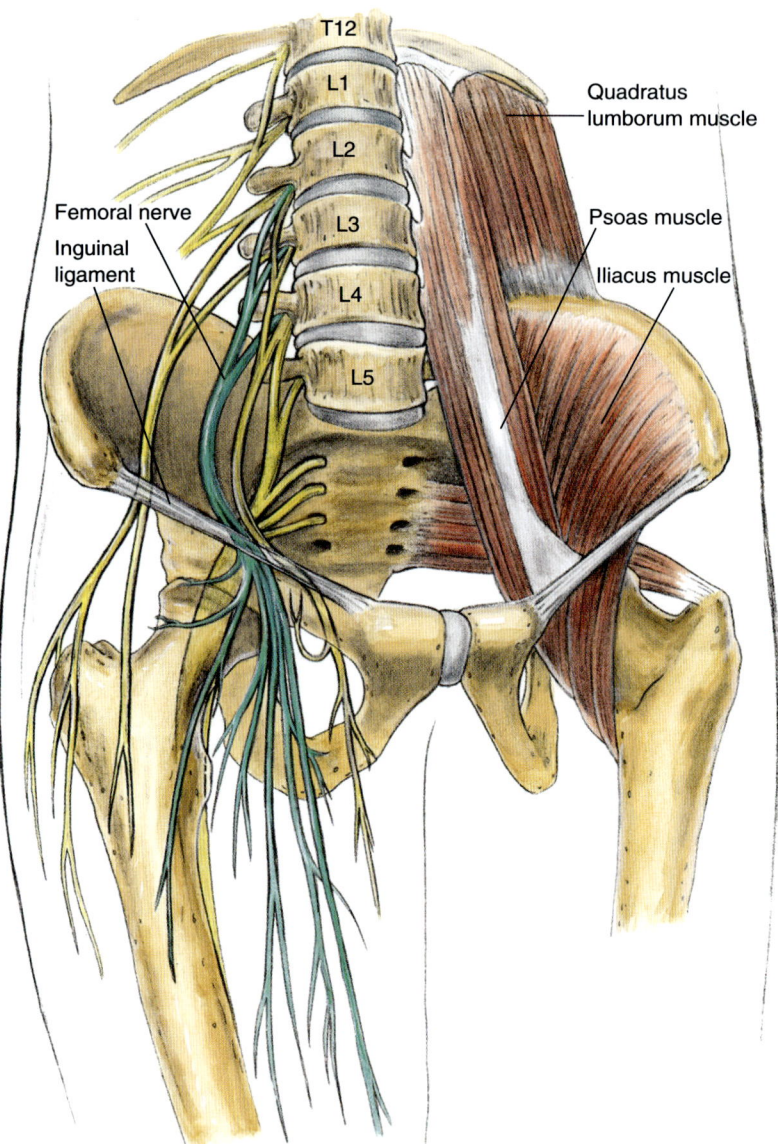

Fig. 15.1 Femoral nerve anatomy: anterior oblique view.

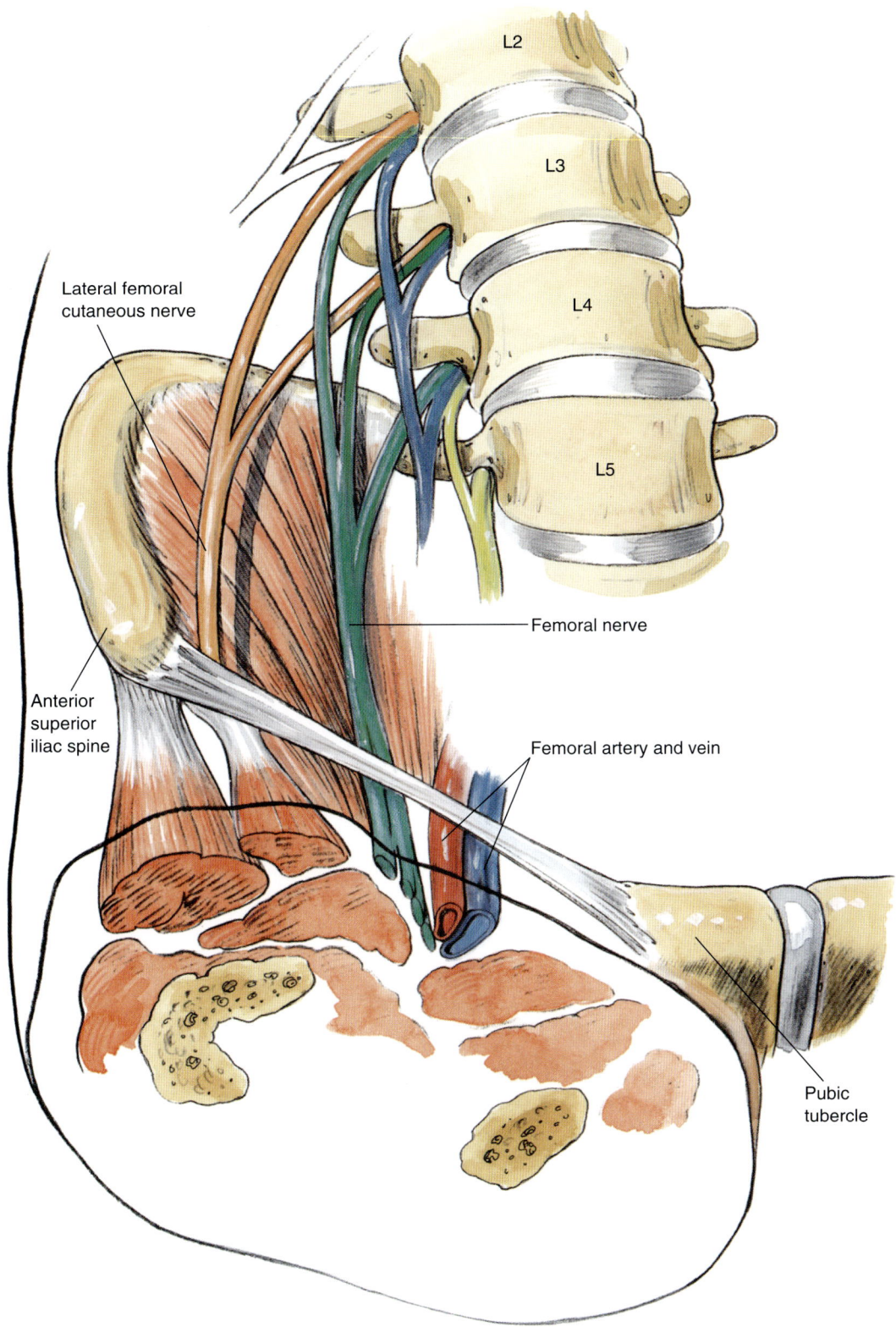

Fig. 15.2 Femoral nerve anatomy: at inguinal ligament.

118 ATLAS OF REGIONAL ANESTHESIA

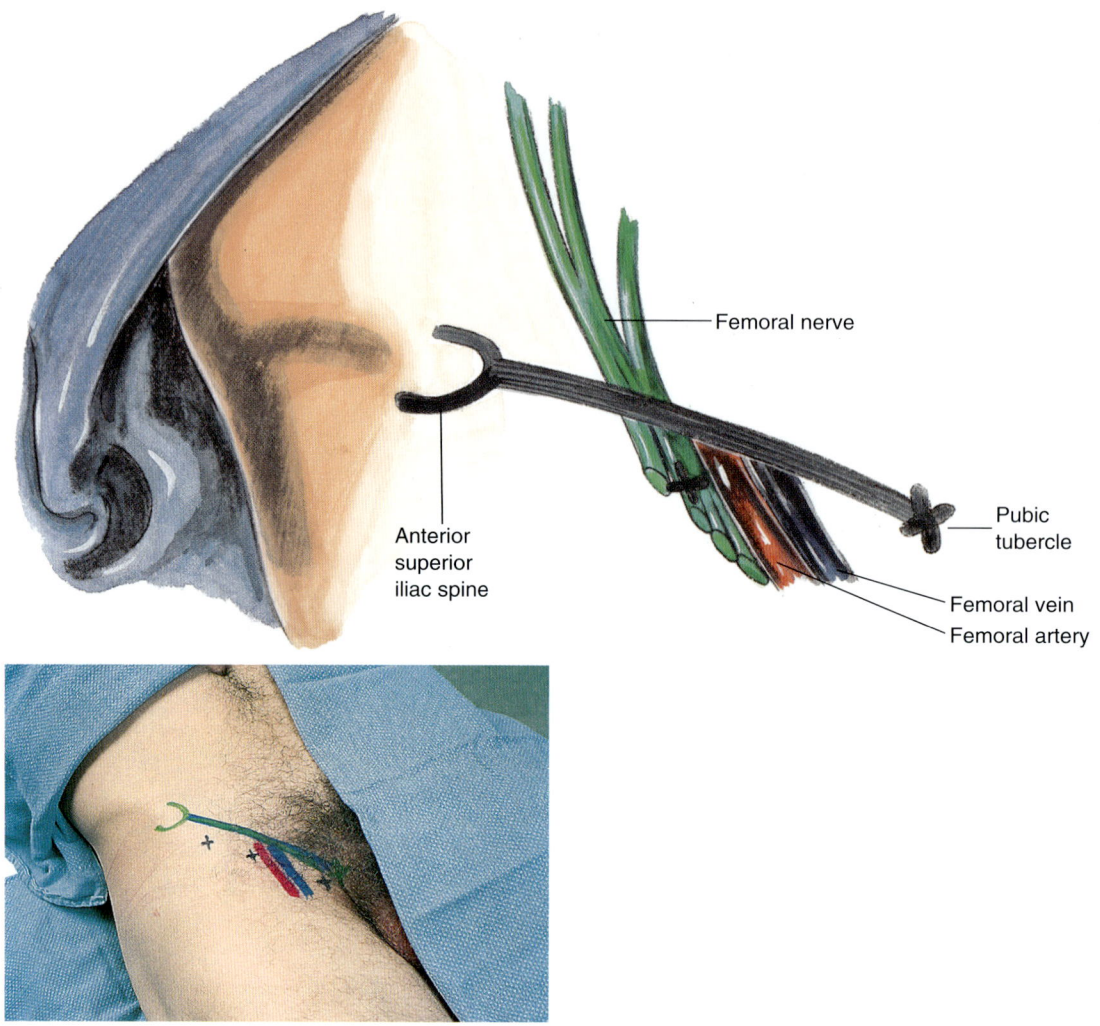

Fig. 15.3 Femoral nerve block: skin markings for needle puncture.

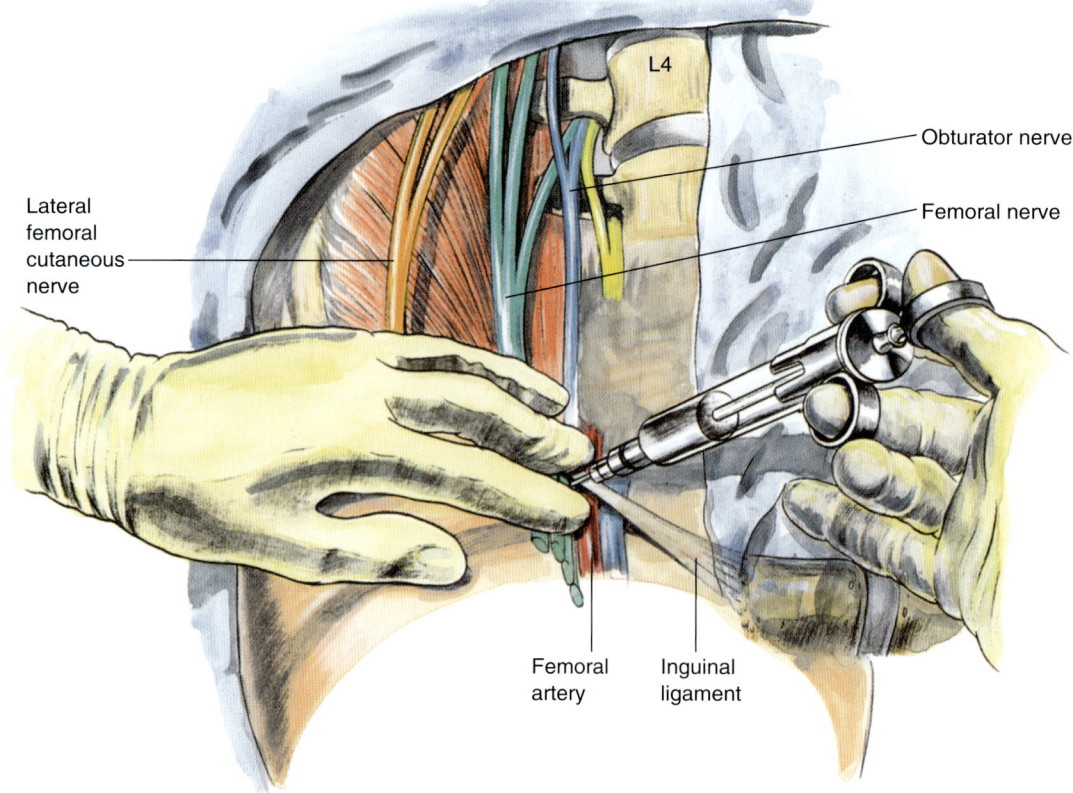

Fig. 15.4 Femoral nerve block: needle puncture.

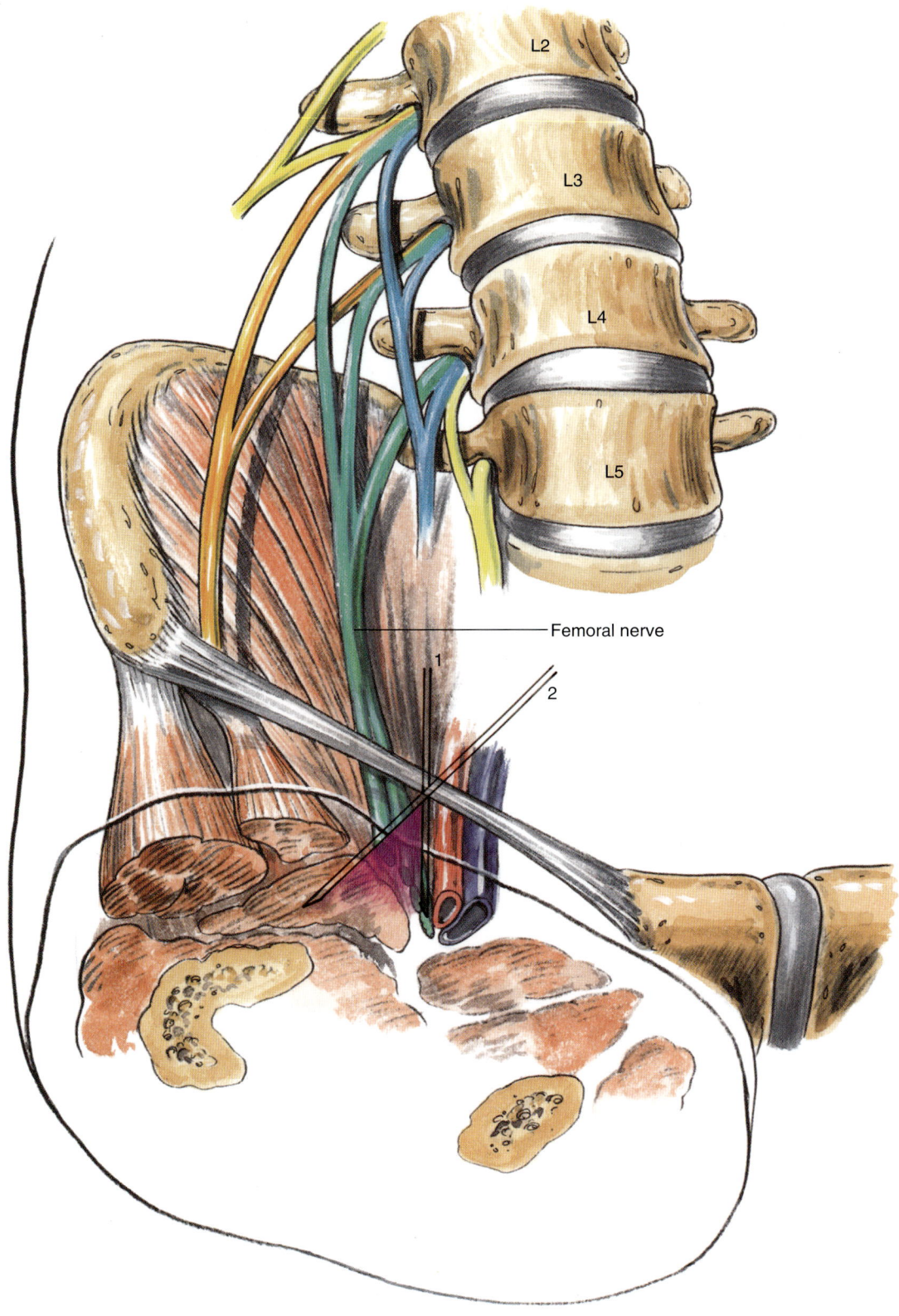

Fig. 15.5 Femoral nerve block: local anesthetic injection. The initial insertion abuts the femoral artery in a perpendicular fashion (*position 1*); a "wall" of local anesthetic is developed by redirecting the needle in a fanlike manner in progressive steps to *position 2*.

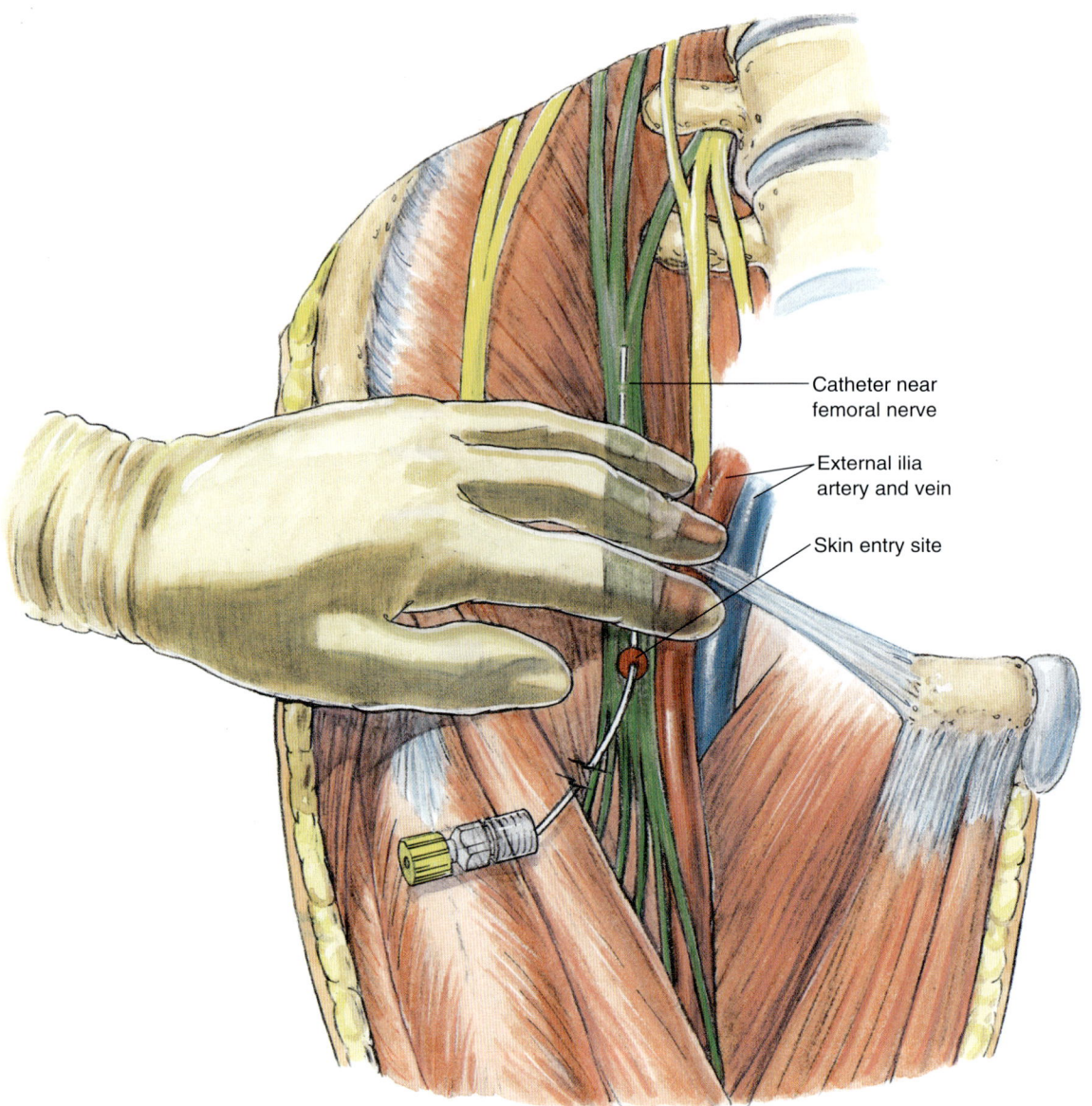

Fig. 15.6 Femoral nerve block: use of continuous catheter.

PEARLS

Because a traditional block is actually a field block, enough "soak time" must be allowed to produce satisfactory anesthesia. When sciatic and femoral blocks are combined, it is often helpful to place the femoral block before the sciatic block, thus allowing extra soak time. Increasingly, patients undergoing surgery on the knee are effectively being offered femoral block as part of the postoperative analgesia regimen. Most often, this is provided as a single-shot technique; however, some practitioners provide the analgesia using a continuous catheter method.

ULTRASONOGRAPHY-GUIDED TECHNIQUE

SONOANATOMY

The femoral nerve is the largest branch of the lumbar plexus and usually consists of the roots of segments L2 to L4. It runs distally to the inguinal region, typically positioned in the groove formed by the iliac and lateral psoas muscles posteriorly and covered by the iliac fascia anteriorly. At this level the iliac fascia, along with the internal aspect of the iliopsoas, thickens to form the iliopectineal band that separates the femoral vein and femoral artery from the nerve. The femoral nerve is often visualized distal to the inguinal ligament within a triangular hyperechoic region lateral to the femoral artery and superficial to the iliopsoas muscle. The nerve may be thin and flat in this region as it may divide into terminal branches. However, it can be visualized as a biconvex or oval hyperechoic structure. Therefore from superficial to deep, the fascia lata is first encountered, then the fascia iliaca, as a hyperechoic line (Figs. 15.7–15.9).

INDICATIONS

- Analgesia for fractured neck/shaft of femur.
- Analgesia after hip joint replacement.

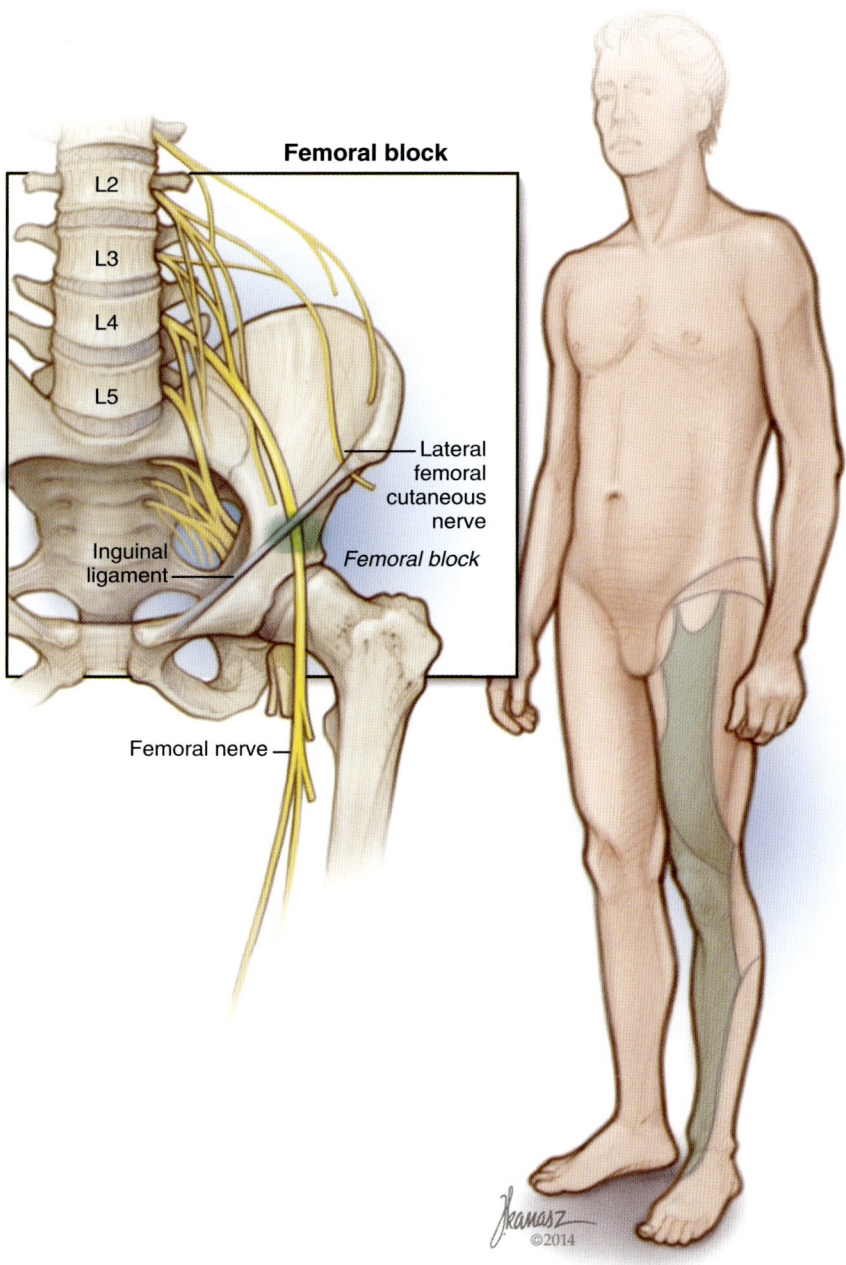

Fig. 15.7 Anatomy of femoral nerve.

122 ATLAS OF REGIONAL ANESTHESIA

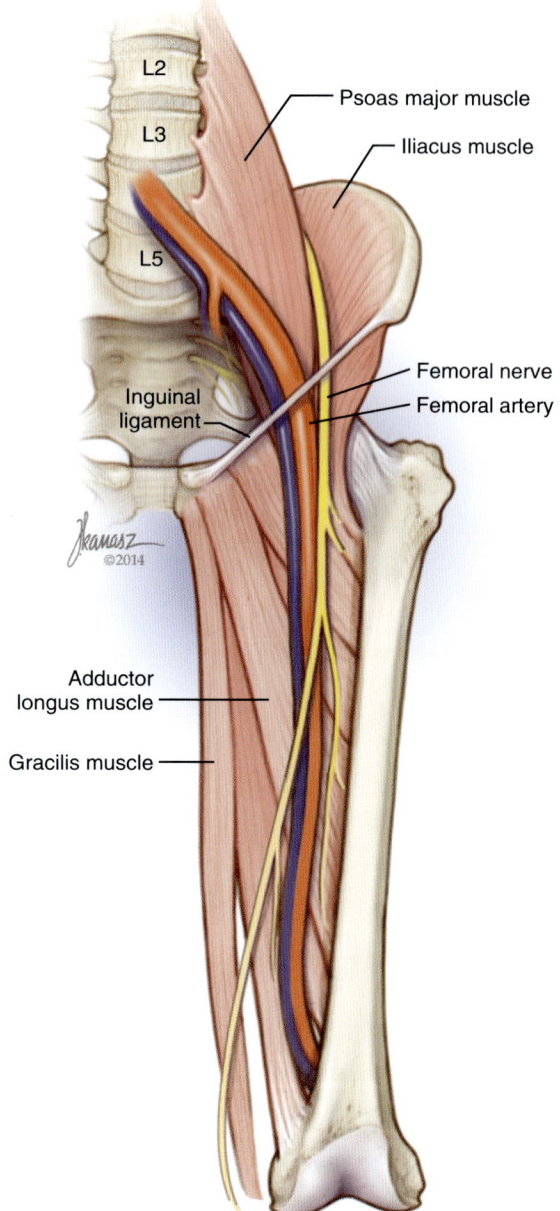

Fig. 15.8 Anatomy of femoral nerve.

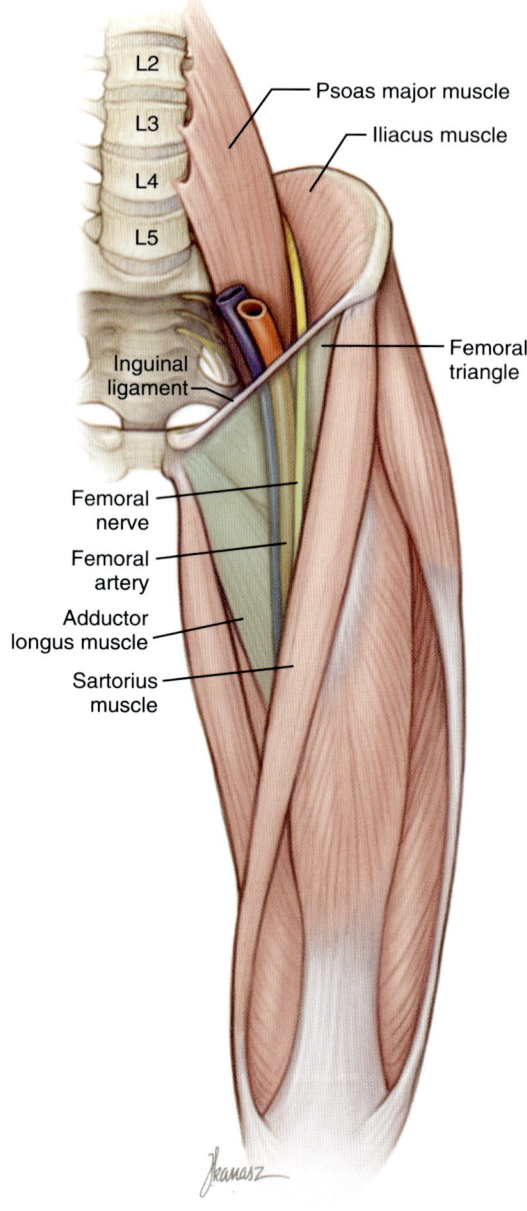

Fig. 15.9 Anatomy of femoral nerve.

- Analgesia after knee joint surgeries, such as total knee arthroplasty or anterior cruciate ligament repair.
- It can be combined with popliteal block to provide anesthesia for lower leg or foot surgeries.

TECHNIQUE

While the patient is in a supine position the ultrasound probe will be parallel to the inguinal crease to obtain the short axis of the nerve within the triangular hypoechoic region. The in-plane technique is most commonly used for this block. In this technique the needle will be inserted in-plane and advanced from lateral to medial in the transverse plane of the image. After piercing the fascia iliaca, inject 2 to 3 mL of saline to ensure the needle tip is beneath the fascia and the saline is spreading lateral to the femoral artery and in the vicinity of the nerve before injecting the local anesthetics (Figs. 15.10–15.15).

KEY POINTS

- High-resolution linear ultrasound (30- to 40-mm footprint) is preferred for the femoral nerve block.
- In some patients, the femoral nerve at the inguinal crease is already branched into superficial and deep divisions along with femoral artery division into superficial and profunda femoris branches. Therefore it is better to scan proximally to place the probe at the common femoral artery in order to ensure blocking the main trunk of the femoral nerve.

Femoral Block 123

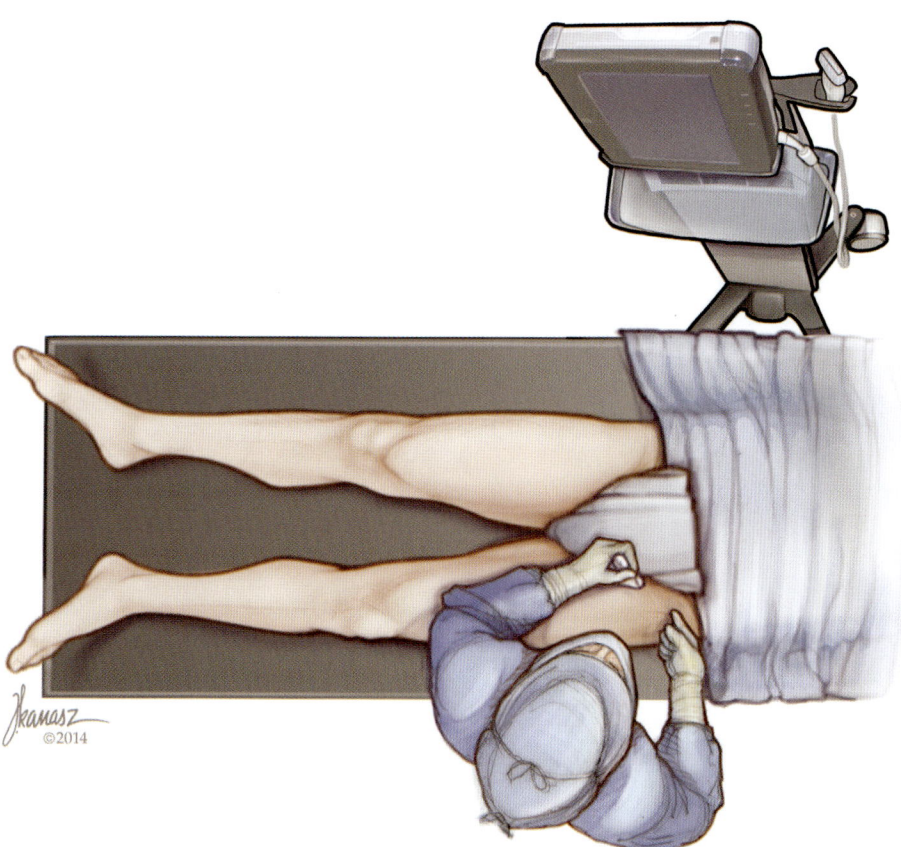

Fig. 15.10. Position of the patient and ultrasound machine.

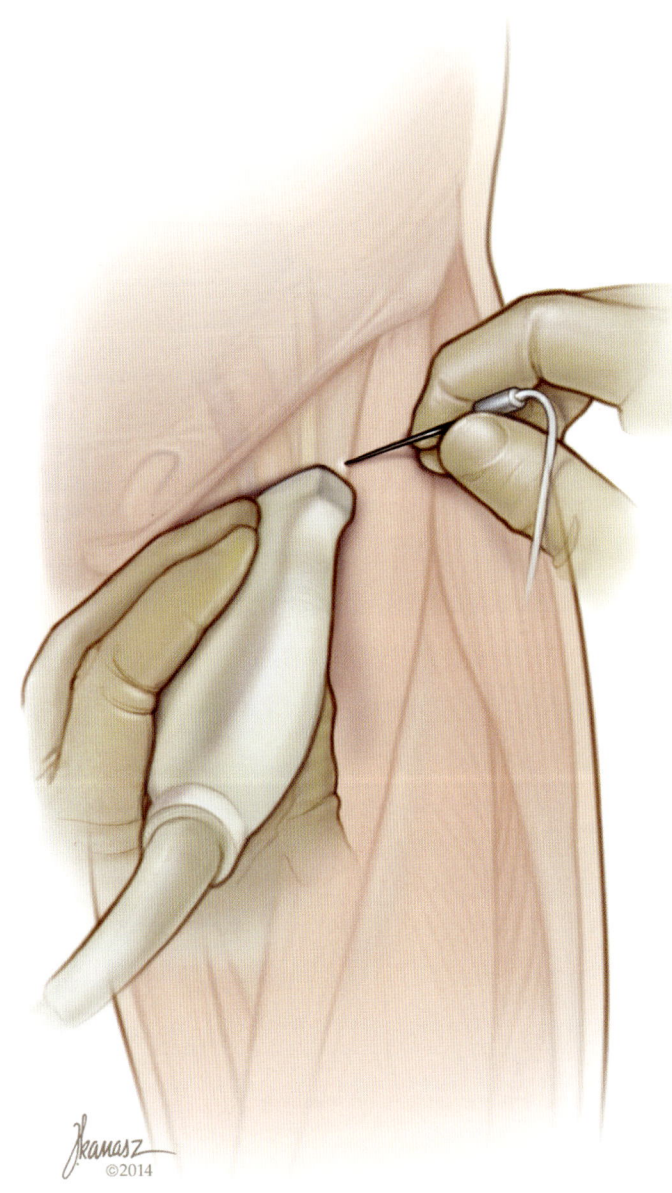

Fig. 15.11 Note the needle in-plane and the needle direction from lateral to medial.

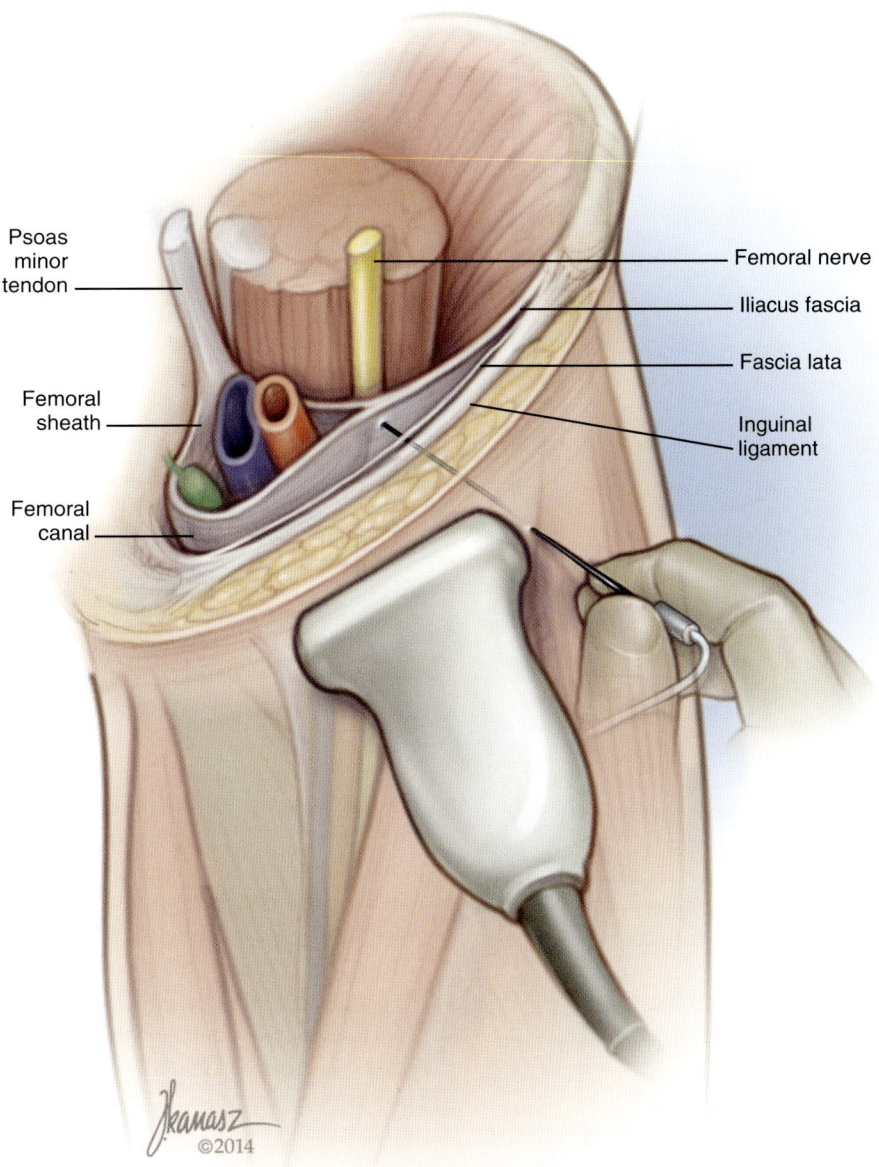

Fig. 15.12 The needle should pierce the iliacus fascia in order to have a successful block.

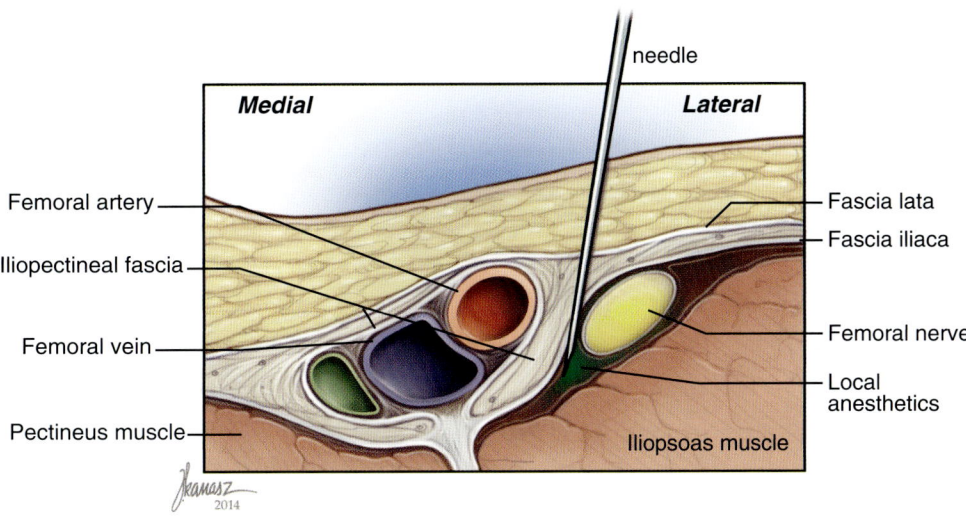

Fig. 15.13 The needle and the local anesthetics are beneath the fascia iliaca.

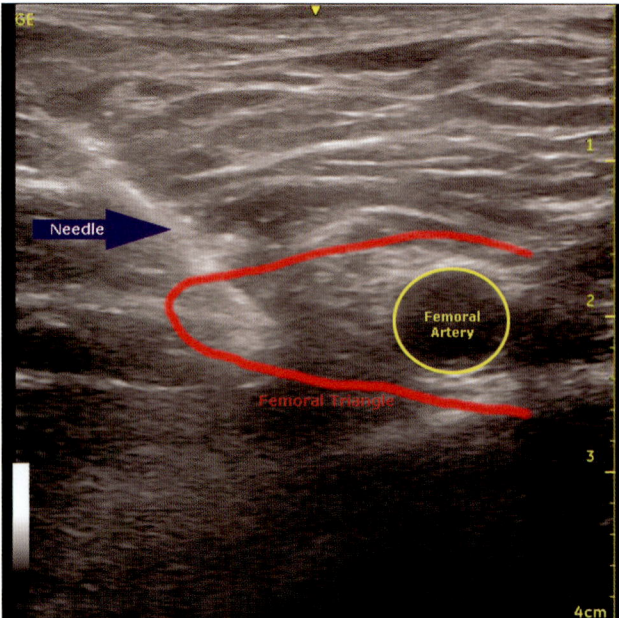

Fig. 15.14 Ultrasound still of femoral block procedure.

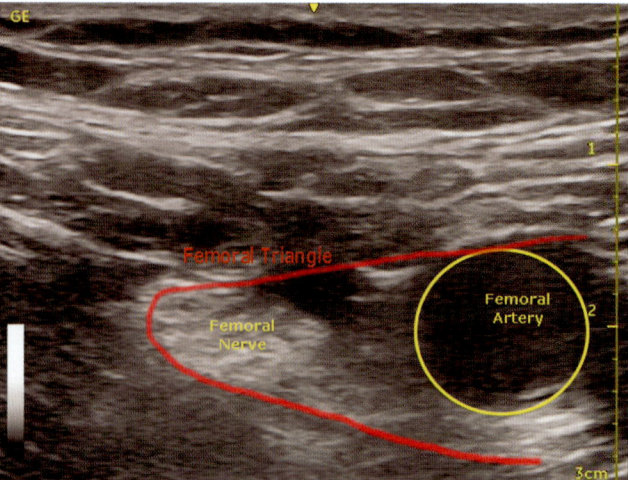

Fig. 15.15 Ultrasound still of anatomy of femoral block.

- For catheter insertion, the Tuohy needle is used. The proper position of the tip of the needle beneath the fascia iliaca can be identified by injecting 2–3 mL of saline, which appears laterally to the artery and in the vicinity of the nerve. Then the catheter will be inserted 3–4 cm beyond the tip of the needle. For further confirmation of the location of the catheter tip, a small volume of air, which appears as a hyperechoic artifact, can be injected through the catheter.

PEARLS

- The femoral nerve can be confused in the short-axis view with inguinal lymph nodes, which also appear hyperechoic.
- If you are not able to identify the femoral nerve, injection in the hyperechoic triangle lateral to the femoral artery will suffice to produce successful block.
- After inserting the catheter through the Tuohy needle, keep the needle in situ and inject through the catheter 2–3 mL of saline or local anesthetic solution to identify the position of the catheter tip. This technique will help modify the catheter position by readjusting the needle and ensuring the catheter position in the vicinity of the nerve.
- The concentration of local anesthetic used in this block usually depends on the aim. For analgesic purposes, ropivacaine 0.1%–0.2% is quite sufficient; however, ropivacaine 0.5% is ideal for anesthetic purposes.

Ultrasound for Fascia Iliaca and Inguinal Region Blocks

16

Mohammed Faysal Malik and Chihiro Toda

Key Points

- A high-frequency linear transducer is preferred for this block.
- The fascia iliaca compartmental block (FICB) can be used as an alternative anterior approach to the lumbar plexus block, targeting the femoral, obturator, and lateral femoral cutaneous nerves.
- The suprainguinal approach to the FICB is associated with better cranial spread of local anesthetic and more complete sensory blockade of the anterior, medial, and lateral thigh compared with the traditional infrainguinal approach.
- The traditional infrainguinal approach required great volumes of local anesthetic to achieve adequate cephalad spread. The suprainguinal approach requires less volume to achieve adequate sensory blockade.

PERSPECTIVE

The fascia iliaca compartmental block (FICB) can be used to provide complete sensory blockade of the medial, anterior, and lateral thigh. This block has been used effectively for postoperative analgesia following hip and knee surgery. It can be used as an alternative to a traditional lumbar plexus block by targeting the femoral nerve, obturator, and lateral femoral cutaneous nerves, which lie deep to the fascia iliaca. It can also provide adequate analgesia for hip and proximal femur fractures as well as for total hip arthroplasty. As with any fascial plane block within the fascia iliacus plane, blockade of the femoral, obturator, and lateral femoral cutaneous nerves is achievable with a large enough volume of local anesthetic. Traditionally, the fascia iliaca block was performed using a 'double pop' technique as the needle traversed the fascia lata and fascia iliaca. This was associated with a significant block failure rate, as high as 10%–37%. However, with advancements in ultrasound and the use of direct needle visualization under continuous ultrasound guidance, the success rate and consequently the popularity of this block is beginning to regain favor.

ANATOMY

The iliacus muscle lies over the ilium. It is a large flat triangular shaped muscle that joins with the psoas major muscle forming the anisotropic hypoechoic iliopsoas muscle. The iliopsoas is covered by the hyperechoic broad ligament and fascia iliaca. The iliopsoas muscle then travels beneath the inguinal ligament, exiting the pelvis, winding around the proximal neck of the femur, and inserts into the lesser trochanter of the hip, functioning as a powerful hip flexor.

The fascia iliaca is located anterior to the iliacus muscle, bound superiorly and laterally by the iliac crest and merges with the overlying psoas muscle fascia medially. The femoral nerve descends through the psoas major muscle passing through its lateral border coursing between psoas and the iliacus muscle deep to the fascia iliaca.

The obturator nerve crosses the iliacus muscle deep to the fascia, innervating the distal medial thigh. The lateral femoral cutaneous nerve emerges from the lumbar plexus and courses inferiorly just lateral to the psoas muscle before crossing the iliacus just deep to the fascia iliaca (Fig. 16.1).

SONOANATOMY

TECHNIQUE

The FICB has been traditionally performed below the level of the inguinal ligament. However, substantial clinical evidence and radiological studies suggest that the infrainguinal approach does not reliably block the femoral, obturator, and lateral femoral cutaneous nerves. Indeed block failure rate has been described as high as 10%–37%.

An alternative technique, the suprainguinal approach has been gaining favor because of improved outcomes in terms of median pain scores in hip fracture patients, and has a more consistent spread of local anesthetic to the lumbar plexus. A recent study identified improved cranial spread of local anesthetic with the suprainguinal approach, compared with a more caudal spread with the traditional infrainguinal injection. The suprainguinal approach has been shown to provide comparable analgesic efficacy to periarticular infiltration for total hip arthroplasty.

Typical injectate volumes include 20 mL of local anesthetic solution such as 0.5% ropivacaine for hip fractures and lower concentrations for postoperative analgesia following hip or knee surgery to minimize motor block.

The patient is positioned supine and a high frequency linear probe is placed in the inguinal crease to identify the femoral artery. Typical depths are 3-4cm from the skin. The probe is moved laterally to identify the sartorius muscle,

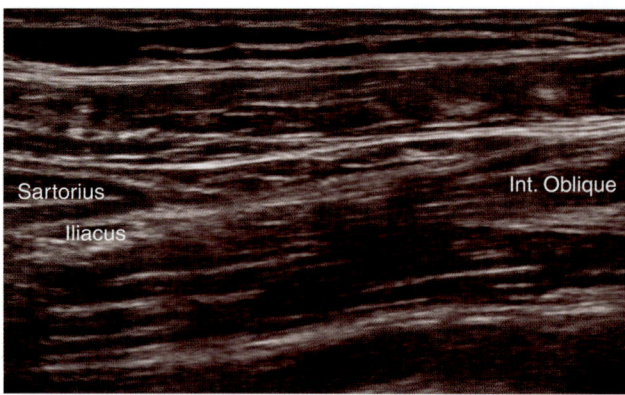

Fig. 16.1 Sonoanatomy of fascia iliaca compartmental block.

which is then traced cephalad to its insertion point over the anterior superior iliac spine (ASIS). The ASIS can be easily identified by its hump-like hypoechoic shadow. Moving the probe 2-3 cm medial to the shadow identifies the iliacus muscle, which covers the ilium. The bright hyperechoic band covering the iliacus is the fascia iliaca.

The probe is then rotated in a slight parasagittal plane such that the medial end is pointing towards the umbilicus. At this position the anterior abdominal muscles may be identified from superficial to deep, as the internal oblique muscle, transversus abdominis, and the fascia iliaca overlying the iliacus muscle. The curve of the ilium will be identified on the inferior caudal side of the ultrasound image with the iliacus muscle overlying it. With this view, the classical "bow-tie" appearance may be appreciated (Fig. 16.2).

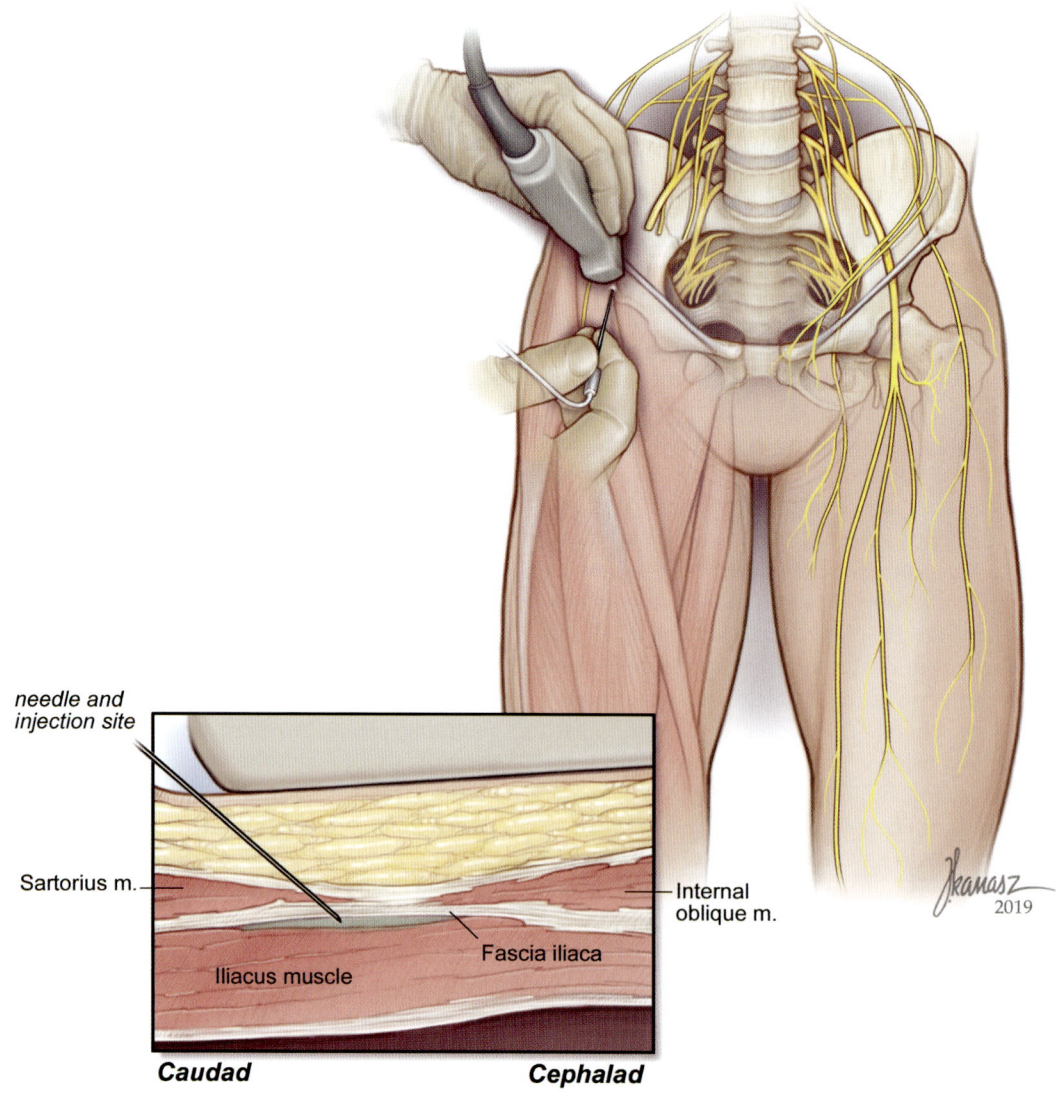

Fig. 16.2 Fascia iliaca compartmental block.

The block needle is inserted and advanced caudad to cephalad such that it traverses the sartorius muscle above the inguinal ligament. It is then advanced in-plane just deep to the fascia iliaca. After piercing the fascia, 1-2 mL of local anesthetic is injected to confirm adequate spread cranially, and peeling of the fascial layers lifting the fascia off the superficial layer of the iliacus muscle. Then 20-30mL of the block solution is deposited superficial to the iliacus muscle and deep to the fascia iliaca. Adequate spread of local anesthetic will expand the space between the iliacus muscle and fascia iliaca in a cephalad direction towards the superior edge of the iliacus muscle. In order to improve the spread of local anesthetic superiorly, the needle tip may be advanced superiorly into the space created by the injectate.

Although the FICB has enjoyed renewed interest and is deemed a safe and effective block, complications that have been described include bladder perforation, and inadvertent puncture of the deep circumflex iliac artery, inferior epigastric artery, external iliac artery, spermatic cord, and hernia contents. Careful use of real-time ultrasound and maintaining an in-plane needle approach should help mitigate these potential complications.

INGUINAL REGION BLOCKS

KEY POINTS

- The ilioinguinal and the iliohypogastric nerves supply the inguinal area, and are the targets of the block.
- It is a superficial block, and a high-frequency linear probe is used for ultrasound guidance.
- The local anesthetic should be given between the muscle layers of abdominal wall near the iliac crest for a successful block.
- The provider should keep in mind that the surgeon may give a local anesthetic intraoperatively as well, and should avoid injecting a total amount of local anesthetic, which would exceed the toxic dose.

INDICATION

The ilioinguinal nerve block provides surgical anesthesia for groin surgery, primarily inguinal herniorrhaphy. It is often combined with iliohypogastric and genitofemoral nerve blocks.

ANATOMY

Innervation of the inguinal region arises from the lumbar plexus nerves. The ilioinguinal and iliohypogastric nerves originate from the first lumbar nerve, and emerge from the upper part or the lateral border of the psoas major muscle. The genitofemoral nerve originates from the first and second lumbar nerves. These peripheral extensions of the lumbar plexus and the twelfth thoracic nerve follow a circular course. As they course anteriorly, they pass near the anterior superior iliac spine. The twelfth thoracic nerve and iliohypogastric nerves run between the internal and external oblique muscles near the anterior superior iliac spine. The ilioinguinal nerve runs between the transverse abdominis muscle and the internal oblique muscle and then penetrates the internal oblique muscle medial to the anterior superior iliac spine. All these nerves continue anteriorly in a medial orientation and become superficial as they terminate in the skin and muscles of the inguinal region. The genitofemoral nerve follows a different course from other nerves, and it often requires supplemental block intraoperatively to make this regional block effective for inguinal herniorrhaphy.

BLOCK TECHNIQUE

Anatomical Landmark Technique The patient is placed in supine position. The anterior superior iliac spine should be identified. A point approximately 3 cm medial and inferior from the anterior superior iliac spine should be marked. After preparing skin, a needle is inserted in a cephalolateral direction. Local anesthetic is injected as the needle is withdrawn through the layers of the abdominal wall. Then the needle should be inserted again at a steeper angle until it penetrates all three muscle layers of the abdominal wall. Ten to 20 mL of local anesthetic is injected as the needle is withdrawn. Patients who are obese or muscled may need another injection. The injection is extended from the previously placed skin wheal toward the umbilicus and creates a subcutaneous field block.

Ultrasound-Guided Technique The patient is placed supine and the anterior superior iliac spine is identified as for the landmark technique. Draw a line from the anterior superior iliac spine to the umbilicus. A high-frequency linear ultrasound probe is placed along the line, superior and medial to the anterior superior iliac spine (Fig. 16.3). The ilioinguinal and iliohypogastric nerves are seen in the fascia plane, either between the internal oblique muscles and transverse abdominis, or between the internal oblique and external oblique muscles. These two nerves are often seen as a hypoechoic structure. Below the transverse abdominis is the peritoneal cavity. It is common to see small blood vessels close to these nerves. Color Doppler is helpful to identify blood vessels. After identifying the anatomy, a needle is inserted in-plane. Ten to 20 mL of local anesthetic is injected into the fascia plane.

MEDICATION

Lower concentrations of intermediate- to long-acting local anesthetics, such as 1% lidocaine, 1% mepivacaine, 0.25% bupivacaine, and 0.2% ropivacaine can be chosen. The anesthesiologist should keep in mind that the surgeon may need an additional injection of local anesthetic intraoperatively, and limit the dose of the initial injection to allow an additional injection without concern of local anesthetic systemic toxicity.

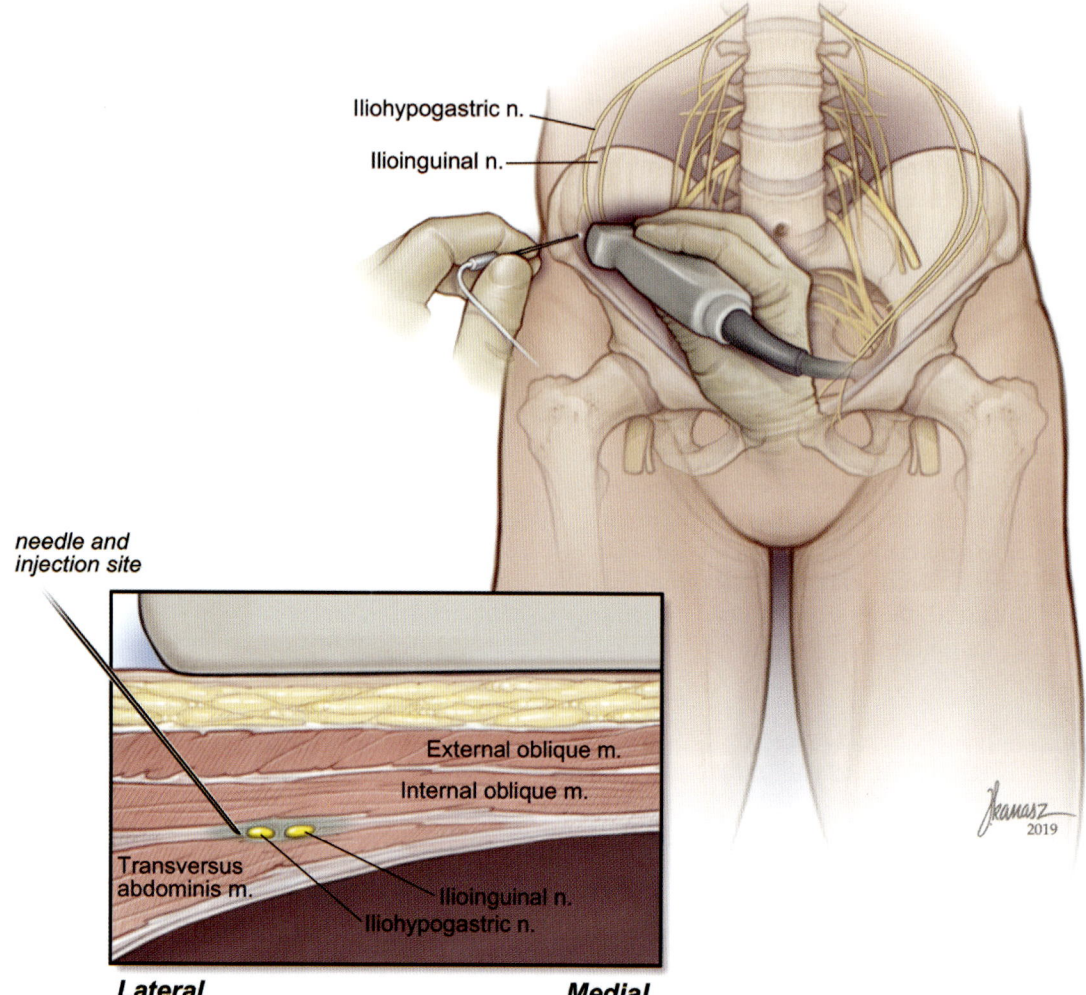

Fig. 16.3 Ilioinguinal-iliohypogastric block.

COMPLICATIONS

The ilioinguinal block is a superficial block and has only a few major complications. These include post block ecchymosis and hematoma formation in the region of the spermatic cord. This may make it difficult for the surgeon to perform an adequate surgical dissection. If a needle is advanced too deep and enters the peritoneal cavity, perforation of the colon could occur.

Lateral Femoral Cutaneous Nerve Block 17

Sanchit Ahuja and Sree Kolli

Key Points

- This block can be used to provide postoperative analgesia following hip surgery, upper lateral thigh skin grafting, and neurolysis for refractory meralgia paresthetica.
- Combined with other lower extremity blocks, it reduces the discomfort from the tourniquet during procedures on the lower leg.
- This is a very superficial block, hence a high-frequency transducer is preferred for this block.

ANATOMY

The lateral femoral cutaneous nerve of the thigh (LFCN) is a pure sensory nerve and a derivative of posterior branches of the lumbar plexus, namely L2 and L3 spinal nerves. It travels downwards along the lateral border of the psoas muscle and continues inferior-lateral towards the anterior superior iliac spine (ASIS), where it angulates acutely and exits in the lower pelvis, under the inguinal ligament, and over the sartorius muscle into the thigh. Near the inguinal ligament the nerve lies beneath the fascia lata. The nerve divides into anterior (main trunk) and posterior branches as it crosses the inguinal ligament. Importantly, it has several distinct patterns of division—the most common being caudal to the inguinal ligament. The anterior branch is roughly 7–10 cm below the ASIS and supplies the skin over the anterolateral aspect of the thigh, while the posterior branch passes through the fascia lata proximal to the division of the anterior branch, and supplies the lateral thigh, from greater trochanter to the midthigh.

LANDMARK TECHNIQUE

With the patient in a supine position, the ASIS is marked and the block needle is inserted at a point 2 cm medial and 2 cm caudal to the ASIS as shown in Fig. 17.1. The needle is advanced until a "pop" is felt as the needle passes through the fascia lata. Local anesthetic is then injected in a fanlike manner from medial to lateral as illustrated in Fig. 17.2.

SONOANATOMY

Under sonogram, the nerve is accessible for visualization before it exits the pelvis. The image of the nerve appears as a hyperechoic rimmed structure seated roughly 0.5–1 cm below the skin surface subfascially (not subcutaneous) and 1–2 cm inferior and medial to the ASIS. It is found within a fat-filled space sandwiched between the two muscles, namely sartorius and the tensor muscle of fascia lata. The orientation of the nerve and its branches is lateral to the sartorius muscle, which is in an oblique and medial position. The nerve can also be confirmed in a sagittal plane by visualization of the deep circumflex iliac artery. In this view, the artery is perpendicular to the course of the nerve and can be seen as a pulsating dot. There are occasions when the nerve has an aberrant course, and in these cases the area under the medial aspect of the inguinal ligament and immediately lateral to the ASIS should be searched.

ULTRASOUND-GUIDED TECHNIQUE

With the patient in a supine position, the ASIS is palpated and the lateral end of a high frequency transducer is positioned immediately inferior to the ASIS, in line with the inguinal ligament—angled slightly in a caudal direction. The inguinal ligament can be seen as a linear hyperechoic structure running from the pubic tubercle to the ASIS. When the probe is moved to a medial-caudad position, the nerve can be visualized in the fat-filled space between the sartorius medially and the tensor muscle of the fascia lata laterally. Once the nerve is found in the transverse plane, it can be traced proximally and distally (Fig. 17.3A-B). Confirmation of the nerve can also be done in a sagittal plane by visualizing deep circumflex vessels (via Doppler), which course parallel to the inguinal ligament and perpendicular to the course of the nerve. It is essential to confirm the nerve by either method as described above, because it is not uncommon to mistake the hyperechoic tendinous part of the sartorius muscle for a nerve. After confirmation, the needle is inserted in a lateral to medial fashion using an in-plane technique, and 5 mL of local anesthetic can be injected subfascially or perineurally.

Another recently described technique involves identifying the LFC nerve in the fat-filled flat tunnel (FFFT), formed by the double layer of the fascia lata between the

132 ATLAS OF REGIONAL ANESTHESIA

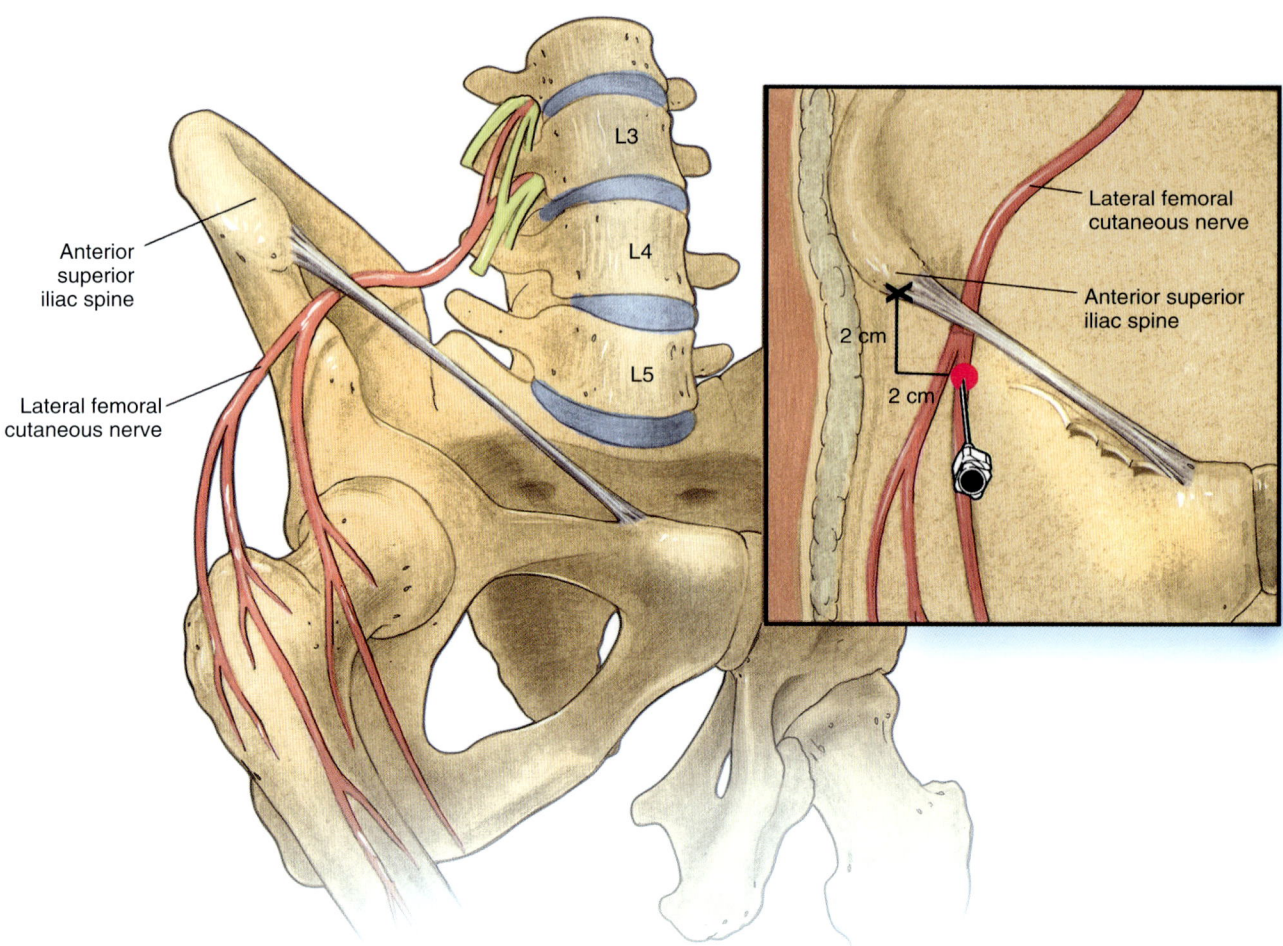

Fig. 17.1 Lateral femoral cutaneous nerve: anatomy.

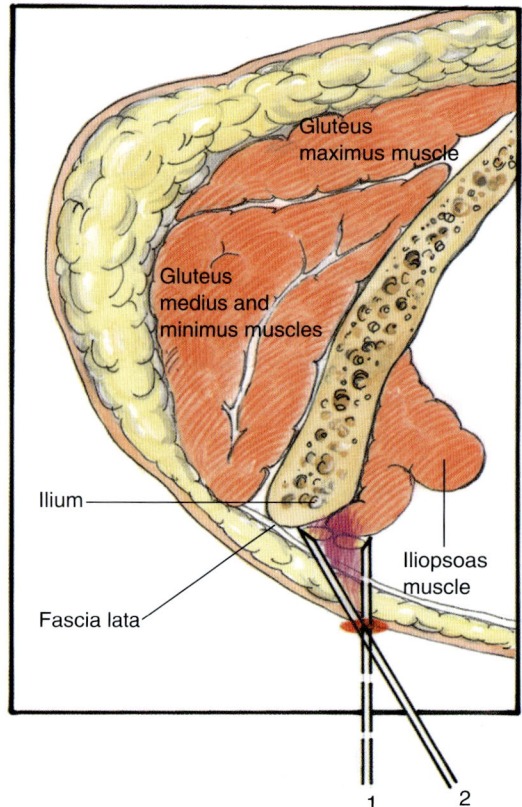

Fig. 17.2 Lateral femoral cutaneous nerve block: technique.

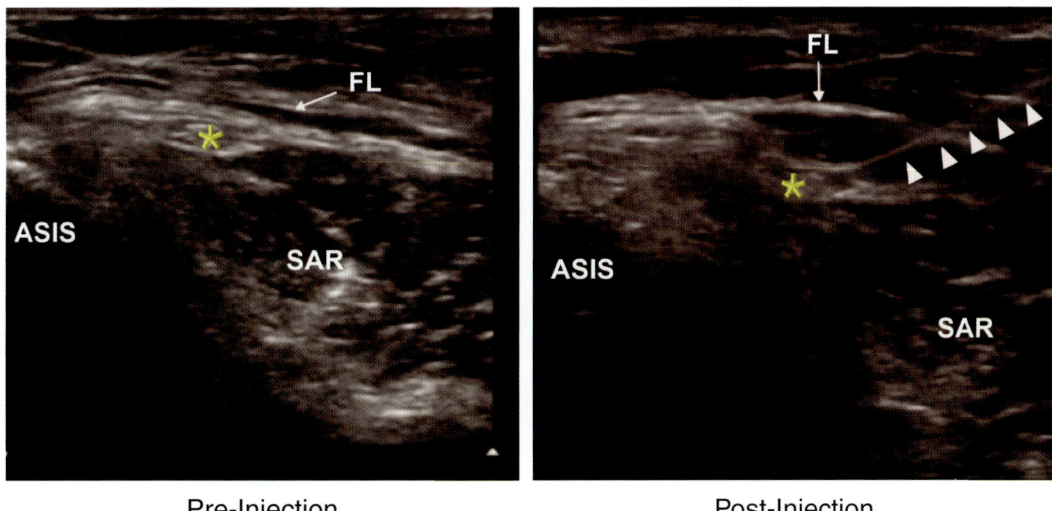

Pre-Injection   Post-Injection

Fig. 17.3 Ultrasound-guided lateral femoral cutaneous nerve block. *ASIS*, Anterior superior iliac spine; *FL,* fascia lata; *SAR,* sartorius; *arrowheads,* needle; *, lateral femoral cutaneous nerve.

sartorius and the tensor muscle of fascia lata, about 10 cm from the ASIS. The needle is inserted out-of-plane into the FFFT and 10 mL of local anesthetic is injected intermittently and simultaneously advancing the needle tip inside the FFFT towards the ASIS, while tracking the needle tip with ultrasonography in real time.

PEARLS

- This block can be used in lieu of lumbar plexus block after hip surgery. However, an injection of a high volume of local anesthetic in the fascia iliaca can spread as far as the anterior and posterior divisions of the femoral nerve.
- The nerve appears as a small hyperechoic structure containing hypoechoic vesicles and must be differentiated from the hyperechoic tendinous part of the sartorius muscle by scanning the course of the nerve. Hydro dissection of fascia iliaca and tensor muscle of fascia lata may also help improve visualization of the nerve.
- It is not uncommon to see variations in the course of the nerve. It is sometimes helpful to locate the nerve distally, between the sartorius and tensor muscle of fascia lata and then trace it up proximally towards the ASIS at the insertion site of the sartorius. Also the deep circumflex artery landmark may be useful.
- Because of the superficial nature of this block, apply light pressure and plenty of ultrasound gel for better nerve visualization.
- Peripheral nerve catheters are not studied with this block.

Obturator Block 18

Loran Mounir-Soliman and David L. Brown

Key Points

- The success of the block depends on the appropriate spread of local anesthetics in the appropriate fascial planes superficially and deeply to the adductor brevis muscle.
- Care should be taken to confirm the spread in the intermuscular fascial planes and not intramuscular.
- Change in adductor strength is the best assessment method for the block since the sensory distribution is variable.
- With a successful block, some residual adductor strength is secondary to the formal innervation to the pectineus, as well as some sciatic innervation to the adductor magnus.

PERSPECTIVE

This block is most often combined with the sciatic, femoral, and lateral femoral cutaneous nerve blocks to allow surgical procedures on the lower extremities. If an operation on the knee using these peripheral blocks is planned, the obturator block is often essential. Another use for this block is in patients who have hip pain. It can be used diagnostically to help identify the cause of pain because obturator nerve block may provide considerable pain relief if the nerve's articular branch to the hip is involved in pain transmission. The block also may be useful in the evaluation of lower extremity spasticity or chronic pain syndromes.

Patient Selection. As with femoral and lateral femoral cutaneous nerve blocks, elicitation of paresthesia is not essential for obturator block. Any patient able to lie supine is a candidate.

Pharmacologic Choice. Motor blockade is most often not necessary for surgical patients receiving obturator nerve block; thus lower concentrations of local anesthetics are appropriate for obturator block: 0.75% to 1.0% lidocaine or mepivacaine, 0.25% bupivacaine, or 0.2% ropivacaine.

PLACEMENT

Anatomy. The obturator nerve emerges from the medial border of the psoas muscle at the pelvic brim and travels along the lateral aspect of the pelvis anterior to the obturator internus muscle and posterior to the iliac vessels and ureter. It enters the obturator canal cephalad and anterior to the obturator vessels, which are branches from the internal iliac vessels. In the obturator canal, the obturator nerve divides into anterior and posterior branches (Fig. 18.1). The anterior branch supplies the anterior adductor muscles and sends an articular branch to the hip joint and a cutaneous area on the medial aspect of the thigh. The posterior branch innervates the deep adductor muscles and sends an articular branch to the knee joint. In 10% of patients, an accessory obturator nerve may be found.

Position. The patient should be supine with the legs in a slightly abducted position. The genitalia should be protected from antiseptic solutions.

Needle Puncture. The pubic tubercle should be located and an "X" marked 1.5 cm caudad and 1.5 cm lateral to the tubercle (Fig. 18.2). The needle is inserted at this point, and at a depth of approximately 1.5 to 4 cm it contacts the horizontal ramus of the pubis. The needle is then withdrawn, redirected laterally in a horizontal plane, and inserted 2 to 3 cm deeper than the depth of the initial contact with bone. The needle tip now lies within the obturator canal (see Fig. 18.2). With the needle in this position, 10 to 15 mL of local anesthetic solution is injected while the needle is advanced and withdrawn slightly to ensure development of a "wall" of local anesthetic in the canal.

POTENTIAL PROBLEMS

The obturator canal is a vascular location; thus the potential exists for intravascular injection or hematoma formation, although these are more theoretical than clinical concerns.

PEARLS

This block, even in trained hands, has a variable success rate. Our experience suggests that one must rely on volume of anesthetic delivered rather than on absolute accuracy of needle position. Fortunately, use of an obturator block with the other lower extremity peripheral nerve blocks is not an absolute requirement for most surgical procedures. If this block is used diagnostically for patients with chronic pain, it is helpful to use a nerve stimulator to guide needle placement. This will minimize diagnostic confusion when pain relief is produced with a small volume of local anesthetic.

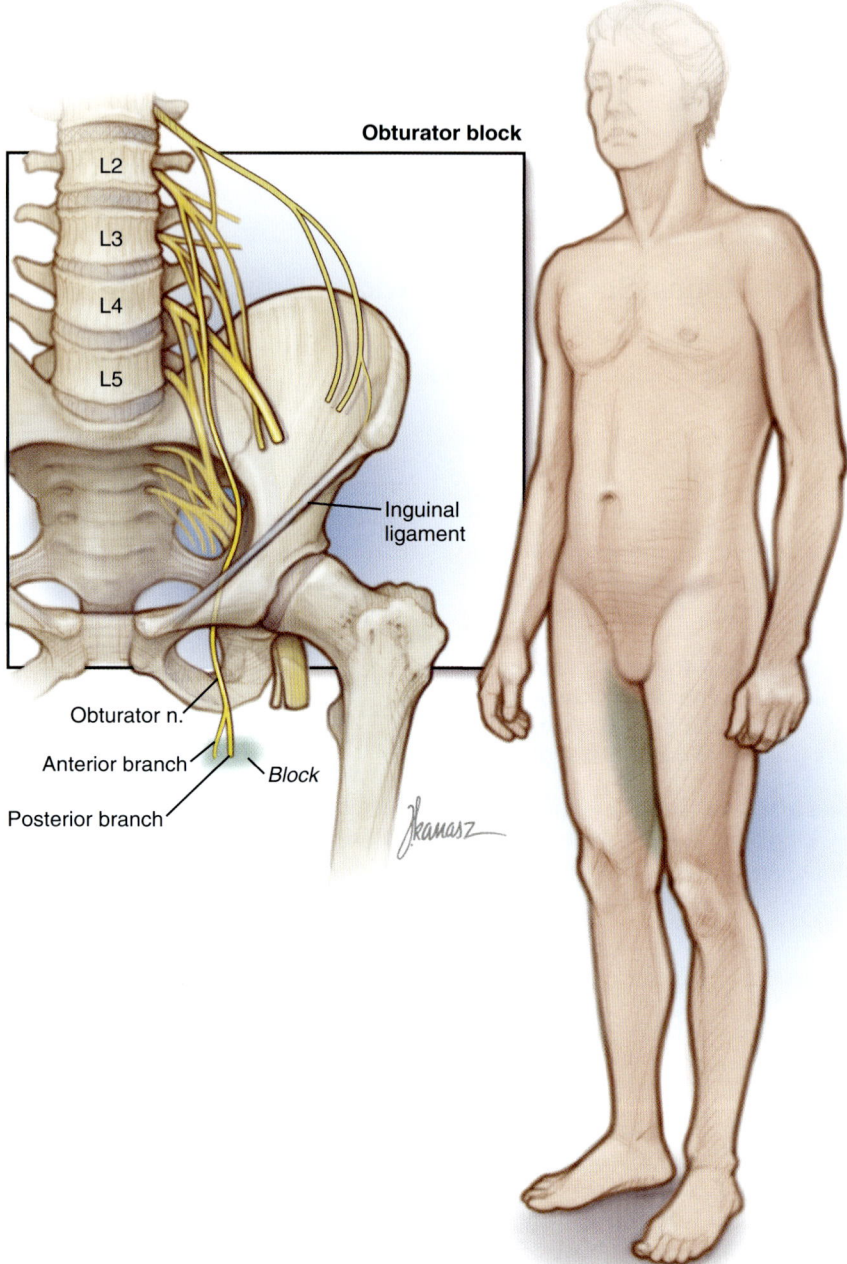

Fig. 18.1 Obturator nerve: functional anatomy.

Large-volume injections (approximately 15 mL) are performed with this block for many surgical procedures.

SONOANATOMY

The obturator nerve is formed from the anterior primary rami of the L2 to L4 roots as a branch of the lumbar plexus within the psoas muscle. The nerve exits the pelvis through the obturator foramen then typically divides into an anterior and posterior branch before entering the thigh. The anterior branch provides sensory supply to a variable area of the medial aspect of the thigh, as well as motor fibers to the adductor muscles. The posterior branch provides primarily motor fibers to the adductor muscles and occasional articular sensation to the medial aspect of the knee joint. Notably, the articular branch of the hip joint provided by the obturator nerve usually originates from the main obturator nerve before division.

In the thigh, the two nerves run within the adductor compartment and medial to the femoral compartment. The anterior branch has a more superficial course between the fascia of the pectineus and adductor brevis muscles, whereas the posterior branch runs at a deeper level between the adductor brevis and adductor magnus muscles (Fig. 18.3).

INDICATIONS

- Avoid adductor muscle contractions during transurethral bladder surgery under spinal anesthesia or when administration of muscle relaxants is undesirable.

Obturator Block   137

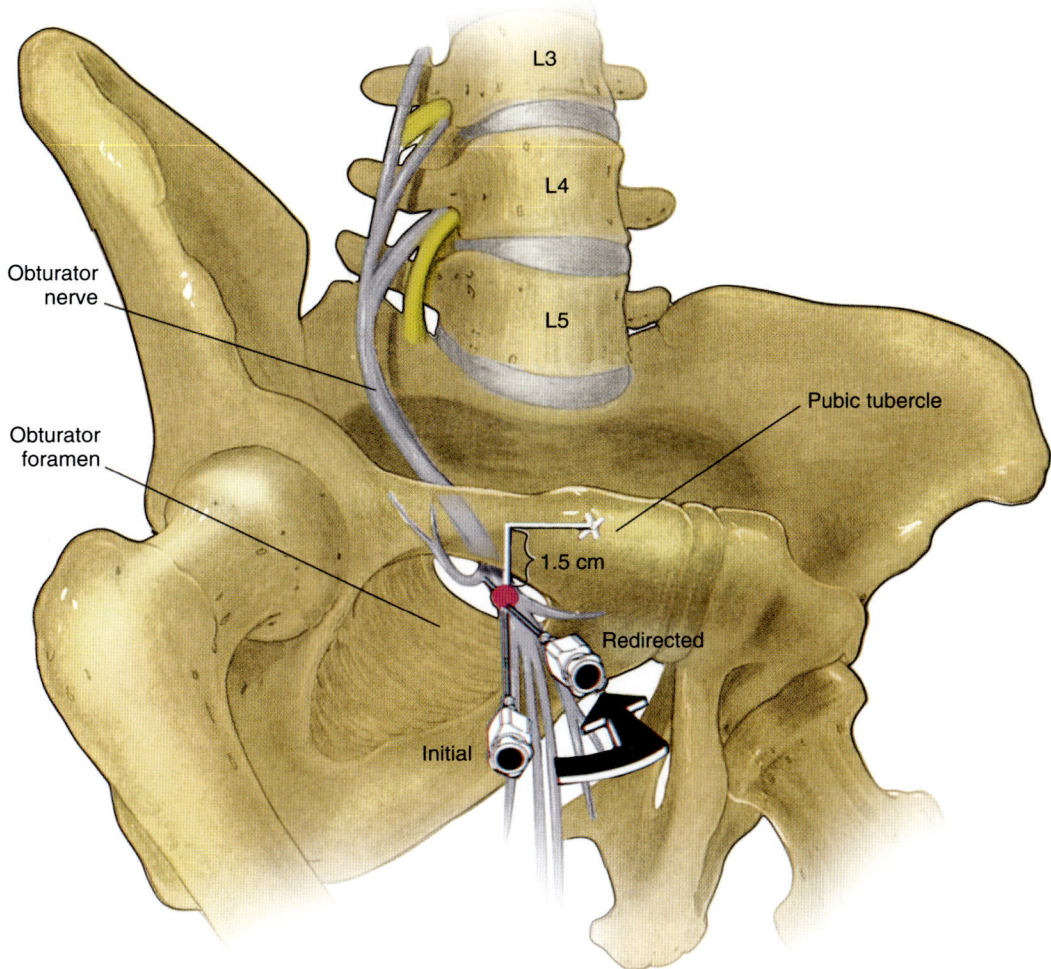

Fig. 18.2 Obturator nerve block: technique.

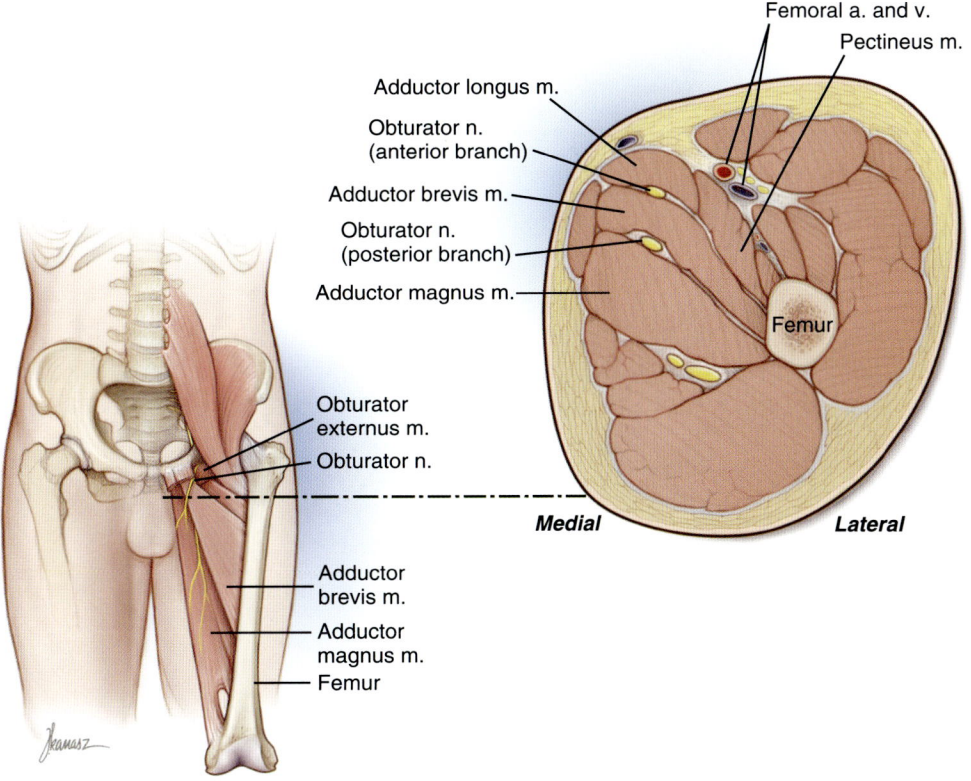

Fig. 18.3 Obturator anatomy.

- Provide complementary analgesia for major knee and thigh surgeries as a reliable alternative to 3-in-1 block, in conjunction with femoral and lateral femoral cutaneous nerve block; 3-in-1 block is a large volume local anesthetic injected near the femoral nerve.

TECHNIQUE

With the patient in the supine position, the thigh is slightly abducted and laterally rotated to better access the adductor compartment on the medial side of the thigh. The ultrasound probe is positioned in a transverse orientation to the thigh (short-axis view to the adductor muscles) (Fig. 18.4). Usually the pectineus muscle is medial to the femoral vessels slightly below the inguinal crease. Moving the probe farther medially to the pectineus muscle identifies the three adductor muscles aligned from superficial to deep: adductor longus, adductor brevis, and adductor magnus. The anterior and posterior branches of the obturator nerve are identified as hyperechoic and "white bands" superficial and deep to the adductor brevis muscle, respectively. Sometimes the nerves are difficult to identify, especially in morbidly obese patients—the goal of the block is to install 10-15 mL of local anesthetic both superficially and deeply into the adductor brevis muscle. The posterior division of the obturator nerve can be blocked by installing the local anesthetic deeper to the adductor brevis in the fascial plane between the adductor brevis and adductor magnus muscles. The anterior branch is blocked superficially to the adductor brevis in the fascial plane between the pectineus or adductor longus and the adductor brevis muscle (known as the *interfascial injection technique*) (Fig. 18.5).

PEARLS

- Both out-of-plane and in-plane approaches of the needle have been used successfully.
- When approaching the needle from the lateral side of the probe (in-plane technique), care must be taken to avoid vascular injury of the femoral or profunda femoris vessel or its branches.
- Separate injection of both branches in the thigh is mandatory because the obturator externus muscle separates both branches.
- Confirmation of the identified nerve-by-nerve stimulation inducing adduction is reassuring but not necessary for successful blocks.

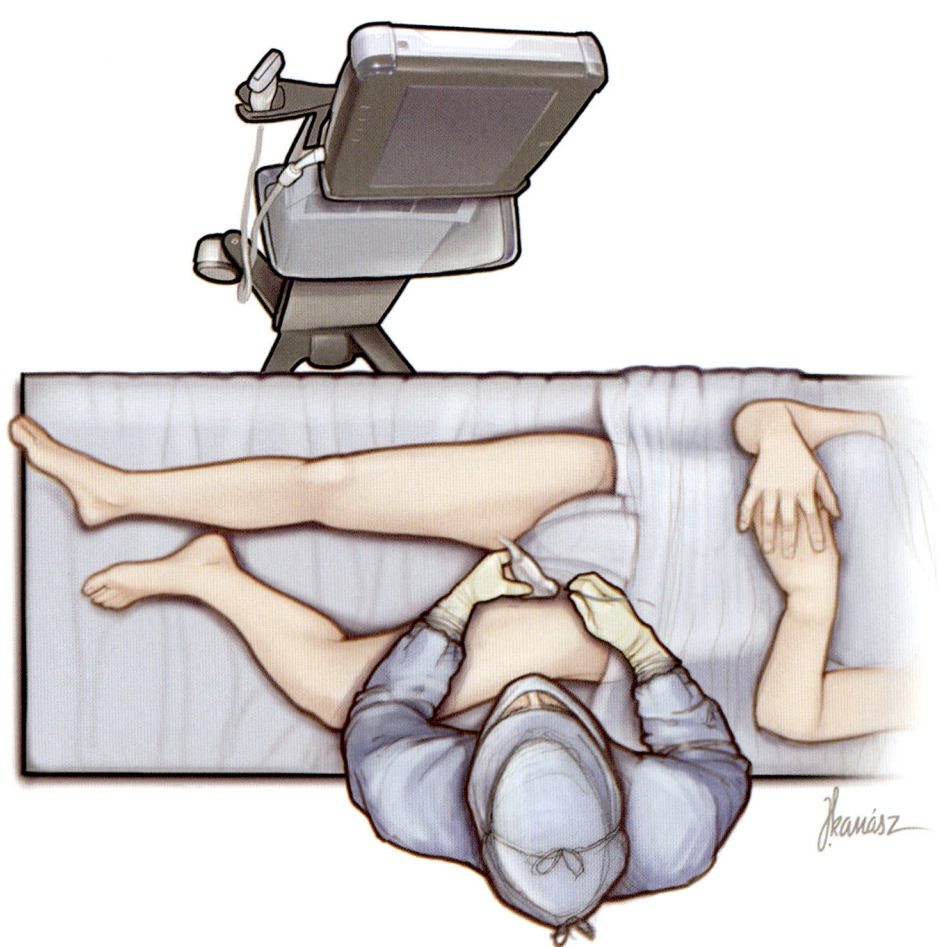

Fig. 18.4 Obturator nerve block: position.

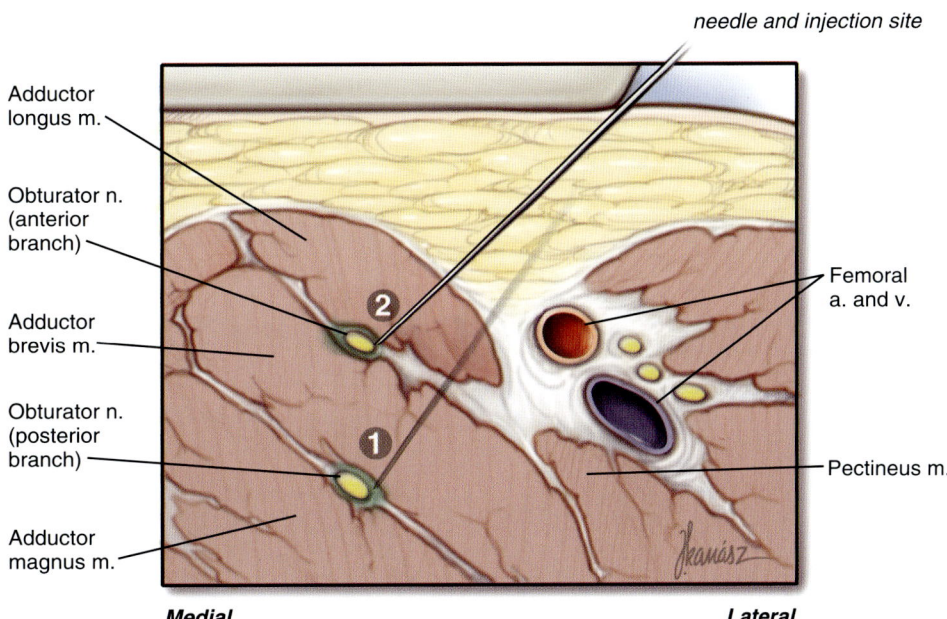

Fig. 18.5 Obturator ultrasound.

Popliteal and Saphenous Block

Maria Yared and David L. Brown

PERSPECTIVE

The nerves blocked in the popliteal fossa—the tibial and peroneal nerves—are extensions of the sciatic nerve. The principal use of this block is for foot and ankle surgery. The addition of a saphenous nerve block improves comfort, because medial lower leg and ankle sensory blockade makes tourniquets and medial ankle surgery more comfortable.

Patient Selection. To use the classic form of this block, the patient must be able to assume the prone position. Elicitation of paresthesia or a motor response is desirable but not essential; however, block effectiveness decreases without these endpoints.

Pharmacologic Choice. The principal use of these blocks is to provide sensory analgesia; thus lower concentrations of a local anesthetic are practical in contrast to situations in which motor blockade is essential. Concentrations of 1% lidocaine, 1% mepivacaine, 0.25% to 0.5% bupivacaine, and 0.2% to 0.5% ropivacaine are effective.

TRADITIONAL BLOCK TECHNIQUE

PLACEMENT

Anatomy. As illustrated in Fig. 19.1, the cephalad popliteal fossa is defined by the semimembranosus and semitendinosus muscles medially and the biceps femoris muscle laterally. Its caudad extent is defined by the gastrocnemius muscles both medially and laterally. If this quadrilateral area is bisected, as shown in Fig. 19.1, the area of interest to the anesthesiologist is the cephalolateral quadrant (hatched area), where both a tibial and common peroneal nerve block is possible. The tibial nerve is the larger of these two nerves; it separates from the common peroneal nerve at the upper limit of the popliteal fossa and sometimes higher. The tibial nerve continues the straight course of the sciatic nerve and runs lengthwise through the popliteal fossa immediately under the popliteal fascia. Inferiorly, it passes between the heads of the gastrocnemius muscles. The common peroneal nerve follows the tendon of the biceps femoris muscle along the cephalolateral margin of the popliteal fossa, as illustrated in Fig. 19.2. After the common peroneal nerve leaves the popliteal fossa, it travels around the head of the fibula and divides into the superficial peroneal and deep peroneal nerves.

Position. The patient is placed in a prone position, and the anesthesiologist stands at the patient's side to allow palpation of the borders of the popliteal fossa.

Needle Puncture. With the patient in the prone position, they are asked to flex the leg at the knee, which allows more accurate identification of the popliteal fossa. Once the popliteal fossa has been defined, it is divided into equal medial and lateral triangles, as shown in Fig. 19.1. An "X" is placed 5–7 cm superior to the skin crease of the popliteal fossa and 1 cm lateral to the midline of the triangles, as shown in Fig. 19.1. Through this site, a 22-gauge, 4- to 6-cm needle is advanced at an angle of 45–60 degrees to the skin while being directed anterosuperiorly (Fig. 19.3). Paresthesia or a motor response is sought; when obtained, 30–40 mL of local anesthetic is injected.

When a saphenous block is added for foot and ankle surgery, the patient's knee is bent at approximately a 45-degree angle and the medial aspect of the leg is exposed. Two primary techniques are used for a saphenous block. A superficial ring of local anesthetic may be injected just distal to the medial surface of the tibial condyle. Often 5–10 mL of local anesthetic is needed. Conversely, a more proximal technique at the cross-sectional level of the superior border of the patella is possible (Fig. 19.4). In this case, a 22- to 25-gauge, 3- to 4-cm needle is inserted immediately deep to the sartorius muscle in the plane between the vastus medialis and the sartorius muscles, and 10 mL of local anesthetic is injected.

POTENTIAL PROBLEMS

Although vascular structures also occupy the popliteal fossa, intravascular injection should be infrequent if the usual precautions are taken. Hematoma formation is possible.

142 ATLAS OF REGIONAL ANESTHESIA

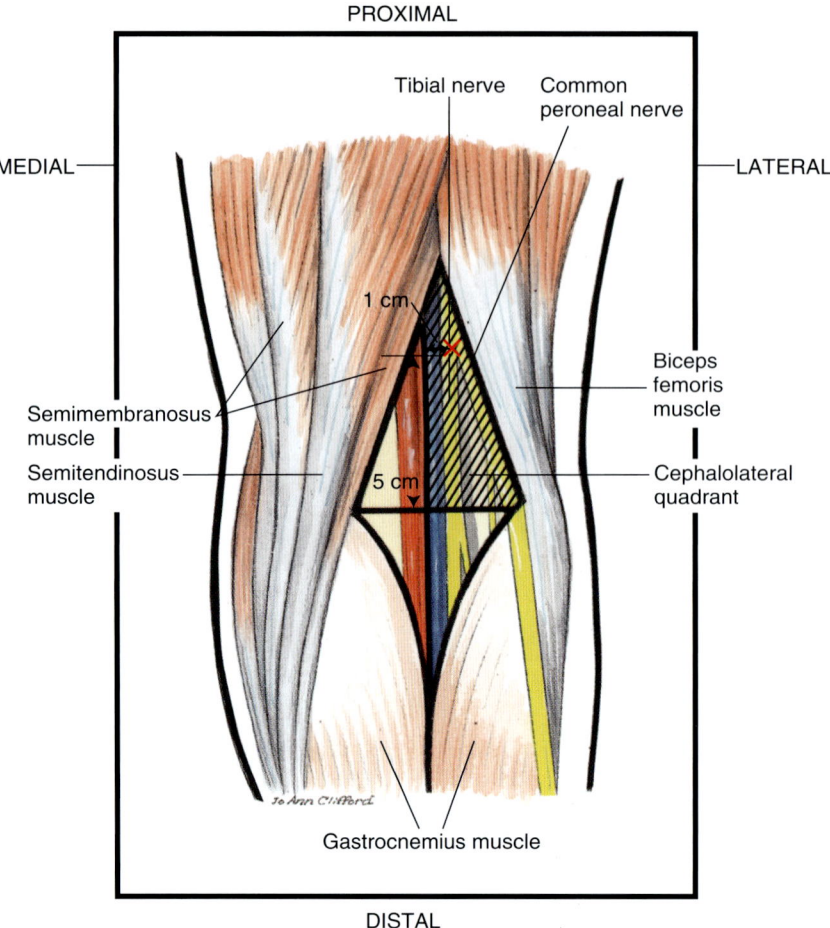

Fig. 19.1 Popliteal fossa: surface anatomy and technique for popliteal block.

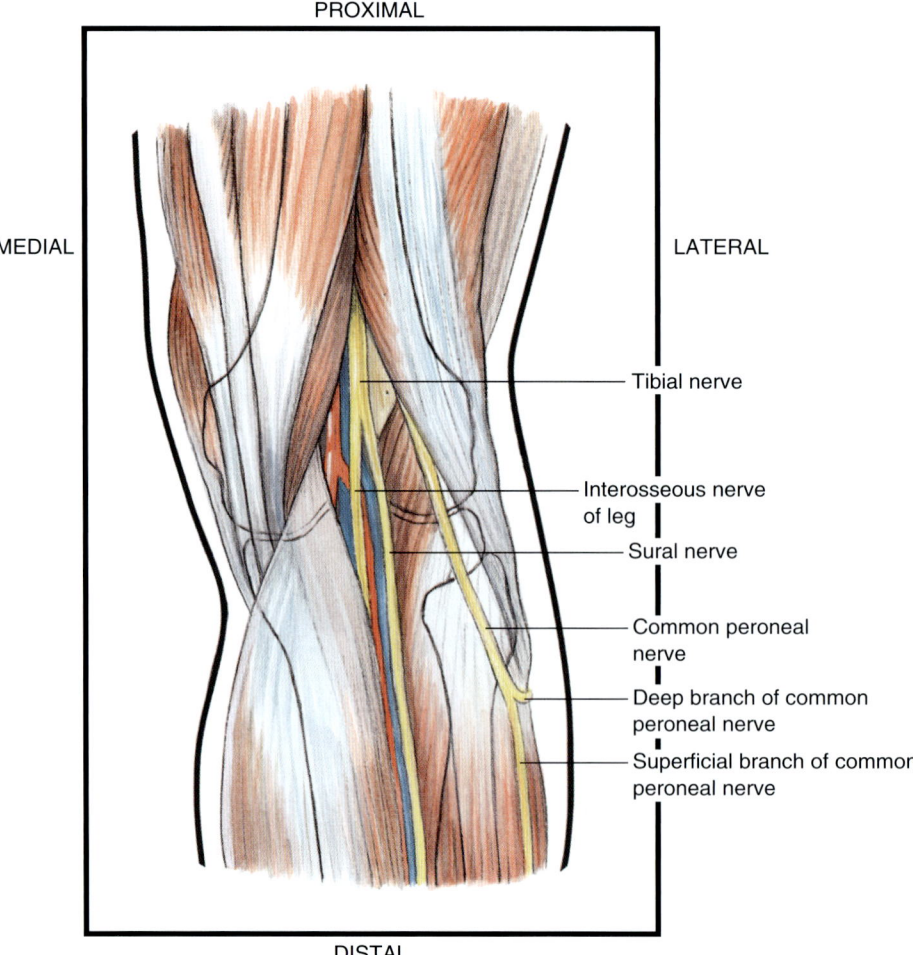

Fig. 19.2 Popliteal fossa: neural anatomy.

Popliteal and Saphenous Block 143

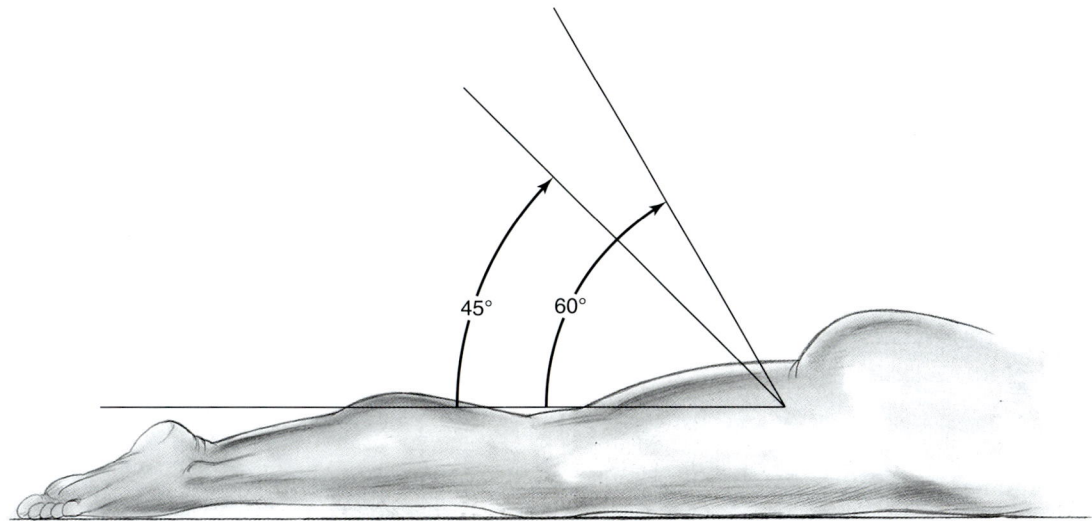

Fig. 19.3 Popliteal fossa: needle angle technique for popliteal block.

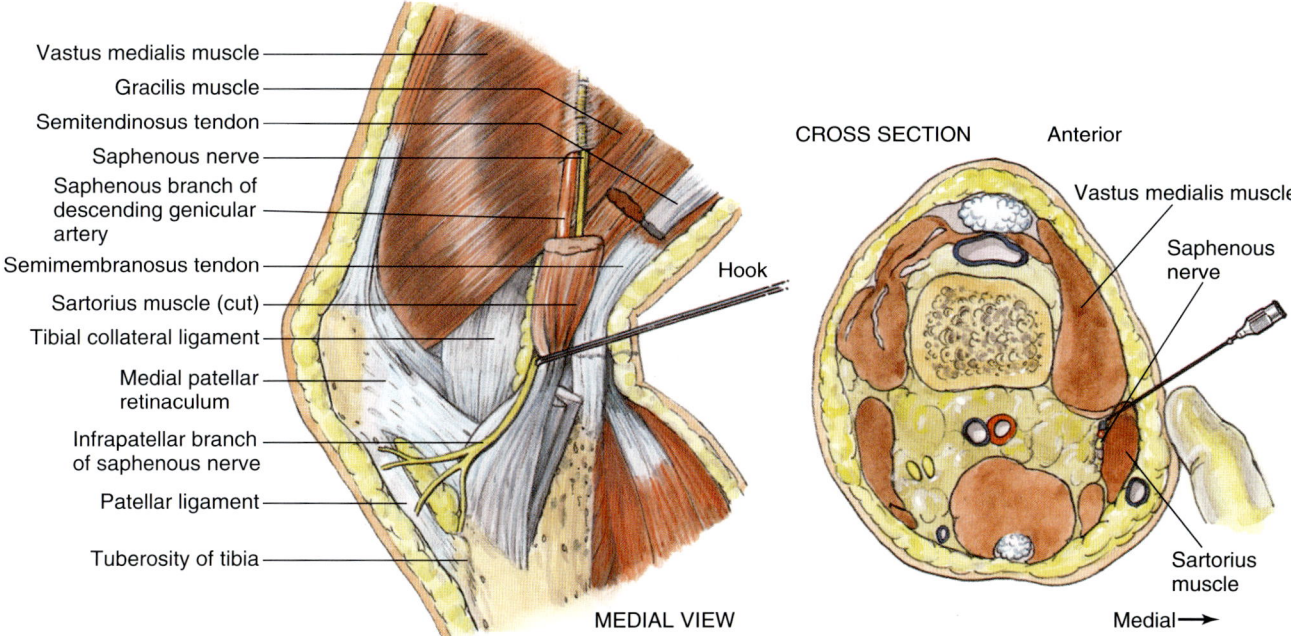

Fig. 19.4 Saphenous nerve block: anatomy and proximal technique.

ULTRASONOGRAPHY-GUIDED TECHNIQUE

SONOANATOMY

The sciatic nerve courses through the popliteal fossa where it is blocked. It is beneficial to use ultrasound for this block because the division of the sciatic nerve into posterior tibial and common peroneal nerves occurs at variable distances from the popliteal crease. The goal is to block the sciatic nerve before it divides and inject the local anesthetic within the epineurium. This allows for a more consistent blockade of both divisions and use of lower volumes of local anesthetic. The same anatomic landmarks that are used for the nerve stimulator-guided technique are also used for the ultrasound-guided block. However, with the ultrasound, the goal is to find the popliteal vessels first (Figs. 19.5 and 19.6).

INDICATIONS

The sciatic nerve block at the popliteal fossa is done when the goal is to block the distal leg and foot (S2 to S4) for the following:

- Tibia or fibula repair
- Achilles tendon repair
- Calf tourniquet pain
- Ankle and toe surgeries
- Below-the-knee amputations
- Posterior knee pain

144 ATLAS OF REGIONAL ANESTHESIA

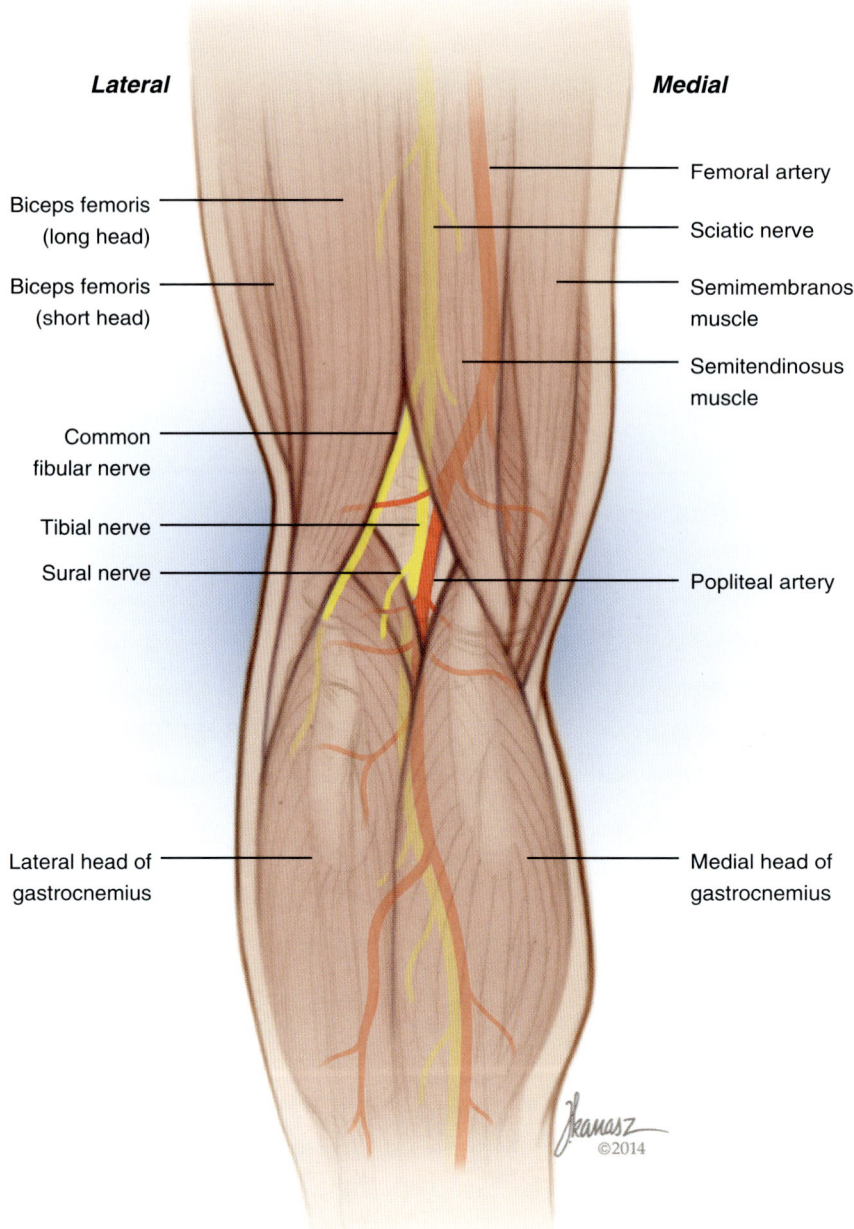

Fig. 19.5 Anatomy of the popliteal fossa.

To have full surgical anesthesia of the area below the knee, one must also block the saphenous nerve, which is the terminal branch of the femoral nerve and innervates the skin of the medial portion of the lower leg.

TECHNIQUE

The popliteal block can be done with the patient in the prone, lateral decubitus, or supine position. We find the prone position to be easiest because it allows us to easily rest and stabilize the hand that is holding the ultrasound probe on the patient's leg, once the desired image has been achieved, especially when placing a nerve catheter (Fig. 19.7). However, if the patient has a cast, external fixation device, or fracture making positioning difficult, then it may be preferable to place the patient lateral decubitus (operative site being superior and placing pillows between the knees), or supine (hip and knee are flexed with blankets serving as a footrest). Whichever approach you decide to use, the ultrasound image will be the same; it is the needle path that changes (Fig. 19.8).

After identifying the popliteal fossa, place the linear ultrasound probe, which is 8–13 MHz, in the transverse position at the crease and ensure that the left side of the screen corresponds to the lateral side of the patient (where the biceps femoris muscle will lie). Then scan medially and laterally to find the popliteal artery, which tends to be about 4 cm deep. The popliteal vein, which is a compressible hypoechoic structure, can be lateral or deep to the artery.

Popliteal and Saphenous Block

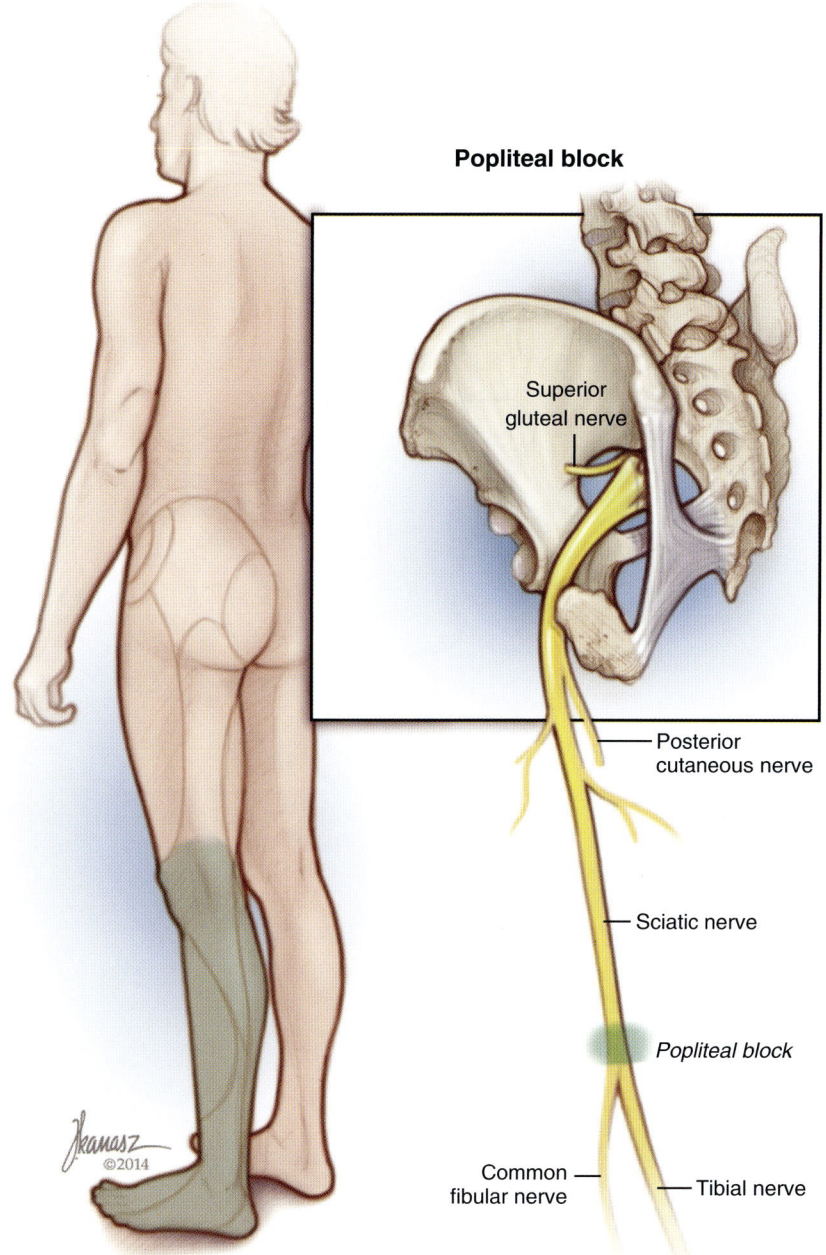

Fig. 19.6 Anatomy of the popliteal block and dermatomal coverage.

The posterior tibial nerve usually lies superficial and lateral to the artery. The posterior tibial nerve will be a hyperechoic oval with a honeycomb interior. Once the posterior tibial nerve is identified, slowly move the ultrasound probe cephalad. Adjust the probe as you scan to maintain a good view of the nerves. As you move cephalad, the popliteal artery tends to course deeper (more anteriorly) and may disappear from the ultrasound view. The common peroneal nerve, usually smaller in size than the tibial nerve, will emerge laterally and move medially to join the posterior tibial nerve until they are enveloped within a common epineural sheath. Their unity forms the sciatic nerve and usually occurs around 5 to 10 cm from the crease, but the distance varies (Fig. 19.9).

We usually prefer the in-line approach when performing this block (Figs. 19.10 to 19.12). For a single-shot nerve block, after the posterior tibial and common peroneal nerves join, we usually move the probe 1 to 2 cm more cephalad to ensure that the injected local anesthetic will surround both nerves. When placing a continuous nerve catheter, we insert a 17-gauge Tuohy needle. Once the tip is located near the 6 o'clock position in relation to the nerve, we insert the catheter through the Touhy needle and follow its trajectory by visualizing the catheter or tissue movement caused by the catheter in order to ensure that it does not migrate. Insert the catheter 5 cm beyond the tip of the Tuohy needle (Fig. 19.11). Please refer to Chapter 20 for a review of the ultrasound-guided adductor canal block.

KEY POINTS

- Use a linear transducer probe (8 to 13 MHz), starting at a depth of 4 cm.
- For a single-shot nerve block, use a 21-gauge, 4-inch or 100-mm needle (stimulating or nonstimulating).

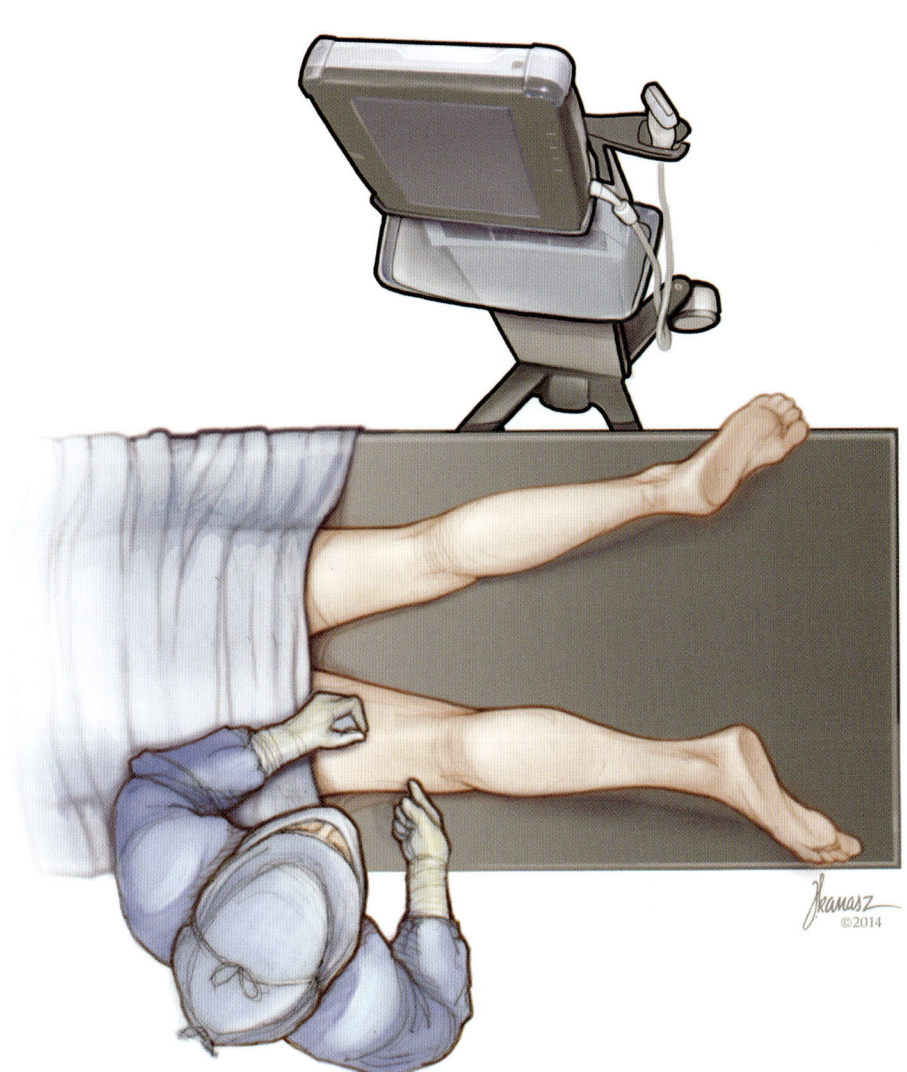

Fig. 19.7 Patient position and ultrasound machine for the popliteal block in prone position.

Popliteal and Saphenous Block 147

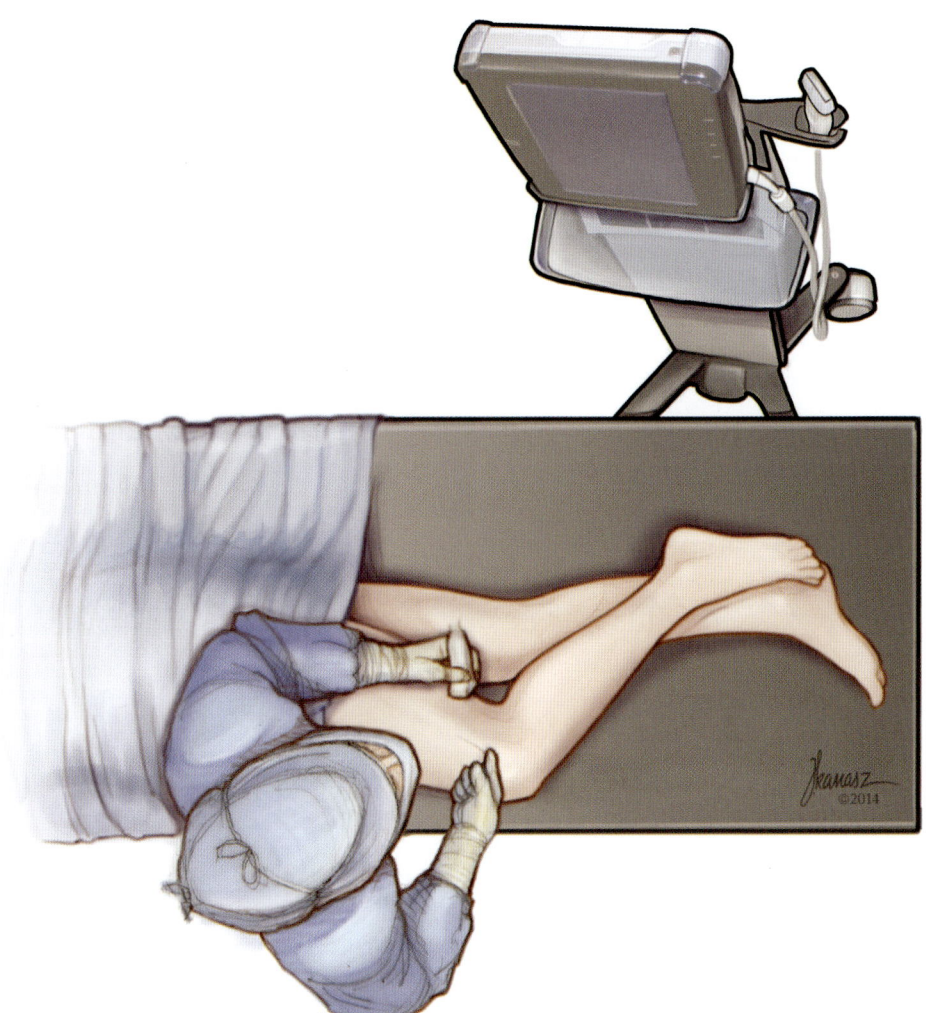

Fig. 19.8 Patient position and ultrasound machine for the popliteal block in lateral position.

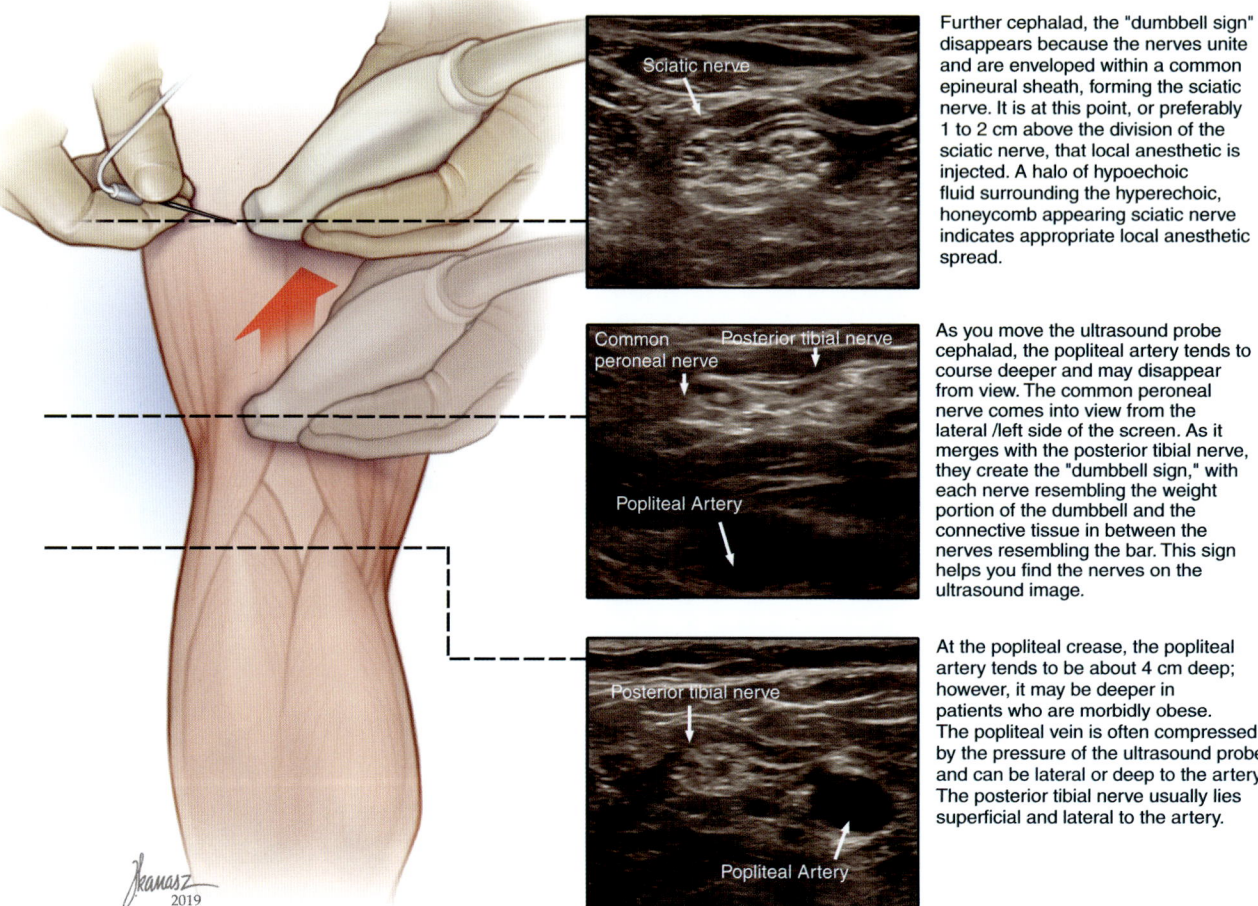

Fig. 19.9 This illustration demonstrates the movement of the ultrasound probe as you move it cephalad from the popliteal crease. Within the popliteal fossa, the popliteal artery and the sciatic nerve's two main terminal branches (posterior tibial and common peroneal nerves) are visualized. One scans proximally/cephalad until the two branches unite together to form the sciatic nerve. Note that the ultrasound probe is in the transverse position; also note the in-plane technique, with the needle directed from lateral to medial, parallel to the ultrasound probe.

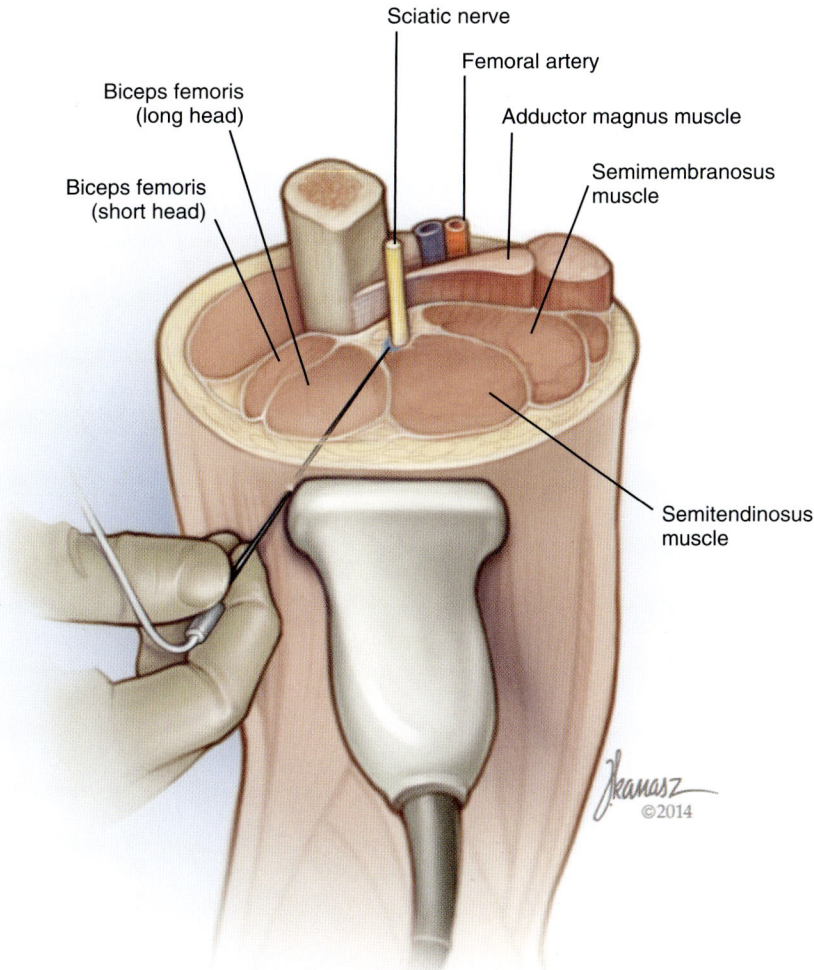

Fig. 19.10 In-plane technique for the popliteal block with needle from lateral to medial.

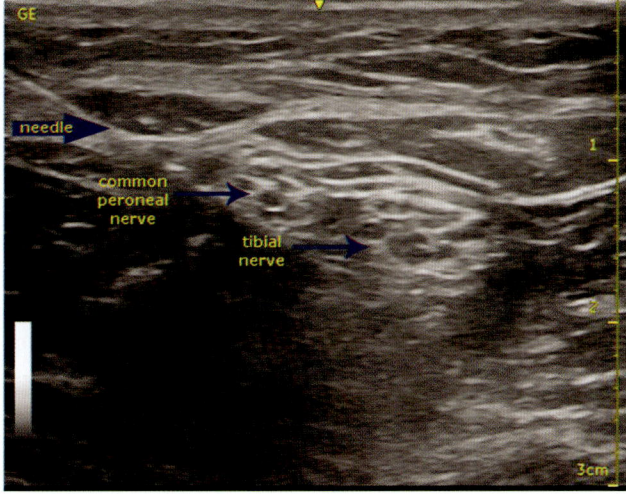

Fig. 19.11 Ultrasound still of popliteal block procedure. Note the needle is in-plane, thus visualizing the entire needle shaft.

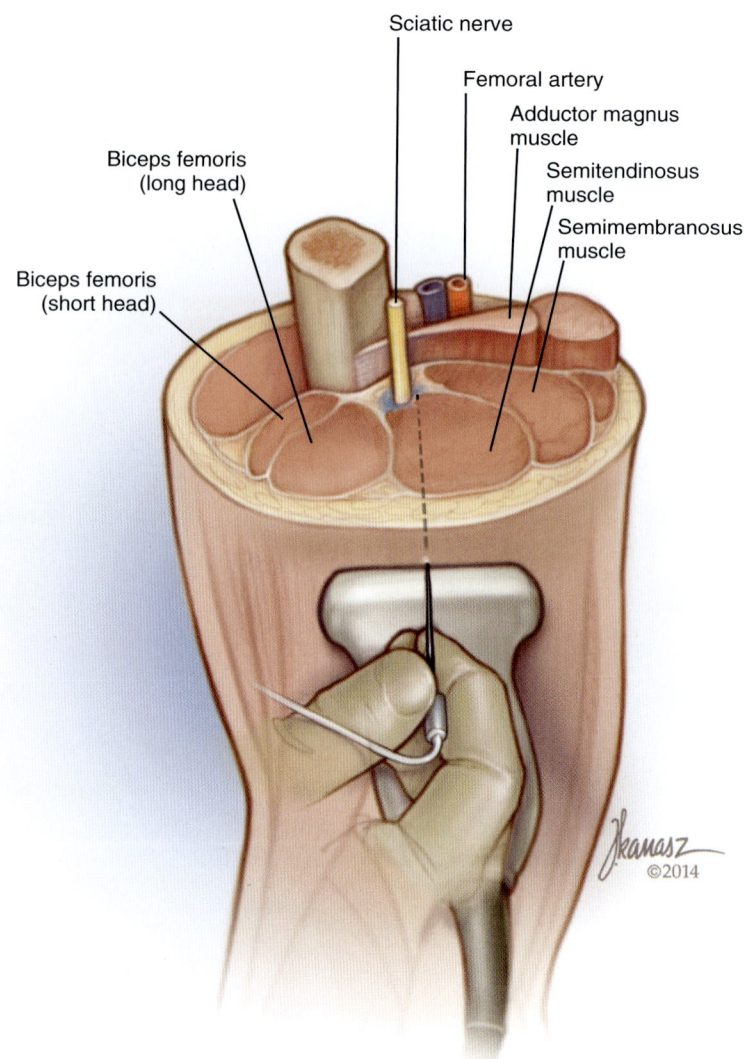

Fig. 19.12 Out-of-plane technique for popliteal block.

- For local anesthetic solution in a single shot nerve block, bupivacaine or ropivacaine 0.5% 20 mL (for ultrasound-guided approach) and 30–40 mL (for anatomic approach alone) can be used.
- For a continuous nerve block, use a 17-gauge, 3.5-inch Tuohy needle with a 20-gauge catheter (stimulating or nonstimulating). You can inject ropivacaine 0.2% or bupivacaine 0.25% 20 mL and use a bag of solution containing ropivacaine 0.2% running at 8 mL per hour with a 12-mL bolus every 60 minutes.
- Confirm local anesthetic injection within the epineurium by tracking the local anesthetic spread proximally and distally from the site of injection around the nerves.
- If you are having trouble finding the artery, use color Doppler (artery pulsates and is hypoechoic).

PEARLS

- If you are having trouble getting a good image of the nerves, try tilting the ultrasound probe caudad to ensure that the ultrasound beams are hitting the nerves at a 90-degree angle.
- As you move the probe cephalad and the nerve tracks deeper, it may be more difficult to visualize the nerve and needle tip despite various attempts at probe manipulation. In this scenario, using the combined technique of ultrasound and nerve stimulation is helpful, or try hydrodissecting with dextrose.
- Muscle tendons may be mistaken for nerves. As you track the course of the tendon cephalad, it will disappear as it turns into muscle. Nerves will stay constant. Furthermore, asking the patient to dorsiflex the ankle will make the nerves rotate or move in relation to their surroundings.

Adductor Canal Block

20

Ehab Farag

Key Points

- A high-frequency transducer is preferred for this block.
- This approach is the most effective and easiest one for saphenous nerve block.
- It can be used in lieu of femoral nerve block after total knee arthroplasty to avoid quadriceps muscle weakness.
- It can be used as a block for the saphenous nerve after surgeries in the medial side of the foot and the ankle.

SONOANATOMY

The saphenous nerve, a terminal branch of the posterior division of the femoral nerve, provides sensory innervation to the medial, anteromedial, and posteromedial aspects of the lower extremity from the distal thigh to the medial malleolus. It travels along the lateral aspect of the superficial femoral artery in the proximal artery within the adductor canal (Hunter's canal). It then crosses over the superficial femoral artery anteriorly just proximal of the lower end of the adductor magnus muscle and runs medially alongside the superficial femoral artery until emerging from the canal with the saphenous branch of the descending genicular artery. After leaving the adductor canal, the saphenous nerve divides into the infrapatellar branch, which provides a sensory branch to the peripatellar plexus of the knee, and the sartorial branch, which perforates the superficial fascia between the gracilis and sartorius muscles and emerges to lie in the subcutaneous tissue below the knee fold. It then descends along the medial tibial border with the saphenous vein giving cutaneous branches to the medial aspect of the leg, ankle, and the forefoot. The nerve to the vastus medialis is also a branch of the posterior division of the femoral nerve. It travels lateral to the superficial femoral artery within the adductor canal sending multiple branches to the vastus medialis, and supplies the anteromedial portion of the knee capsule.

The adductor canal is an aponeurotic tunnel in the middle third of the thigh. It courses between the anterior–medial compartment of the thigh and is covered by strong aponeurosis, the vastoadductor membrane. The canal contains the superficial femoral artery, vein, saphenous nerve, nerve to the vastus medialis, and the terminal nerve endings of the posterior branch of the obturator nerve.

The short-axis ultrasound image of the adductor canal at the midthigh usually shows the sartorius muscle and the saphenous nerve as a hyperechoic structure, which lies lateral to the artery and anterior to the vein. The vastus medialis muscle lies laterally to the saphenous nerve, and the adductor longus and adductor magnus muscles are on its medial side (Figs. 20.1 and 20.2).

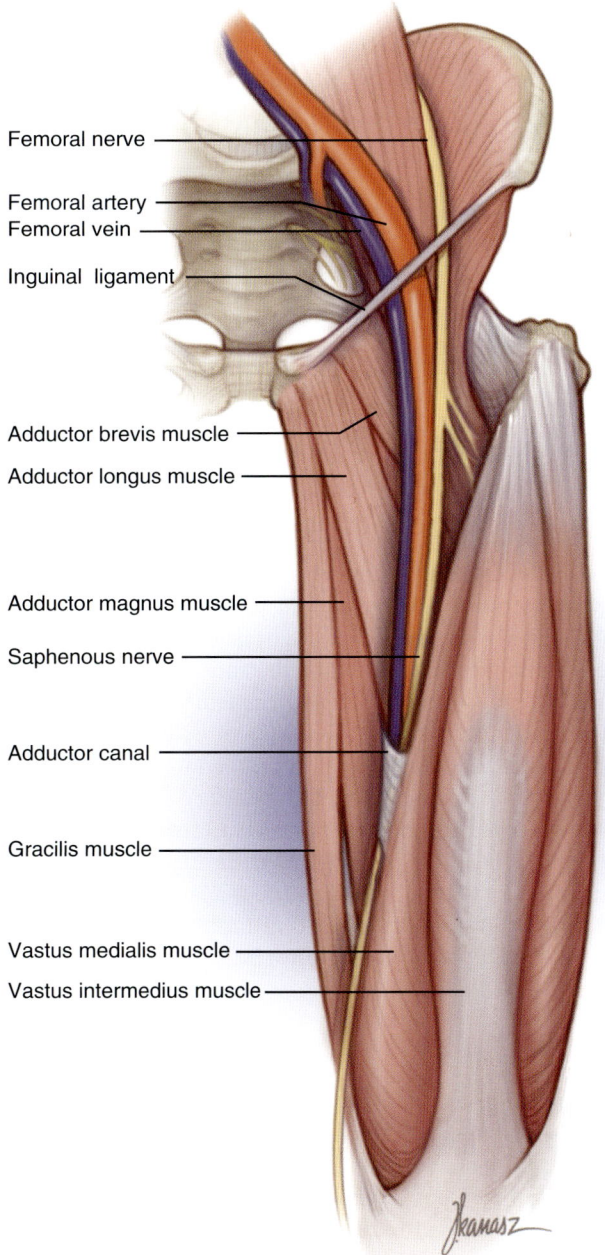

Fig. 20.1 Anatomy of the adductor canal.

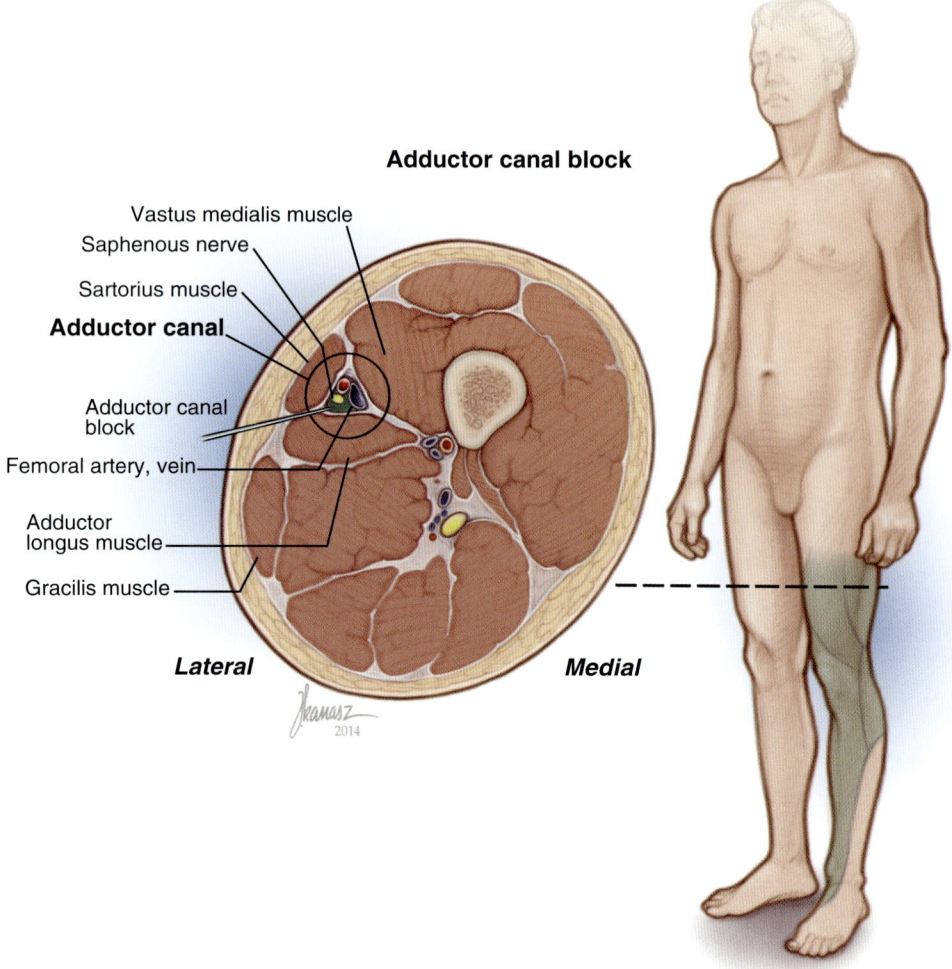

Fig. 20.2 Cross-sectional anatomy of the adductor canal.

TECHNIQUE

At the midthigh level, approximately halfway between the superoanterior iliac spine and the patella, a high-frequency linear ultrasound transducer will be placed in the transverse cross-sectional view to obtain the short-axis view of the adductor canal and its contents. The femoral artery will be identified underneath the sartorius muscle with the vein just underneath the artery. The saphenous nerve usually appears at this position lateral to the artery as a hyperechoic structure. The block needle is usually inserted in-plane from the lateral side of the transducer, through the sartorius muscle, with the tip of the needle placed lateral to the artery. After careful aspiration, 20 mL of local anesthetic will be injected lateral to the artery (Figs. 20.3 through 20.6).

PEARLS

- This block is very useful as an alternative to the femoral nerve block after total knee arthroplasty to avoid quadriceps weakness. However, an injection of a high volume of local anesthetic in the adductor canal can spread as far as the anterior and posterior divisions of the femoral nerve to induce quadriceps weakness. Moreover, it has been demonstrated that there is no boundary between the apex of the femoral triangle and the adductor canal.
- The saphenous nerve block via the adductor canal approach can be successfully used to block the medial sides of the foot and the ankle after foot and ankle surgeries, either as a solo block or in addition to the popliteal nerve block.
- In morbidly obese patients, it can be difficult to identify the adductor canal and the femoral artery at the midthigh level. Therefore we usually identify the femoral artery at the inguinal crease and follow it distally into the adductor canal.
- The combination of vastoadductor membrane and vessel sheaths within the adductor canal can appear as hyperechoic structures resembling the saphenous nerve during ultrasound imaging. However, placing the needle tip through the vastoadductor membrane, within the adductor canal, may result in the successful localization of the saphenous nerve.
- For catheter insertion, with the Tuohy needle placed just lateral to the artery and the saphenous nerve, the catheter will be inserted 5–8 cm through the needle. To correctly position the catheter tip, the catheter will be slowly withdrawn while injecting 10 mL of normal saline under ultrasound guidance, until an

Adductor Canal Block

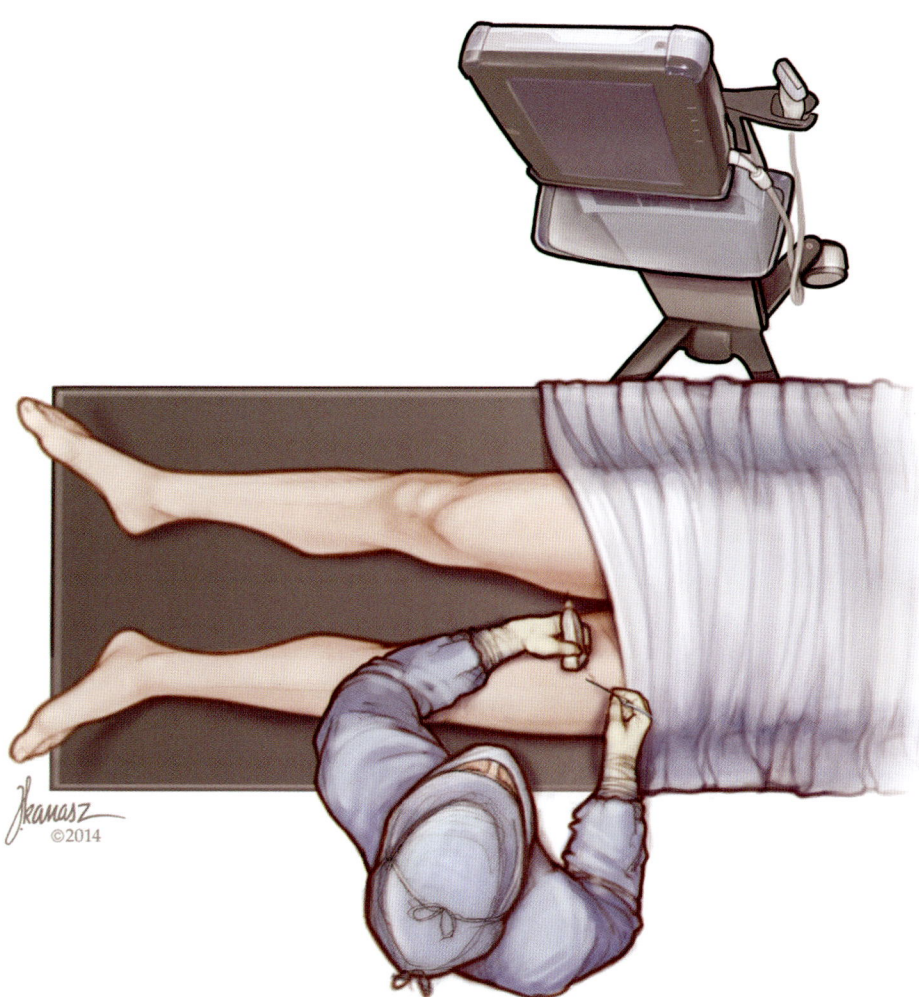

Fig. 20.3 Position for the patient and the ultrasound machine.

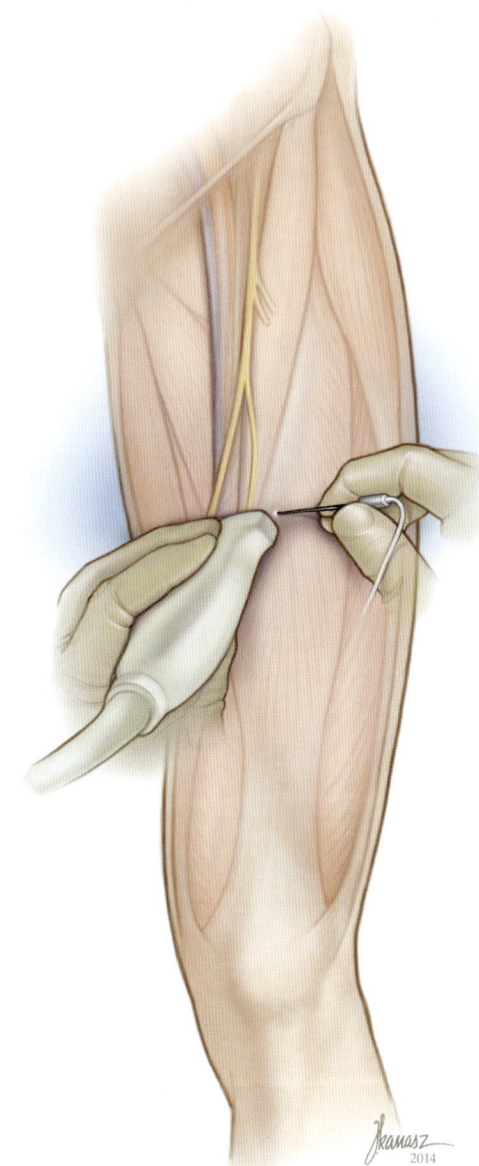

Fig. 20.4 In-plane technique with needle direction from lateral to medial.

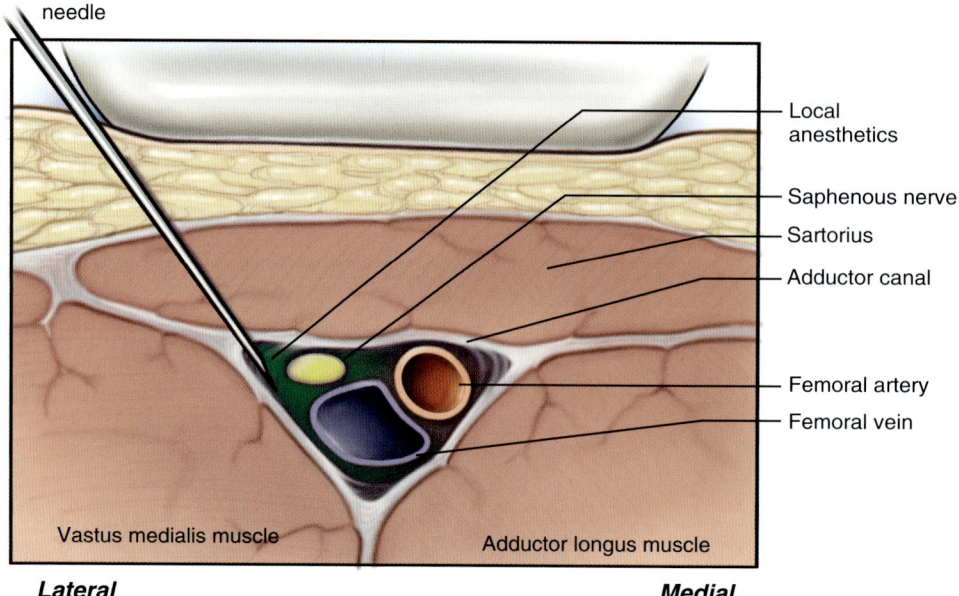

Fig. 20.5 Position of the needle with local anesthetic in the adductor canal. Note there should be separation of the artery from the fascia by the local anesthetic.

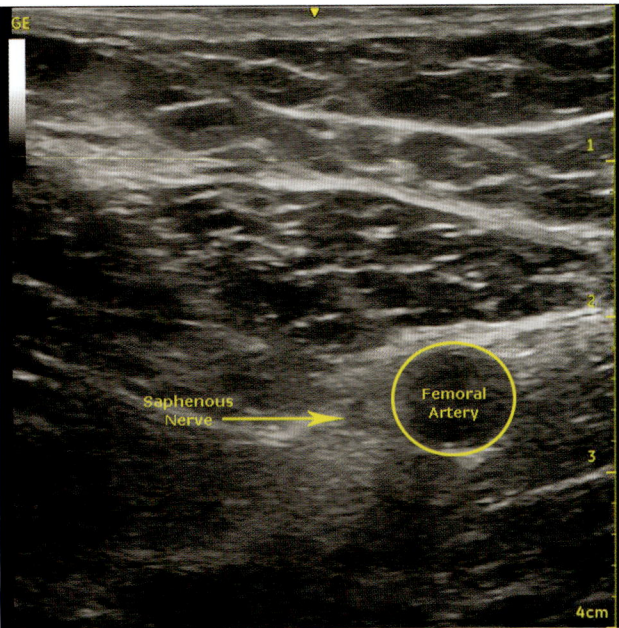

Fig. 20.6 Ultrasound image of adductor canal.

expansion between the fascia that separates the sartorius muscle from the adductor canal and the vessels is visualized. After negative aspiration for blood through the catheter, the local anesthetic can be injected.

- Because the femoral artery lies above the vein in the adductor canal, the author usually applies firm pressure with the ultrasound transducer to occlude the vein for better nerve visualization and to decrease the incidence of inadvertent vascular injection.

Ankle Block 21

Maria Yared and David L. Brown

PERSPECTIVE

This block is often used for surgical procedures carried out on the foot, especially for those not requiring high lower-leg tourniquet pressure.

Patient Selection. The ankle block is principally an infiltration block and does not require elicitation of paresthesia. Thus patient cooperation is not mandatory. Although the block is most efficient for the anesthesiologist if the patient can assume both the prone and supine positions, this is not essential.

Pharmacologic Choice. Because motor blockade is not often needed for procedures carried out during ankle block, lower concentrations of local anesthetics may be used. Practical choices are 1% lidocaine, 1% mepivacaine, 0.25%–0.5% bupivacaine, and 0.2%–0.5% ropivacaine. Many physicians suggest that epinephrine not be used during ankle block, especially if injection is circumferential.

TRADITIONAL BLOCK TECHNIQUE

PLACEMENT

Anatomy. The peripheral nerves requiring block are derived from the sciatic nerve, with the exception of a terminal branch of the femoral nerve—the saphenous nerve. The saphenous nerve is the only branch of the femoral nerve below the knee; it courses superficially anterior to the medial malleolus, providing cutaneous innervation to an area of the medial ankle and foot. The remaining nerves requiring block at the ankle are terminal branches of the sciatic nerve—the common peroneal and tibial nerves. The tibial nerve divides into the posterior tibial and sural nerves, which provide cutaneous innervation as outlined in Figs. 21.1 and 21.2. The common peroneal nerve divides into its terminal branches—the superficial and deep peroneal nerves—in the proximal portion of the lower leg. Their cutaneous innervation is also illustrated in Fig. 21.2. Fig. 21.3 identifies the locations of these nerves in a cross-sectional view at the level of ankle block.

Needle Puncture: General. It is often helpful (although not necessary) to have the patient in the prone position initially to facilitate block of the posterior tibial and sural nerves. Once these two nerves have been blocked, the patient assumes the supine position so that block of the saphenous and peroneal nerves can be carried out. The block can be performed with the patient in the supine position if the lower leg is placed on a padded support, and this position facilitates appropriate intravenous sedation.

Needle Puncture: Posterior Tibial Nerve. With the patient in the prone position, the ankle to be blocked is supported on a pillow. A 22-gauge, 4-cm needle is directed anteriorly at the cephalad border of the medial malleolus, just medial to the Achilles tendon, as shown in Fig. 21.3. The needle is inserted near the posterior tibial artery, and if paresthesia is obtained, 3–5 mL of local anesthetic is injected. If paresthesia is not obtained, the needle is allowed to contact the medial malleolus, and 5–7 mL of local anesthetic is deposited near the posterior tibial artery.

Needle Puncture: Sural Nerve. The sural nerve is blocked with the patient positioned as for the posterior tibial nerve block. As illustrated in Fig. 21.3, the sural nerve is blocked by inserting a 22-gauge, 4-cm needle anterolaterally immediately lateral to the Achilles tendon at the cephalad border of the lateral malleolus. The sural nerve (lateral ankle) is found in a more superficial position relative to the malleolus than is the tibial nerve (medial ankle). If paresthesia is not obtained, the needle is allowed to contact the lateral malleolus, and 5–7 mL of local anesthetic is injected as the needle is withdrawn.

Needle Puncture: Deep Peroneal, Superficial Peroneal, and Saphenous Nerves. After the patient assumes the supine position, the anterior tibial artery pulsation is located at the superior level of the malleoli. A 22-gauge, 4-cm needle is advanced posteriorly and immediately lateral to this point (see Figs. 21.3 and 21.4). An alternative is to insert the needle between the tendons of the anterior tibial and the extensor hallucis longus muscles. Approximately 5 mL of local anesthetic is injected into this area to block the deep peroneal nerve. From this midline skin wheal, a 22-gauge, 8-cm needle is advanced subcutaneously laterally and medially to the malleoli, injecting 3–5 mL of local anesthetic in each direction. These lateral and medial approaches block the superficial peroneal and saphenous nerves, respectively.

158 ATLAS OF REGIONAL ANESTHESIA

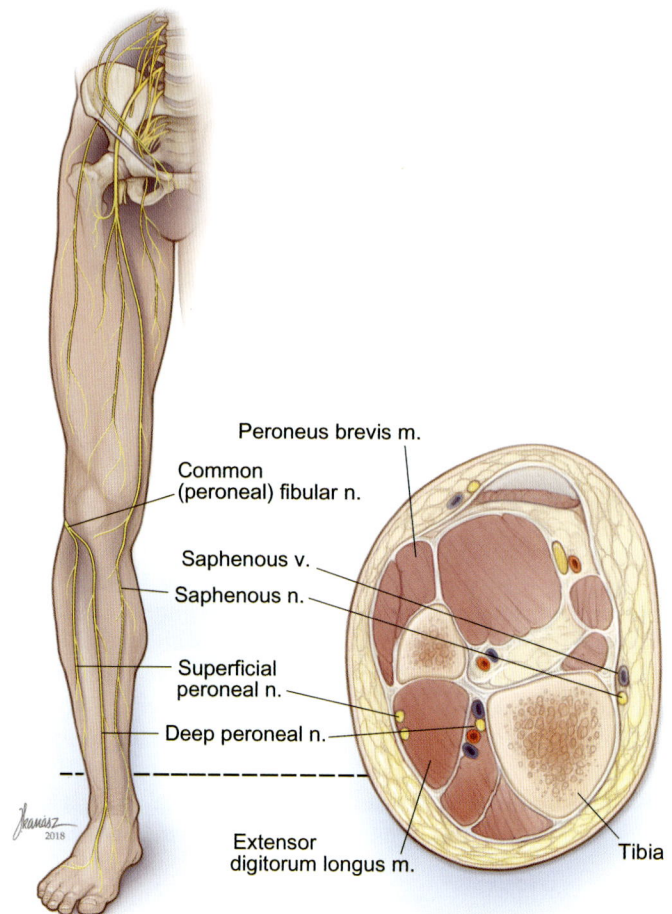

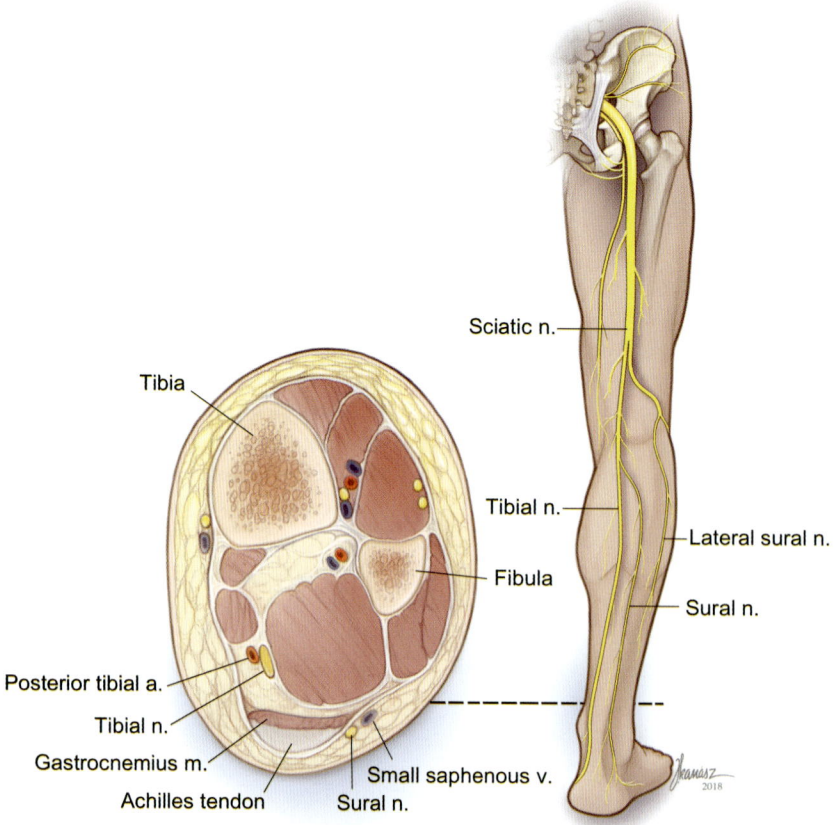

Fig. 21.1 Image of the anterior and posterior leg showing the course of the nerves as well as a cross section of the leg showing the location of the nerves in relationship to arteries, veins, muscles, and bones. The tibia is medial and anterior, and the fibula is lateral.

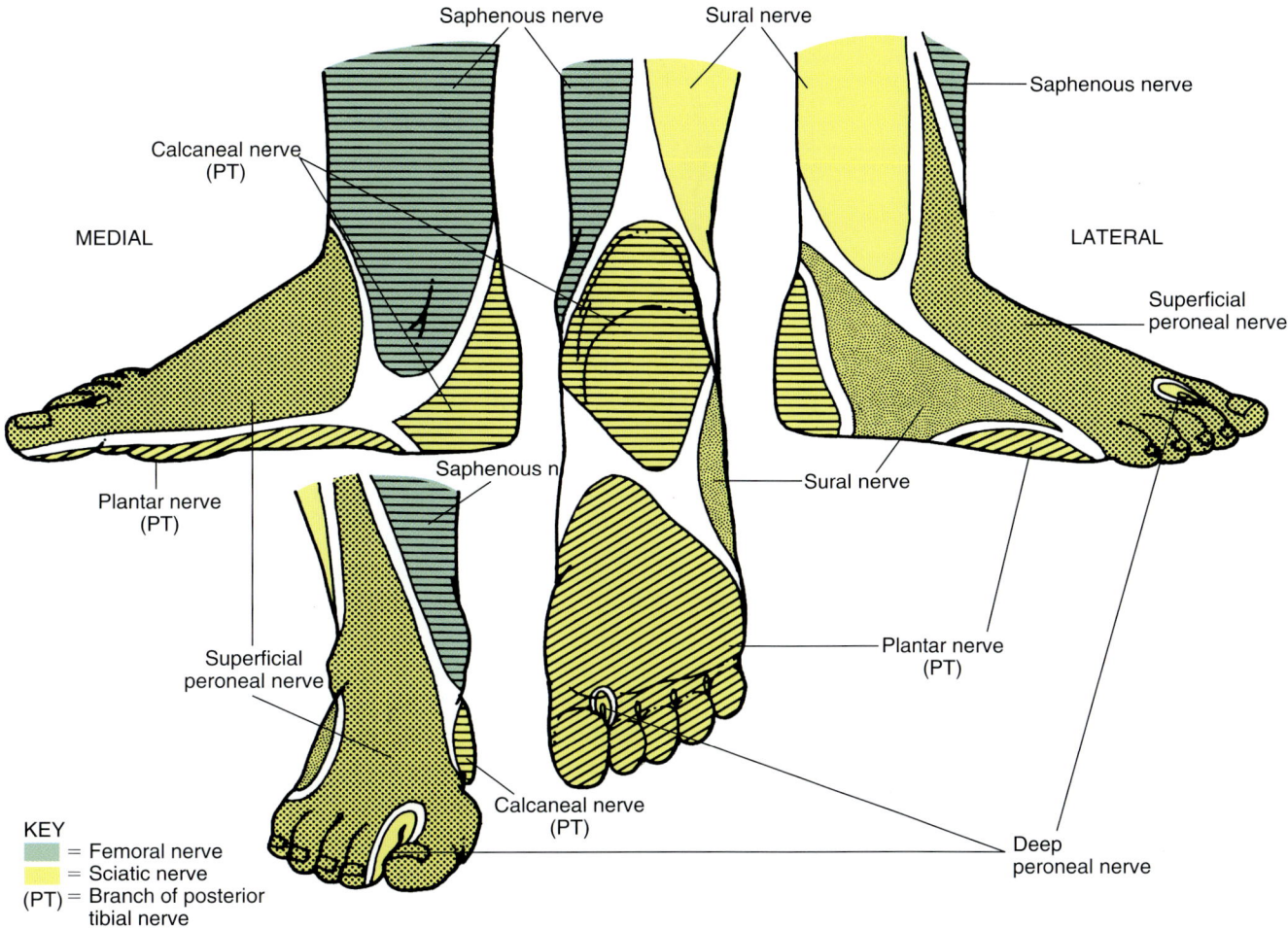

Fig. 21.2 Ankle block: peripheral innervation.

ULTRASONOGRAPHY-GUIDED TECHNIQUE

SONOANATOMY

Ankle blocks have a variable success rate because of the variable positions of the nerves and multiple branches of the superficial nerves. The tibial and deep peroneal nerves supply deep structures of the foot and therefore must be blocked beneath the deep fascia of the ankle. Under ultrasound guidance, these two nerves are hyperechoic but small and may be difficult to visualize or distinguish from tendons; thus identifying the associated artery or muscle is beneficial. The recommendation is to block these first since subcutaneous injection of the superficial nerves can change the appearance of structures under ultrasound. The remaining nerves supply sensory innervation to the skin and can be blocked superficially by making a circular wheal from the lateral Achilles tendon to the medial Achilles tendon. As a reminder, the distal end of the tibia forms the medial malleolus while the distal end of the fibula forms the lateral malleolus of the ankle.

INDICATIONS

- Toe and metatarsal foot surgeries (amputation, debridement, podiatric surgery) that do not require calf tourniquet pressure.
- It does not block the ankle itself.
- Preserves motor function of the leg thus not impacting postoperative ambulation.

TECHNIQUE

The ankle block can be done using anatomical landmarks as described earlier in the chapter and/or under ultrasound guidance. There are five nerves to the ankle, two that are deep beneath the fascia of the ankle—tibial and deep peroneal nerves—and three superficial ones—sural, saphenous, and superficial peroneal nerves. If the superficial/sensory nerves are difficult to visualize under ultrasound, which is not uncommon, block them subcutaneously, making a skin wheal, using anatomic landmarks.

When performing the ankle block under ultrasound, the patient can be positioned supine with a footrest or pillow under the calf. While performing the block, the leg may need to be rotated internally or externally as needed depending on the nerve being blocked. It may be efficient for the proceduralist to walk around the foot as the block is performed. The entire foot should be cleaned and a linear transducer used. The needle can be in-plane or out-of-plane depending on the patient's position. These nerves are so small that injecting 3–5 mL of local anesthetic per nerve is usually effective.

Tibial Nerve This is the largest of the five nerves at the level of the ankle. Because of its extensive coverage, a successful

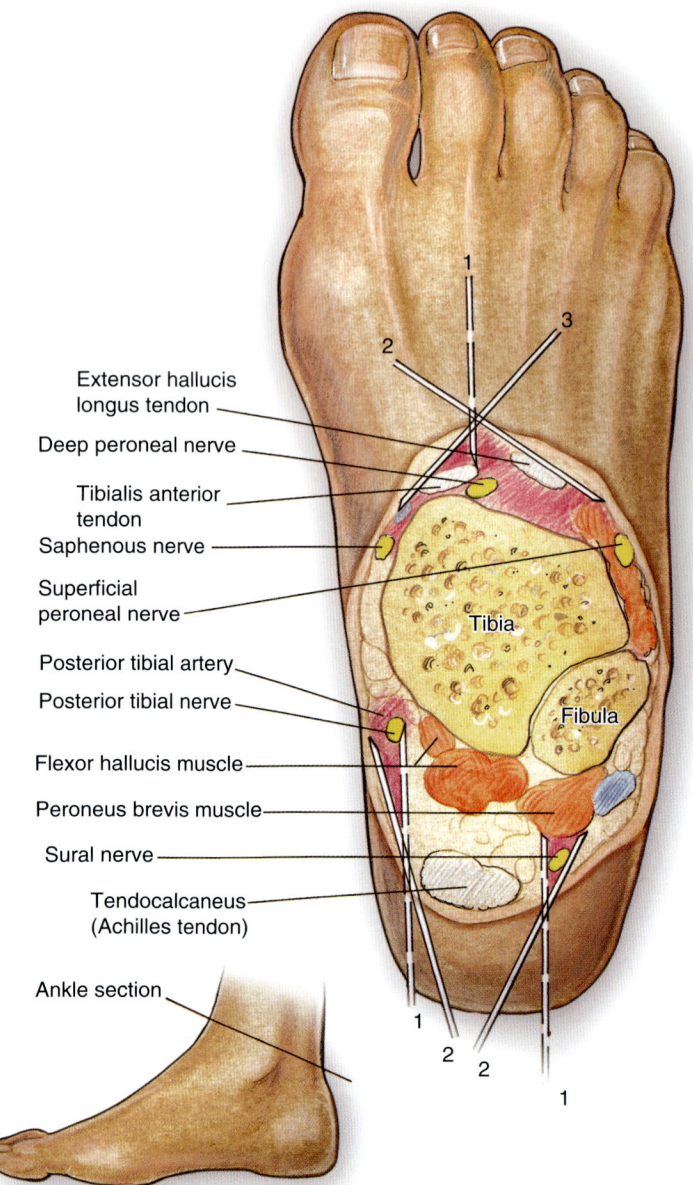

Fig. 21.3 Ankle block: cross-sectional anatomy and technique.

block of this nerve is essential for surgical anesthesia of the foot; using a combination of anatomic landmarks, ultrasound, and neurostimulation (note plantarflexion of the toes) will maximize the chance of a successful block.

To block this nerve, the foot may need to be externally rotated. A linear ultrasound transducer (high frequency 10–15 MHz) is placed transversely just proximal/cephalad to the medial malleolus. Behind the medial malleolus, identify the posterior tibial artery (with or without help of color Doppler), and the nerve is posterior to the artery, about halfway between the medial malleolus and the Achilles tendon (Fig. 21.5). The nerve is hyperechoic with a honeycomb pattern. The tibialis posterior tendon, flexor digitorum longus tendon, and flexor hallucis longus tendon are also in the vicinity and can be distinguished from the nerve by tracking the tendons and seeing them turn into a muscle; they also move with ankle flexion.

Deep Peroneal Nerve
The deep peroneal nerve is a branch of the common peroneal nerve; it innervates the ankle extensor muscles, the ankle joint, and the web space between the first and second toes. The linear ultrasound transducer probe is placed transversely/horizontally at the intermalleolar level of the ankle across the anterior surface of the tibia and extensor retinaculum. The nerve is on the surface of the tibia and lateral to the dorsalis pedis artery (also referred to as the anterior tibial artery) the majority of the time, although occasionally it is located medial to it (Fig. 21.6). It is a small nerve and may be difficult to identify; thus local anesthetic injection around the artery may create enough contrast to make the nerve visible. Another landmark is created when dorsiflexing the toes. Local anesthetic is injected, 2–4 mL, on both sides of the artery. From this landmark on the tibia, the needle can be advanced laterally towards the lateral malleolus to block the superficial peroneal nerve and then advanced medially towards the medial malleolus to block the saphenous nerve; as the needle is moved, it should stay at the level of the ankle, making an imaginary horizontal line across the upper borders of both malleoli, while avoiding the great saphenous vein.

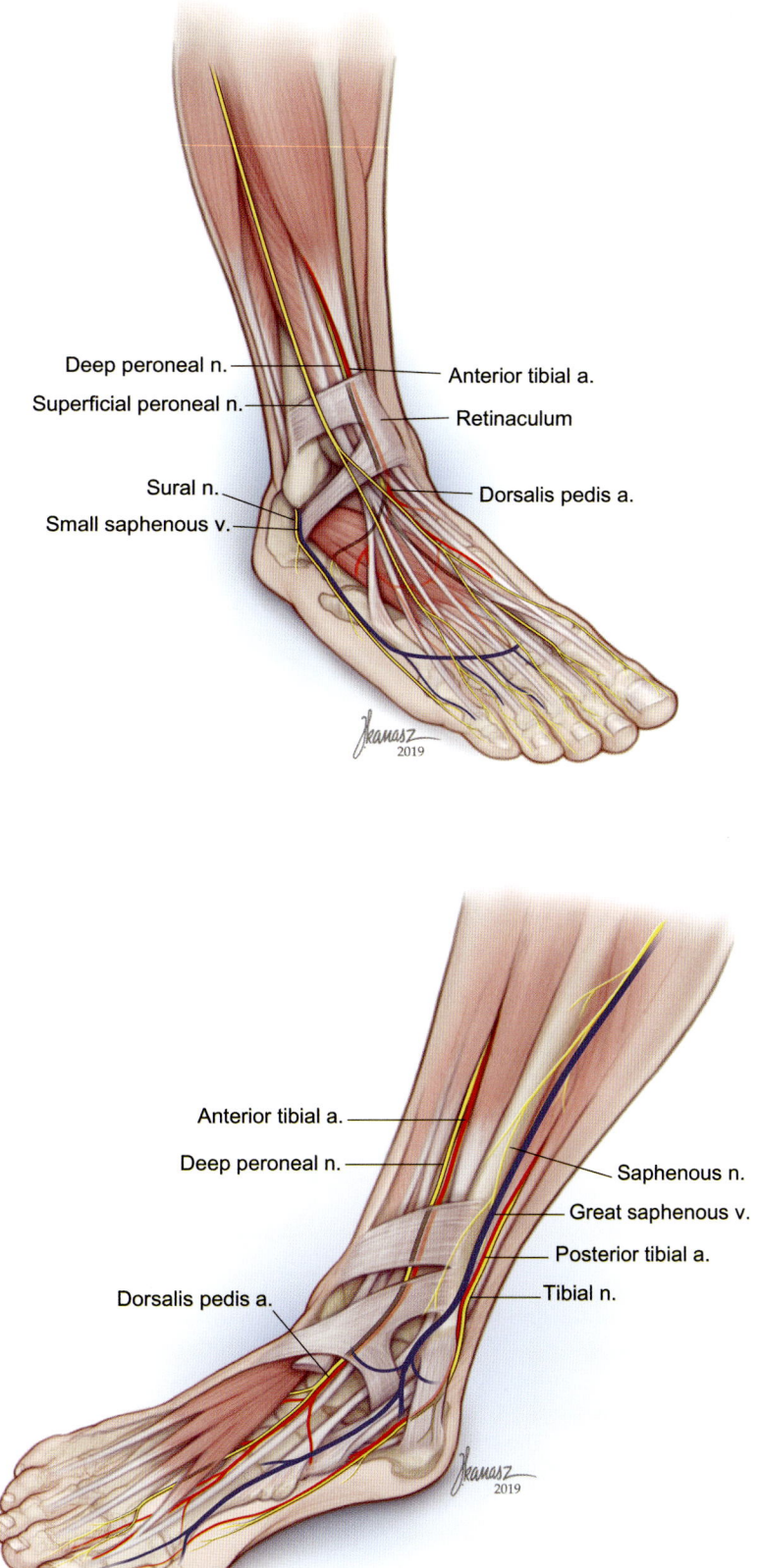

Fig. 21.4 Image of the lateral and medial ankle showing the course of the nerves in relationship to arteries and veins.

Superficial Peroneal Nerve Under ultrasound guidance, the linear transducer probe is placed transversely on the lower leg 5–10 cm above the lateral malleolus. Although this nerve is hyperechoic, it is small and may have already branched and be difficult to see in the subcutaneous tissue superficial to the fascia. Thus the probe may have to be moved cephalad, 10–20 cm from the ankle along the anterolateral surface of the leg, to find the nerve prior to its division into branches. The superficial peroneal nerve can be visualized in the intermuscular septal groove created

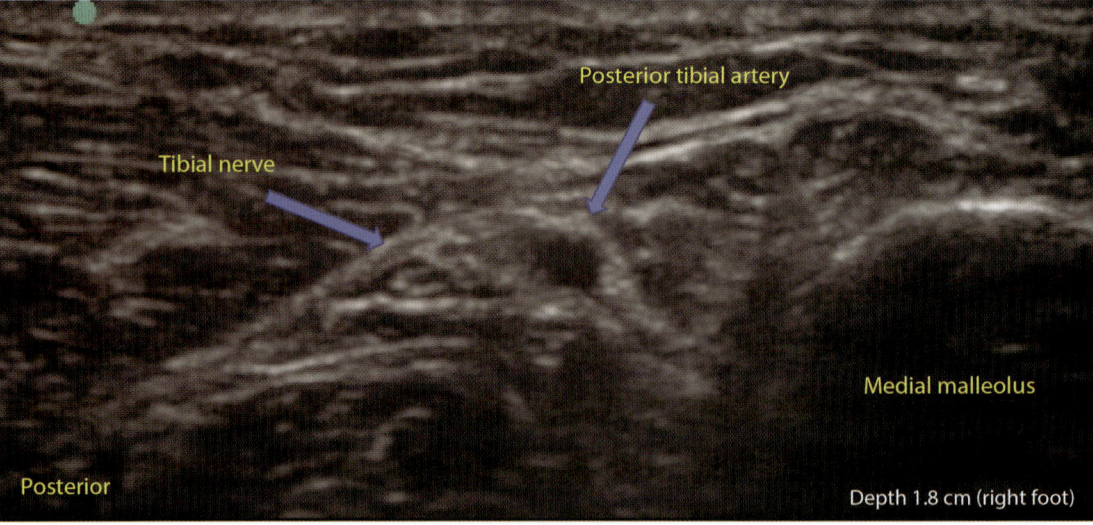

Fig. 21.5 Ultrasound still of the tibial nerve and surrounding anatomy.

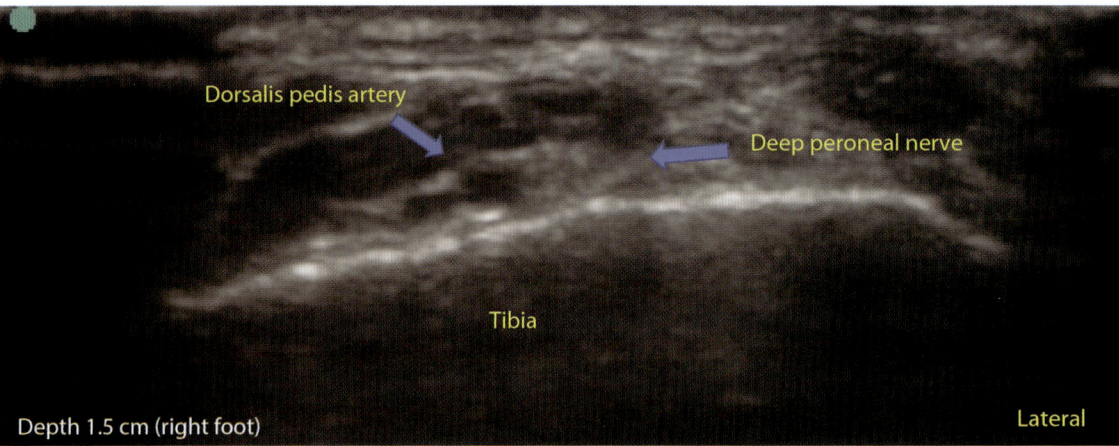

Fig. 21.6 Ultrasound still of the deep peroneal nerve and surrounding anatomy.

by the extensor digitorum longus and peroneus brevis muscle (Fig. 21.7). At this level, the nerve is now deep to the fascia but lying above the muscles. The nerve can be blocked at this level or traced back distally and blocked at the ankle.

Saphenous Nerve Again the linear transducer probe is placed transversely on the lower leg. The saphenous nerve is best seen 10–15 cm cephalad and anterior to the medial malleolus. It can be tracked, traveling down the medial leg with the great saphenous vein. A calf tourniquet can help increase the size of the vein. The nerve is anterior to the saphenous vein and superficial to the medial malleolus (Fig. 21.8).

Sural Nerve The linear transducer probe is placed just cephalad to the lateral malleolus and the nerve is near the small saphenous vein, which can be easily compressed/collapsed by the pressure exerted on the transducer by the proceduralist. The nerve is between the superior border of the lateral malleolus and the Achilles tendon (Fig. 21.9). If needed, the nerve can be traced along the posterior aspect of the leg, midline, and superficial to the gastrocnemius muscles. A calf tourniquet can also help increase the size of the vein.

KEY POINTS

- Use a linear transducer probe (8–18 MHz), starting at a depth of 2 cm.
- Use a 22- to 25-gauge, 4-inch or 100-mm needle (stimulating or nonstimulating) and 10 mL syringes to ease injection effort.
- Either bupivacaine or ropivacaine 0.5% 20–30 mL without epinephrine may be used. Avoid epinephrine since circumferential injections might cause vasoconstriction and ischemia.
- Three 10-mL syringes are needed to block all five nerves, injecting about 5 mL per nerve.
- Low risk of systemic complications. However, patient may have residual paresthesias. Small nerves are more sensitive to intraneural injections. Preferable not to repeat deep nerve injections.
- Bleeding risk is mainly from the greater saphenous vein located at the level of the medial malleolus.
- This block should not be chosen if high tourniquet pressures are required to carry out the surgical procedure.

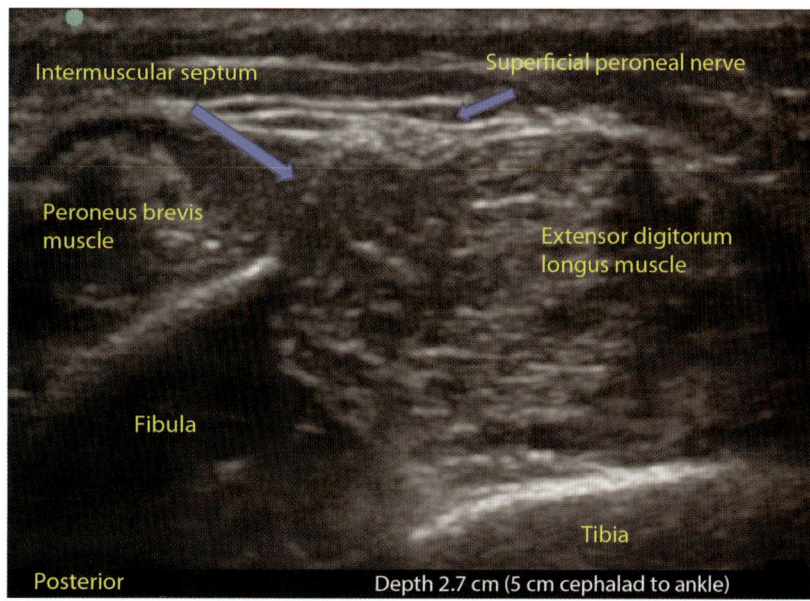

Fig. 21.7 Ultrasound still of the superficial peroneal nerve and surrounding anatomy.

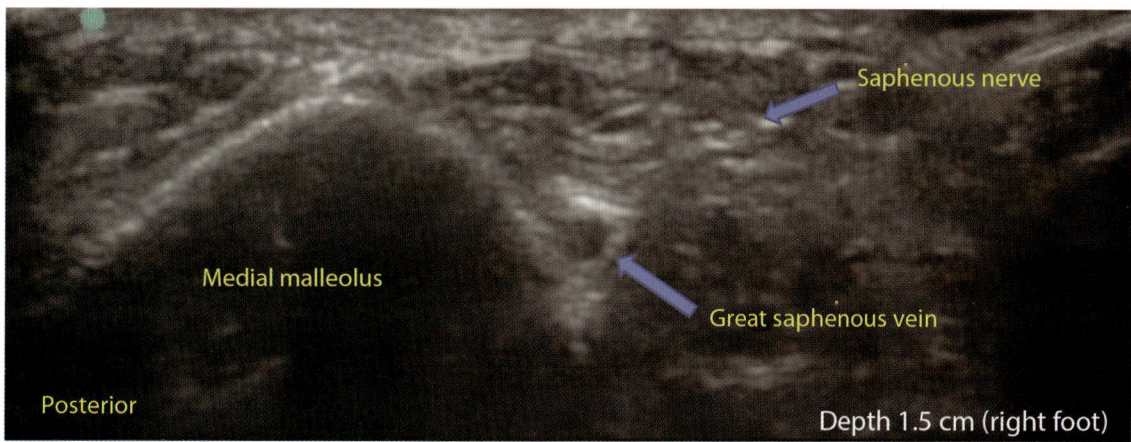

Fig. 21.8 Ultrasound still of the saphenous nerve and surrounding anatomy.

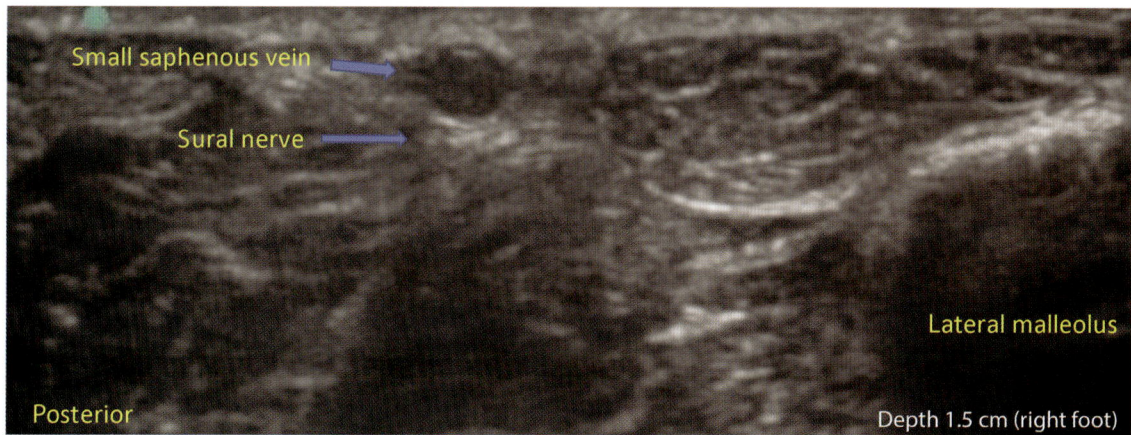

Fig. 21.9 Ultrasound still of the sural nerve and surrounding anatomy.

PEARLS

- Patients should be adequately sedated during this block because it is primarily a "volume" block requiring several different needle insertions and superficial injection of local anesthetic, which can be uncomfortable. An alert patient is not essential for the block.
- When injecting local anesthetic to block superficial nerves, make sure to see a wheal to ensure that the needle is in the correct superficial plane.
- Both the posterior tibial and deep peroneal nerves are deep to fascia.
- When used for outpatient foot surgery, ankle block allows most patients to walk with assistance, thus facilitating earlier discharge from the surgery center.

SECTION 4
Head and Neck Blocks

Retrobulbar (Peribulbar) Block

22

David L. Brown

KEY POINTS

- The most common complication of the retrobulbar block is hematoma formation, which can be minimized by using a needle shorter than 31 mm or performing a peribulbar approach.
- Sudden apnea may happen secondary to unexpected spinal anesthesia—related to injection within the optic nerve sheath.
- Additional block of the facial nerve is essential to produce an immobile eye by blocking the orbicularis oculi muscle.

PERSPECTIVE

This block is performed more often by ophthalmologists than by anesthesiologists. The combination of retrobulbar anesthesia and block of the orbicularis oculi muscle allows most intraocular surgery to be performed. This regional block is most useful for corneal, anterior chamber, and lens procedures.

Patient Selection. Patients who require retrobulbar (peribulbar) anesthesia are principally older patients who are undergoing ophthalmic operations.

Pharmacologic Choice. If retrobulbar block is used, 2–4 mL of local anesthetic is all that is required to produce adequate retrobulbar anesthesia. Conversely, if the peribulbar approach is chosen (i.e., the needle tip is not purposely inserted through the cone of extraocular muscles), slightly larger volumes—4–6 mL—may be necessary. Almost any of the local anesthetic agents are applicable, with many ophthalmic anesthetists using combinations of bupivacaine and lidocaine.

PLACEMENT

Anatomy. Sensation to the eye is provided by the ophthalmic nerve through the long and short posterior ciliary nerves. Autonomic innervation is provided by the same nerves, and sympathetic fibers traveling with the arteries and parasympathetic fibers carried by the inferior branch of the oculomotor nerve provide additional autonomic innervation. Because the innervation of the orbicularis oculi muscle is through the facial nerve, blockade of these fibers is required to ensure a quiet eye during ophthalmic operations. The ciliary ganglion, measuring approximately 2–3 mm in length, lies deep in the orbit just lateral to the optic nerve and medial to the lateral rectus muscle. From this ganglion, the long and short ciliary nerves extend forward in the orbit. Immediately posterior to the ciliary ganglion, the ophthalmic artery can be found at the lateral side of the optic nerve as it crosses superior to it and passes forward medially (Fig. 22.1).

Position. Patients are placed in the supine position and are instructed to maintain their primary gaze directly ahead, not "up and in" as in earlier recommendations. With the globe in primary gaze, the optic nerve position minimizes potential intraneural injection. The anesthesiologist is positioned for the injection as illustrated in Fig. 22.2.

Needle Puncture. While the patient's gaze is directed cephalad and opposite to the site of injection, a 27-gauge, 31-mm, sharp-beveled needle is inserted at the inferolateral border of the bony orbit and directed toward the apex of the orbit, as illustrated in Fig. 22.3. The needle should be oriented so that the bevel opening faces toward the globe. A "pop" may be appreciated as the needle tip traverses the bulbar fascia and enters the orbital muscle cone. Before 2–4 mL of local anesthetic is injected, careful needle aspiration should be carried out. After retrobulbar block, 5–10 minutes should be allowed to pass before the operation is started. This helps avoid operating on patients who develop retrobulbar hematomas. During these 5–10 minutes, the anesthesiologist can apply gentle pressure to the globe, principally to facilitate lowering the intraocular pressure. If a peribulbar technique is chosen, needle insertion begins like that used for retrobulbar (inferotemporal) injection; however, the operator inserts the needle parallel and lateral to the lateral rectus muscle and bulbar fascia rather than making an effort to puncture it. Many practitioners also now suggest making a second injection of 3–5 mL for a peribulbar block either in the superomedial orbit or at the extreme medial side of the palpebral fissure. To complete the local block for ocular surgery, the orbicularis oculi muscle must be blocked to produce an immobile eye. This is carried out by blocking the facial nerve fibers that innervate the muscle.

There are many ways of performing blocks of these facial nerve fibers, and the method illustrated in Fig. 22.4 is the

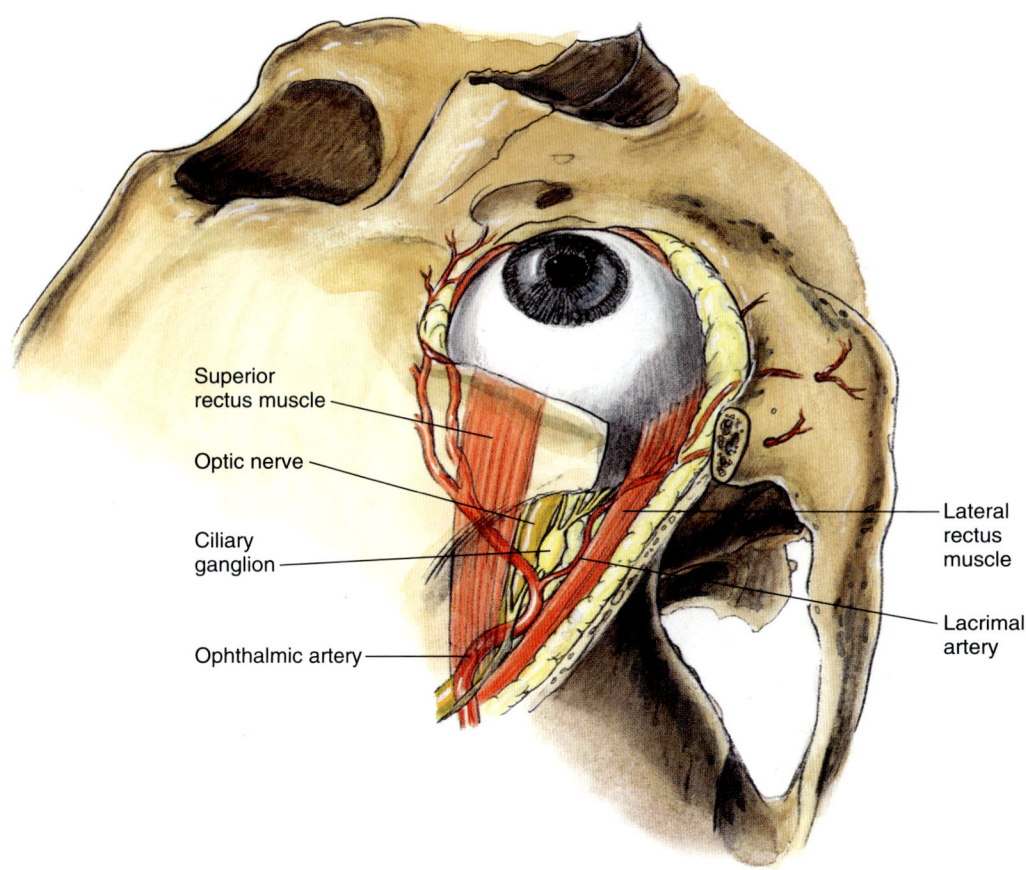

Fig. 22.1 Orbital anatomy.

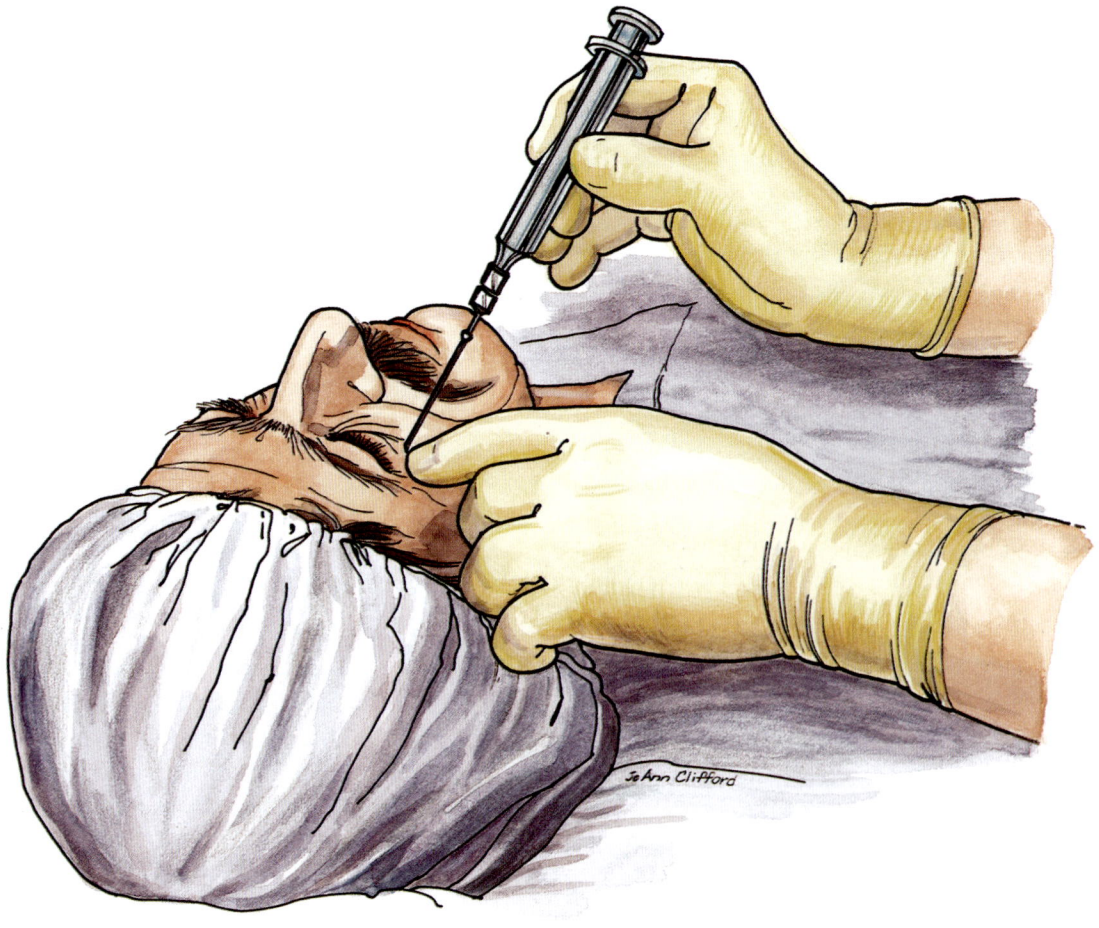

Fig. 22.2 Retrobulbar (peribulbar) block: position.

Retrobulbar (Peribulbar) Block

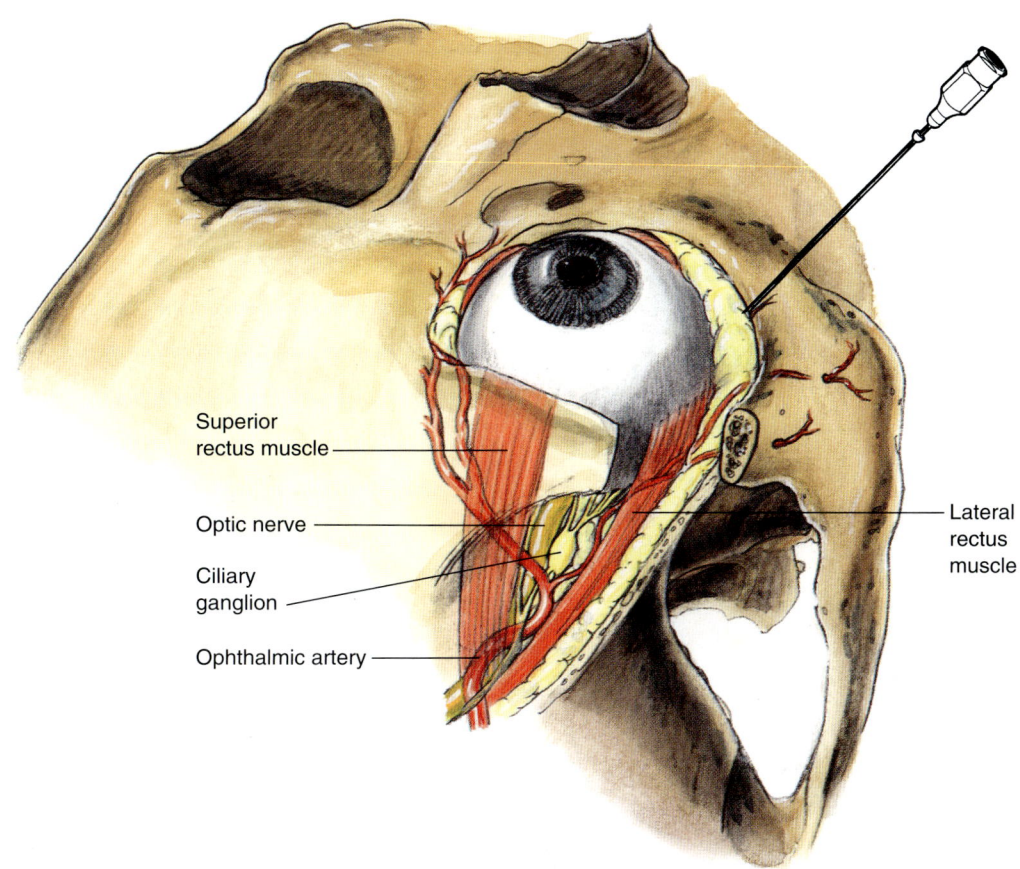

Fig. 22.3 Retrobulbar (peribulbar) block: needle puncture.

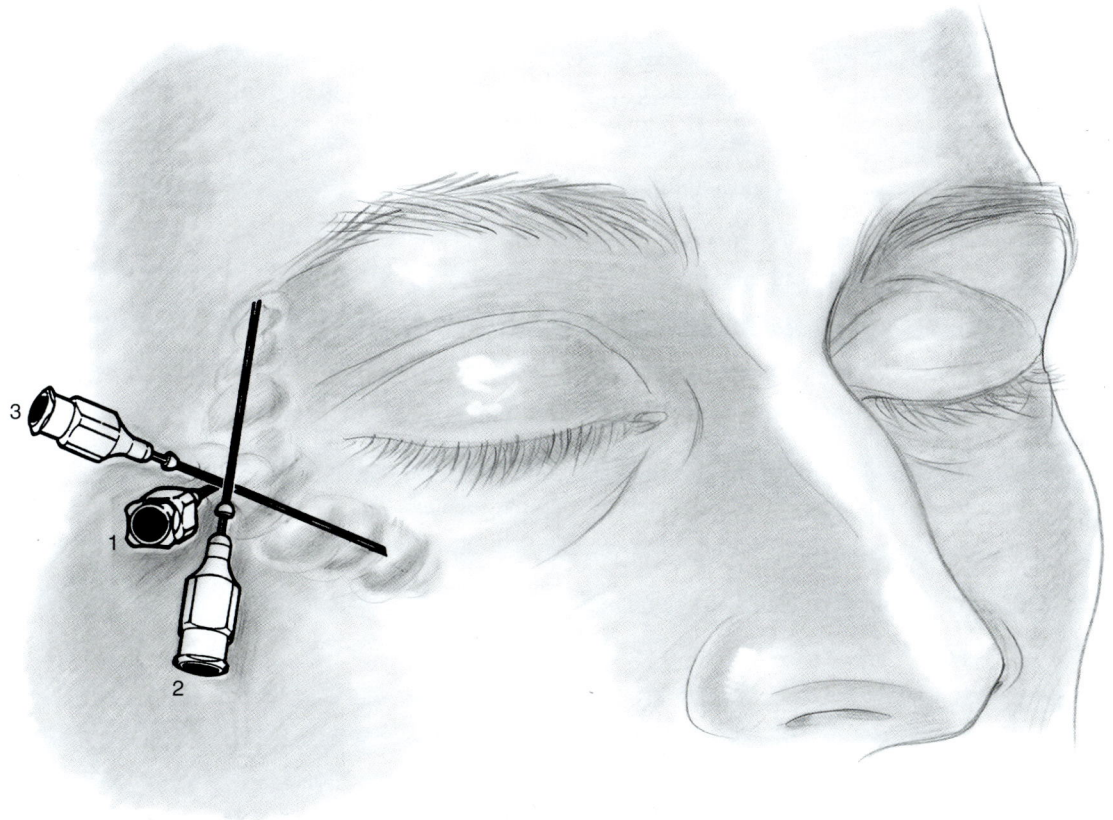

Fig. 22.4 Regional block of orbicularis oculi muscle: van Lint method.

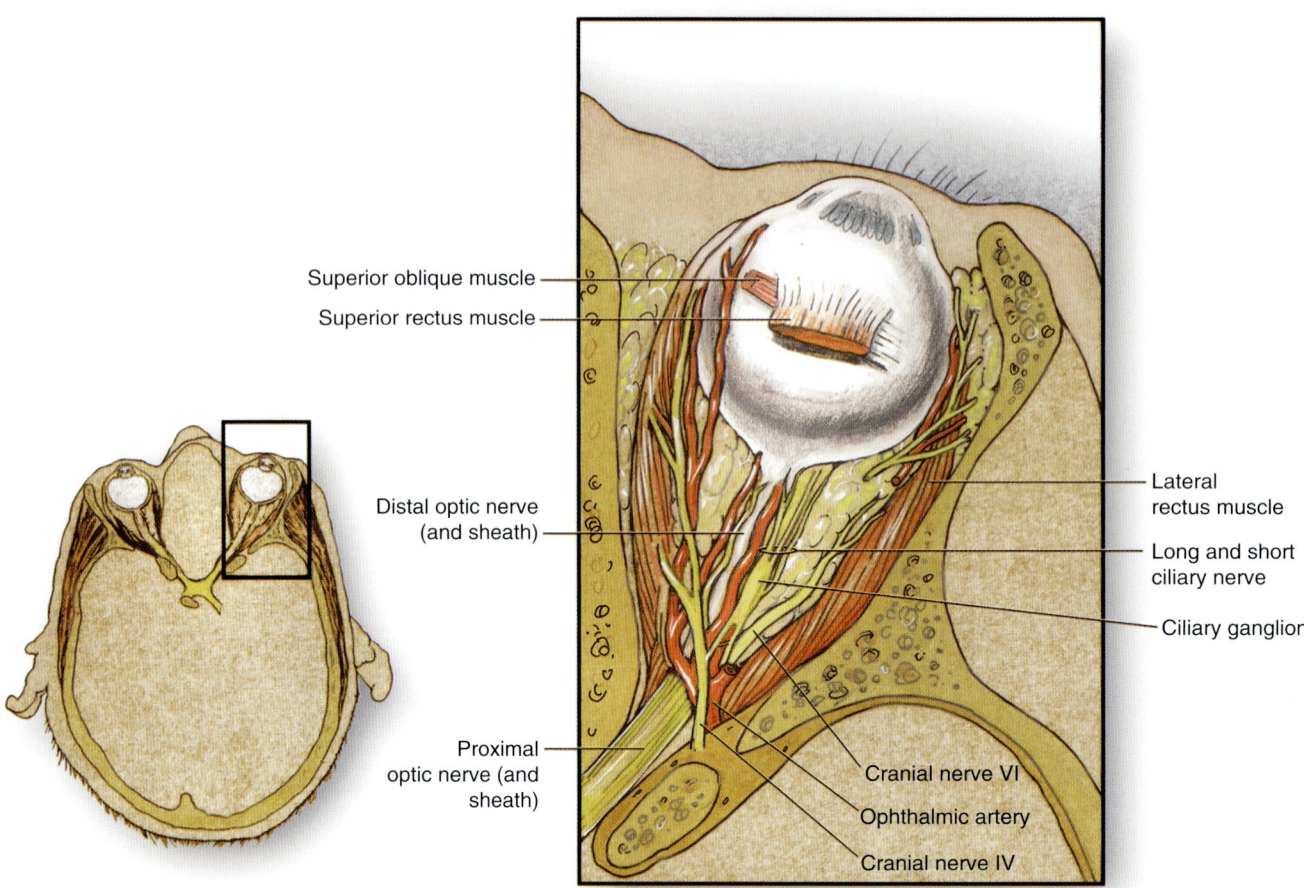

Fig. 22.5 Orbital functional anatomy.

example of the van Lint block. In this block, a 25-gauge, 4-cm needle is inserted at *needle position 1* until the lower inferolateral orbital rim is reached. When the needle tip contacts the bony surface, 1 mL of local anesthetic is injected. Through this skin wheal, the needle is repositioned along the lateral and inferior margins of the orbit (*needle positions 2 and 3*), and 2–3 mL of local anesthetic is injected along each needle path.

POTENTIAL PROBLEMS

The most common complication with retrobulbar block is hematoma formation. This can be minimized by using a needle shorter than 31 mm. Hematoma formation is more likely if a longer needle is used and the needle tip rests in the vicinity of the ophthalmic artery as it crosses the optic nerve. Hematoma can also be minimized by using a peribulbar approach. Other complications that can accompany retrobulbar block include local anesthetic toxicity, development of the oculocardiac reflex, and cases of sudden apnea and obtundation after retrobulbar injection. The latter two results are probably related to injection within the optic nerve sheath, resulting in unexpected spinal anesthesia, or intravascular injection affecting the respiratory centers in the midbrain, as illustrated in Fig. 22.5.

PEARLS

If anesthesiologists carry out retrobulbar anesthesia, they must work with ophthalmologists who are supportive and willing to share this part of their practice. Theoretically, many of the complications of retrobulbar anesthesia can be avoided if peribulbar block is carried out. This can be produced by placing the needle along the muscular cone of extraocular muscles rather than within the muscular cone. Although slightly larger volumes of local anesthetic are required with this technique, most of the major complications can be avoided.

Cervical Plexus Block

23

Jacob Ezell and Samantha Stamper

Key Points

- A high-frequency transducer is preferred for this block due to the shallow nature of the cervical plexus.
- This approach is for the superficial cervical plexus nerve block, which aims to spare the motor components and avoid serious complications that are more associated with the deep cervical plexus block.
- This block can be used for surgeries such as a carotid endarterectomy, superficial neck surgery, lymph node dissection, vascular access surgery, and excision of thyroglossal duct cysts or brachial cleft cysts.

SONOANATOMY

The cervical plexus, which originates from the anterior rami of the cervical vertebrae 2 to 4, provides sensory innervation to the ipsilateral neck, jaw, occiput, and anterior supraclavicular area (Fig. 23.1). It begins at the level of the first cervical vertebra, anterior to the levator scapulae and middle scalene muscles before piercing the platysma muscle near the posterior border of the sternocleidomastoid muscle. The cervical plexus divides into four terminal cutaneous branches: the lesser occipital nerve, greater auricular nerve, transverse cervical nerve, and supraclavicular nerve (Fig. 23.2). Before the cutaneous branches, the cervical plexus also divides to supply motor innervation to the phrenic nerve, the ansa cervicalis (innervation to the geniohyoid and infrahyoid muscles), components of the accessory nerve to sternocleidomastoid and trapezius muscles, and direct branches to the prevertebral muscles of the neck. The location of the division of the motor and sensory components is at the posterior border of the sternocleidomastoid. The fascia planes at this location allow for selective sensory blockade without compromising the neck and accessory muscles. Several authors use these planes to divide the cervical plexus block into superficial, intermediate, and deep blocks. This chapter focuses on the superficial cervical plexus block to target only the sensory portion of the nerve. This technique to correctly place a superficial cervical plexus block is easy, safe, and provides most anesthetic goals. For this nerve block technique, local anesthetic should be injected above the deep cervical fascia.

TECHNIQUE

The posterior border of the sternocleidomastoid muscle should be located. This can be a challenge in obese patients. For those in whom identification of the sternocleidomastoid muscle is difficult, asking the patient to raise his or her head off the bed can help identify the muscle belly. Drawing a line between the mastoid process and the clavicular head of the sternocleidomastoid can also identify the posterior border. Halfway along this line approximates the fourth cervical vertebra and site of injection.

Using ultrasound, with the patient in a supine or sitting position, the head is turned slightly away from the operative site. With the probe in a transverse, short-axis position, a small collection of nodules are identified (dark oval structures) deep to the sternocleidomastoid border at the posterior border of the halfway point of the sternocleidomastoid (Fig. 23.3). The nerves lie above the prevertebral fascia. Attention is given to avoid injection below the prevertebral fascial plane in order to avoid a motor block. Ideally, local anesthetic is injected below the sternocleidomastoid next to the cervical plexus between the cervical fascia and posterior border of the sternocleidomastoid. By advancing the needle in an in-plane fashion, approximately 5–10 mL can be used for this block following careful aspiration (Fig. 23.4A,B). In the illustration, the needle passes lateral to the sternocleidomastoid muscle to pierce the cervical fascia but does not penetrate below the deeper prevertebral fascia. Classically this block is performed without ultrasound but by using a superficial, fanning-needle injection just below the border of the posterior sternocleidomastoid.

PEARLS

- The block described is very useful and easily performed, even without ultrasound; however, the deep cervical plexus block is considered an advanced procedure and can have serious or even life-threatening complications.
- Visualization of the cervical plexus is not required for a successful block placement. Proper identification of the posterior border of the sternocleidomastoid and injection immediately posterior to this muscle will result in a successful block.
- If identification of the fascial planes proves difficult near C4, scanning caudad to the level of the sixth cervical vertebra may elucidate tissue planes.

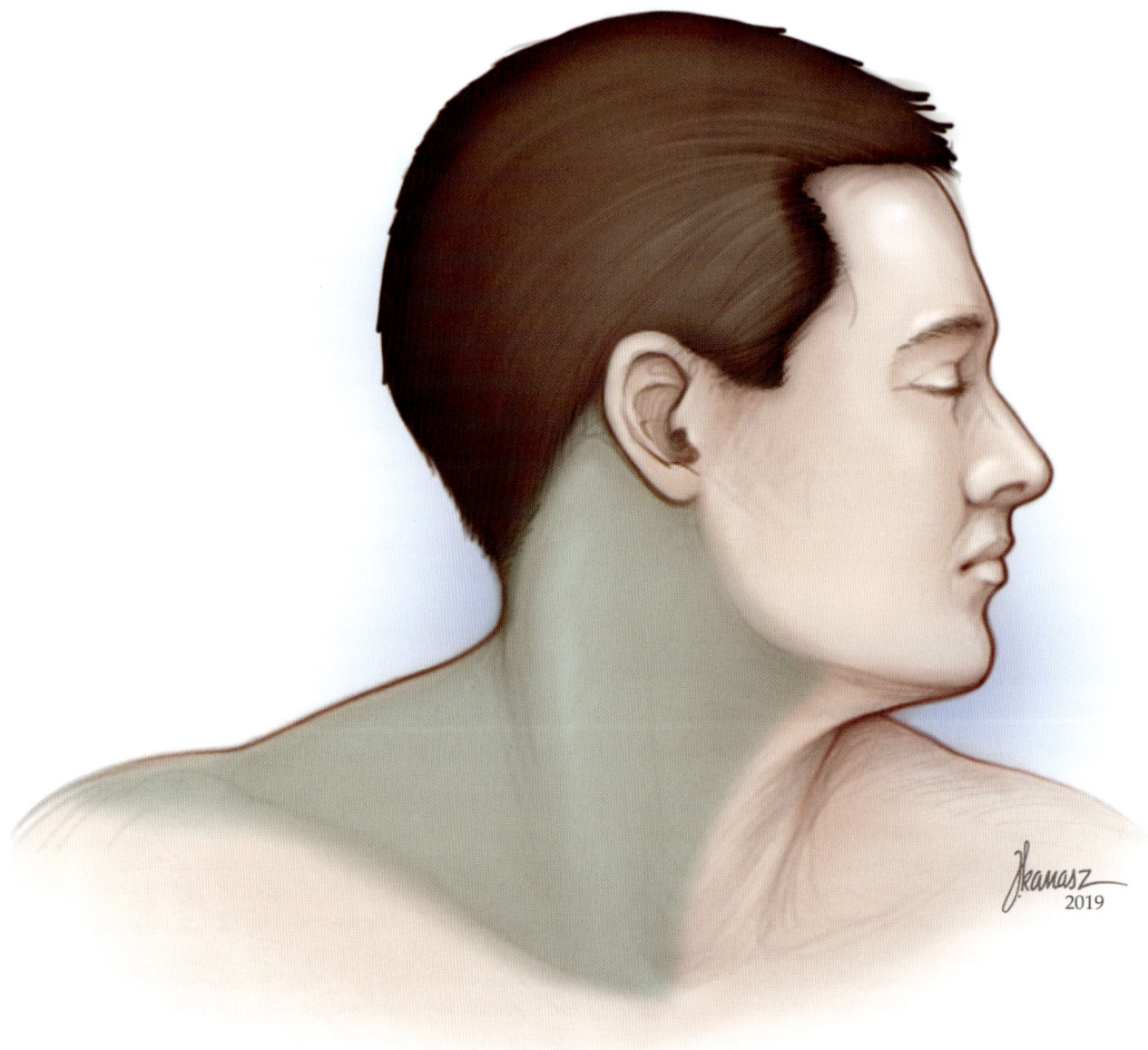

Fig. 23.1 A representation of the sensory distribution of the cervical plexus.

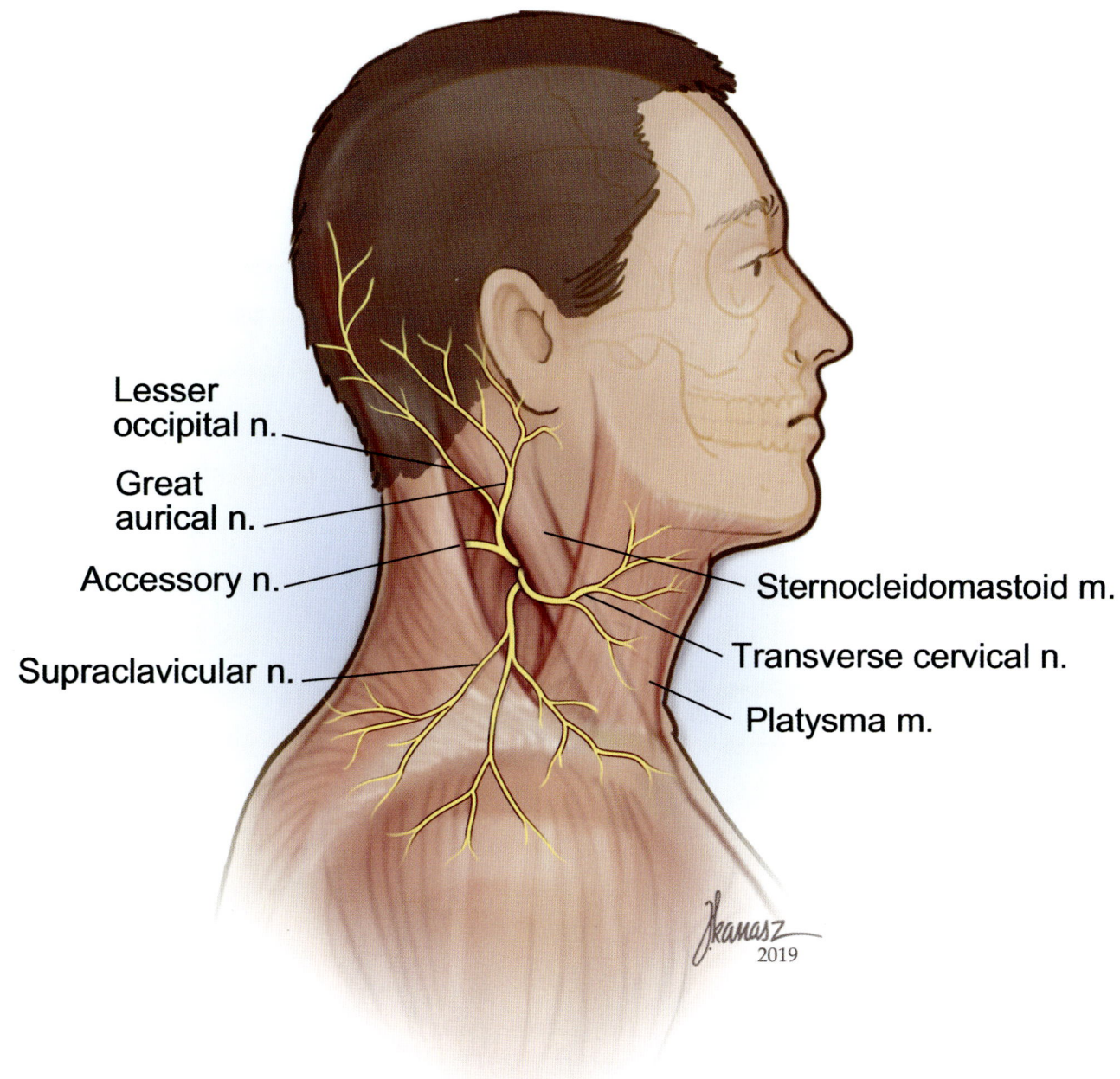

Fig. 23.2 The anatomy of the cervical plexus is seen as it emerges from the posterior border of the sternocleidomastoid muscle.

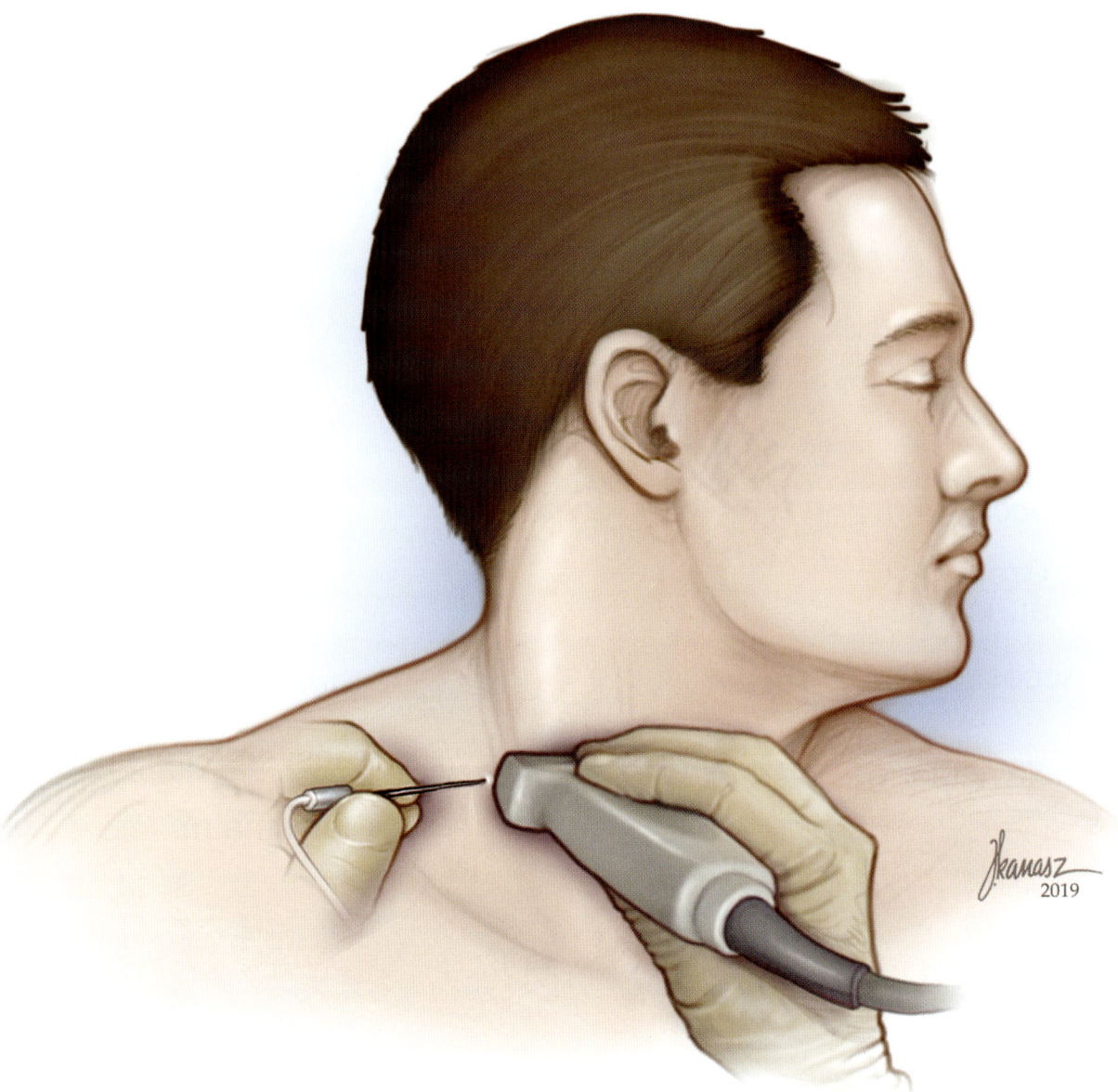

Fig. 23.3 Proper positioning of the patient showing the preferred technique to perform a right-sided cervical plexus block.

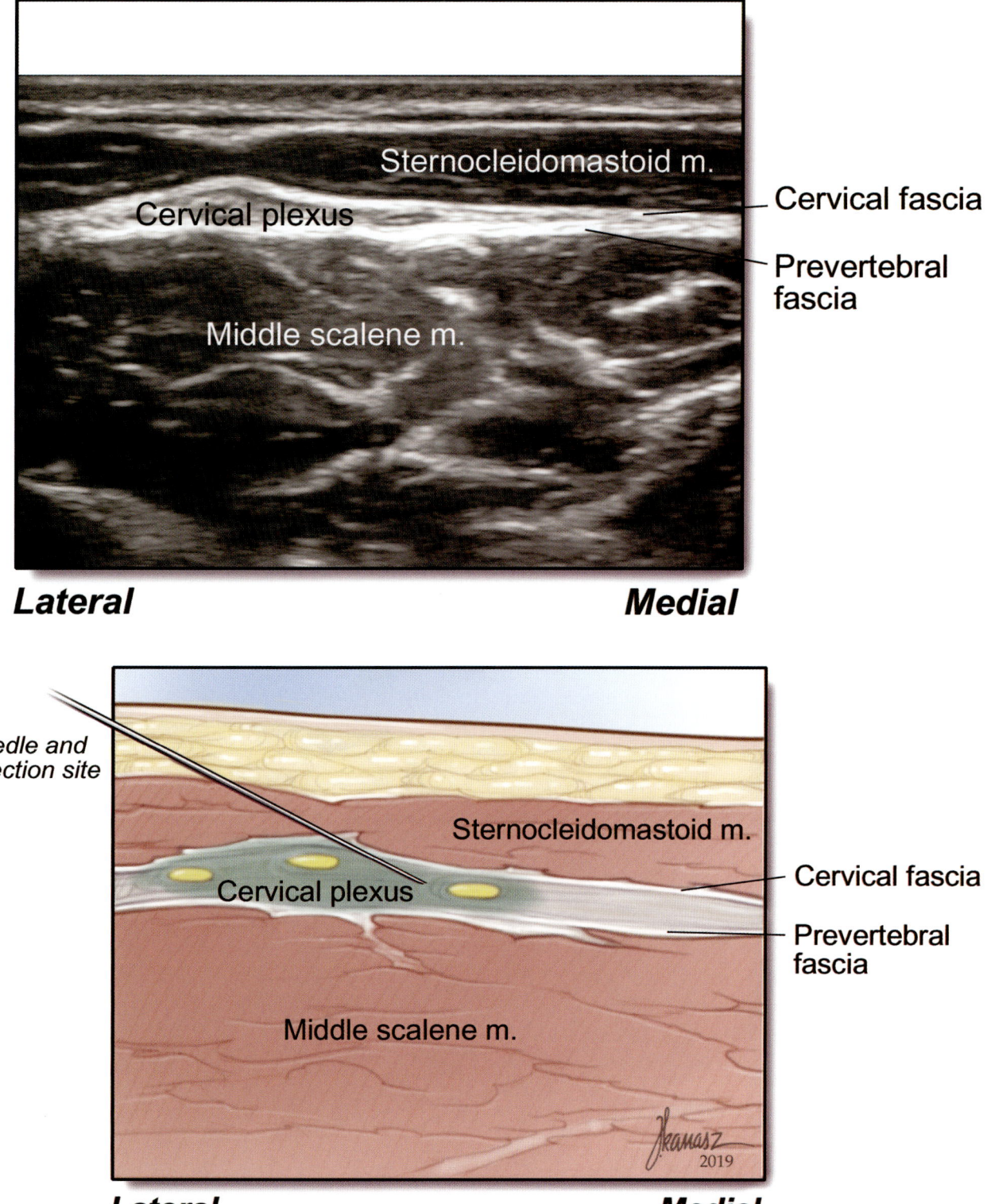

Fig. 23.4 **(A)** A comparison of an actual ultrasound image and **(B)** an illustrated example.

Stellate Ganglion Block

24

Vicente Roqués-Escolar and Ana Isabel Sánchez-Amador

Key Points

- Used for treatment or diagnosis of complex regional pain syndromes as well as upper limb vascular syndromes.
- Ultrasound appears to allow a more effective and precise sympathetic block.
- Long-lasting local anesthetics with steroid are commonly used.
- C7 transverse process and longus colli muscle must be located with a high-frequency linear transducer (6-13 MHz).
- The needle should be directed in-plane from lateral to medial towards the prevertebral fascia located over the longus colli muscle and below the carotid artery.
- A total of 5 mL of local anesthetic is then injected with real time visualization of spread, avoiding intravascular injection.

PERSPECTIVE

This is also called a cervicothoracic sympathetic block and has been used since the 1920s for treatment or diagnosis of complex regional pain syndrome. It has also been used to treat refractory angina, phantom limb pain, vascular insufficiency, and other pain and vascular syndromes.

Stellate ganglion blocks have traditionally been performed blindly by palpating the anterior tubercle of the transverse process of C6 (Chassaignac tubercle) and infiltrating as much as 20 mL of local anesthetic. This method has a relatively high failure rate, with numerous significant and even potentially fatal adverse effects.

Ultrasound allows for a more effective and precise sympathetic block with the use of a small injectate volume. It may also improve the safety of the procedure by real-time visualization of vascular structures and soft tissue structures.

Indications.

Pain Syndromes	Vascular Insufficiency
Complex regional pain syndrome type I and II	Raynaud's syndrome
Refractory angina	Scleroderma
Phantom limb pain	Frostbite
Herpes zoster	Obliterative vascular disease Vasospasm Trauma Emboli
Angina	Hyperhidrosis

Pharmacologic Choice. Even during diagnostic use of stellate ganglion block, it is often desirable to produce a long-lasting block. Therefore a solution of 0.25% bupivacaine or 0.2% ropivacaine with epinephrine is often used. Steroid coadjutants are frequently added in this technique.

Thermal and pulsed radiofrequency have been successfully used in some cases and can be considered an option in the treatment of these patients to prolong the effects of the blockade.

PLACEMENT

Anatomy. The sympathetic chain is each of the pair of ganglionated longitudinal cords of the sympathetic nervous system, situated on either side of the vertebral column. The sympathetic trunk travels from the base of the skull to the coccyx, just lateral to the vertebral bodies. The cervical portion of the chain extends from the base of the skull to the first rib, below which it becomes continuous with the thoracic part of the chain. In the neck, the cervical sympathetic chain lies embedded in the deep fascia between the carotid sheath and the prevertebral layer of deep fascia. The cervical sympathetic chain is composed of three ganglia: superior cervical ganglion, immediately below the skull; middle cervical ganglion, at the level of carotid cartilage; and inferior cervical ganglion, between the first rib and the transverse process of the seventh cervical vertebra. In most people, the inferior cervical ganglion is fused with the first thoracic ganglion and forms the stellate ganglion (Fig. 24.1A,B).

Position. The patient is placed in the supine position with the neck slightly extended and the head rotated slightly to the opposite side of the block. This is often facilitated by removing the patient's pillow before positioning.

Ultrasound-guided injection technique. A high-frequency linear transducer (6-13 MHz) is placed at the level of C6 to allow visualization of the anterior and posterior tubercle of the transverse process. At that level the longus colli muscle, prevertebral fascia, carotid artery, jugular vein, thyroid gland, trachea, and esophagus must be located.

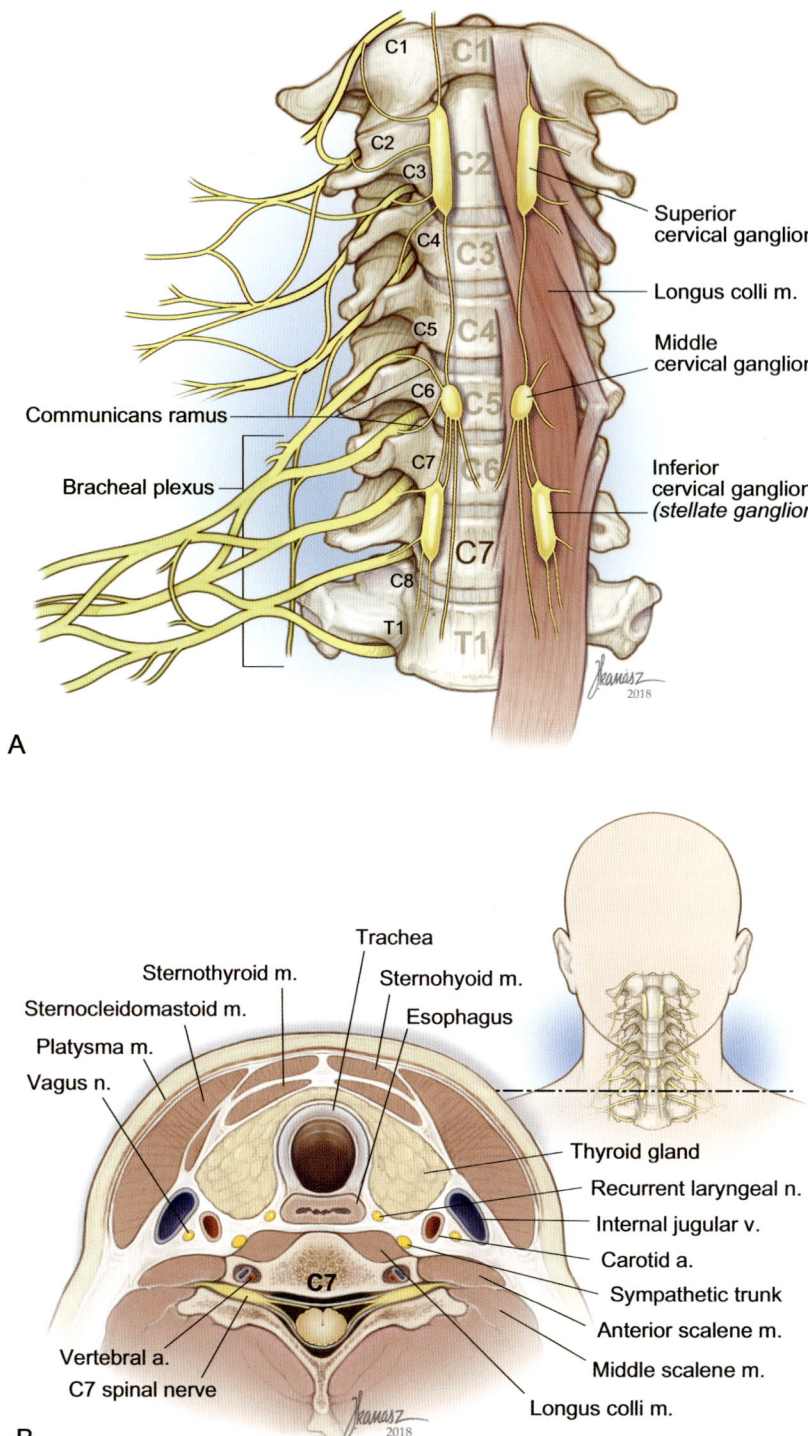

Fig. 24.1 (A) Stellate ganglion block: sympathetic chain anatomy. (B) Cross-sectional anatomy at C7 level.

The transducer is slightly displaced caudally until the C7 transverse process is located with a single posterior tubercle and C7 root that will constitute the middle trunk by itself. At that point, the vertebral artery and vein must be identified. For the lateral approach over this scanning plane, the needle should be directed in-plane from lateral to medial towards the prevertebral fascia located over the longus colli muscle and below the carotid artery (Fig. 24.2). A total of 5 mL of local anesthetic is then injected with real-time visualization of spread, avoiding intravascular injection.

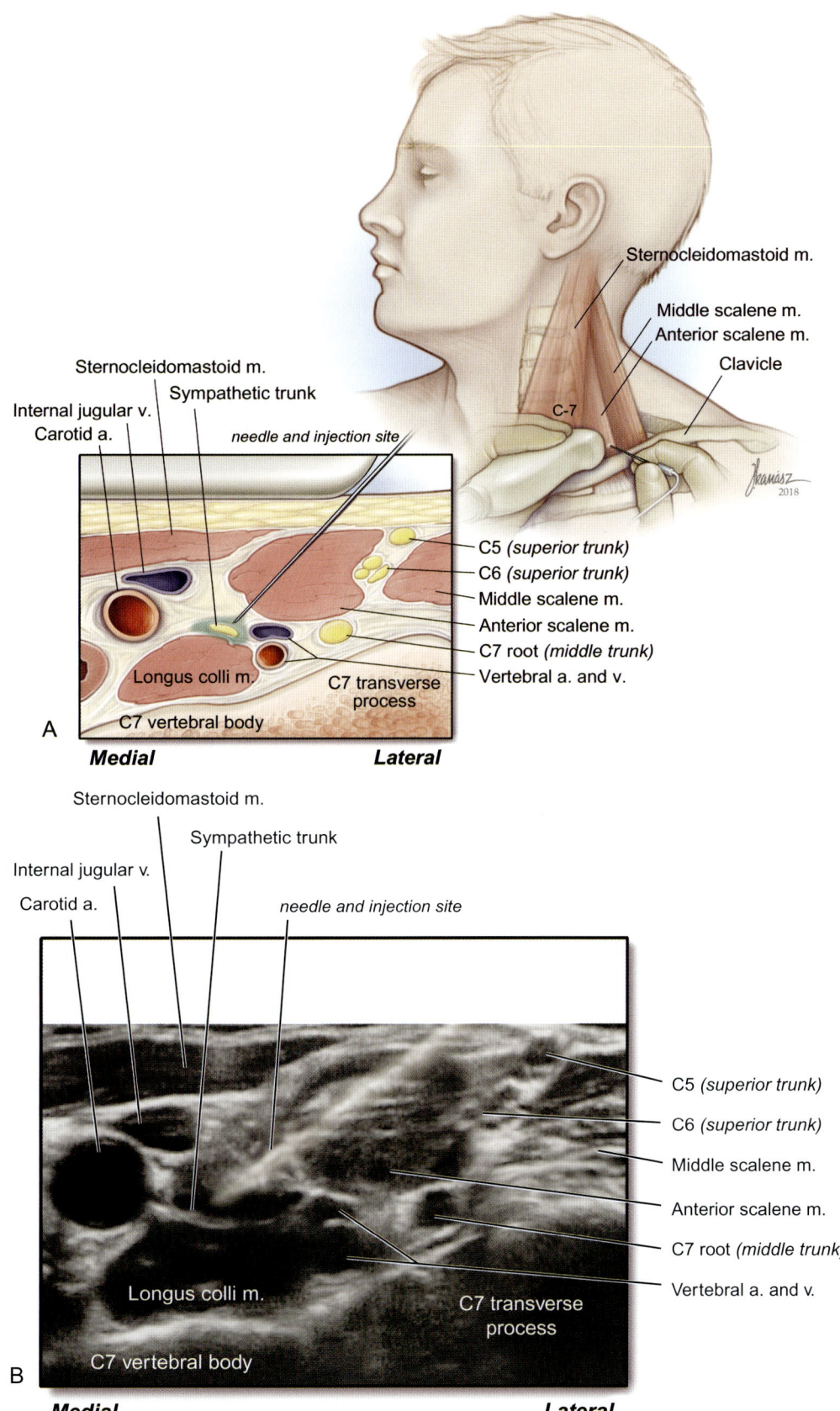

Fig. 24.2 Ultrasound-guided stellate ganglion block. (A) Transducer position and needle insertion point. Axial cross-section over C7 level. (B) Sonoanatomy for ultrasound-guided stellate ganglion approach.

POTENTIAL COMPLICATIONS

Complications have been described due to malposition of the needle:
- Hematoma caused by carotid, jugular, or vertebral artery trauma.
- Neural injury in case of vagus or brachial plexus root trauma.

Complications due to the spread of local anesthetic:
- Intravascular injection.
- Neuraxial or brachial plexus spread.
- Phrenic nerve or recurrent laryngeal nerve palsy.
- Infection caused by esophageal perforation or meningitis.

PEARLS

- Possible postprocedural effects should be explained to the patient including ptosis, miosis, blurred vision, enophthalmos, anhidrosis, facial and conjunctival flushing, upper extremity numbness or weakness and sense of dyspnea, dysphagia, or a lump in the throat.
- It is crucial to identify potential dangerous structures such as the vertebral artery and vein, esophagus, trachea, and brachial plexus roots prior to puncture.
- A constant and real-time view of the needle trajectory and distribution of the local anesthetic over the longus colli muscle should be maintained all the time.

SECTION 5
Airway Blocks

Airway Block Anatomy 25

David L. Brown

> **Key Point**
> - Block of the glossopharyngeal nerve is required for manipulations of the posterior third of the tongue and pharyngeal wall. Structures more distal in the airway to the epiglottis will require block of vagal branches.

If there is one set of regional blocks that an anesthesiologist should master, it is airway blocks. Even those anesthesiologists who prefer to use general anesthesia for the majority of their cases will be faced with the need to provide airway blocks before anesthetic induction in patients who may have airway compromise, trauma to the upper airway, or unstable cervical vertebrae. As illustrated in Fig. 25.1, innervation of the airway can be separated into three principal neural pathways: trigeminal, glossopharyngeal, and vagus. If nasal intubation is planned, some method of anesthetizing the maxillary branches from the trigeminal nerve will need to be carried out. Because manipulations involve the pharynx and posterior third of the tongue, glossopharyngeal block will be required. Structures more distal in the airway to the epiglottis will require block of vagal branches.

Specific glossopharyngeal nerves that are of interest to anesthesiologists who undertake airway anesthesia are the pharyngeal nerves, which are primarily sensory to the pharyngeal mucosa; the tonsillar nerves, which provide sensation to the mucosa overlying the palatine tonsil and contiguous parts of the soft palate; and sensory branches to the posterior third of the tongue. The glossopharyngeal nerve exits the skull through the jugular foramen in close contact with the spinal accessory nerve. As the glossopharyngeal nerve exits the jugular foramen, it is also in close contact with the vagus nerve, which likewise travels within the carotid sheath in the upper portion of the neck.

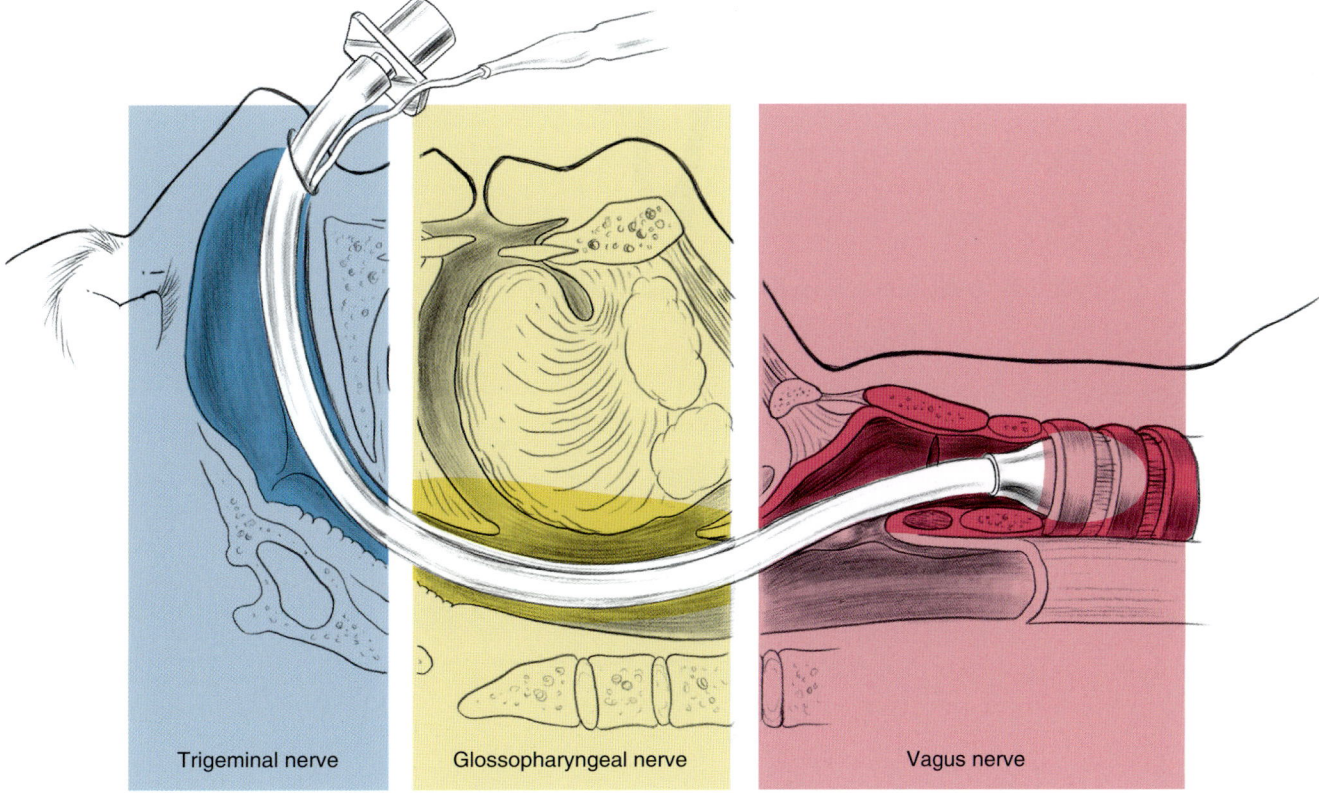

Fig. 25.1 Airway blocks: simplified functional anatomy.

The vagus nerve supplies innervation to the mucosa of the airway from the level of the epiglottis to the distal airways through both the superior and the recurrent laryngeal nerves, as illustrated in Figs. 25.2 and 25.3. Although the vagus is primarily a parasympathetic nerve, it also contains some fibers from the cervical sympathetic chain, as well as motor fibers to laryngeal muscles. The superior laryngeal nerve provides sensation to the surfaces of the epiglottis and to the airway mucosa to the level of the vocal cords. It provides innervation to the mucosa after entering the thyrohyoid membrane just inferior to the hyoid bone between the greater and the lesser cornua of the hyoid. This mucosal innervation is carried out through the internal laryngeal nerve, a branch of the superior laryngeal nerve.

The superior laryngeal nerve also continues as the external laryngeal nerve along the exterior of the larynx; it provides motor innervation to the cricothyroid muscle.

The recurrent laryngeal nerve is a branch of the vagus nerve that ascends along the posterolateral margin of the trachea after looping under the right subclavian artery as it leaves the vagus nerve on the right, or around the left side of the arch of the aorta, lateral to the ligamentum arteriosum on the left. The recurrent nerves ascend and innervate the larynx and the trachea caudal to the vocal cords. This anatomy is illustrated in Figs. 25.2 through 25.4. Fig. 25.5 shows a sagittal magnetic resonance image with an interpretive illustration of airway innervation keyed to the colors used in Fig. 25.1.

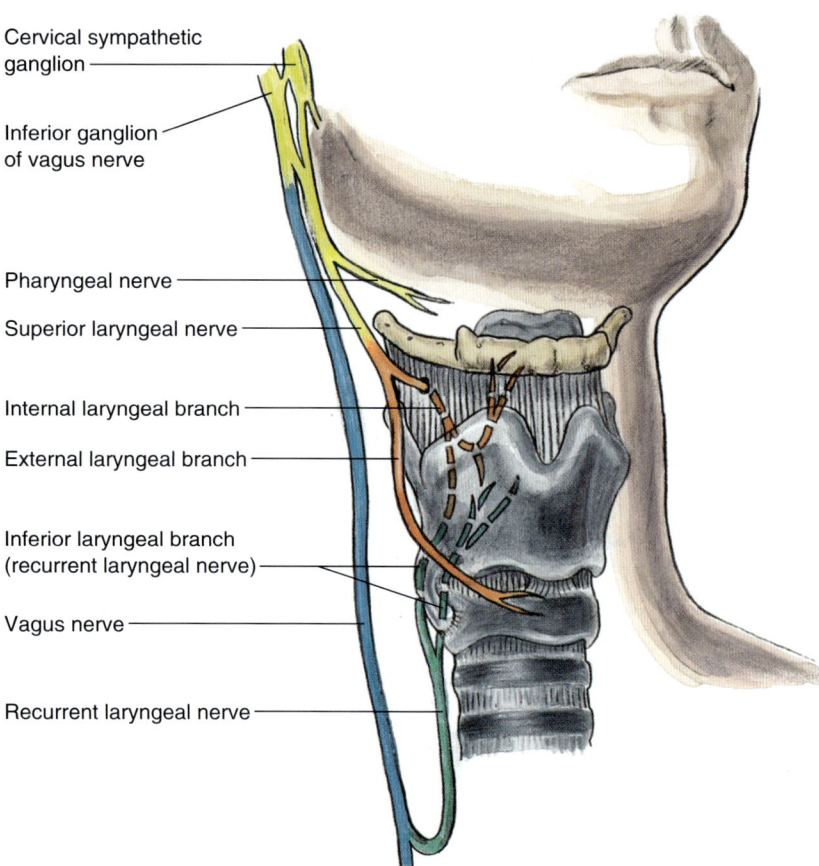

Fig. 25.2 Airway blocks: anatomy of laryngeal innervation.

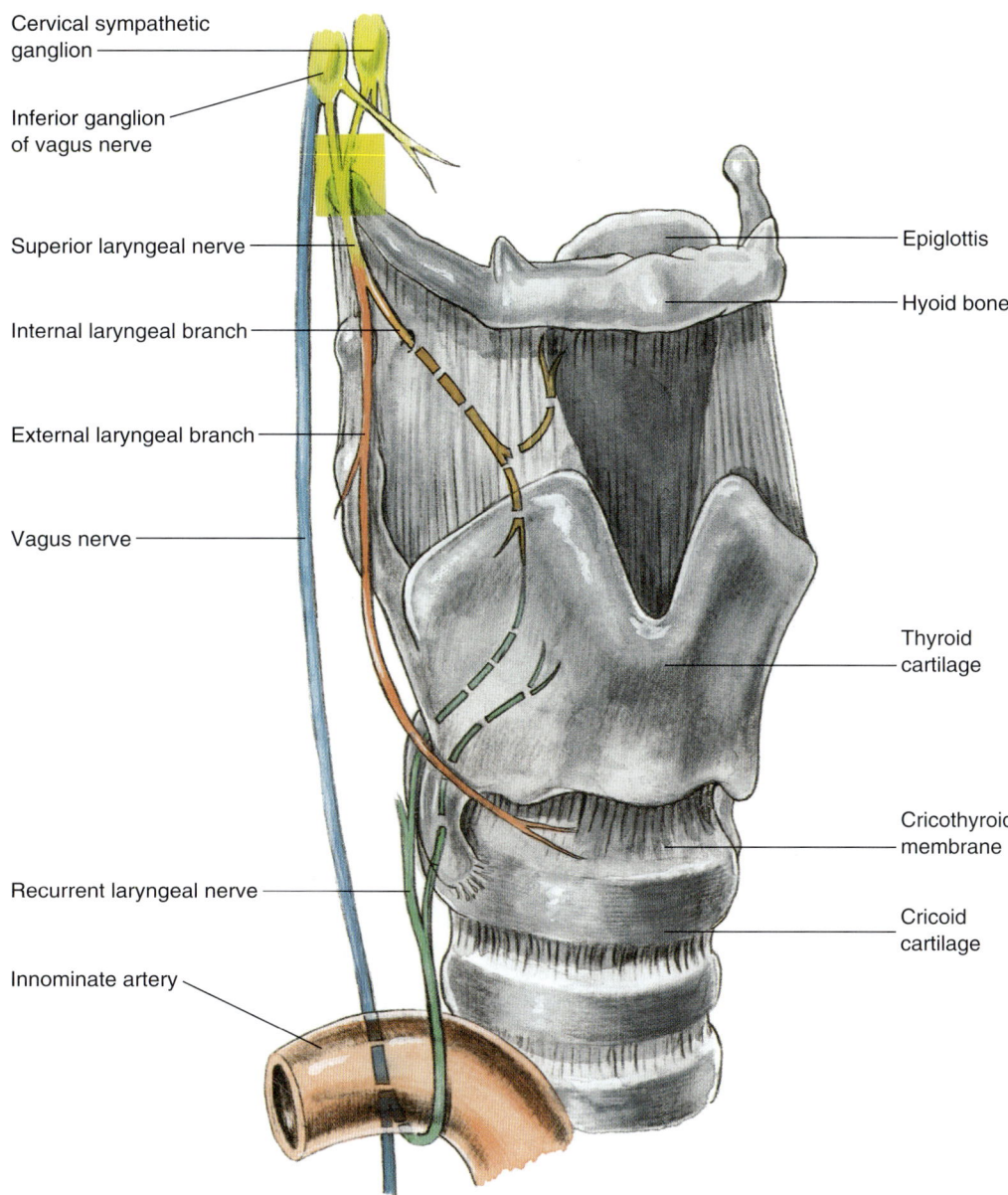

Fig. 25.3 Airway blocks: anatomy of laryngeal, vagal, and sympathetic connections.

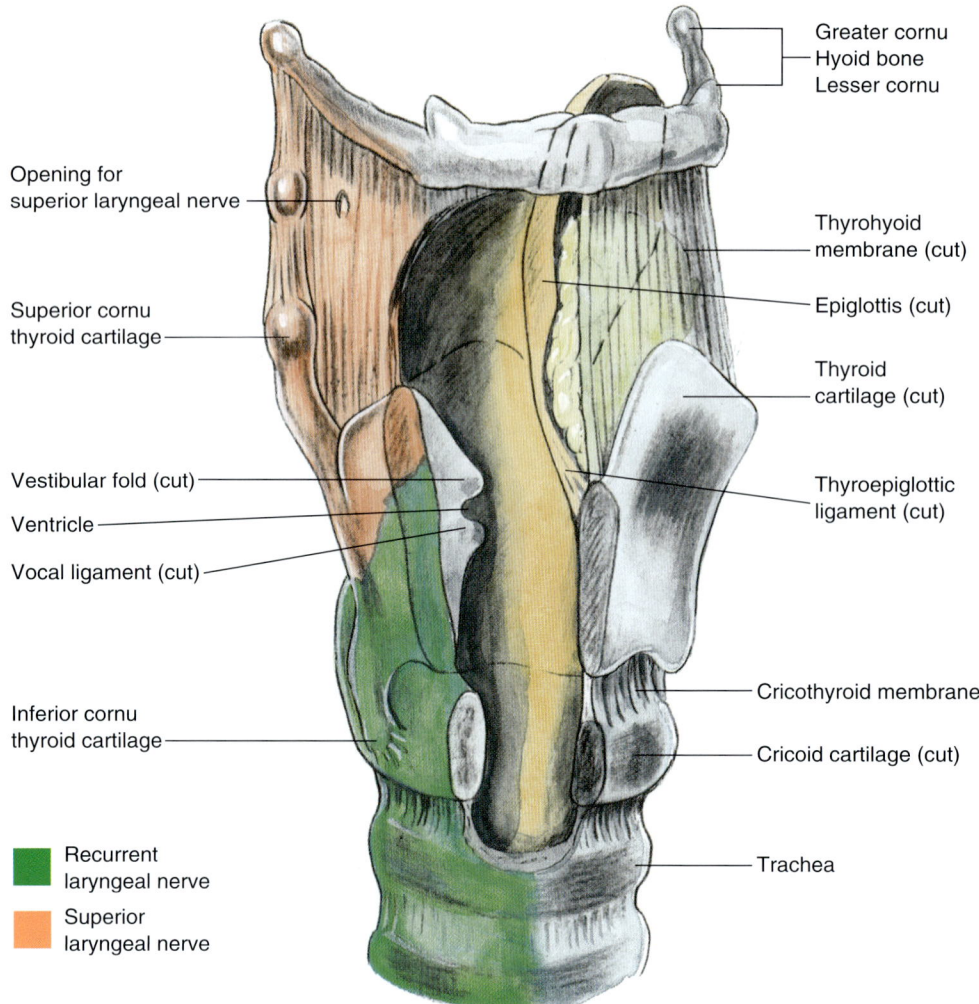

Fig. 25.4 Airway blocks: anatomy of laryngeal structures and simplified innervation.

Airway Block Anatomy 187

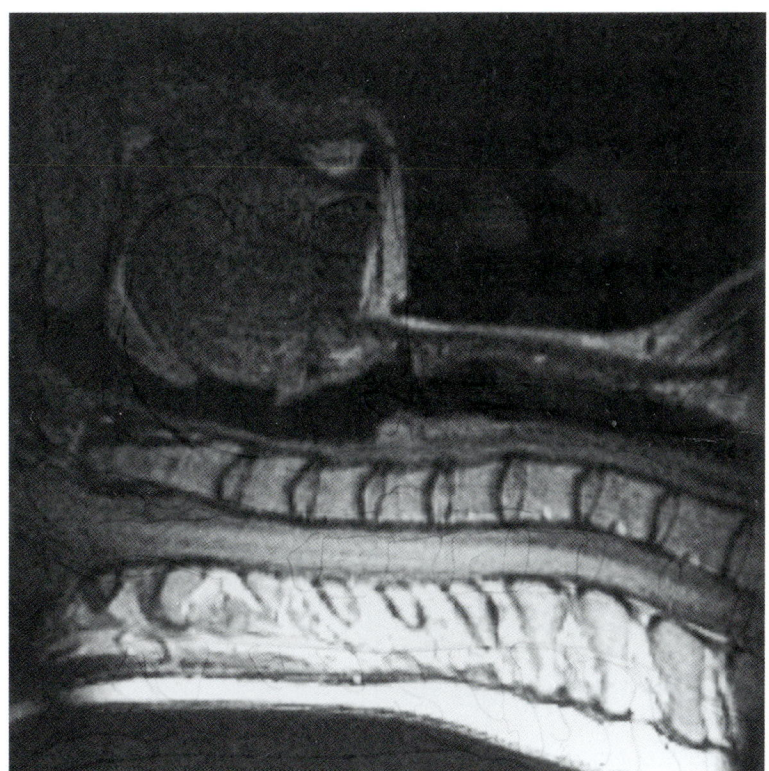

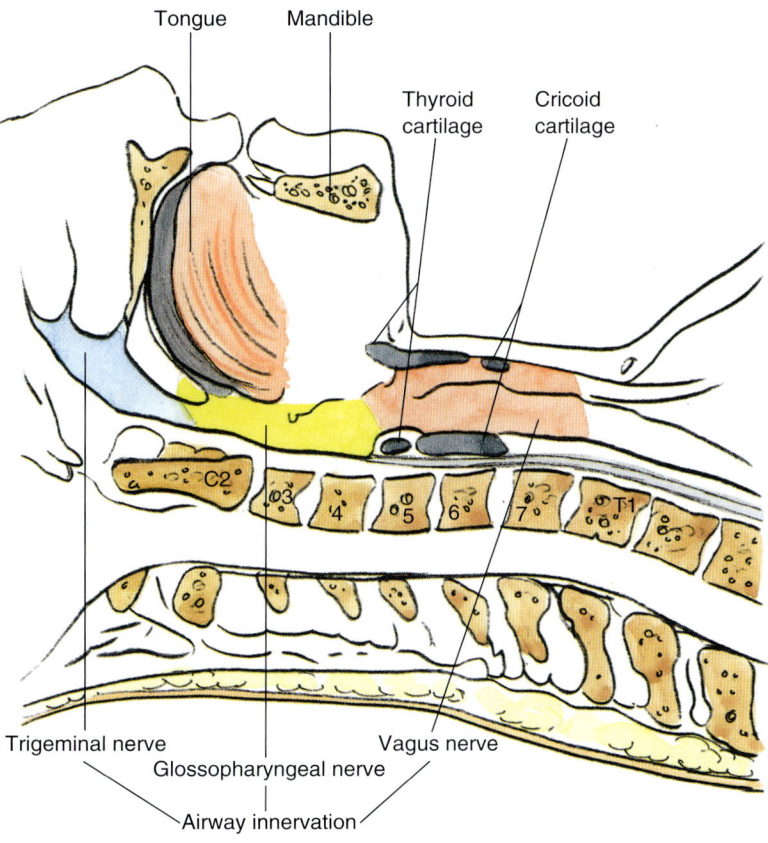

Fig. 25.5 Airway blocks: sagittal anatomy on magnetic resonance imaging and an interpretive line drawing.

Glossopharyngeal Block

26

David L. Brown

Key Points

- The distal branches of the glossopharyngeal nerve are located submucosally immediately posterior to the palatine tonsil, deep to the posterior tonsillar pillar.
- Glossopharyngeal blocks can be achieved from an intraoral approach or externally next to the styloid process.
- Bending the tip of the needle helps positioning the needle submucosally in posttonsillar be when performing the intraoral approach.

PERSPECTIVE

Glossopharyngeal block is useful for anesthesia of the mucosa of the pharynx and soft palate, as well as for eliminating the gag reflex that results when pressure is applied to the posterior third of the tongue.

Patient Selection. Glossopharyngeal block can be used in most patients who need atraumatic, sedated, spontaneously ventilating, "awake" tracheal intubation.

Pharmacologic Choice. The local anesthetic chosen for glossopharyngeal block does not need to provide motor blockade. Lidocaine (0.5%) is an appropriate choice of local anesthetic.

PLACEMENT

Anatomy. The glossopharyngeal nerve exits from the jugular foramen at the base of the skull, as illustrated in Fig. 26.1, in close association with other structures of the carotid sheath, vagus nerve, and styloid process. The glossopharyngeal nerve descends in the neck, passes between the internal carotid and the external carotid arteries, and then divides into pharyngeal branches and motor branches to the stylopharyngeus muscle, as well as branches innervating the area of the palatine tonsil and the posterior third of the tongue. These distal branches of the glossopharyngeal nerve are located submucosally immediately posterior to the palatine tonsil, deep to the posterior tonsillar pillar.

Position. Glossopharyngeal block can be carried out intraorally or in a peristyloid manner. If the block is to be carried out intraorally, the patient must be able to open the mouth, and sufficient topical anesthesia of the tongue must be provided to allow needle placement at the base of the posterior tonsillar pillar. If the block is to be carried out in a peristyloid manner, the patient does not need to be able to open the mouth.

Needle Puncture: Intraoral Glossopharyngeal Block. After topical anesthesia of the tongue, the patient's mouth is opened widely and the posterior tonsillar pillar (palatopharyngeal fold) is identified by using a no. 3 Macintosh laryngoscope blade. An angled 22-gauge, 9-cm needle (see comment in Pearls section) is inserted in the caudad portion of the posterior tonsillar pillar. The needle tip is inserted submucosally and then, after careful aspiration for blood, 5 mL of local anesthetic is injected. The block is repeated on the contralateral side (Fig. 26.2).

Needle Puncture: Peristyloid Approach. The patient lies supine with the head in a neutral position. Marks are placed on the mastoid process and the angle of the mandible, as illustrated in Fig. 26.3. A line is drawn between these two marks, and at the midpoint of that line the needle is inserted to contact the styloid process. To facilitate styloid identification, a finger palpates the styloid process with deep pressure and, although this can be uncomfortable for the patient, the short 22-gauge needle is then inserted until it impinges on the styloid process. This needle is then withdrawn and redirected off the styloid process posteriorly. As soon as bony contact is lost and aspiration for blood is negative, 5–7 mL of local anesthetic is injected. The block can then be repeated on the contralateral side.

POTENTIAL PROBLEMS

Both the intraoral and the peristyloid blocks have few complications if careful aspiration for blood is carried out. In the peristyloid approach, the glossopharyngeal nerve is closely related to both the internal jugular vein and the internal carotid artery. In the intraoral approach, the terminal branches of the glossopharyngeal nerves are closely related to the internal carotid arteries, which lie immediately lateral to the needle tips if they are correctly positioned.

PEARLS

A frequent problem with the intraoral glossopharyngeal block is finding a needle to use for the block. This problem can be easily overcome by using a 22-gauge disposable

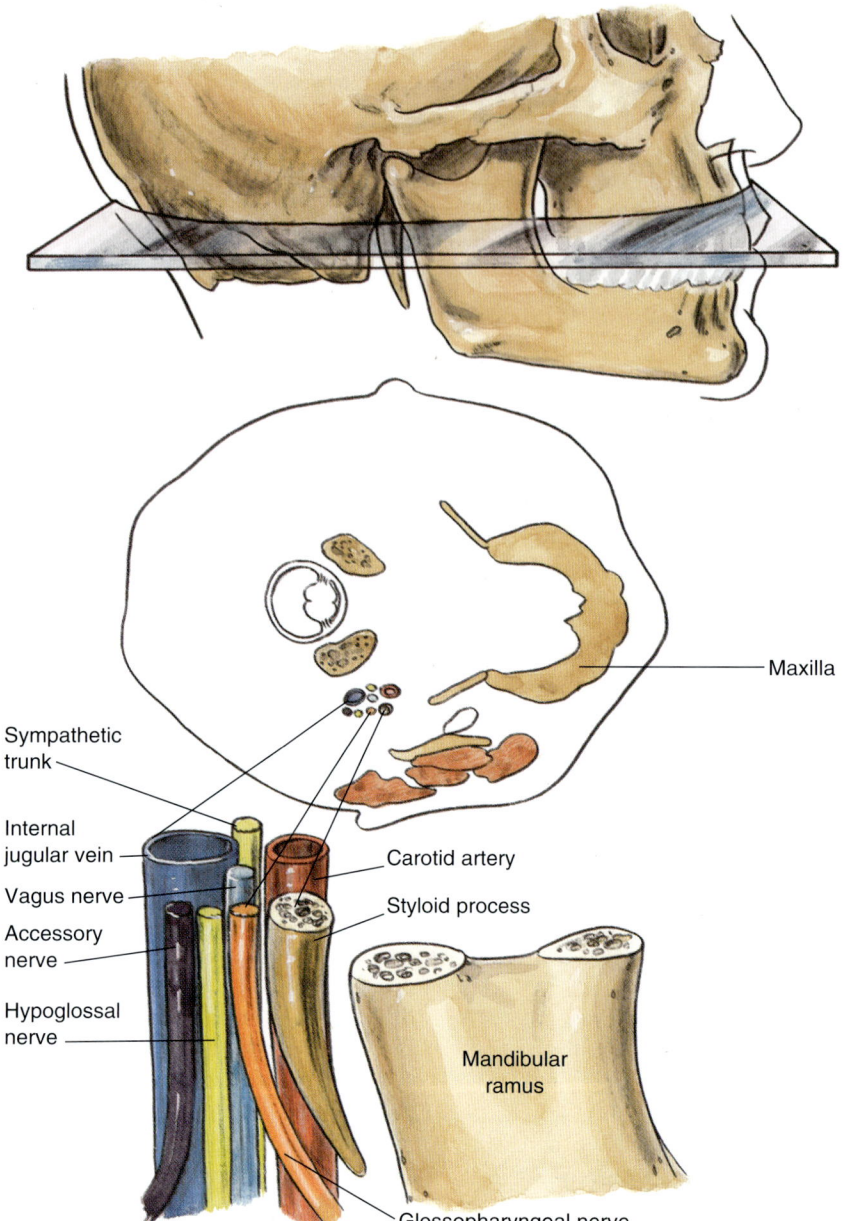

Fig. 26.1 Glossopharyngeal block: cross-sectional view of peristyloid anatomy with detail.

spinal needle. In an aseptic manner, the stylet should be removed from the disposable spinal needle and discarded. Subsequently, using the sterile container in which the 22-gauge spinal needle was packaged, the distal 1 cm of the needle is bent to allow more control during submucosal insertion.

This block is underused when airway anesthesia is needed for sedated, spontaneously ventilating, "awake" patients requiring tracheal intubation. The author believes that the block is effective in further reducing the gag reflex that results from pressure on the posterior third of the tongue, even after adequate topical mucosal anesthesia has been obtained.

Glossopharyngeal Block

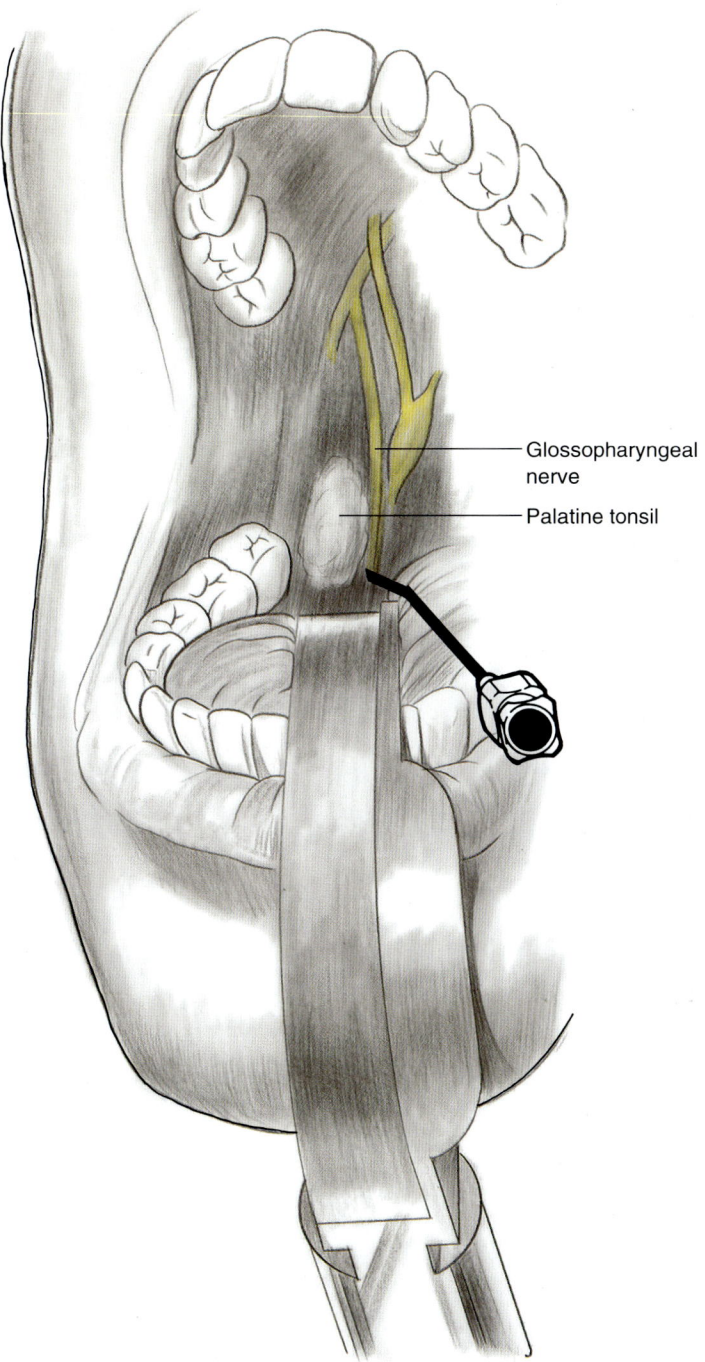

Fig. 26.2 Glossopharyngeal block: intraoral anatomy and technique.

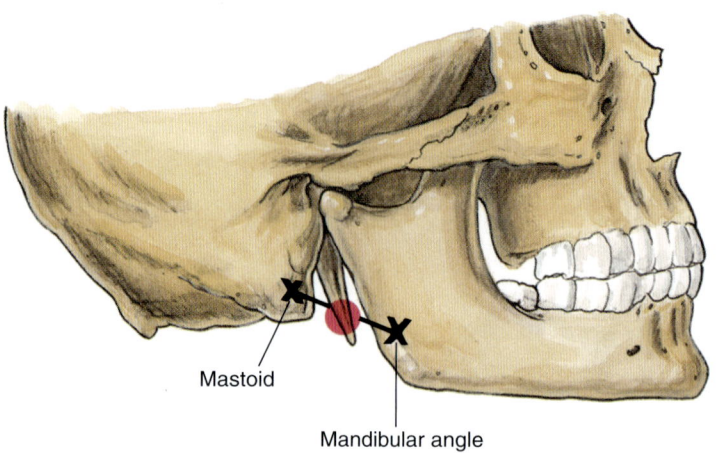
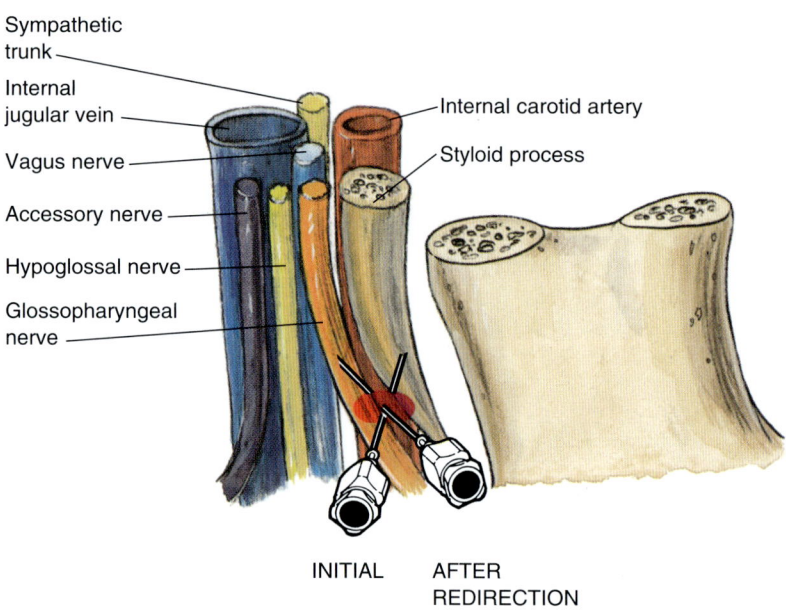

Fig. 26.3 Glossopharyngeal block: peristyloid technique.

Superior Laryngeal Block

27

David L. Brown

Key Points

- The superior laryngeal nerve is blocked at the lower border of the hyoid bone.
- A small 25-gauge, short needle is used to reduce the risk of intravascular or intralaryngeal injections.

PERSPECTIVE

The superior laryngeal nerve block is one of the methods of providing airway anesthesia. Block of the superior laryngeal nerve provides anesthesia of the larynx from the epiglottis to the level of the vocal cords.

Patient Selection. This block may be appropriate for any patient requiring tracheal intubation before anesthetic induction.

Pharmacologic Choice. Lidocaine (0.5%) is an appropriate local anesthetic for this block.

PLACEMENT

Anatomy. The superior laryngeal nerve is a branch of the vagus nerve. After it leaves the main vagal trunk, it courses through the neck and passes medially, caudal to the greater cornu of the hyoid bone, at which point it divides into an internal branch and an external branch. The internal branch is the nerve of interest in superior laryngeal nerve block, and it is blocked where it enters the thyrohyoid membrane just inferior to the caudal aspect of the hyoid bone (Fig. 27.1).

Position. The patient is placed supine with the neck extended. The anesthesiologist should displace the hyoid bone toward the side to be blocked by grasping it between the index finger and the thumb (Fig. 27.2). A 25-gauge, short needle is then inserted to make contact with the greater cornu of the hyoid. The needle is "walked off" the caudal edge of the hyoid and advanced 2–3 mm so that the needle tip rests between the thyrohyoid membrane laterally and the laryngeal mucosa medially. Two to 3 mL of the drug is then injected; an additional 1 mL is injected while the needle is withdrawn.

POTENTIAL PROBLEMS

It is possible to place the needle into the interior of the larynx with this approach, although that should not result in long-term problems. If the block is carried out as described, intravascular injection should be infrequent despite the presence of the superior laryngeal artery and vein, which pierce the thyrohyoid membrane with the internal laryngeal nerve.

PEARLS

One helpful maneuver when performing this block is to firmly displace the hyoid bone toward the side to be blocked, even if it causes the patient some minor discomfort. The discomfort usually can be minimized by using appropriate amounts of sedation. If a three-ring syringe is used, the sedation, coupled with an efficient block, provides an acceptable experience for both patient and anesthesiologist.

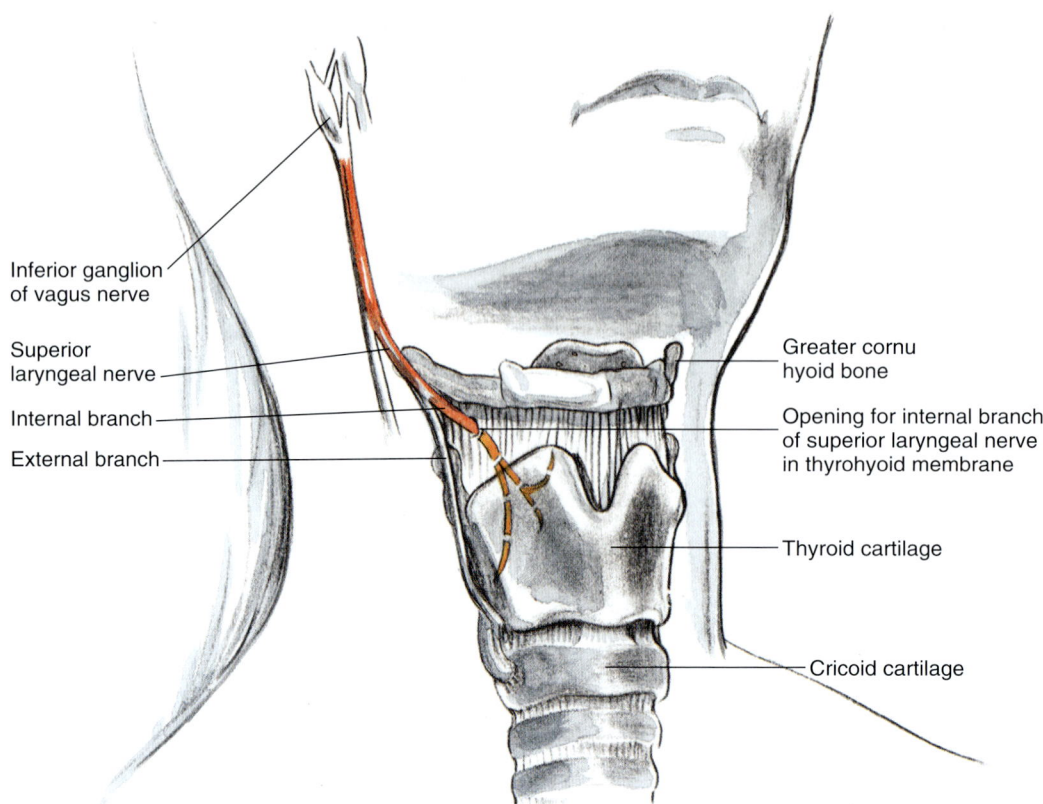

Fig. 27.1 Superior laryngeal nerve block: anatomy.

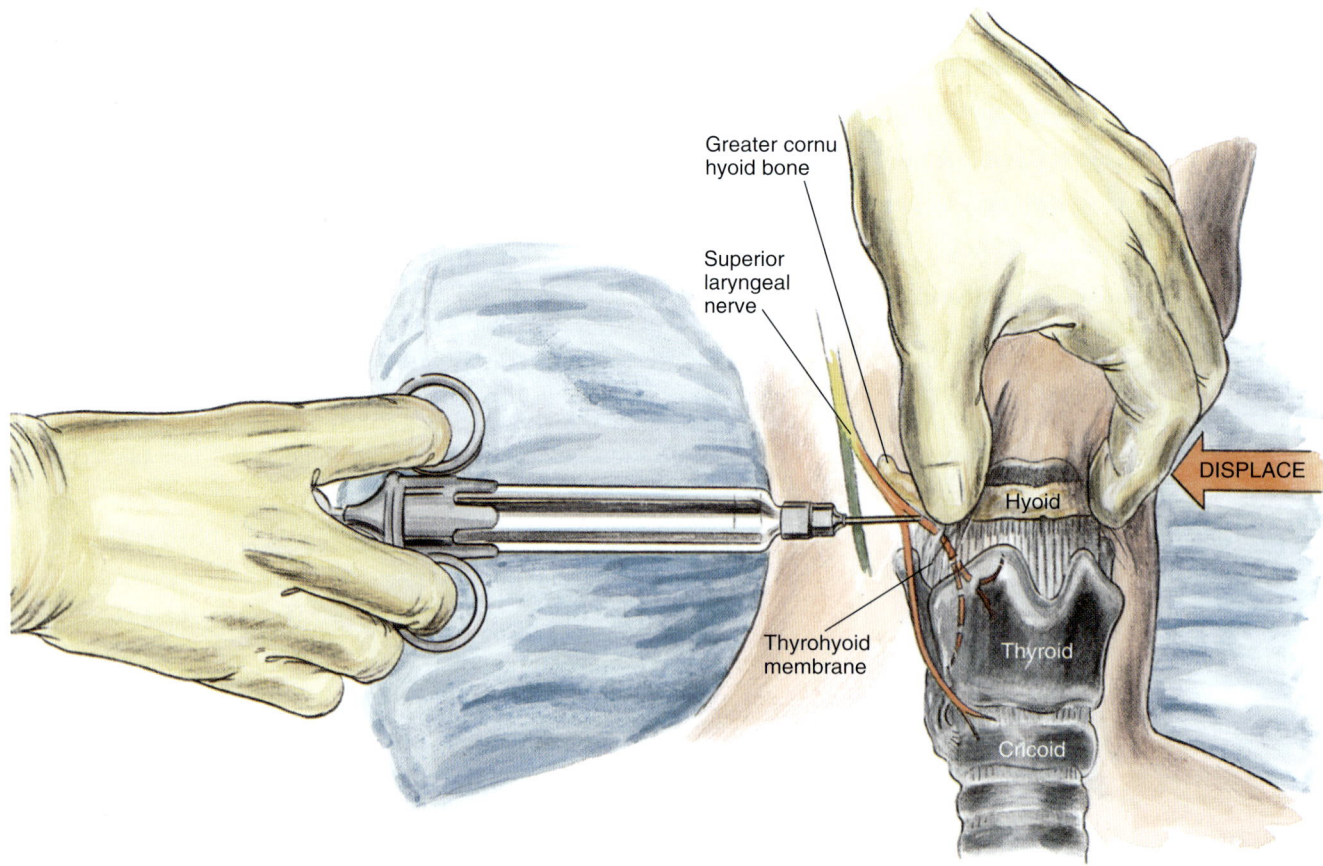

Fig. 27.2 Superior laryngeal nerve block: technique.

Translaryngeal Block

28

David L. Brown

Key Points

- It is a useful block in providing topical anesthesia to the laryngotracheal mucosa innervated by branches of vagus nerve.
- Injection through the cricothyroid membrane results in the solution being spread onto the tracheal structures and coughed onto the more superior laryngeal structures.
- Air should be aspirated freely before injecting the local anesthetics.

PERSPECTIVE

This block, like all airway blocks, can be useful in sedated, spontaneously ventilating, "awake" patients requiring tracheal intubation.

Patient Selection. Any patient is a candidate in whom it is desirable to avoid the Valsalva-like straining that may follow awake tracheal intubation (in which the patient is sedated and spontaneously ventilating).

Pharmacologic Choice. The local anesthetic most often chosen for this block is 3–4 mL of 4% lidocaine. When multiple airway blocks are administered, the anesthesiologist should be aware of the total dose of local anesthetic used.

PLACEMENT

Anatomy. Translaryngeal block is most useful in providing topical anesthesia to the laryngotracheal mucosa innervated by branches of the vagus nerve. Both surfaces of the epiglottis and laryngeal structures to the level of the vocal cords receive innervation through the internal branch of the superior laryngeal nerve, a branch of the vagus. The distal airway mucosa also receives innervation through the vagus nerve but through the recurrent laryngeal nerve. Translaryngeal injection of local anesthetic is helpful in providing topical anesthesia for both of these vagal branches because injection below the cords through the cricothyroid membrane results in the solution being spread onto the tracheal structures and coughed onto the more superior laryngeal structures (Fig. 28.1).

Position. The patient should be in a supine position, with the pillow removed and the neck slightly extended. As illustrated in Fig. 28.2, the anesthesiologist should be in position to place the index and third fingers in the space between the thyroid and the cricoid cartilages (cricothyroid membrane).

Needle Puncture. The cricothyroid membrane should be localized, the midline identified, and the needle, 22-gauge or smaller, inserted into the midline until air can be freely aspirated. When air can be freely aspirated, 3 mL of local anesthetic is rapidly injected. The needle should be removed immediately because it is almost inevitable that the patient will cough at this point. Conversely, a needle-over-the-catheter assembly (intravenous catheter) can be used for the block. Once air has been aspirated, the inner needle is removed and the injection is performed through the catheter.

POTENTIAL PROBLEMS

This block can result in coughing, which should be considered in patients in whom coughing is clearly undesirable. The midline should be used for needle insertion because the area is nearly devoid of major vascular structures. The needle does not need to be misplaced far off the midline to encounter significant arterial and venous vessels.

PEARLS

This block is most effective after the patient has been appropriately sedated. There has long been a belief that this block should be used cautiously, if at all, in patients at high risk for gastric aspiration. The author's belief is that the block is more frequently misused by not being applied in appropriate situations than by being applied when the patient is at risk for gastric aspiration.

Another hint is to perform the local anesthetic injection after asking the patient to forcefully exhale. This forces the patient to initially inspire before coughing, making distal airway anesthesia predictable.

196 ATLAS OF REGIONAL ANESTHESIA

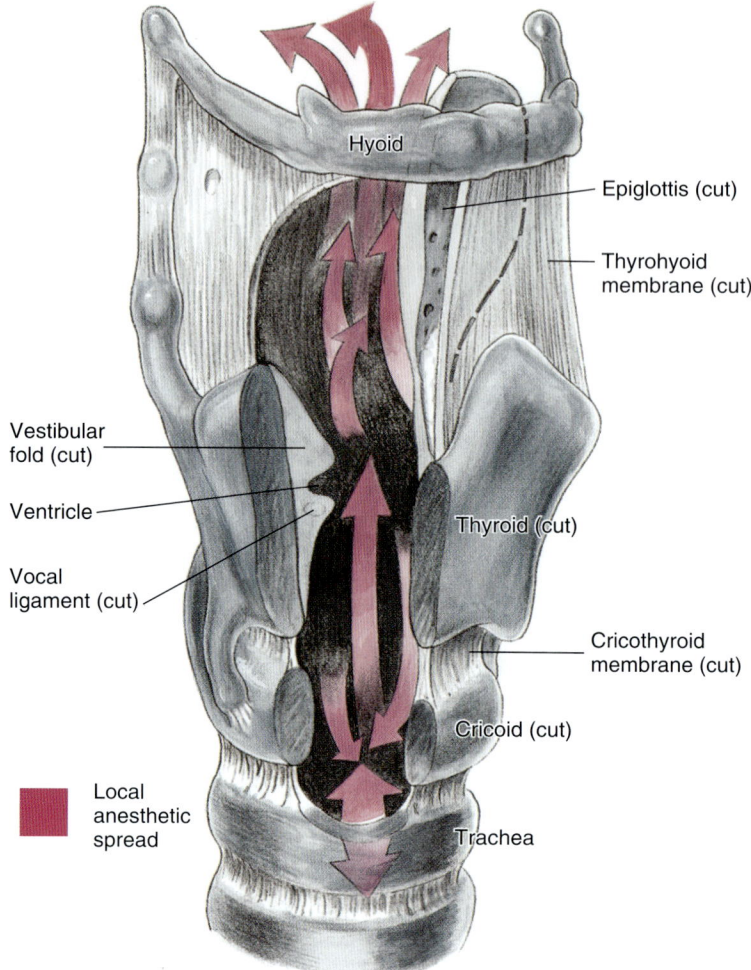

Fig. 28.1 Translaryngeal block: anatomy and local anesthetic spread.

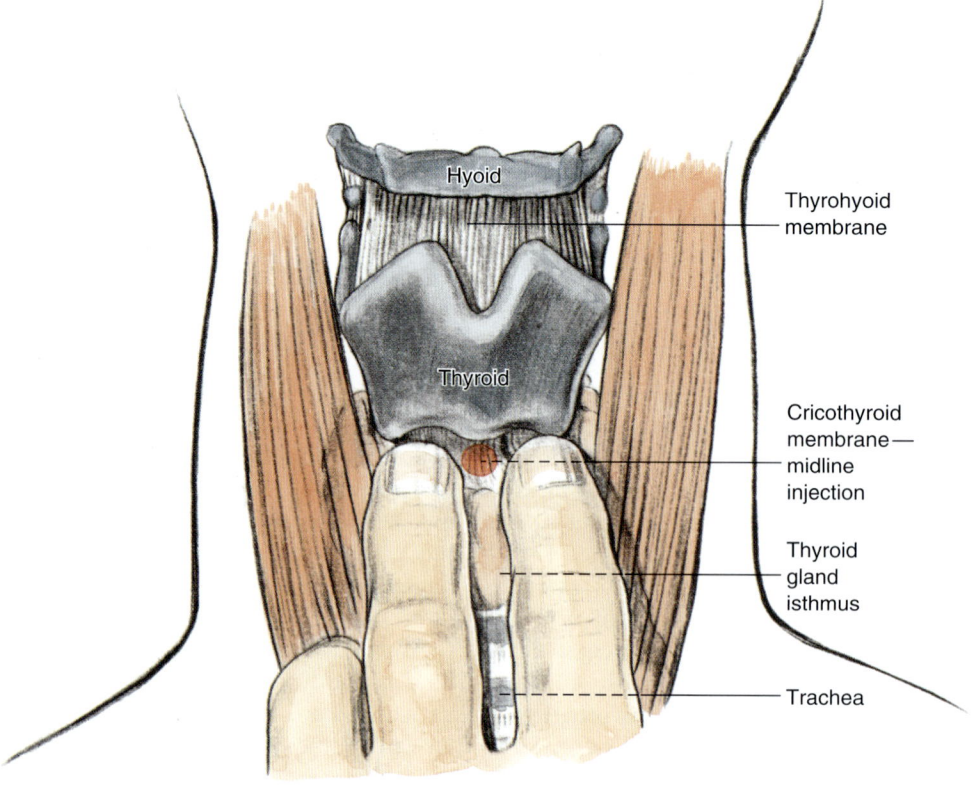

Fig. 28.2 Translaryngeal block: anatomy and technique.

Section 6
Truncal Blocks

Truncal Block Anatomy

David L. Brown

Key Points

- Thoracic and lumbar somatic innervation extends from the chest and axilla to the toes.
- Paravertebral block has an advantage over neuraxial block in its ability to avoid widespread interruption of the sympathetic nervous system.
- Major somatic nerves are the ventral rami of the thoracic and lumbar nerves.
- The dorsal rami of the spinal nerves provide innervation to dorsal midline structures.

A number of regional anesthetic techniques rely on block of the thoracic or lumbar somatic (paravertebral) nerves. As illustrated in Fig. 29.1, thoracic and lumbar somatic innervation extends from the chest and axilla to the toes. Although few major surgical procedures can be carried out under somatic block alone, appropriate use of somatic block with long-acting local anesthetics provides unique and useful analgesia. Also, when even longer-acting local anesthetics become available, possibly some form of thoracic or lumbar somatic nerve block, such as intercostal or paravertebral nerve block, will be able to provide even more useful postoperative analgesia. This is approaching clinical relevance with thoracic paravertebral use during care of patients undergoing breast surgery.

One of the advantages that somatic (paravertebral) block has over neuraxial blocks is the ability to avoid widespread interruption of the sympathetic nervous system. As shown in Fig. 29.2, the major somatic nerves are the ventral rami of the thoracic and lumbar nerves. In addition, as shown in the inset in Fig. 29.2, the nerves contribute preganglionic sympathetic fibers to the sympathetic chain through the white rami communicantes and receive postganglionic neurons from the sympathetic chain through gray rami communicantes. These rami from the sympathetic system connect to the spinal nerves near their exit from the intervertebral foramina. The dorsal rami of these spinal nerves provide innervation to dorsal midline structures. The medial branch of the dorsal primary ramus supplies the dorsal vertebral structures, including the supraspinous and intraspinous ligaments, the periosteum, and the fibrous capsule of the facet joint.

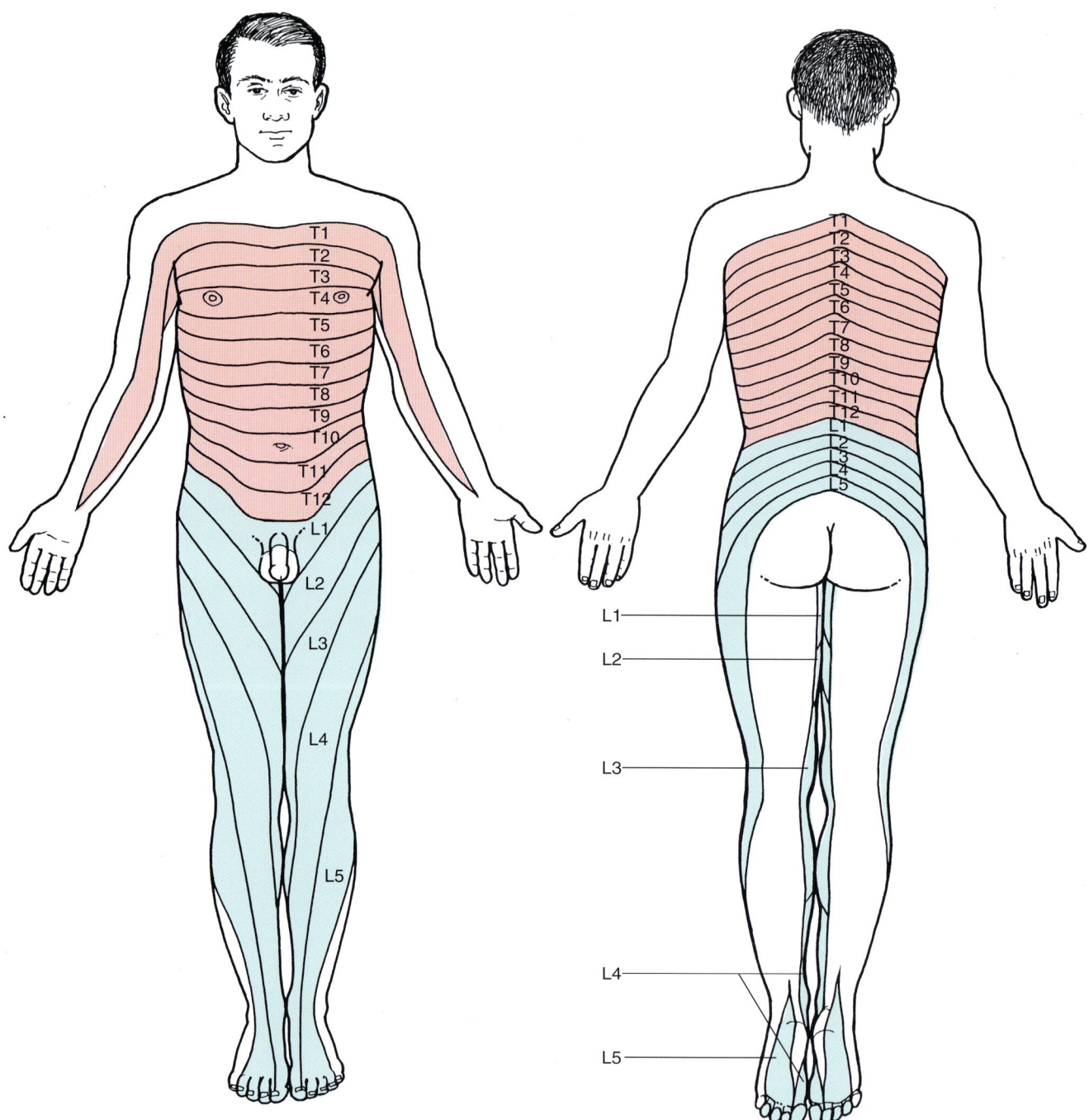

Fig. 29.1 Truncal anatomy: dermatomes.

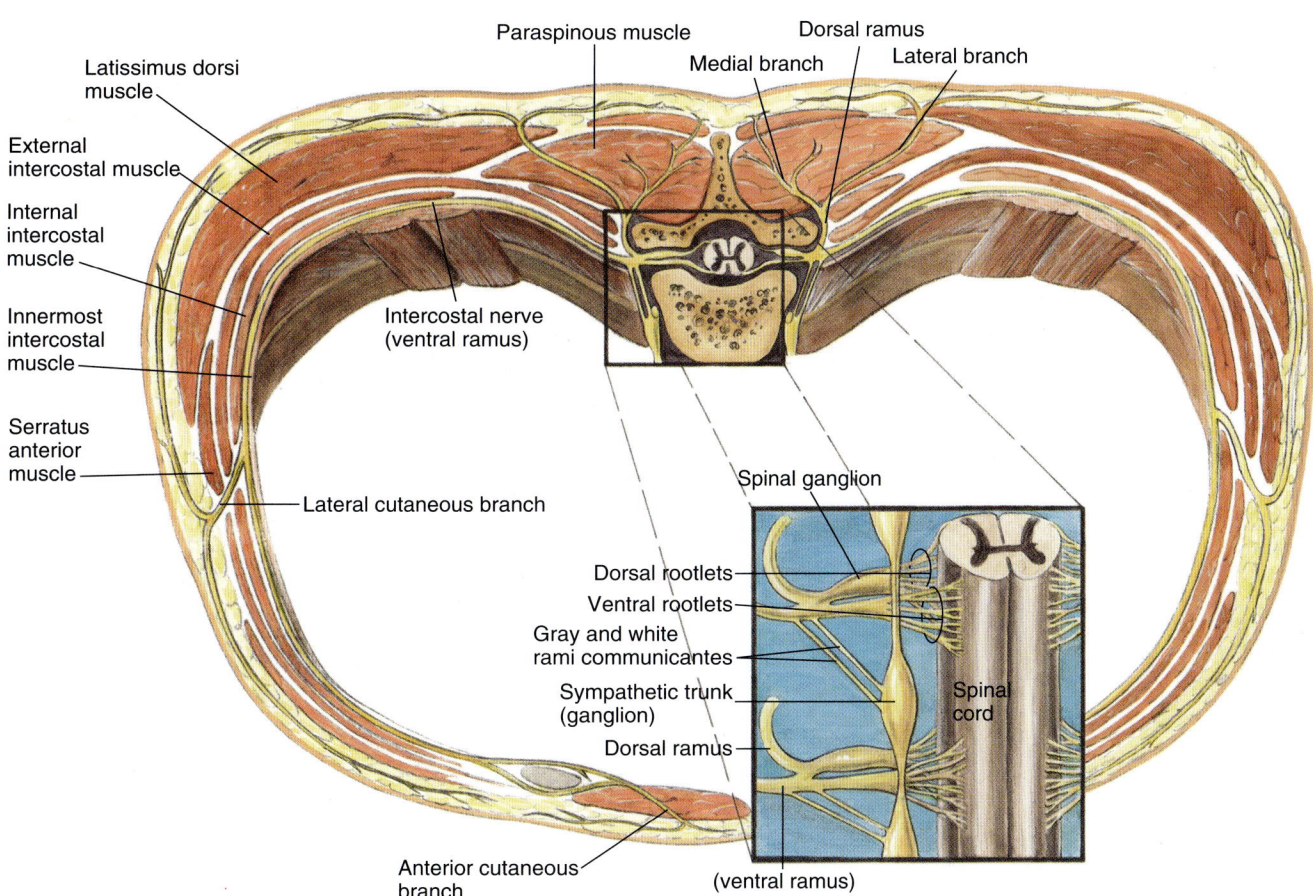

Fig. 29.2 Truncal anatomy: cross-sectional view.

PECS and Pecto-Intercostal Blocks

30

Loran Mounir-Soliman

Key Points

- Anterior chest wall blocks are used as alternatives to thoracic epidurals and paravertebral blocks for breast surgeries and procedures involving the anterior chest walls.
- Serratus plane blocks and supraclavicular blocks may be required for more extensive surgeries.
- Pectoralis major, pectoralis minor, and serratus anterior muscles are the main landmarks for the PEC blocks at the level of the fourth and fifth ribs.
- Bilateral pecto-intercostal blocks are required for sternal wound incisions.
- All fascial plane blocks need ultrasound guidance, skill with ultrasound-guided procedures, and larger volume of local anesthetics.

PERSPECTIVE AND BACKGROUND

The introduction of ultrasound to regional anesthesia allowed identification of various interfascial planes between the different muscles, including the chest wall musculature. Some of the interfascial planes (between the investing fascias of the muscles) are considered neurovascular potential spaces, hosting the different nerves and vessels supplying the chest wall. Along the course of the intercostal nerves, they branch and communicate with the adjacent intercostal nerves as well as other pectoral nerves when crossing between those different interfascial planes.

The ventral rami of the thoracic spinal nerves (T2–T9) pierce the intercostal muscles giving lateral and anterior cutaneous branches that further divide into posterior, anterior, medial and lateral branches, providing sensory innervations to the anterior and lateral aspects of the chest wall including the breast (T4–5–6). The apex of the axilla is innervated by the intercostobrachial nerve, a branch of T2 spinal nerve. These multiple divisions of the spinal nerves communicate with the branches of the adjacent spinal nerves through the neurovascular planes existing between the muscles of the chest wall, mainly pectoralis major, pectoralis minor, and serratus anterior muscles, bounded by the fascial layers covering the muscles (interfascial planes). Those planes also host branches of the brachial plexus along their course in the chest; mainly medial pectoral nerve (C8–T1), lateral pectoral nerve (C5–7), long thoracic nerve (C5–7), and thoracodorsal nerve (C6–8) (Figs. 30.1–30.4).

PECS 1 BLOCK

Injection of local anesthetics in the interval between the pectoralis major and minor muscles at the level of the third to fourth rib is viewed as PECS 1 block. Along this plane, the medial (C8–T1) and lateral pectoral (C5–7) nerves can be anesthetized by injecting a relatively large volume of local anesthetics. This block targets surgeries involving the pectoralis major muscle; for example, expander insertion, port-a-cath placement, and implantable cardiac devices (Fig. 30.5).

PECS 2 BLOCK

For more extensive surgeries of the anterior chest wall including mastectomies, sentinel node biopsies, and axillary dissections, blockade of the intercostal nerves, intercostobrachial nerves, as well as long thoracic nerves, is necessary. It is achieved through injection of the local anesthetics at a deeper level between the pectoralis minor and serratus anterior muscle at the level of the fourth to fifth ribs (PECS 2 block). Typically, PECS 1 block is performed as part of the PECS 2 block through the same entry point during the passage of the needle between the pectoralis major and pectoralis minor muscles (Fig. 30.6).

PECTO-INTERCOSTAL BLOCK

For a sternal wound, the anterior cutaneous branches of the intercostal nerves can be blocked by infiltrating local anesthetics in the fascial plane between the pectoralis major and intercostal muscles on both sides of the sternum (pecto-intercostal block) (Figs. 30.7 and 30.8).

ULTRASOUND-GUIDED INJECTION TECHNIQUE

The patient is usually positioned supine for the PECS and pecto-intercostal blocks with the anesthesiologist standing at the head of the patient. Ideally, the ultrasound machine should be facing the anesthesiologist across from the patient, to allow him to view the screen as well as the needle entry point and needle direction within the same visual field.

PECS 1 and 2. A high frequency, linear probe is best suited for these superficial blocks to better identify the different fascial planes and borders of the chest wall muscles. Scanning

204 ATLAS OF REGIONAL ANESTHESIA

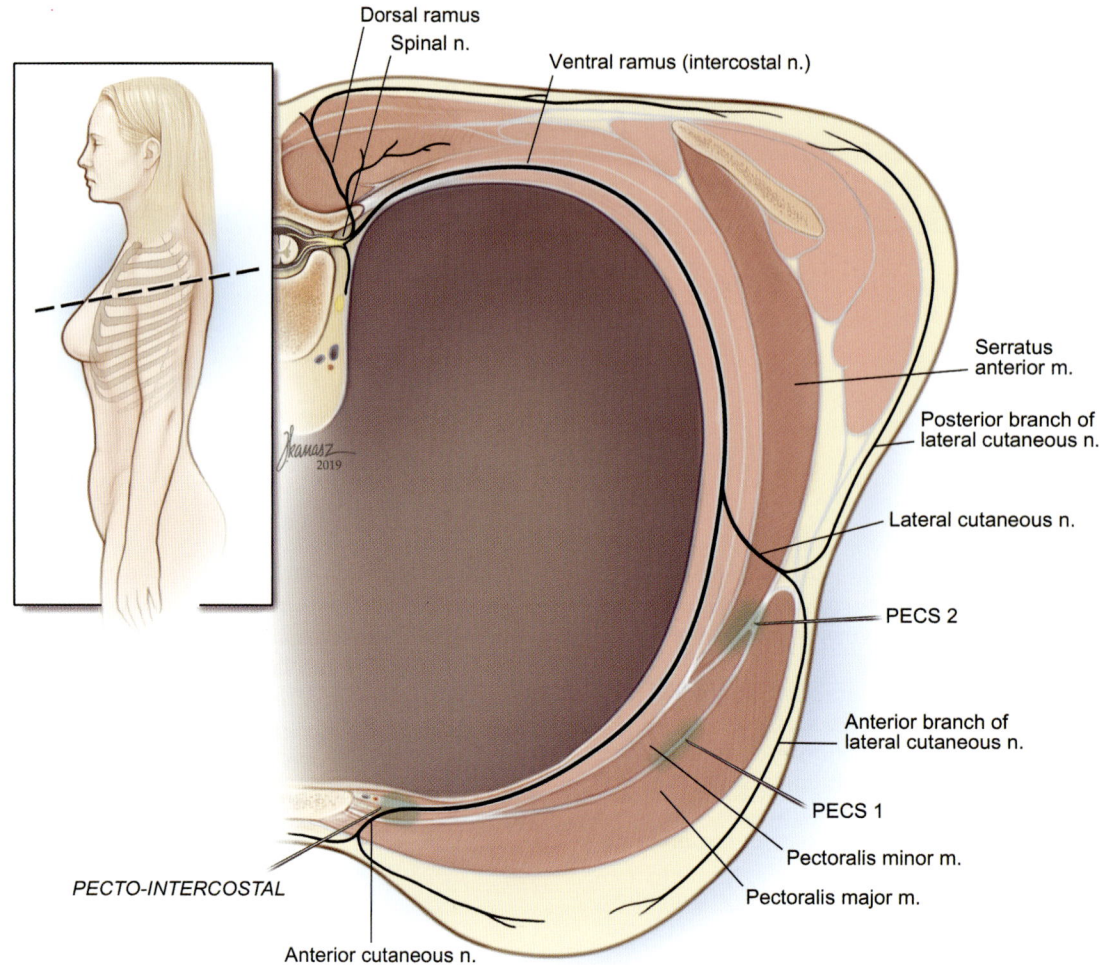

Fig. 30.1 Cross section showing the muscles of the chest wall, indicating the correct interfascial planes for PECS 1 and 2 blocks.

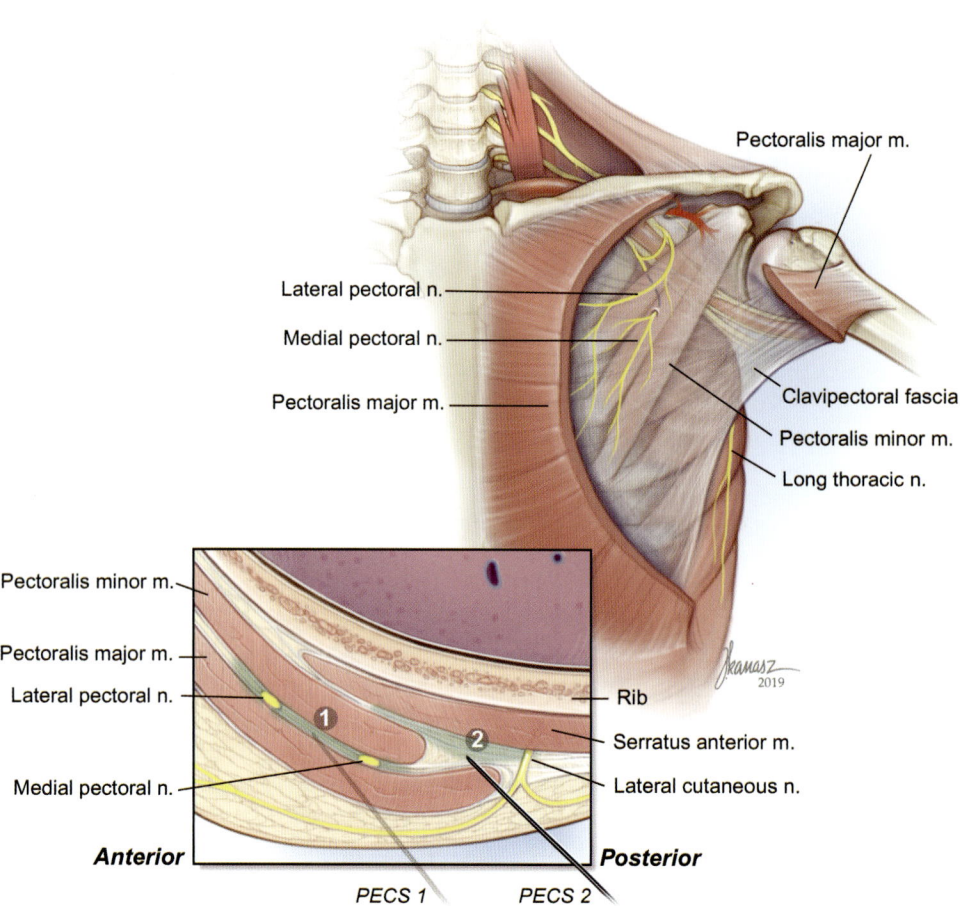

Fig. 30.2 Anatomy of the anterior chest wall with a cross section showing the correct interfascial planes for PECS 1 and 2.

PECS and Pecto-Intercostal Blocks 205

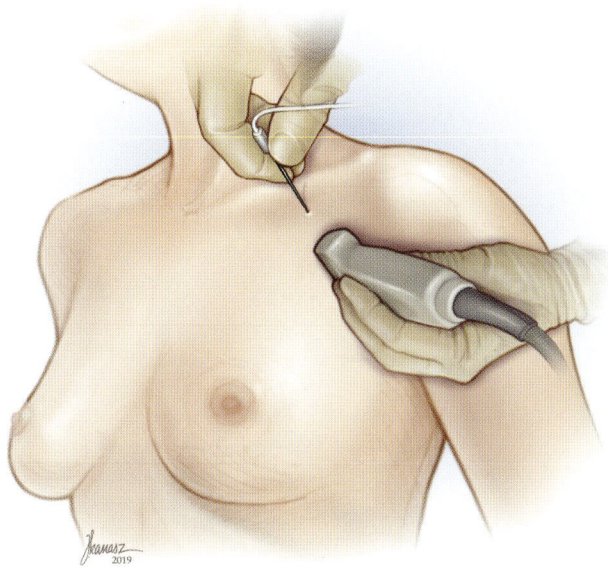

Fig. 30.3 Probe position for PECS 1,2. Note the in-plane technique for the block

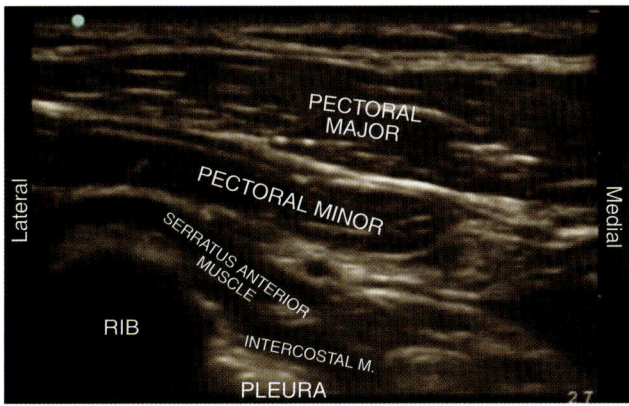

Fig. 30.4 Ultrasound image for the PECS 1 and 2 shows the muscles.

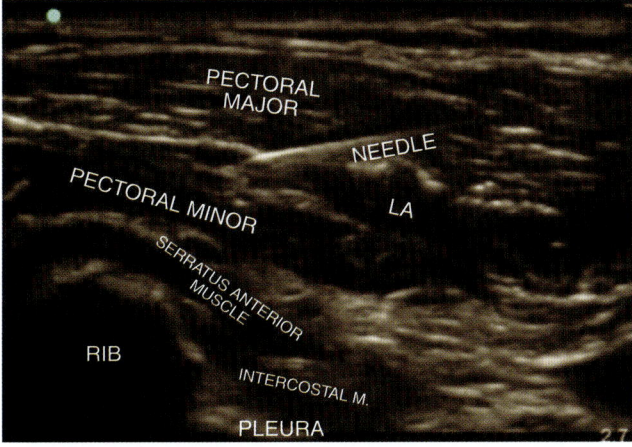

Fig. 30.5 Ultrasound image for the PECS 1 shows the position of the needle deep to the pectoralis major muscle.

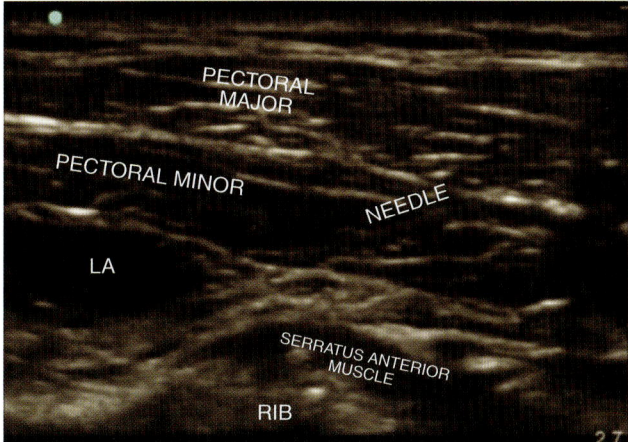

Fig. 30.6 Ultrasound image of the PECS 2 shows the position of the needle and the local anesthetics deep to the pectoralis minor muscle.

is started by placing the probe parallel to the long axis of the body (cephalo-caudad direction) medial to the coracoid process, visualizing the axillary artery and the cords of the brachial plexus surrounding it deep to the pectoralis major muscle. At this point, tilting the probe medially will allow visualization of the second rib and pleura. Scanning caudad will enable viewing of the pectoralis minor deeper to pectoralis major, especially when angulating the leading edge of the probe slightly lateral at the same time towards the axilla and lateral edge of the pectoralis muscle (see Fig. 30.2). By counting down the ribs, the interval between the third and fourth ribs, in addition to the fourth and fifth ribs is identified. The probe is usually turned oblique to the long axis of the body to allow the needle path from a cephalo-medial to a caudal and lateral direction. The target of infiltration of local anesthetics is between the pectoralis minor and serratus (PECS 2), followed by the interval between the pectoralis major and pectoralis minor (PECS 1) at those two levels. It is easier to perform the deeper block first when doing both blocks with a single needle path. That will also avoid obliteration of the deeper fascial ultrasound identification if air is accidentally injected during the first injection. Care should be taken to avoid vascular punctures of the multiple small branches of the thoracoacromial vessels hosted within the same targeted planes (neurovascular fascial planes) (Figs. 30.4–30.6).

Pecto-intercostal. The probe is placed an inch lateral and parallel to the long axis of the sternum in a longitudinal orientation. The level of injection is typically at the level of the midsternum. With this view, multiple ribs can be visualized with the intercostal muscles between them and the pleural underneath both. The pectoralis major muscle is the only muscle covering the ribs and the intercostal muscles. The interfascial interval between the pectoralis muscle and the underlying ribs and intercostal muscles is the target of infiltration of local anesthetics, in order to block the anterior cutaneous branches for sternal incisions. Care should be taken to avoid vascular injuries of the branches of the internal thoracic artery (Figs. 30.7 and 30.8).

POTENTIAL COMPLICATIONS

Intramuscular hematoma and pleural puncture can be possible complications of this block, however these are rare. Care should be taken to visualize the needle the whole time it is advanced underneath the ultrasound beam to avoid vascular or pleural puncture.

Multiple encounters of the surface of the ribs are unnecessary, can be painful to patients, and should be minimized.

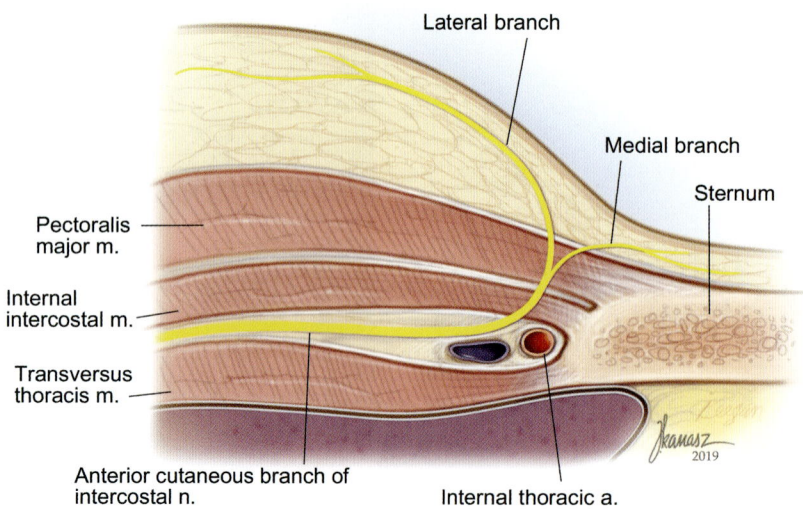

Fig. 30.7 Cross section showing the anatomical course of the anterior cutaneous branches of the intercostal nerves.

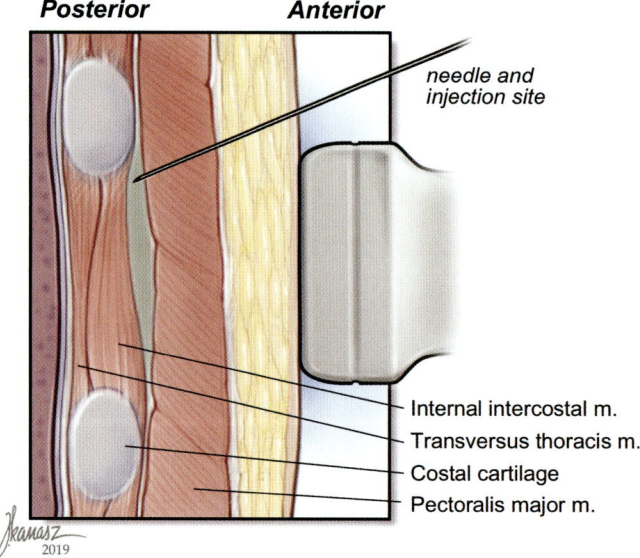

Fig. 30.8 Anatomy and needle position for the pecto-intercostal block. Note the needle and local anesthetics deep to pectoralis major and superficial to the intercostal muscles.

PEARLS

- Injection of local anesthetics underneath the pectoralis major high up in the chest (at the level of the second rib) can lead to an accidental block of the brachial plexus.
- Like most fascial plane blocks, the target is not a specific nerve as much as it is a plexus of nerves formed by the communication of multiple branches. The injection of a large volume (20-30 mL) is necessary to have a wider spread and block most of those branches. Care should be taken to calculate the maximum dose of local anesthetics injected to avoid systemic toxicity.
- Combining PECS blocks to the serratus anterior block may be necessary to cover anterior and anterolateral chest wall incisions.
- For continuous infusion techniques, intermittent bolus programming may provide better spread and more effective block.
- The area immediately below the clavicle and the upper part of the breast is supplied by the supraclavicular nerve (C3–4), and nerve to subclavius (C5–6). The typical injection for PECS 1 and 2 blocks does not provide coverage to this area. Separate injection of the supraclavicular nerve (superficial injection above the clavicle) and nerve to subclavius (superficial injection below the clavicle) may be needed as a supplement if the incision extends high up in the chest towards the clavicle.
- Original hydrodissection can be achieved by saline to limit the total dose of local anesthetics used.

Serratus Anterior Block

Loran Mounir-Soliman

Key Points

- Serratus anterior block is indicated for anterolateral chest wall incisions, targeting the lateral and postcutaneous branches of upper and middle thoracic dermatomes.
- The block has been used for different thoracoscopic and open chest wall incisions as well as chest tube placements and rib fractures.
- The long thoracic nerve is included in the serratus anterior block.
- Injection of the local anesthetic either superficial or deep to the serratus anterior muscle leads to similar results clinically.
- The optimal point of injection should be posterior to the midaxillary line at the level of fifth or sixth ribs. This allows better identification of the muscle as well as better spread of the medication.

RELEVANT ANATOMY

The serratus anterior muscles originate from the anterior surface of the first to eighth ribs at the lateral chest wall and insert along the entire anterior length of the medial border of the scapula, as well as the ventral aspect of its inferior angle. It consists of multiple serrated tendinous projections connecting the ribs, with the costal margin of the scapula pulling the scapula forward around the chest (protraction), especially when pushing forwards. It also helps with upward rotation of the scapula, adding to the trapezius muscle action. The muscular serrations are thinner at its origin (anteriorly) and get bigger along its course posteriorly.

The serratus anterior receives its nerve supply from the long thoracic nerve, also called nerve to serratus anterior; it originates from the roots of the brachial plexus (C5–C7). Its injury results in "winging" of the scapula. It has multiple sensory and motor branches and typically runs in a course between the middle and posterior axillary lines.

Anterior to the anterior axillary line, the serratus anterior muscle is covered by the pectoralis muscles. Along its dorsal course starting at the level of the fifth rib, the serratus anterior is covered by the latissimus dorsi muscle. Accordingly, posterior to the midaxillary lines, there are two potential fascial planes: superficial and deep to the serratus muscle. Superficial to the serratus anterior, the fascial plane is bounded by the deep surface of the latissimus dorsi, and deep to the serratus the plane is bounded by the ribs and intercostal muscles.

The lateral and posterior cutaneous branches of T2–T9 intercostal nerves, along with the long thoracic nerve, travel across those two fascial planes: superficial and deep to the serratus anterior muscle posterior to the midaxillary line. Clinical results indicate that injection of local anesthetic along both planes results in similar outcomes; mainly blocking upper and midthoracic dermatomes of the lateral chest wall (Fig. 31.1).

ULTRASOUND-GUIDED INJECTION TECHNIQUE

Typically, a high-frequency linear probe is used for the serratus anterior block to better identify the superficial and deep boundaries of the muscle. However, a curvilinear probe can be more useful in morbidly obese patients to allow deeper penetration and broader visual window. The patient is positioned laterally with the side to be blocked, uppermost. Transverse scanning along the course of the serratus muscle posteriorly at the level of the fifth rib identifies the muscle starting in the midaxillary line. The size of the muscle varies according to its position along the chest wall, being larger posteriorly. Tilting the probe from side to side can also change the viewable section of the muscle according to the trajectory of the beam. The muscle is identified by its position just on top of the ribs, distinguished from the intercostal muscles located between the costal hyperechoic lines. As the probe moves posteriorly, the beam will encounter the large latissimus dorsi muscle, superficial to the serratus anterior. The needle is inserted in-plane from anterior to posterior (however, it can be introduced from the dorsal side of the probe, if needed). The local anesthetic is injected in one of two fascial planes: superficial to the serratus anterior (deep to the latissimus dorsi), or deep to the serratus anterior, lifting the muscle of the ribs and intercostal muscles. As mentioned previously, clinical results have been reported to be similar since the long thoracic nerve and the branches of the intercostal nerves run across both planes. It is the author's practice to install half of the volume in each plane, starting with the deeper one first, for wider spread.

The optimal level of injection is at the posterior axillary line at the level of the fifth or sixth rib to allow more coverage of the lateral and posterior cutaneous branches.

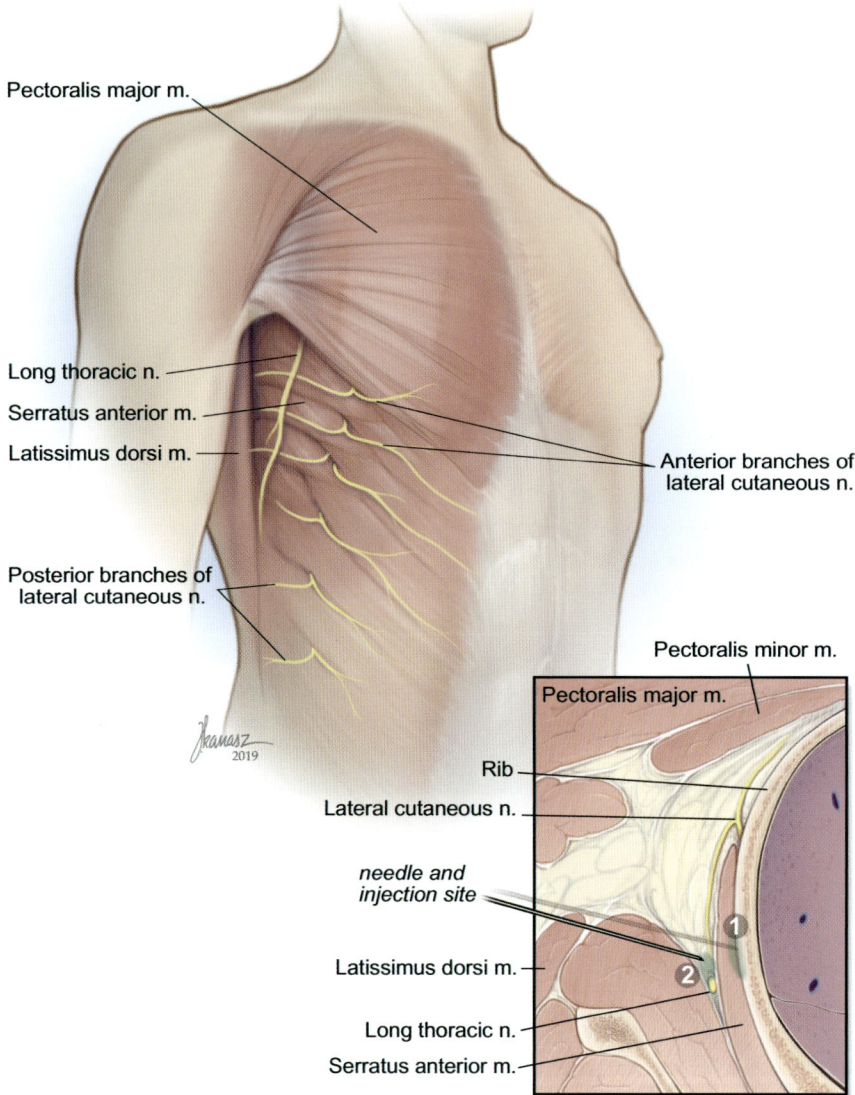

Fig. 31.1 Anatomy of the anterior chest wall showing the sensory distribution of serratus anterior block.

The single-shot technique, as well as continuous indwelling catheter, have been described for this block (Figs. 31.2–31.4).

POTENTIAL COMPLICATIONS

Intramuscular hematoma, as well as pleural puncture, can be possible complications of this block, but are rare. Care should be taken to visualize the needle the entire time it is advanced below the ultrasound beam to avoid vascular or pleural puncture.

Multiple encounters of the surface of the ribs are unnecessary, can be painful to patients, and should be minimized.

PEARLS

- The serratus anterior block is usually a superficial block going 2–3 inches deep in most patients. Accordingly, there is no need to use a needle longer than 3–4 inches in length.
- Like most fascial plane blocks, the target is not a specific nerve as much as it is a plexus of nerves formed by the communication of multiple branches. The injection of a large volume (20–30 mL) is necessary to have a wider spread and block most of those branches. Care should be taken to calculate the maximum dose of local anesthetic injected to avoid systemic toxicity.
- Combining PECS blocks to the serratus anterior block may be necessary to cover anterior and anterolateral chest wall incisions.
- For continuous infusion techniques, intermittent bolus programming may provide better spread and more effective block.

Serratus Anterior Block 209

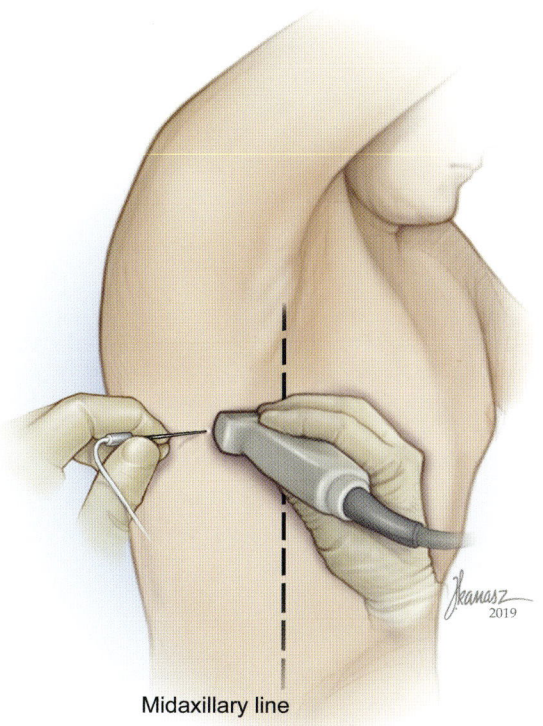

Fig. 31.2 Ultrasound probe position. Note the in-plane technique of the block.

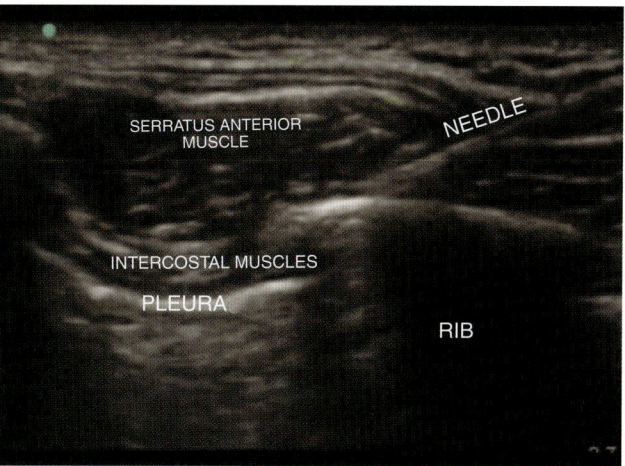

Fig. 31.4 Ultrasound image of the serratus anterior block with the needle deep to serratus anterior muscle but superficial to the intercostal muscles. The injection of local anesthetic is between the serratus anterior and intercostal muscles. Note, the pleura is always visualized when performing the block to avoid pneumothorax or injury to the lung.

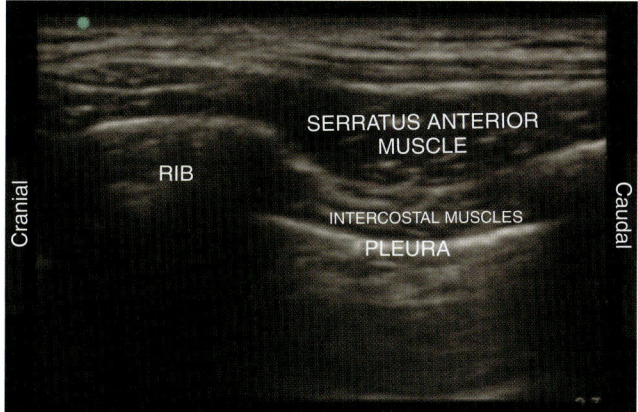

Fig. 31.3 Ultrasound image of the serratus anterior block showing the serratus anterior and intercostal muscles. It is very important to visualize the pleura when performing the block as shown in the figure.

Ultrasound for Intercostal Block

32

Ehab Farag and Rajeev Krishnaney Davison

Key Points

- Intercostal nerves supply major parts of the skin and musculature of the chest and abdominal wall.
- Intercostal nerve block is now commonly performed for treatment of acute and chronic pain conditions affecting the thorax and upper abdomen.
- Intercostal nerve block provides excellent analgesia for chest trauma such as rib fractures and after chest and upper abdominal surgeries.
- Ultrasound provides the safest and most successful way for intercostal nerve blocks.
- The online technique is the preferred way for performing the block.

SONOANATOMY

There are three layers of intercostal muscles: external, internal, and innermost intercostal muscles, which are all incomplete, thin layers of muscle and tendinous fibers. The neurovascular bundle lies between the internal and innermost intercostal muscles in the costal groove. Of note, the neurovascular bundle lies midway between the ribs in the majority of cases. The use of ultrasound allows the visualization of the pleura and the different layers of the intercostals. The pleura will be easily identified as a hyperechoic line that glides with respiration (sliding sign).

TECHNIQUE

A linear probe with high resolution (6–13 Hz) is used for the technique. The patient can be placed in prone position, sitting position, or lateral position with the side to be blocked facing upward. The angle of the rib, which is 6–7.5 cm from the spinous process or on the lateral edge of the paraspinal muscle, is the common site of injection as the rib is the thickest at this site and the intercostal nerve has not yet branched. The probe is usually placed in the short axis to the ribs, so the two consecutive ribs are in view. The probe can also be placed in the long axis of the consecutive ribs, the author's preferred technique. Both in-plane and out-of-plane techniques could be used for intercostal nerve block. The author prefers the in-plane technique as the complete needle path can be visualized. The needle is advanced under real time ultrasound guidance until the tip is positioned between intercostal and innermost intercostal muscles. After proper positioning of the needle 4–5 mL of local anesthetic is usually injected for each intercostal space (Figs. 32.1A,B–32.3).

PEARLS

- The preferred local anesthetic for this block is either 0.2% ropivacaine for sensory block or 0.5% for surgical block.
- The pleura should be observed at all times when performing the technique.
- After performing the block, ultrasound can be used to scan for the possible complication of pneumothorax.
- Pneumothorax can be diagnosed by absence of the sliding sign and/or comet-tail artifacts that appear as vertical lines to the pleura.

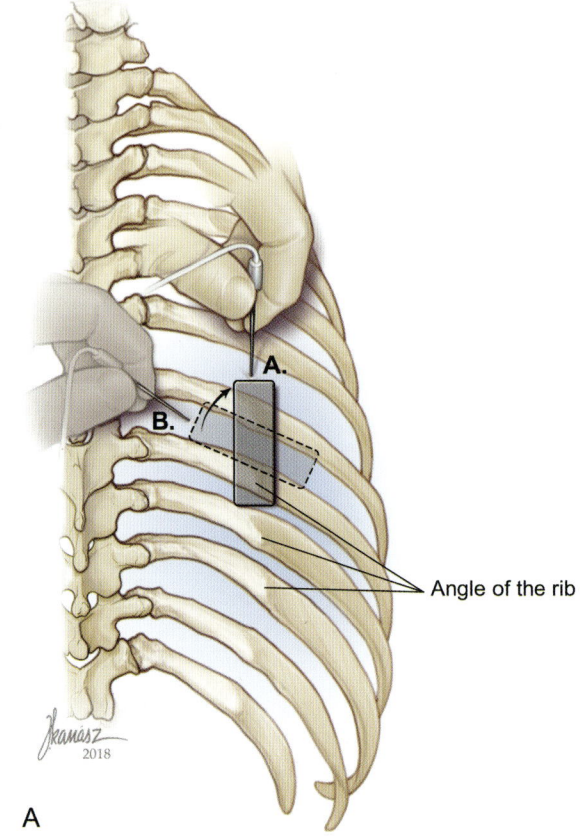

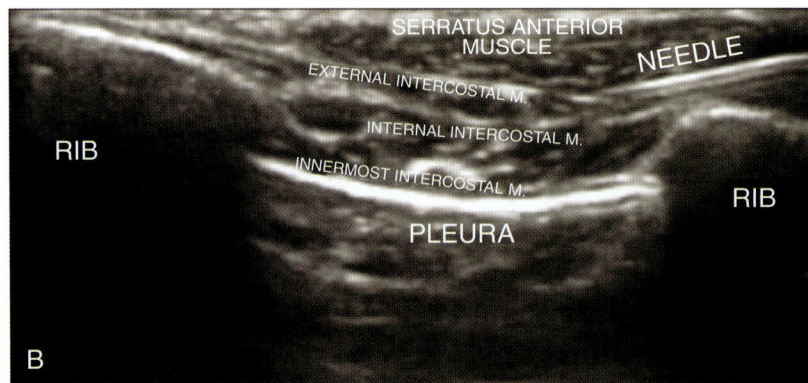

Fig. 32.1 (A) The position of the ultrasound probe at the angle of the ribs is either at short axis *(A, across the ribs)* or at long axis *(B, parallel to the ribs)*. Note that in-plane technique is preferred. (B) Ultrasound image of the intercostal block shows the three intercostal muscles and the pleura.

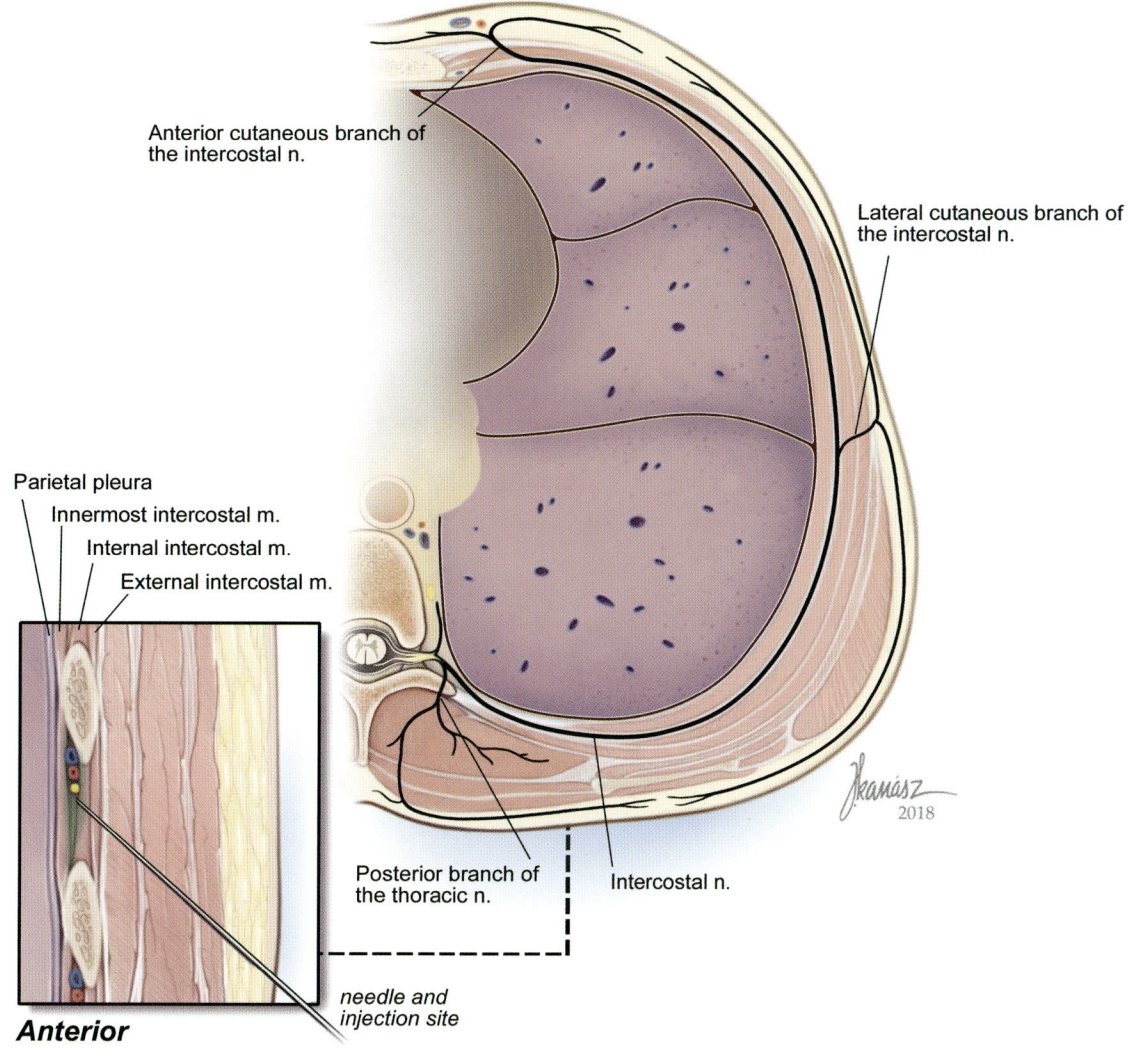
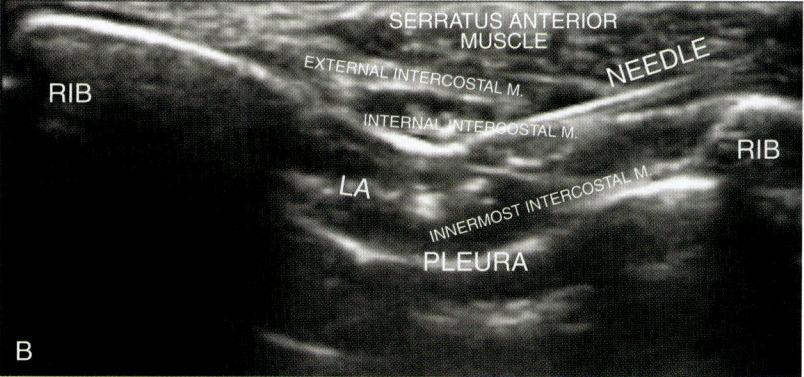

Fig. 32.2 **(A)** Needle position and injection is between internal intercostal and innermost intercostal muscles. **(B)** Ultrasound image of intercostal block shows the position of the needle and local anesthetic distribution between internal intercostal and innermost intercostal muscles.

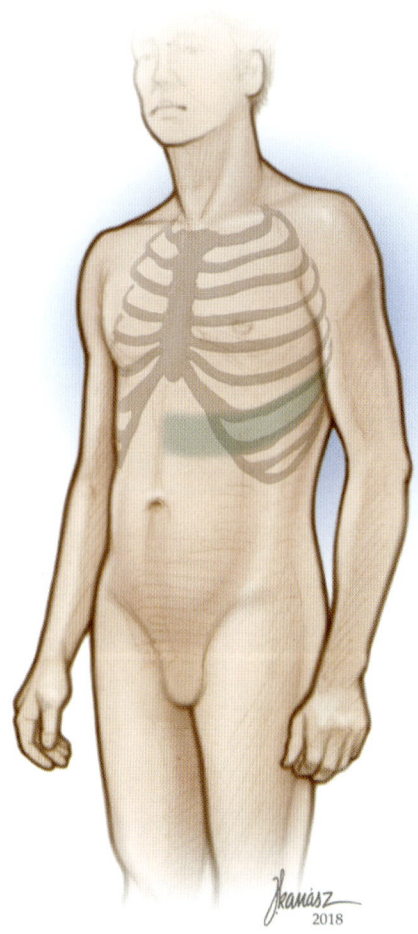

Fig. 32.3 The distribution of analgesia after intercostal block.

Paravertebral Block 33

Ehab Farag

Key Points

- The thoracic paravertebral block, with or without catheter, can be used in lieu of thoracic epidural catheter for unilateral procedures and for breast surgeries.
- Pneumothorax is the major complication of this block.
- When performing the block and the injection, make sure the needle tip always remains visible in the plane.

INDICATIONS

- Thoracic paravertebral catheter can be used in lieu of thoracic epidural analgesia for unilateral procedures like thoracotomies, nephrectomies (either partial or radical), rib fractures, and breast surgeries.
- This block is used in cases where epidural catheter is difficult or epidural analgesia failed, for unilateral procedures.
- Bilateral paravertebral blocks, with or without catheter insertion, can be used for bilateral procedures taking care to avoid the development of bilateral pneumothoraces and local anesthetic overdose toxicity.

CONTRAINDICATIONS

- The same contraindications exist as with epidural catheter insertions regarding the use of anticoagulants and antiplatelet drugs.
- Pneumothorax is the main complication of thoracic paravertebral block, with or without catheter insertion. Therefore, inexperience performing regional anesthesia using ultrasound is considered a relative contraindication for thoracic paravertebral block.

SONOANATOMY

The thoracic paravertebral space lies adjacent to the thoracic spine bodies and contains the spinal nerves as they emerge from the intervertebral foramina, the anterior divisions (intercostal nerves), the posterior divisions, and the rami communicantes. The thoracic paravertebral space is sandwiched between the parietal pleura anteriorly and the superior costotransverse ligament posteriorly. The vertebral body, intervertebral disc, and intervertebral foramen form the medial boundary. The thoracic paravertebral space is connected to the level above and below, with the caudad limit being the origin of the psoas major at T12.

The thoracic paravertebral space can be scanned in both the transverse (intercostal) and paramedian approaches. In the transverse approach, the probe is aligned in the space between two adjacent ribs overlying the transverse process. In this approach, the external intercostal muscle, internal intercostal membrane that binds medially with the costotransverse ligament, and the parietal pleura can be viewed. The landmarks in this scan are the bony reflections from the transverse process, with its dropout shadow, and the pleural reflection, which moves with respiration.

In the paramedian (longitudinal) approach, the probe lies in the paramedian plane of the transverse processes. The main landmarks in this approach are reflections and dropout from the tips of the transverse processes. The external intercostal muscle and costotransverse ligament lie between the transverse processes. The parietal pleura lie deep to these layers and can be recognized by their movement with respiration as evidenced in ultrasound by characteristic sliding and comet tails signs (Fig. 33.1).

TECHNIQUE

The linear ultrasound probe (50-mm footprint) is usually used for this block. In the transverse approach, the probe is aligned over the long axis of the rib; then it is moved medially to visualize the transverse process. By toggling (tilting) the probe, the external intercostal muscle, internal intercostal membrane that binds medially with the costotransverse ligament, and the parietal pleura can be identified. The needle is introduced in-plane at the lateral end of the probe from the lateral to medial direction. The needle tip should be positioned just deep to the costotransverse ligament in the paravertebral space. Local anesthetic spread should cause displacement of the pleura anteriorly.

In the paramedian (longitudinal) approach, the linear ultrasound probe (50-mm footprint) or curvilinear probe can be used for this approach. However, the author prefers to use the linear probe for this block. First, the technician

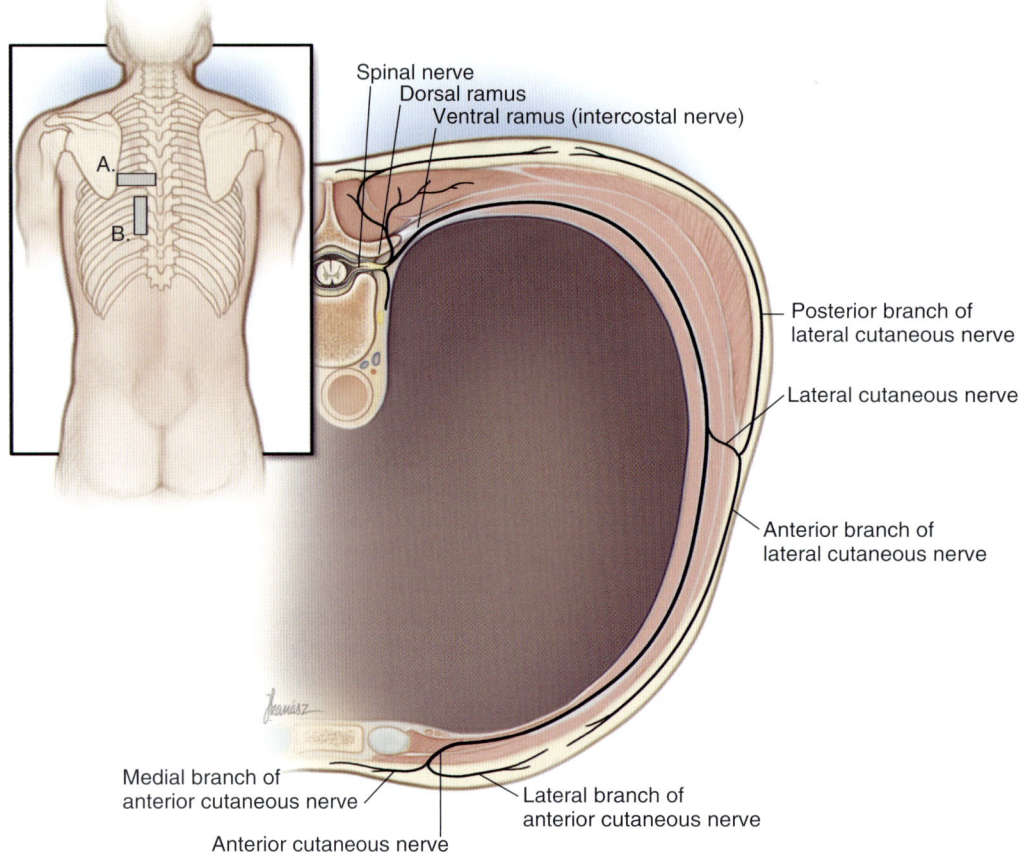

Fig. 33.1 Anatomy of paravertebral space.

scans the spinous process and then moves the probe laterally to visualize the transverse process. The probe then will be rotated through 90 degrees to lie 2.5 cm lateral to the spine over the desired thoracic levels. The needle is introduced in-plane at the lower end of the probe. For better needle visualization, the probe can be rotated to lie oblique to the spine rather than parallel to it. As in the transverse approach, the needle tip should be positioned just deep to the costotransverse ligament in the paravertebral space. Injecting local anesthetic will displace the pleural anteriorly. In both techniques the catheter can be inserted via Tuohy needle (Figs. 33.2–33.5).

PEARLS

- Patients may be positioned in the sitting, lateral decubitus (surgical side up), or prone position during the block.
- The parietal pleura appear as a glittering hyperechoic structure between the transverse processes.
- The presence of lung sliding, which is the to and fro movement of the lung caused by respiration, and comet tail signs rule out pneumothorax after thoracic paravertebral block.
- Patients with lung hyperventilation, as in chronic obstructive lung disease, are at higher risk of developing pneumothorax.
- The costotransverse ligament can be mistakenly identified as parietal pleura, and the injection of local anesthetic superficial to the ligament will result in block failure. Optimizing the image depth and gain will help with proper identification of the pleura and the costotransverse ligament. Furthermore, asking the patient to take a deep breath will identify the visceral and parietal pleura. The latter maneuver will cause a visible movement of the visceral and parietal pleura over each other (sliding sign).
- The paramedian approach is the preferred one for catheter insertion, as theoretically it decreases the incidence of placing the catheter in the epidural space.
- The continuous thoracic paravertebral catheter infusion rate is 5–10 mL per hour of 0.2% ropivacaine. However, for paravertebral block without catheter insertion, 5 mL of 0.2% or 0.5% ropivacaine is injected at each level.
- Pneumothorax is the major complication of this block. Injections into the root canal and epidural or spinal blockade are other possible complications.

Paravertebral Block 217

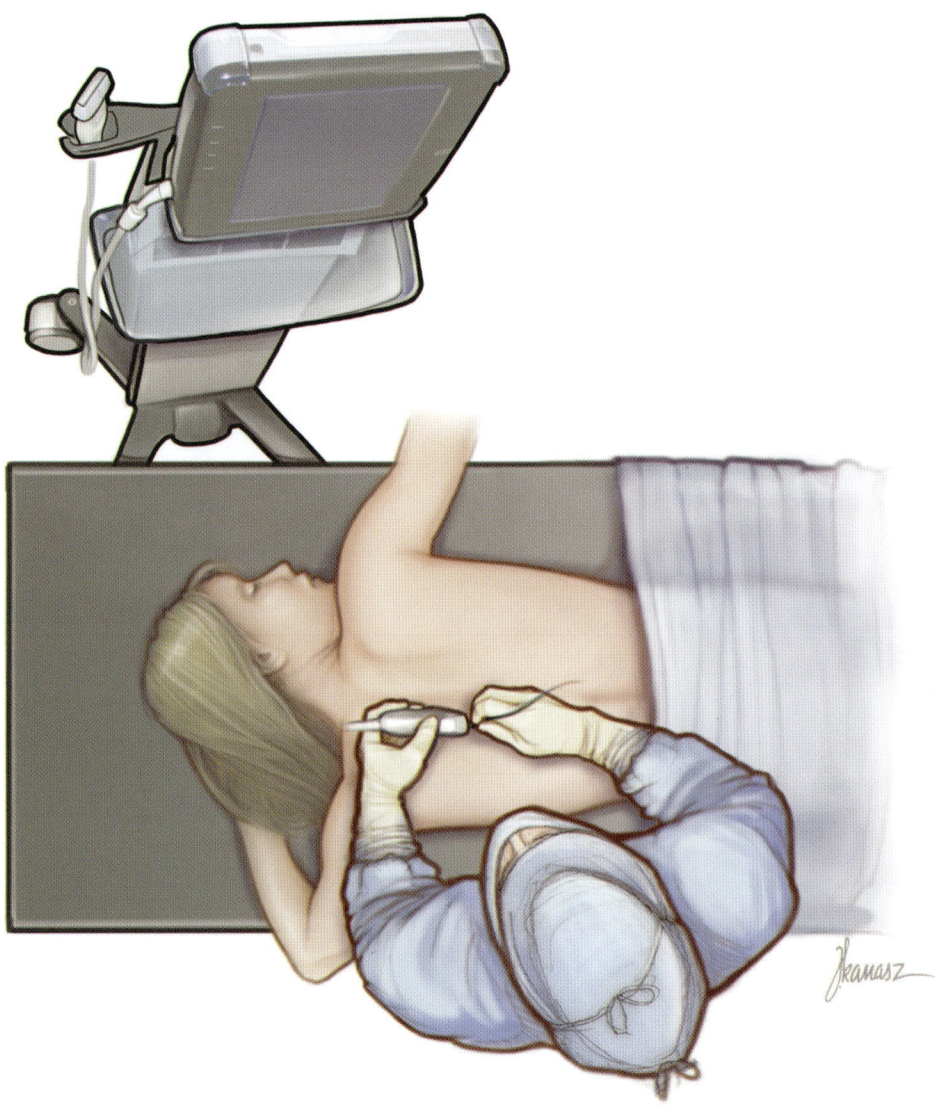

Fig. 33.2 Patient positioned with ultrasound machine for paravertebral block.

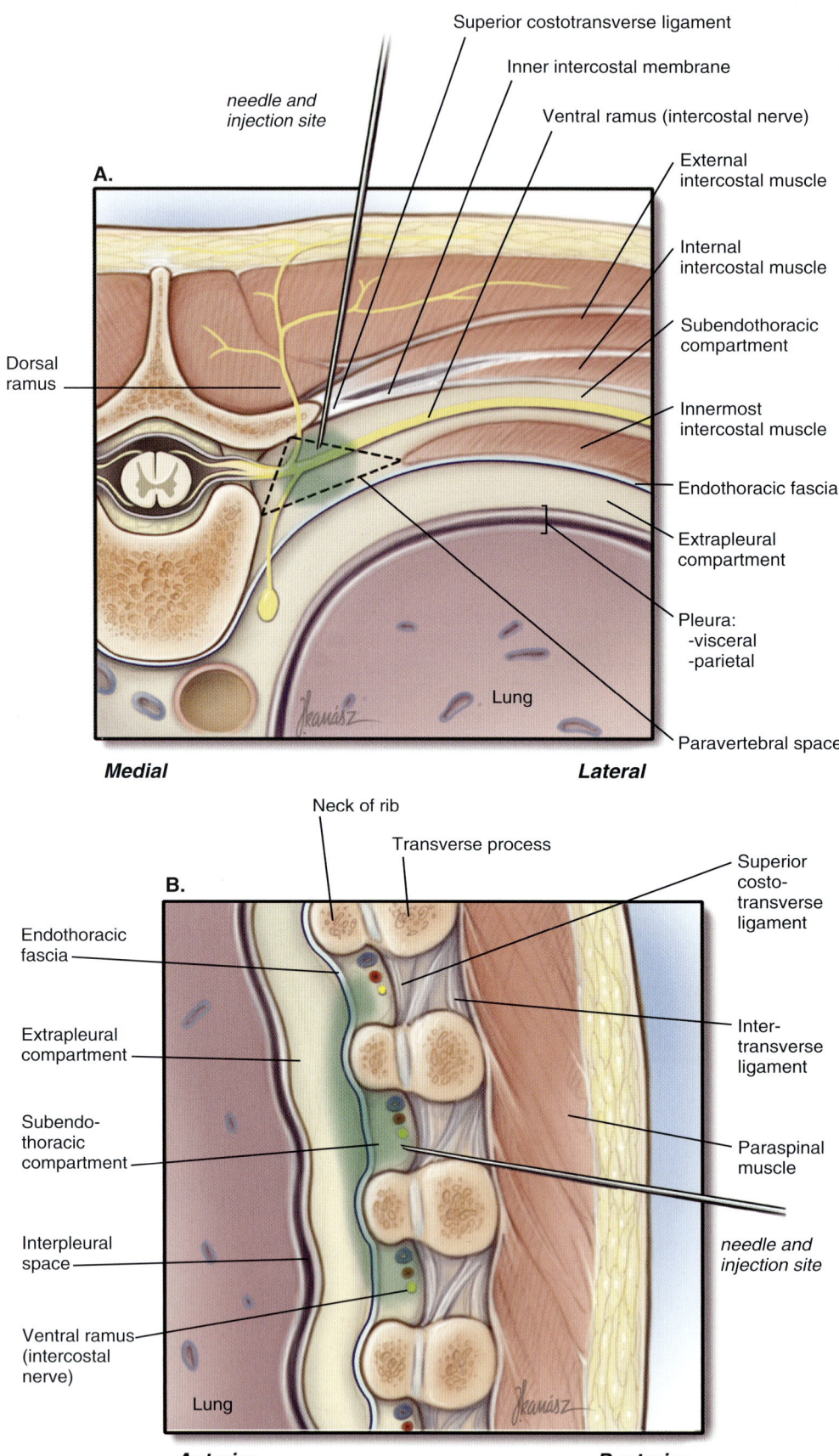

Fig. 33.3 (A) Transverse intercostal technique for paravertebral block. Note the internal intercostal membrane binds medially with the costotransverse ligament. (B) Paramedian (longitudinal) approach for paravertebral block.

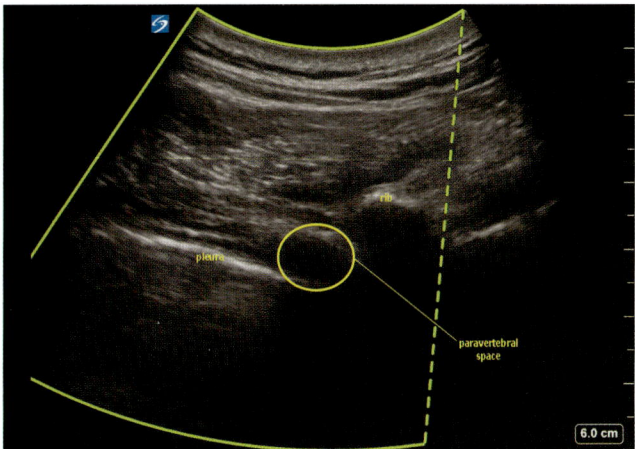

Fig. 33.4 Transverse approach for paravertebral block.

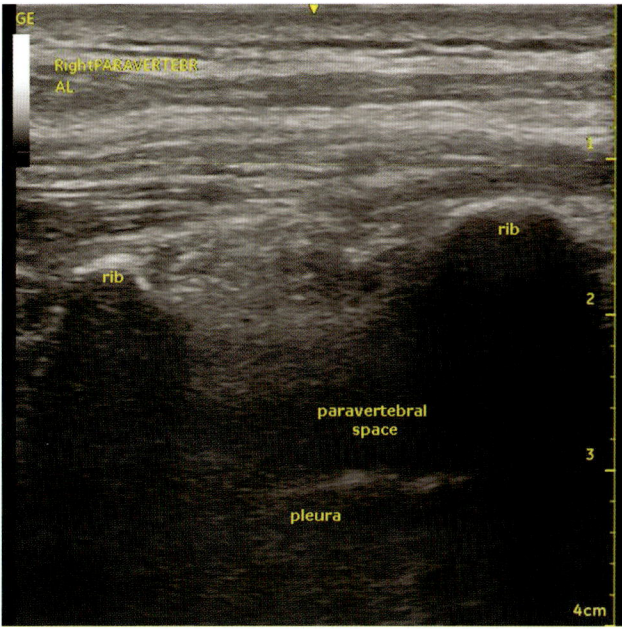

Fig. 33.5 Paramedian (longitudinal) approach for paravertebral block.

Erector Spinae Plane Block

34

Vicente Roqués-Escolar and Mauricio Forero

KEY POINTS

- The erector spinae plane block (ESPB) is actually used for acute and chronic thoracoabdominal pain syndromes, although its indication has been described for the treatment of pain in other locations.
- It is advisable to use a high frequency transducer (7–12 MHz).
- Clear identification of the transverse process is mandatory prior to infiltration or catheter insertion.
- Injection volumes ranging from 20–40 mL of a long-lasting local anesthetic are commonly used.
- Local anesthetic injected over the transverse process and beneath the erector spinae muscle spreads cranial and caudal to achieve multiple vertebral levels and reaches the paravertebral space.

PERSPECTIVE

The ESPB was first described by Forero et al in 2017, and was initially applied in the management of thoracic neuropathic pain. Actually, there are more than 100 reports published, most of which demonstrated efficacy for acute and chronic thoracoabdominal pain syndromes.

The ESPB is an interfacial plane block whereby local anesthetic is injected within a plane beneath the erector spinae muscle, to achieve multimodal analgesia for thoracic or abdominal surgery. Its analgesic effect appears to be the result of local anesthetic diffusion into the paravertebral space, affecting both the dorsal and ventral ramus of the thoracic spinal nerves.

Clinical results indicate that local anesthetic injected over the transverse process and beneath the erector spinae muscle spreads cranial and caudal to achieve multiple vertebral levels and reaches the paravertebral space to anesthetize dorsal and ventral ramus as well as the rami communicantes, which supply the sympathetic chain. The exact pathway by which the local anesthetic reaches the spinal nerves is still undefined. Between the erector spinae plane and paravertebral space, we can find a series of anatomical structures that conceptually are given the name of "intertransverse connective tissue complex". This complex is a layer composed of multiple separate structures (intertransverse and costotransverse ligaments, levator costarum, rotator costarum, external intercostal muscles, and fat). As such, there may well be perforations that allow local anesthetic to diffuse through into the paravertebral space.

Indications

Spine region	Indications
High Thoracic T2 or T3	Chronic shoulder pain syndrome
	Postsurgical shoulder pain
Mid Thoracic T4 to T6	Rib fracture (midpoint of level of ribs fracture)
	Open thoracotomy and VATS lobectomy (T5)
	Rescue after TE failure for thoracic surgery (T5)
	Cardiac surgery-sternotomy (T5)
	Breast surgery with axillary lymph node dissections (T3)
	Chronic postherpetic neuralgia (level of segment involved)
	Chronic postthoracotomy pain (level of segments involved)
	Metastatic ribs cancer (level of segments involved)
Low Thoracic T7 to T12	Nephrectomies (T8)
	Hysterectomies (T10)
	Laparoscopic ventral hernia repair with mesh (T7)
	Laparotomies (T7)
	Chronic postherpetic neuralgia (level of segment involved)
	Chronic abdominal pain syndrome (T7 to T10)
	Chronic pelvic pain syndrome (T10)
Lumbar (L4)	Vertebral surgery (midpoint of levels involved)
	Postsurgical hip replacement pain management (L4)

TE, Thoracic epidural anesthesia; VATS, video assisted thoracoscopic surgery.

Pharmacologic Choice. Long acting local anesthetics (bupivacaine, levobupivacaine, or ropivacaine) are used at concentrations of 0.5% (unilateral) or 0.25% (bilateral), with 2.5 μg/cc of epinephrine. Further studies are necessary to determine the optimal dosing of both single-shot and continuous techniques.

The exact volume and concentration of local anesthetic to be used in ESPB is not well established. Injection volumes ranging from 20–40 mL are commonly used.

Following the administration of 20 mL initial bolus, a catheter can be inserted for long lasting analgesia. For unilateral infusions the local anesthetic recommended is bupivacaine 0.2% and for bilateral infusions is 0.125%, at a rate between 8–12 mL per catheter per hour. Usually 12 mL per hour provides sensory block to around 6 spinal levels. As pressure during injections may be an important factor for its effectiveness, PCA (patient controlled analgesia) programmed intermittent boluses have been suggested as a better option than continuous infusions.

Anatomy. The back plays a major role in how the entire body functions. By virtue of its attachments to the vertebral column, the back integrates the activity of the lower limbs, upper limbs, spine, and pelvis.

The muscles of this region can be easily divided into two major groups:

- **The extrinsic back muscles** functionally belong to the upper limbs, but are situated on the posterior aspect of the trunk also known as "immigrant" muscles (trapezius, rhomboid, latissimus dorsi, and serratos posterior inferior muscles) (Fig. 34.1A).
- **The intrinsic back muscles** act specifically on the vertebral column. The erector spinae muscle is included in this group (Fig. 34.1B).

The ESPB targets the erector spinae plane, which lies in the chest wall between the anterior surface of the erector spinae muscles and the posterior surface of the spinal transverse processes.

The erector spinae are not just one muscle, but a bundle of muscles and tendons. Actually, the erector spinae muscle consists of three columns of muscles (the iliocostalis, longissimus, and spinalis muscles) each running parallel on either outer side of the vertebral column. This muscular column is encased in a retinaculum (a complex sheet of blended aponeurosis and fascia) that extends from the sacrum to the skull base (Fig. 34.2A,B).

Each spinal nerve splits into a dorsal and ventral ramus as it exits from the intervertebral foramen. The dorsal ramus travels posteriorly through the costotransverse process and gets into the erector spinae muscle. The ventral ramus travels laterally as the intercostal nerve, running deep to the internal intercostal membrane.

Position. Depending on the operator's and patient's comfort, sitting, lateral decubitus, or a prone position is chosen.

Ultrasound guided injection technique. A high-frequency linear transducer (7–12 MHz) is used. For high BMI (body mass index; person's weight in kilograms divided by his or her height in meters squared) or low thoracic and lumbar region a curvilinear transducer (2–6 MHz) is advised.

Initially, place the probe in transverse orientation over the spinous process in the midline, and transverse process laterally (axial view). The tip of the transverse process, costotransverse joint, and rib are well-defined as a hyperechoic structure superficial and lateral to the lamina. This axial view allows marking our target (transverse process tip) over the skin of the patient to posteriorly rotate the transducer in a cranial-caudal orientation (sagittal-paramedian view). It is important to keep the tip of the target transverse process on the middle of the ultrasound screen.

As the transducer moves lateral or medial, the acoustic shadows generated by the costotransverse joint, rib, or lamina respectively can be observed. Clear identification of the transverse process is mandatory prior to infiltration or catheter insertion. The transverse process will be more superficial, blunter, and wider, while the rib will be deeper, rounder, and thinner (Fig. 34.3).

Cranial-caudal in-plane approach is preferred to facilitate diffusion of local anesthetic. The needle insertion point is 1 to 1.5 cm away from the ultrasound probe. Once the tip of the needle approaches the transverse process in its distal end, hydrodissection of normal saline is used to ensure spread anterior to the anterior fascia of erector muscle and posterior to the transverse process. Following confirmation of appropriate cranial-caudal spread, the total volume of local anesthetic is deposited (Fig. 34.4).

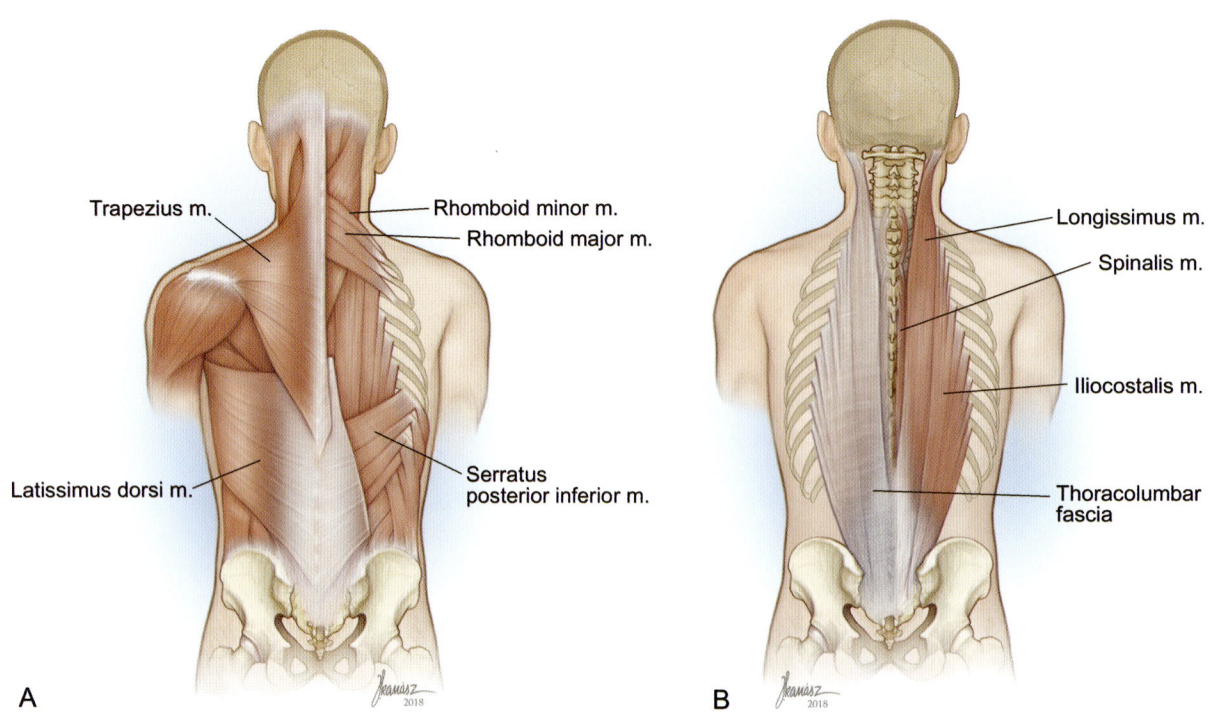

Fig. 34.1 (A) The extrinsic back muscles: trapezius, rhomboid major and minor, latissimus dorsi and serratus posterior inferior muscles. (B) The intrinsic back muscles: longissimus, spinalis, and iliocostalis muscles and thoracolumbar fascia.

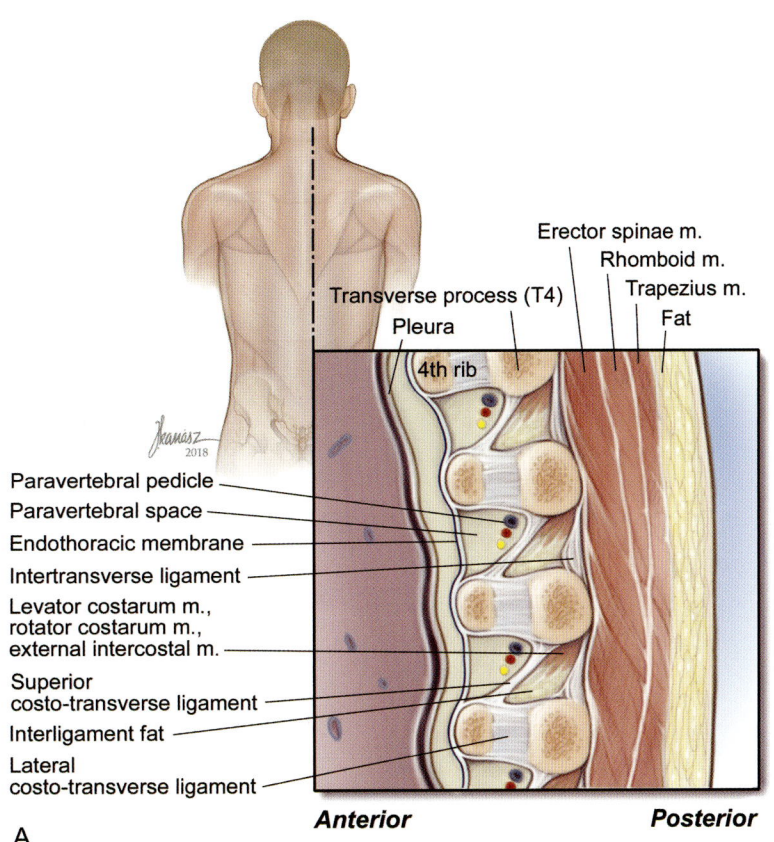

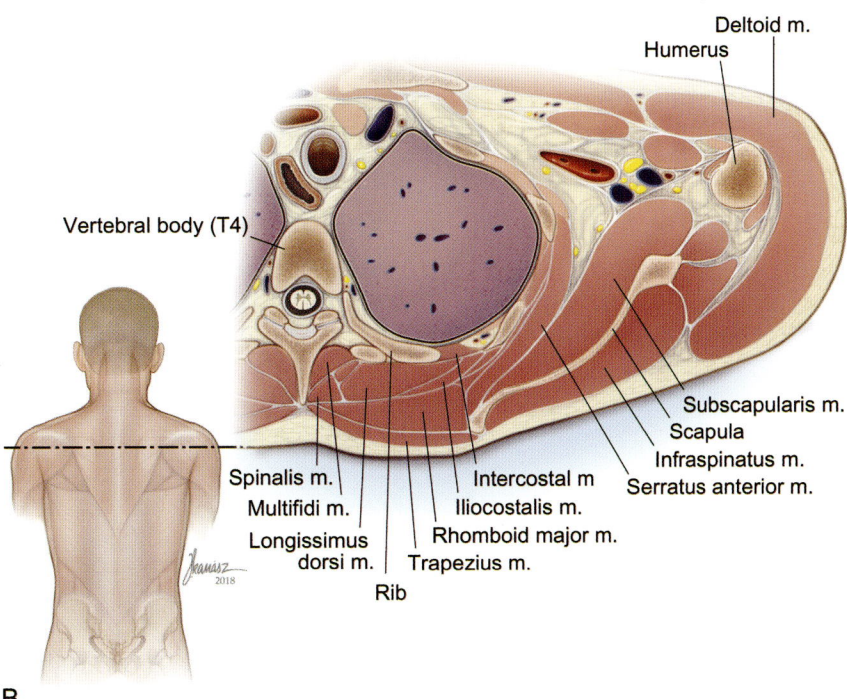

Fig. 34.2 (A) Sagittal paramedian cross section of posterior wall of thorax. (B) Axial cross section at T4 level.

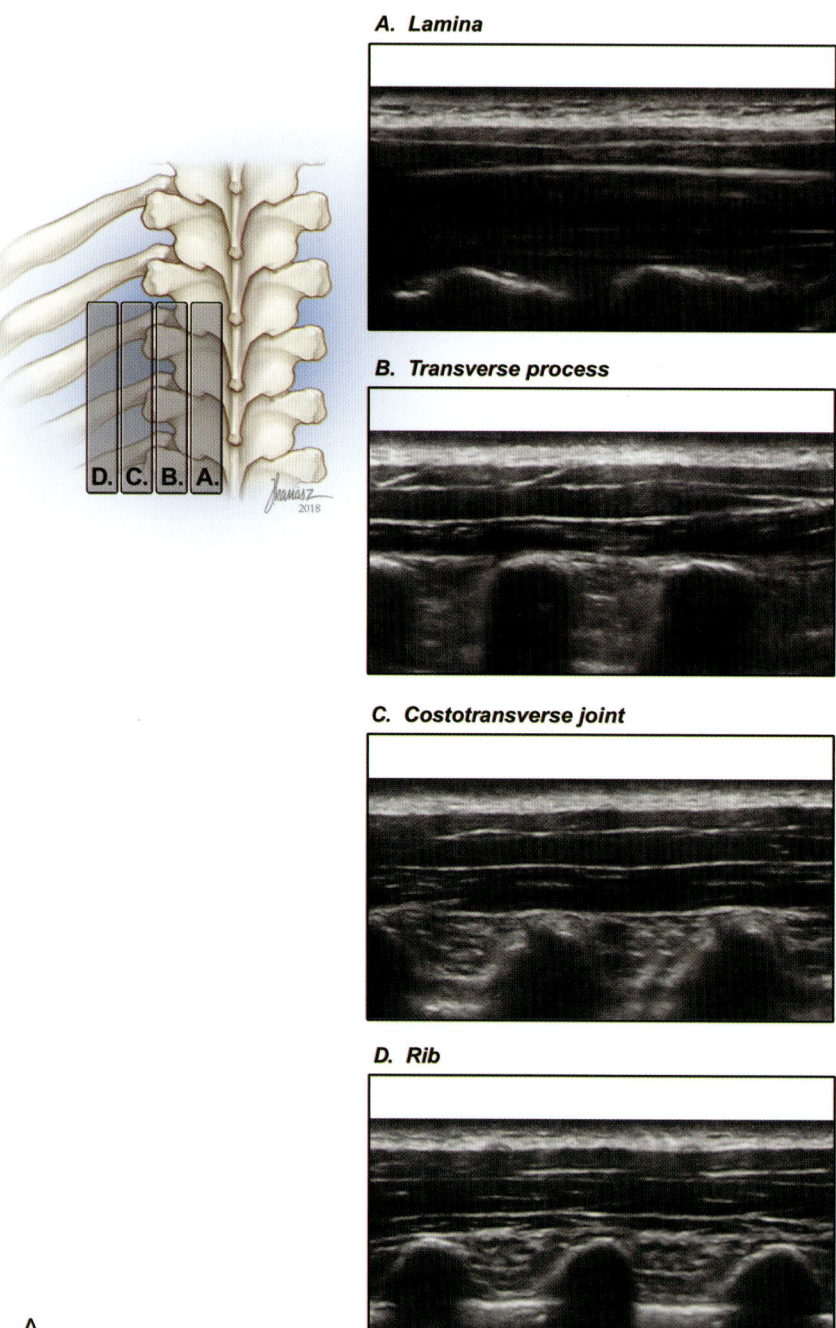

Fig. 34.3 Sonoanatomy of anatomical structures in sagittal paramedian scanning for erector spinae plane block.

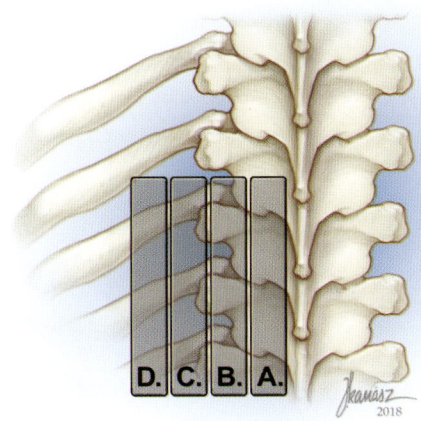
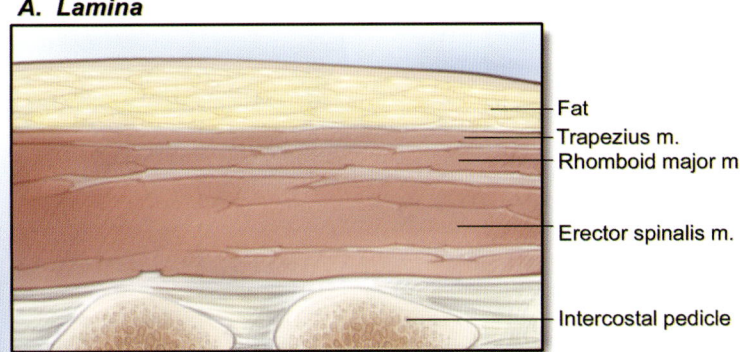

A. Lamina
- Fat
- Trapezius m.
- Rhomboid major m.
- Erector spinalis m.
- Intercostal pedicle

B. Transverse process
- Fat
- Trapezius m.
- Rhomboid major m.
- Erector spinalis m.
- Intertransverse ligament
- Costotransverse ligament
- Paravertebral space
- Intercostal pedicle
- Pleura

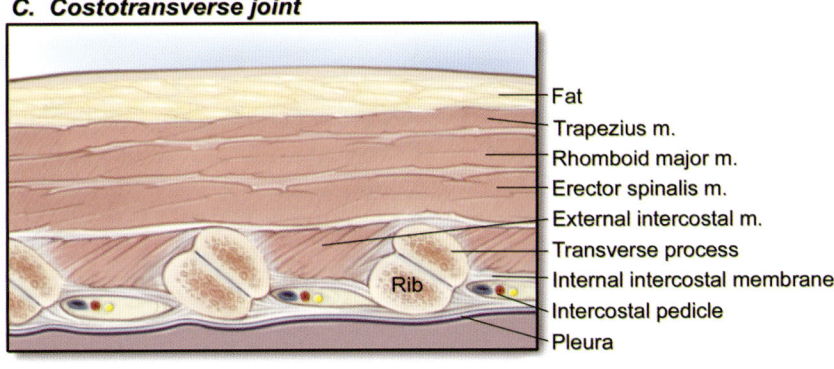

C. Costotransverse joint
- Fat
- Trapezius m.
- Rhomboid major m.
- Erector spinalis m.
- External intercostal m.
- Transverse process
- Internal intercostal membrane
- Intercostal pedicle
- Pleura

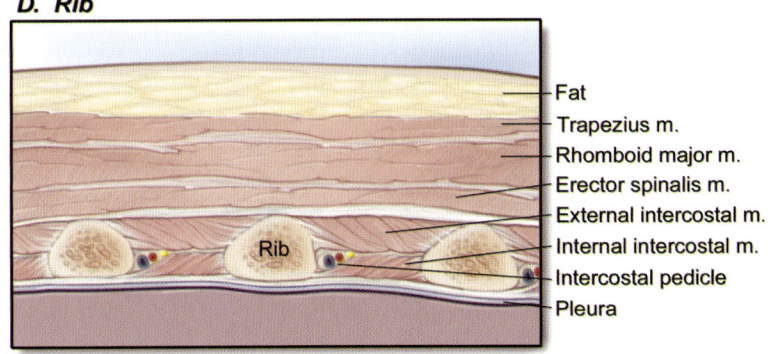

D. Rib
- Fat
- Trapezius m.
- Rhomboid major m.
- Erector spinalis m.
- External intercostal m.
- Internal intercostal m.
- Intercostal pedicle
- Pleura

B

Fig. 34.3—cont'd

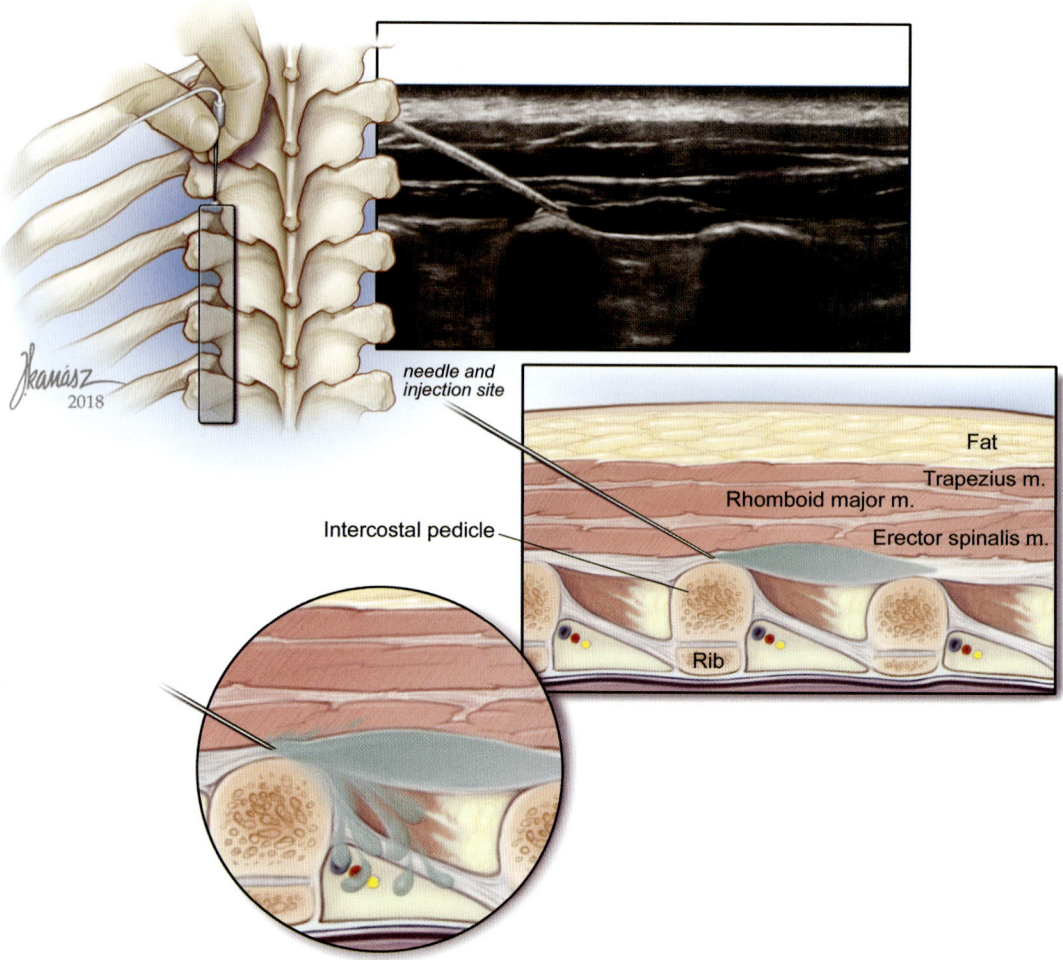

Fig. 34.4 In-plane approach, from cranial-caudal in sagittal paramedian view.

POTENTIAL COMPLICATIONS

No complications have been reported, although the high volumes and doses of local anesthetic used are associated with high plasma levels that could facilitate local anesthetic toxicity.

PEARLS

- When scanning you can find the transverse process tip moving either from medial to lateral (from lamina to transverse process) or from lateral to medial (from rib to transverse process). It is probably easier moving from lamina, which is a flat and deeper bony structure to lateral, where the transverse process will be identified clearly as more superficial bony flat structure.
- The needle must be aligned with the axis of the ultrasound probe. Place the target transverse process in the middle of the ultrasound screen, then make sure that your needle entry point is 1–1.5 cm away from the ultrasound to avoid a steep angle of the needle.
- The ESP block's success fully depends on the appropriate spread of the local anesthetic during the injection. Careful and detailed hydrodissection ensures that the injectable is located between the most anterior fascia layer of the erector muscle and the transverse process. After appropriate hydrodissection using low volumes as 5 mL of normal saline, the spread must be seen in a cranial and caudal direction in at least three spinal levels. After confirmation of appropriate spread, the total of injectable must be delivered in aliquots of 3 mL following safety maneuvers during injection to avoid intravascular depositions.
- If a catheter is inserted, we recommend placing it after an initial single shot bolus (usually 20 mL) to open up the space.

Rectus Sheath Block and Catheter in Adults

Jacob Ezell, Junaid Mukhdomi, Samantha Stamper and John Seif

Key Points

- A high-frequency transducer is preferred for this block.
- The rectus sheath block provides periumbilical somatic analgesia from the levels T9–T11 and is used for surgeries involving a periumbilical incision.
- The block is performed at or slightly above the level of the umbilicus to avoid injury to the deep epigastric artery.
- Direct visualization of the nerves is not required to perform a successful rectus sheath nerve block; instead, identification of the fascial plane is paramount.
- The branches of the thoracolumbar nerves do not cross midline; therefore in order to provide a bilateral block, a right and left rectus abdominis block is performed.

SONOANATOMY

The rectus abdominis muscle receives sensorimotor innervation through thoracolumbar spinal segmental nerves from spinal levels T7–L1. These nerves travel in the fascial plane between the internal oblique and the transversus abdominis muscles to the anterior abdominal wall.

At the lateral border of the rectus abdominis, the aponeuroses of the external oblique, internal oblique, and transversus abdominis muscle combine to form the linea semilunaris. At this lateral aspect, the thoracolumbar spinal segmental nerves pierce through the rectus abdominis muscle and create a nerve plexus to provide motor and sensation to the rectus abdominis muscles (Fig. 35.1). The common aponeurosis splits into an anterior and posterior aponeurosis that encase the rectus abdominis muscle and nerve plexus in a sheath.

The rectus sheath is composed of an anterior and posterior aponeurosis that bind the rectus abdominis muscle and form the rectus sheath. At midline, the anterior and posterior aponeuroses of the right and left rectus abdominis muscles combine to form the linea alba, a thick fibrous band of fascia. The thoracolumbar spinal nerves do not cross the linea alba; therefore a rectus sheath block requires a bilateral block or two separate catheters to be performed.

It is important to note the deep epigastric artery provides blood supply to the rectus abdominis muscle and enters the muscle body at the level of the arcuate ligament. To avoid this, the block should always be performed at or above the level of the umbilicus. Beneath the rectus sheath the peritoneal cavity can be appreciated with the presence of abdominal contents, which can usually be observed during the block.

TECHNIQUE

With the patient in a supine position, a high-frequency, linear ultrasound probe is placed in a transverse position just lateral to the umbilicus (Fig. 35.2). The lens-shaped rectus abdominis muscle is identified below the ultrasound transducer with attention to identify and avoid the deep epigastric artery during the procedure (Fig. 35.3). The authors recommend sliding the probe lateral from this position to identify the linea semilunaris. This location allows for a more direct visualization of the posterior rectus sheath and a more superficial access to the posterior fascial plane (Fig. 35.4). Direct identification of the intercostal nerves is not required in order to complete a successful rectus sheath block.

In this position, the block needle is inserted in plane from the lateral side of the transducer at a 45-degree angle, through the anterior abdominal fascia and rectus abdominis muscle body. When the needle tip is near to the posterior rectus sheath, an aspiration test followed by injection of a small amount of local anesthetic or saline can elucidate the exact location of the needle tip. For placement of catheters, the authors recommend using normal saline for this step in order to conserve local anesthetic for ultrasound visualization of local anesthetic spread through the nerve catheter after placement. If intramuscular, the needle is carefully advanced 1–2 mm followed by an aspiration test and injection until a satisfactory position is obtained.

Once confirmed, 10–20 mL of local anesthetic is injected after aspiration. During injection, advancement of the needle under direct ultrasound visualization separates the rectus abdominis from the posterior fascial sheath, to create a lens-shaped space and ensure coverage of intercostal nerves, while avoiding displacement of the needle as the rectus abdominis muscle is separated from the posterior fascial sheath. The authors recommend optimizing this space prior to attempting catheter insertion.

Upon placement of a catheter, a negative aspiration, injection of local anesthetic through the catheter, and visualization of an expanding cavity confirms correct placement.

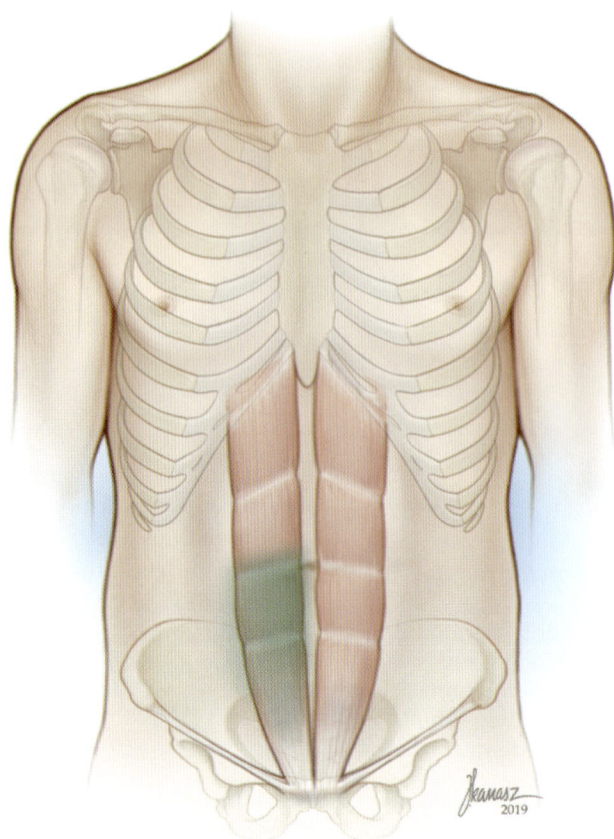

Fig. 35.1 A representation of the sensory distribution of the T9–T11 thoracolumbar spinal nerves in the rectus abdominis muscle.

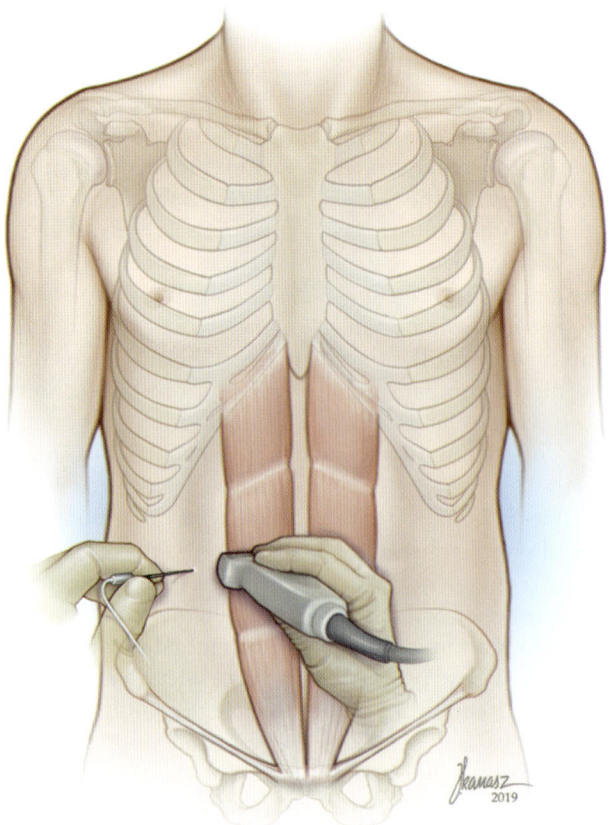

Fig. 35.2 A depiction of the preferred orientation to perform a rectus sheath block.

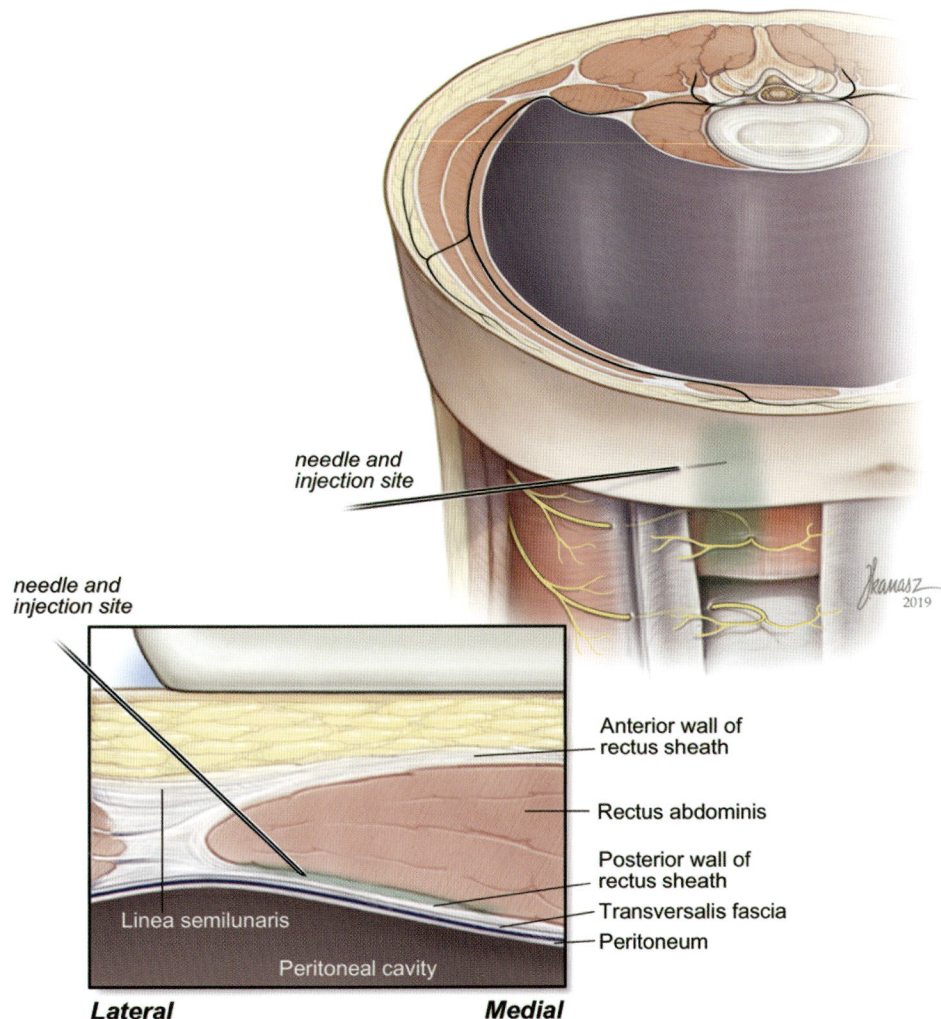

Fig. 35.3 A coronal section showing the path the thoracoabdominal nerves travel to the rectus abdominis muscle. Next to it is an illustration of an ultrasound image at the level of the umbilicus and the anterior and posterior rectus sheath components encasing the muscle.

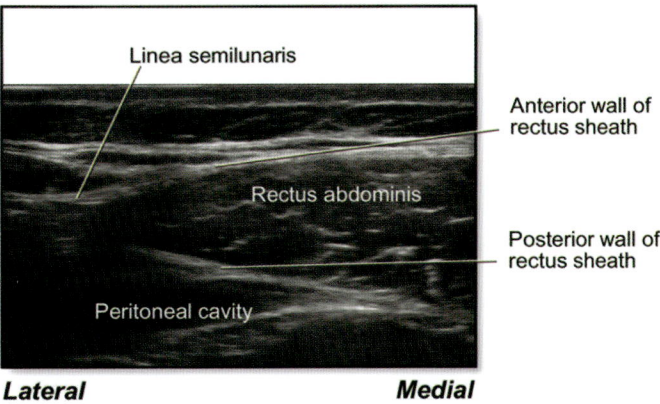

Fig. 35.4 An ultrasound image showing an ideal image to perform a successful block.

PEARLS

- The block needle should be inserted from the lateral side of the transducer at a 45-degree angle or shallower in order to avoid penetration through the peritoneum.
- Normal saline should be used for placement of rectus sheath catheters in order to conserve local anesthetic for direct ultrasound visualization through the catheter when placed.
- Once proper needle insertion is observed under ultrasound (rectus abdominis separating from posterior rectus sheath), 10–20 mL of local anesthetic can be injected after a negative aspiration.
- During injection, advancement of the needle into the newly formed lens-shaped space using direct ultrasound visualization separates the rectus abdominis from the posterior fascial sheath to ensure coverage of the intercostal nerves.

Transversus Abdominis Plane Block (Classic Approach)

36

Loran Mounir-Soliman

Key Points

- The transversus abdominis plane (TAP) block is a tissue plane block depending on adequate spread of local anesthetics through the plane—accordingly a minimum volume of 20 mL is usually needed for effective block.
- Frequent, small, incremental injections of saline while advancing the needle can identify the progress of the needle tip through the various tissue planes.
- When performed appropriately, the TAP block is very safe and devoid of major complications and can be placed safely in anesthetized patients.
- For midline incisions, bilateral blocks are needed; the rectus sheath block may be considered as an alternative.

RELEVANT ANATOMY

The ventral rami of the lower six thoracic nerves (T7 to L1) emerge through the intervertebral foraminae to pass through the corresponding intercostal spaces, and enter a fascial plane between the transversus abdominis and the internal oblique muscles of the abdominal muscular wall (known as the TAP) accompanied by blood vessels. They follow the curvilinear course of this neurovascular plane to reach the anterior abdominal wall as far as the semilunar line at the lateral border of the rectus abdominis muscle (Fig. 36.1).

The abdominal wall consists of three muscle layers: the external oblique, the internal oblique, and the transversus abdominis muscles and their associated fascial sheaths. The three muscles, as well as the parietal peritoneum, are innervated by the ipsilateral ventral rami of T7 to L1. The external oblique and the anterior lamella of the internal oblique aponeurosis pass anteriorly to the rectus muscle, forming the anterior rectus sheath. The aponeuroses from the posterior lamella of the internal oblique muscle and the transversus abdominis muscle pass posteriorly to the rectus muscle, forming the posterior layer of the sheath. At this point, the ventral rami of the lower thoracic nerves are located between the posterior rectus sheath and the rectus muscle. They run medially within the sheath before perforating the muscle anteriorly, forming the anterior cutaneous branches. Along their course through the TAP, the lower thoracic spinal nerves give origin to the lateral cutaneous branches posterior to the midaxillary line. Within the TAP, the nerves communicate with each other, forming neural plexuses in close proximity to the vessels in this neurovascular plane.

TECHNIQUE

A linear, high-frequency probe (8–12 MHz) is usually used for optimal identification of the different muscle layers and their corresponding fascial sheaths. However, a curvilinear, lower-frequency probe (2–5 MHz) may be used in obese patients. The block can be performed in the supine or lateral position, with the side to be blocked upwards, and a wedge beneath the lower side in order to stretch the flank on the upper side. The lower costal margin and the iliac crest are identified, and the probe is placed in a transverse orientation between the two bony landmarks at the midaxillary line. The probe is moved both cephalad and caudad to get the best view of the three muscles. Scanning too medially may only show two muscle layers because the external oblique muscle forms an aponeurosis; also, scanning more posteriorly may encounter the large latissimus dorsi muscle, which may confuse the view of the muscles.

The fascial layers appear as hyperechoic structures under ultrasound, giving the muscles their characteristic multiple striations.

A blunt needle is introduced from the posterior edge of the probe with the in-plane technique (parallel to the ultrasound beam) and advanced in a medial anterior direction through the skin, subcutaneous fat, and external and internal oblique muscles to reach the interfascial layer between the internal oblique and transversus abdominis muscles (TAP). The endpoint of the needle should be superficial to the transversus abdominis muscle. Deeper to this muscle, there is a layer of preperitoneal fat separating it from the peritoneum and the bowels, which are often identified by their peristaltic movements. A blunt needle is preferred to appreciate the tactile "pop" when crossing each fascial layer. The intramuscular location of the needle within the internal oblique muscle is identified by retraction of the needle when it is released, as well as swelling of the muscle with injection instead of separation from the transversus abdominis.

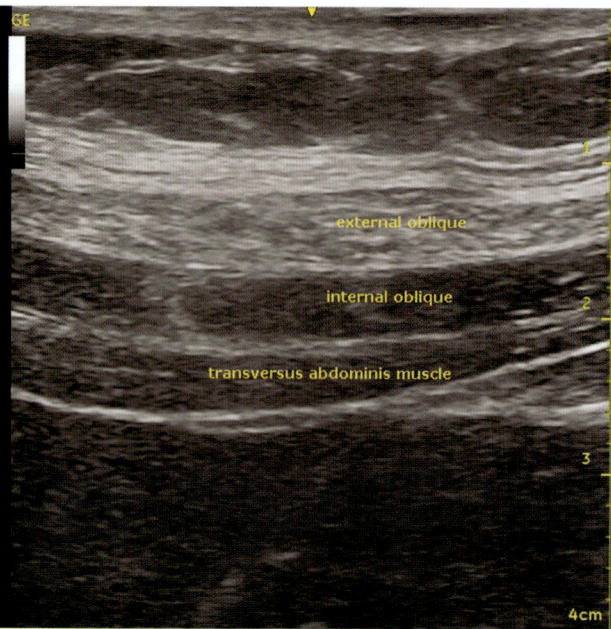

Fig. 36.1 Ultrasound still of anatomy of TAP block.

INDICATIONS

- The TAP block can potentially provide unilateral analgesia to the skin, muscles, and parietal peritoneum of the anterior abdominal wall, although the extent of the block has been reported to be variable in different studies.
- Bilateral blocks have been used for midline and transverse incisions.
- Classical TAP has been reported to provide adequate analgesia following caesarian section, hysterectomy, hernia repair, kidney transplant, colostomy closure, and multiple other lower abdominal surgeries.
- Both single-shot and continuous catheters have been used successfully.
- The TAP block has been used for patients with chronic abdominal pain to identify somatic pain originating from the abdominal muscular wall and the parietal peritoneum versus visceral pain, which is transmitted via sympathetic innervation instead.

PEARLS

- Placement of the needle as far posteriorly as possible (by the midaxillary line or behind) has the theoretical advantage of blocking the lateral cutaneous branches before they exit the TAP.
- The internal oblique muscle is usually identified as the largest muscle among the three abdominal muscles.
- The transversus abdominis muscle sometimes shows as a hypoechoic band that can be confused with the underlying preperitoneal fatty layer. The peristaltic movements of the bowels within the preperitoneal fatty layer can identify it from the muscular layer.
- An out-of-plane technique can be more suitable in obese patients when the needle path is not easily seen.

Subcostal Transversus Abdominal Plane Block

37

Ehab Farag

Key Points

- The subcostal transversus abdominal plane (TAP) approach is very useful for supraumbilical procedures.
- The most cephalad sensory dermatomal spread is T8.
- The bilateral continuous catheter infusion can be used in the upper abdominal surgeries where epidural analgesia is contraindicated or failed.
- The key for the success of this technique is the proper identification of the fascial plane between the transversus abdominis and rectus abdominis muscles.

SONOANATOMY

There are four paired muscles of the anterolateral abdominal wall: the anterior rectus abdominis muscles and, from deep to superficial, the three lateral muscles: transversus abdominis, internal oblique, and external oblique muscles. It is only in the lateral abdomen that the three fleshy muscle bellies overlie one another because medially they become an aponeurosis. Under ultrasound the rectus abdominis can be easily identified, and by moving laterally, the transversus abdominis muscle will appear beneath the rectus abdominis muscle. The transversus abdominis has two key features on ultrasound imaging. It is usually darker (more hypoechoic) than other muscles, and it passes beneath the rectus abdominis muscle (Fig. 37.1).

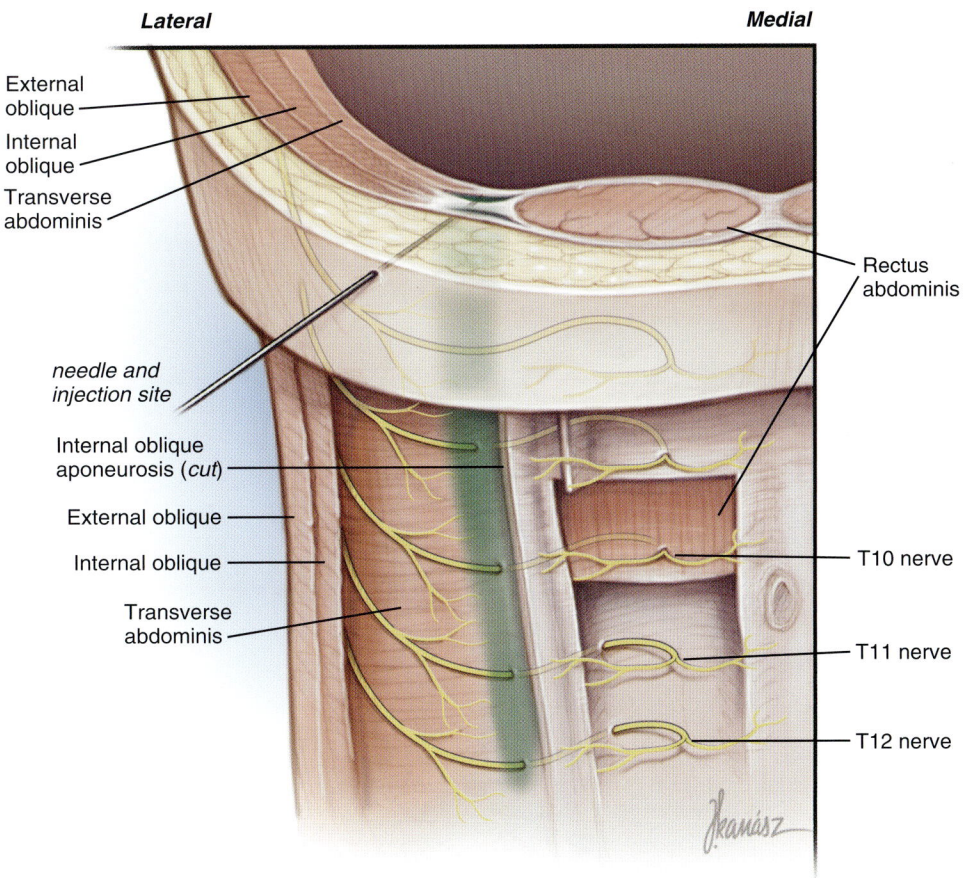

Fig. 37.1 Anatomy of anterior abdominal wall.

TECHNIQUE

The linear ultrasound probe will be placed over the anterior abdominal wall immediately inferior and parallel to the costal margin. The rectus abdominis muscle will be identified medially, and then the probe will be moved laterally until the transversus abdominis muscles are also identified. Further lateral movement of the ultrasound probe will demonstrate the lateral abdominal wall muscles (external and internal obliques and transverse abdominis muscles) to provide further confirmation of sonographic anatomy. Using the in-plane approach, the needle will be inserted from the posterolateral position and advanced anteromedially until its tip is in the fascial plane between the rectus abdominis and transverse abdominis muscles. The author usually injects 20 mL of ropivacaine 0.5% in each side of the bilateral block (Figs. 37.2–37.4).

INDICATION

- Used in supraumbilical procedures.
- Bilateral continuous subcostal TAP can be used in lieu of epidural analgesia for midline supraumbilical procedures.

PEARLS

- When performing the procedure on the right side, care should be taken not to injure the liver, especially in patients with hepatomegaly or a thin patient.
- For the single-shot technique, the author prefers to use 22-gauge needles; however, in the continuous catheter technique, the author inserts the catheter via a 17- to 18-gauge Tuohy needle.

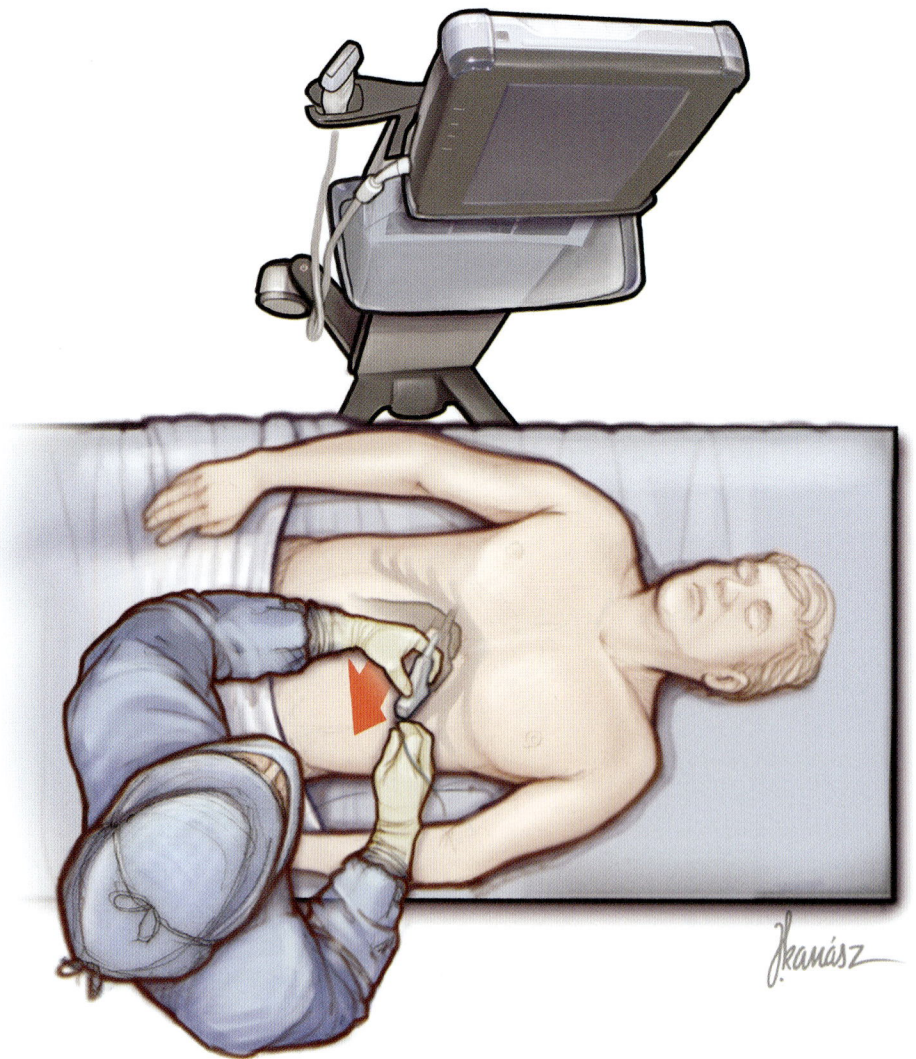

Fig. 37.2 Position of the patient and the ultrasound machine. Note the probe position is immediately inferior and parallel to the costal margin. Moving the probe laterally will visualize the rectus abdominis and transverse abdominis muscles.

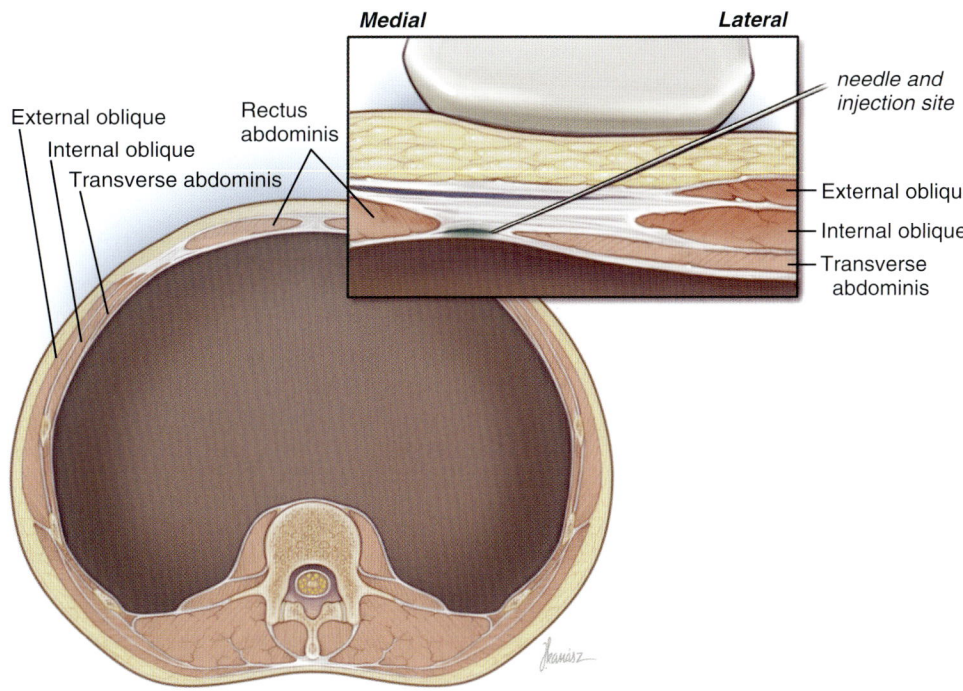

Fig. 37.3 In-plane technique for the subcostal TAP block. The needle direction is from lateral to medial.

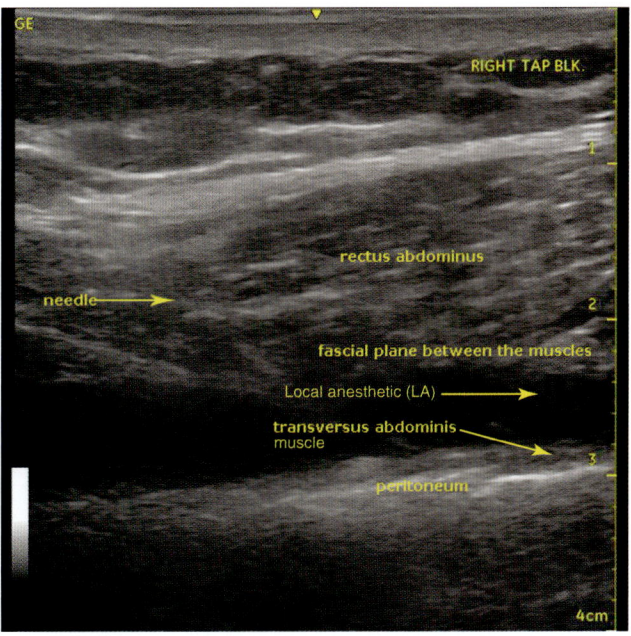

Fig. 37.4 Ultrasound image of subcostal TAP block with needle.

Quadratus Lumborum Block 38

Hesham Elsharkawy and Ehab Farag

Key Points

- Quadratus lumborum (QL) block is a novel approach for managing postoperative pain in patients undergoing abdominal and hip surgeries.
- The sensory dermatomal coverage of the QL block can extend from T7 to L2.
- There is currently no general consensus on the mechanism of action of QL blockade.
- This is a "tissue plane" block and thus requires a large volume of local anesthetic to obtain a reliable block.

SONOANATOMY

The ultrasound probe is placed in the posterior axillary line between the iliac crest and the costal margin (Fig. 38.1). The transversalis fascia (TF) covers the peritoneal surface of the transversus abdominis muscle and continues posteromedially covering the anterior side of the investing fascia of both the quadratus lumborum (QL) and psoas major (PM) muscles. The QL muscle is generally visualized as hypoechoic relative to the hyperechoic PM muscle located anteromedial to the QL muscle.

The QL muscle surrounded by the thoracolumbar fascia (TLF) is the target of the injection, not the muscle itself. The three-layered model of TLF is comprised of anterior, middle, and posterior layers. The posterior layer surrounds the erector spinae muscles; the middle-layer of the TLF passes between the erector spinae muscles and the QL muscle; and the anterior layer is thin and lies anterior to both the QL and PM muscles. The anterior layer of the TLF turns posterior between the QL and the psoas and attaches to the anterior aspect of each transverse process (Fig. 38.2).

At the L3–L4 level, the transverse process of the third or fourth lumbar vertebrae, erector spinae muscle, PM muscle, and the QL muscle can be identified as the so-called "Shamrock sign".

The external oblique muscle abuts the latissimus dorsi muscle. The internal oblique, with the transversus abdominis muscles, forms the aponeurosis of the middle thoracolumbar fascia (lateral raphe) posterior to the QL muscle (Fig. 38.2).

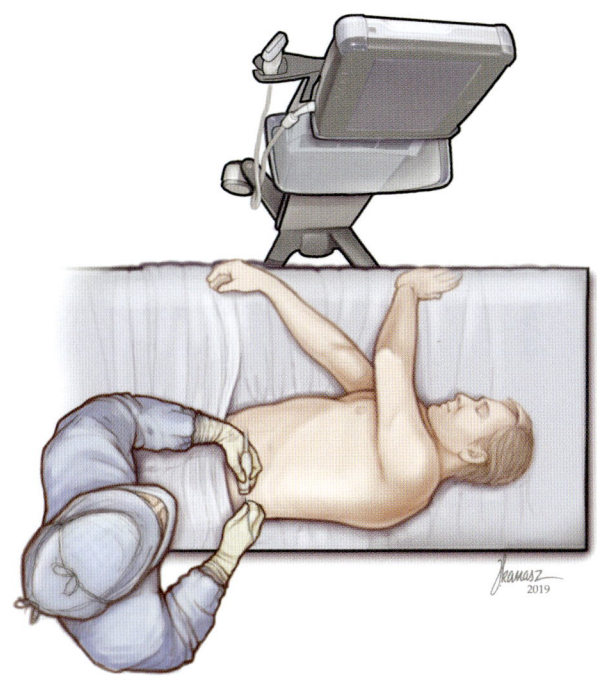

Fig. 38.1 Patient in the lateral decubitus position for QL Blocks.

TECHNIQUES (FIG. 38.3–38.8)

- *Lateral QL* (Previously referred as QL 1 block) The needle can be directed from anterior to posterior towards the junction of tapered transversus abdominis muscle and QL muscle; local anesthetic (LA) will then be deposited in the lateral border of QL muscle at the junction of the transversalis fascia and penetrate the aponeurotic attachment of the transversus abdominis muscle (lateral raphe) (Fig. 38.3–38.4).
- *Posterior* (Previously referred as QL 2 block) By advancing the needle more posteriorly, local anesthetic can be deposited posterior to the lateral edge of the QL muscle, between the QL muscle and the erector spinae and latissimus dorsi muscles (Fig. 38.3–38.4).
- *Anterior* (Previously referred as transmuscular, QL 3 block) The needle can be advanced either posteriorly through the erector spinae muscle, or anteriorly through the latissimus dorsi muscle, and then

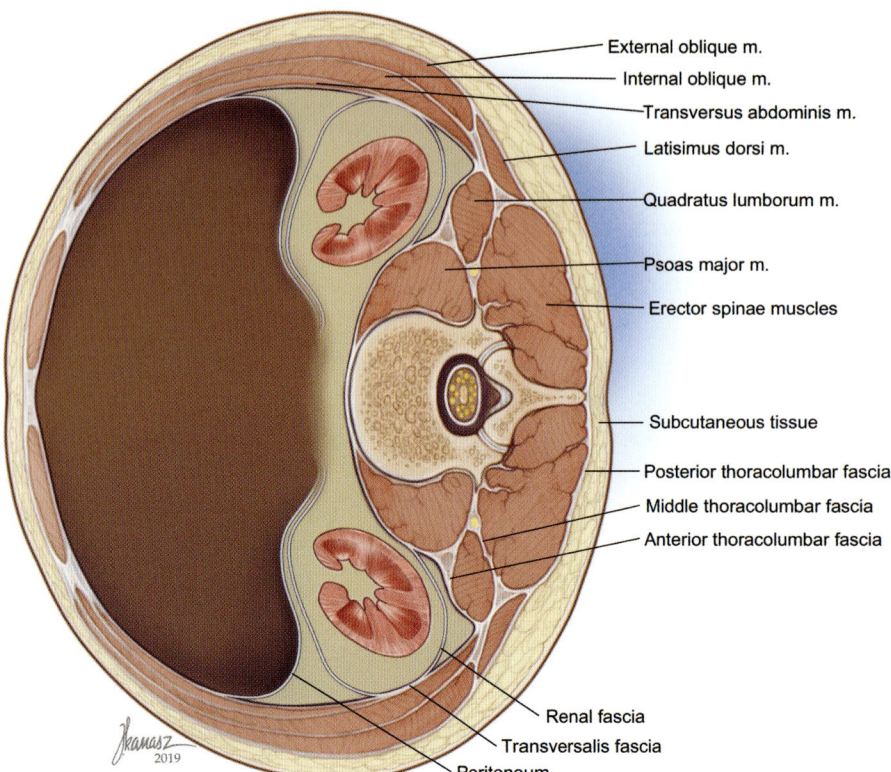

Fig. 38.2 A schematic illustration of cross section showing the quadratus lumborum muscle with the different layers of the thoracolumbar fascia. (three layers model).

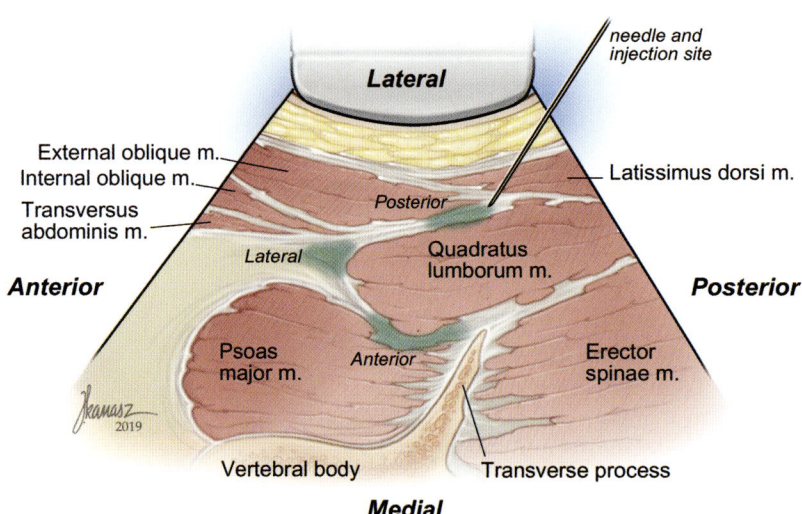

Fig. 38.3 A schematic illustration showing the different sites of injection of local anesthetics in relation to the quadratus lumborum muscle.

through the muscle (transmuscular approach) to deposit the local anesthetic in the fascial plane between the QL and PM muscles (Fig. 38.3–38.4).

- **The subcostal** (Paramedian oblique sagittal) The ultrasound transducer is positioned lateral to the lumbar spinous process at the L1–L2 level. Using a curvilinear transducer with the orientation marker of the ultrasound directed cranially, the probe is slightly tilted medially. The needle is advanced in the plane with ultrasound in a caudal to cephalad direction, through the latissimus dorsi, and QL muscles; then LA is deposited anterior to the QL muscle, between the QL muscle and the anterior layer of the thoracolumbar fascia (ATLF)/transversalis fascia, observing spread in cephalad direction close to

Quadratus Lumborum Block 239

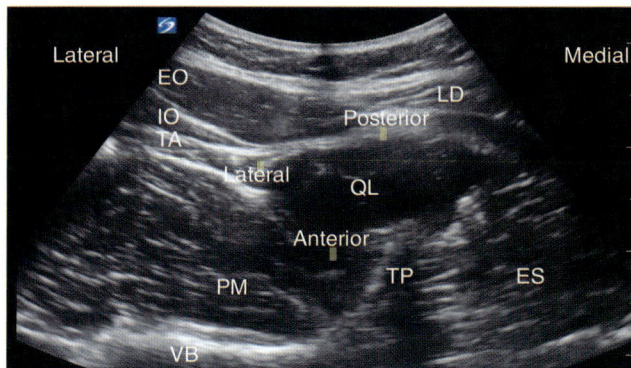

Fig. 38.4 Ultrasound still showing the different sites of injection in relation to the Quadratus Lumborum muscle. *EO*, External Oblique; *IO*, Internal oblique; *TA*, Transversus Abdominus; *LD*, Latissimus Dorsi; *QL*, Quadratus Lumborum; *PM*, Psoas Major; *VB*, Vertebral body; *TP*, Transverse process; *ES*, Erectror Spinae.

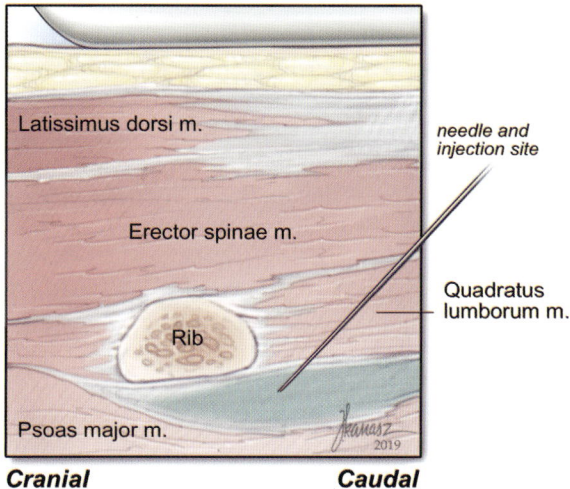

Fig. 38.5 Schematic representation of the subcostal approach

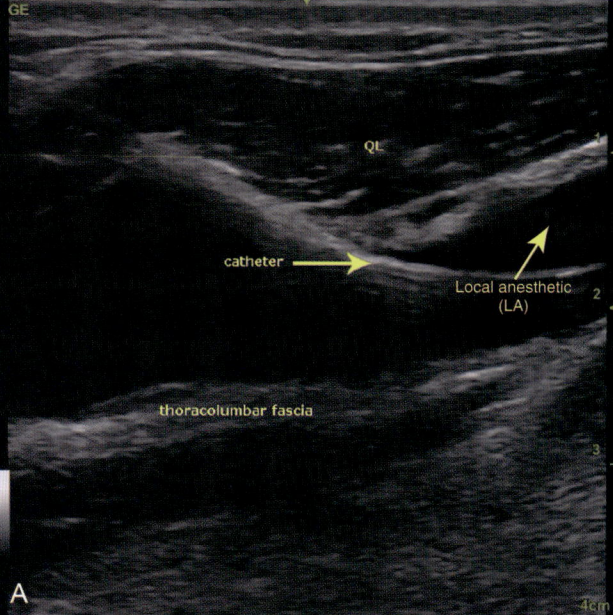

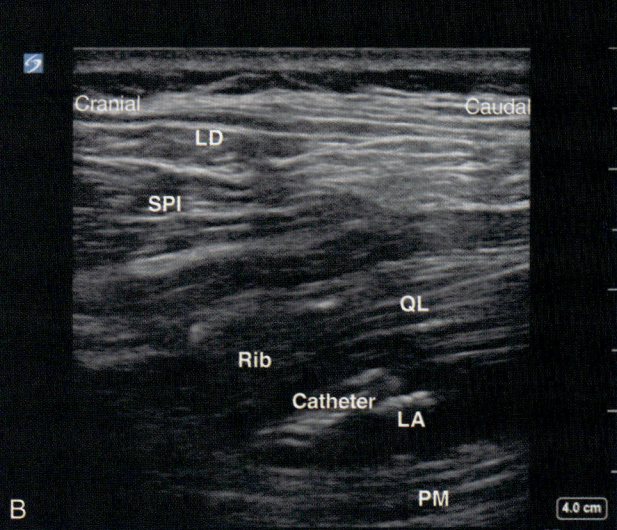

Fig. 38.6 Ultrasound picture of the local anesthetics spread and catheter placement through the subcostal approach. (A) Between the Quadratus Lumborum and Thoracolumbar fascia (B) Between the Quadratus Lumborum and psoas major *SPI*, serratus posterior inferior; *LD*, Latissimus Dorsi; *QL*, Quadratus Lumborum; *LA*, Local Anesthetics; *PM*, Psoas Major

the last rib, a lunar shaped distribution of local anesthetic with anterior displacement of the ATLF (Fig. 38.5–38.6).

- **The suprailiac anterior** Above the iliac crest a curvilinear transducer is placed in a transverse orientation with slight medial and caudal angulation to obtain a transverse oblique view at the L5 transverse process. The ultrasound probe is further tilted so the lateral end of the ultrasound probe is more cranial than the medial side of the probe to avoid the acoustic shadow of the iliac crest. The needle is advanced in-plane in a lateral-to-medial direction, through the latissimus dorsi and QL muscle, to position the tip between the QL and psoas major muscles close to the transverse process. Spread is deemed appropriate when the injectant is seen between QL and PM muscles and tracked medially towards the L5 transverse process (Fig. 38.7–38.8). This approach blocks T10 to L3 nerve territories and has clinical utility for analgesia in hip surgery. (Fig. 38.7–38.8).

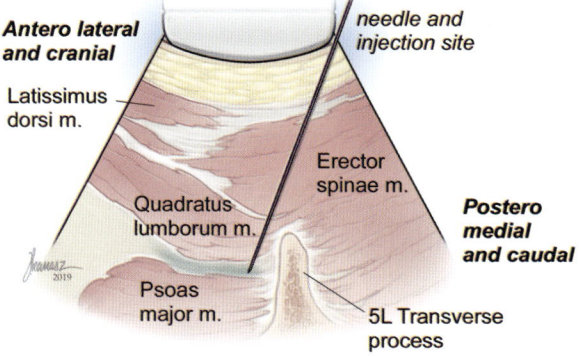

Fig. 38.7 Schematic representation of the local anesthetic site through the Suprailiac Anterior approach.

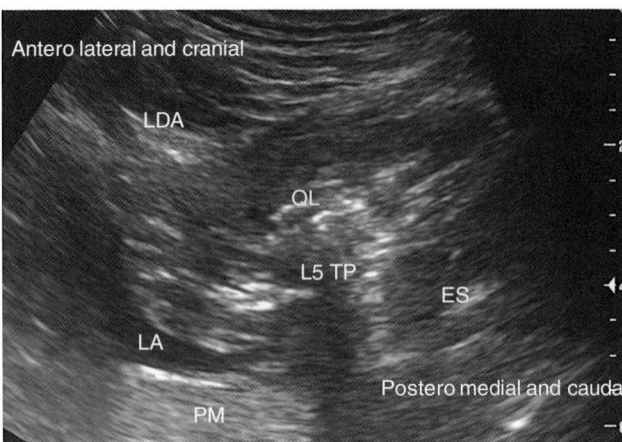

Fig. 38.8 Ultrasound picture of the local anesthetic spread through the Suprailiac Anterior approach. L 5 *TP*, Acoustic shadow; *QL*, Quadratus Lumborum; *PM*, Psoas Major; *LDA*, Latissimus Dorsi Aponeurosis; *ES*, Erector Spinae; *LA*, Local Anesthetics.

PEARLS

- The QL muscle is attached to the transverse process, which once identified provides orientation for the operator.
- If the QL muscle is small and difficult to delineate, the ipsilateral hip joint is abducted and laterally flexed towards the same side of the block to contract the QL muscle; this temporarily thickens the QL muscle.
- While performing the block especially with the subcostal approach, it is common to visualize the lower pole of the kidney and lower lobe of the liver and spleen; great caution should be taken to avoid any visceral injury.
- The QL muscle acts like a bed for the kidney, which helps to identify the QL muscle.
- Apply color Doppler before insertion of the needle to detect the abdominal branches of the lumbar arteries on the posterior aspect of the quadratus lumborum muscle or any other vessels close to the transverse process, and on the intended track of the needle.
- The tactile feedback (as pops) when encountering different fascial planes is not accurate in QL blocks due to the complexity of the anatomical planes, multilayered components of the TLF muscle, and the approach angle; therefore the visual confirmation using ultrasound and hydrodissection should be used.
- With the anterior QL block, the local anesthetic is deposited in the plane between the QL and psoas major muscle. Both during administration of and subsequent to administration of the local anesthetic solution, the transducer should be moved from the transverse to the longitudinal position. With the curvilinear probe in the longitudinal position, the local anesthetic can be seen to spread cephalad from the iliac crest to the 12th rib.
- The usual initial dose is 0.3 mL/kg of ropivacaine 0.2%. However, higher doses up to 0.6 mL/kg can cover more dermatomes.

SECTION 7
Neuraxial Blocks

39 Ultrasound-Assisted Neuraxial Blocks

Loran Mounir-Soliman

Key Points

- Prepuncture ultrasound scanning is helpful to determine the midline, the depth from the skin, the desired level, and rotation of the spine.
- There are limited outcome data on the real-time guidance with ultrasound for neuraxial blocks.
- The available evidence suggests that the use of ultrasound may improve the success rate from the first attempt, reduce the number of attempts, and improve patient comfort.
- The use of ultrasound for epidural access is a technically advanced procedure. It requires adequate experience with ultrasound scanning and ultrasound guidance of the needle at deep levels with a less-than-optimal angle of incidence.
- Thorough understanding of the neuraxial anatomy and conceptual visualization of the different echogenic structures are necessary for ultrasound scanning of the epidural space.

RELEVANT SONOANATOMY OF THE SPINE

There are a couple of challenges for ultrasound imaging of the spine and the neuraxial structures. The depth of the spine makes it less than optimal for the ultrasound beams to produce higher-resolution images. Also, the osseous structure of the laminae and articular processes conceal the underlying neuraxial structures of interest to perform the blocks. Accordingly, it is important to have a visual appreciation of the spine outline when scanning for neuraxial blocks.

In general, scanning the vertebrae demonstrates three hyperechoic levels: the spinous process, the lamina, and the articular facet joint with the transverse process.

The spinous processes reflect the most superficial hyperechoic shadow closest to the skin. Careful scanning, cephalad and caudad to the spinous process, reveals an acoustic window representing the interspinous space occupied with the less echogenic interspinous ligaments. Careful examination of the deeper layer of the ligamentous structure shows the ligamentum flavum as a slightly more hyperechoic layer separated from another hyperechoic layer—the posterior dura—by the epidural space. The spinal canal underneath represents the next anechoic layer deeper to the posterior dura. On the deeper side of the spinal canal (anterior), the anterior dura with the postlongitudinal ligament form a hyperechoic structure called the *anterior complex*.

With the aforementioned echogenic characteristics of the neuraxial structures in mind, scanning the different levels of the spine leads to different views. These views also depend on the scanning plane and orientation of the ultrasound beam. These are the main planes for scanning the spine:

- **Median sagittal plane**: A longitudinal scan along the midline where the beam of the ultrasound is parallel to the long axis of the spine on top of the spinous processes (unless the spine is scoliotic).
- **Paramedian sagittal plane**: A longitudinal scan parallel to the long axis of the spine but off the midline. The beams are usually on top of the transverse processes or the laminae, with the articular joints (facets) between the adjacent spines.
- **Paramedian sagittal oblique plane:** Another longitudinal plane that is similar to the paramedian sagittal plane with the probe tilted medially to direct the beams toward midline. The ultrasound beams usually travel across the laminae with the intervertebral foraminae in between. Access to the ligaments, dura, and spinal canal are usually accessed with the beam within the interlaminar windows.
- **Transverse axial view**: A transverse view where the beam of the ultrasound is perpendicular to the long axis of the spine. With this orientation, the ultrasound probe can be on top of the vertebra where the beams cross the spinous process, lamina, and transverse process. If the beam is steered cephalad or caudad by sliding the probe or tilting it, an interspinous (acoustic) window is obtained. The ligaments, epidural space, and spinal canal can be visualized through this window.

TECHNIQUE

Except for the caudal block, the neuraxial scanning requires a low-frequency (2–5 MHz) curvilinear probe to see the depth of the target structures. In addition to the ability to scan deeper structures, the curved probe provides a divergent beam, giving a wider field of vision and helping to scan the different anatomic structures in a single view compared with the limited field of vision produced by the linear probe. The disadvantage of the curved probe is a lack of spatial resolution at deeper levels, making viewing the needle a challenge when performing the block. Scanning the spine for procedures can be performed in sitting, lateral, and prone positions depending on the level of the procedure to be performed.

CAUDAL EPIDURAL BLOCK

Because the sacral hiatus is a relatively superficial structure, a high-frequency linear probe (6–13 MHz) is usually used for caudal scanning. The block is performed in the prone position with a pillow under the pelvis. The ultrasound probe is placed in a transverse orientation (axial scan) to scan the sacral cornua as two hyperechoic, reversed U-shaped structures. The sacrococcygeal ligament connecting both cornua, forming the superficial boundary of the sacral hiatus, appears as a hyperechoic band. The anterior boundary of the sacral canal is formed by the posterior surface of the sacrum, which appears as another hyperechoic linear structure anterior (deep) to the sacrococcygeal ligament. The sacral hiatus appears as a hypoechoic space between these two described hyperechoic lines. With this view, the needle can be introduced in the middle of the probe, perpendicular to the ultrasound beams, out of the plane approach, and targeting the sacral hiatus (Fig. 39.1).

With the sacral hiatus and the sacrococcygeal ligament identified, the ultrasound probe can be rotated 90 degrees to the median sagittal plane scan. A long-axis view of the sacrococcygeal ligament and the sacral bony surface are reidentified with the sacral hiatus between them. The needle is introduced with an in-plane approach from the caudal end of the probe to be able to visualize the whole length of the needle. Crossing the tip of the needle into the sacrococcygeal membrane into the sacral canal is associated with a "pop" feeling, especially when using a blunt needle. The sacral bony structure impedes the ultrasound beams, making it hard to see the tip of the needle or the spread of the injection in the sacral canal (Figs. 39.2–39.4).

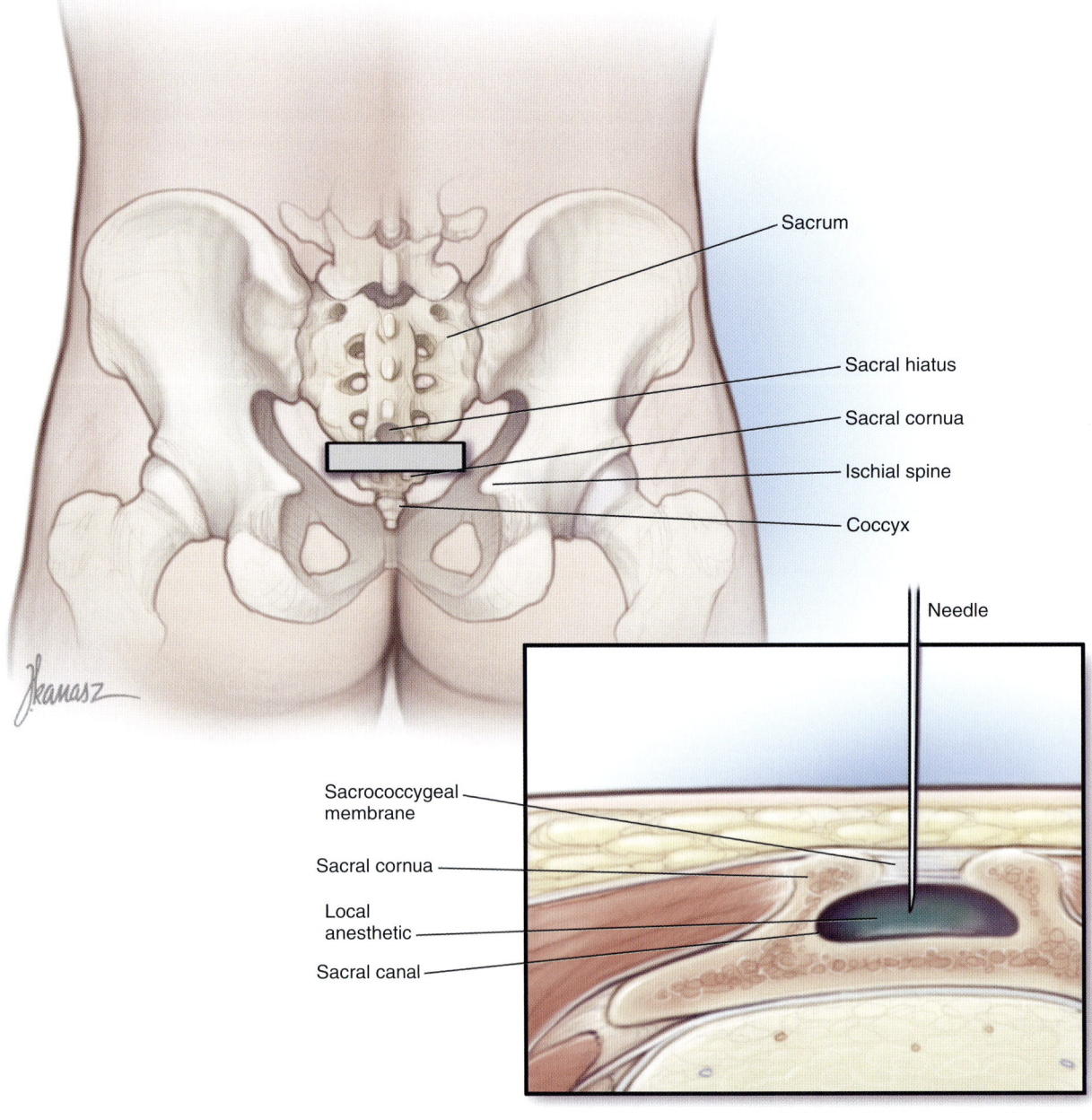

Fig. 39.1 Transverse approach to the caudal block. The needle is introduced in out-of-plane direction in the middle of the probe targeting the sacral hiatus.

Ultrasound-Assisted Neuraxial Blocks 245

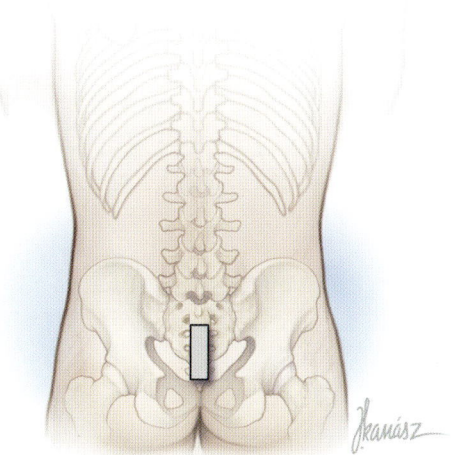

Fig. 39.2 Median approach of caudal block. Note the probe is in long-axis view of the sacrococcygeal ligament.

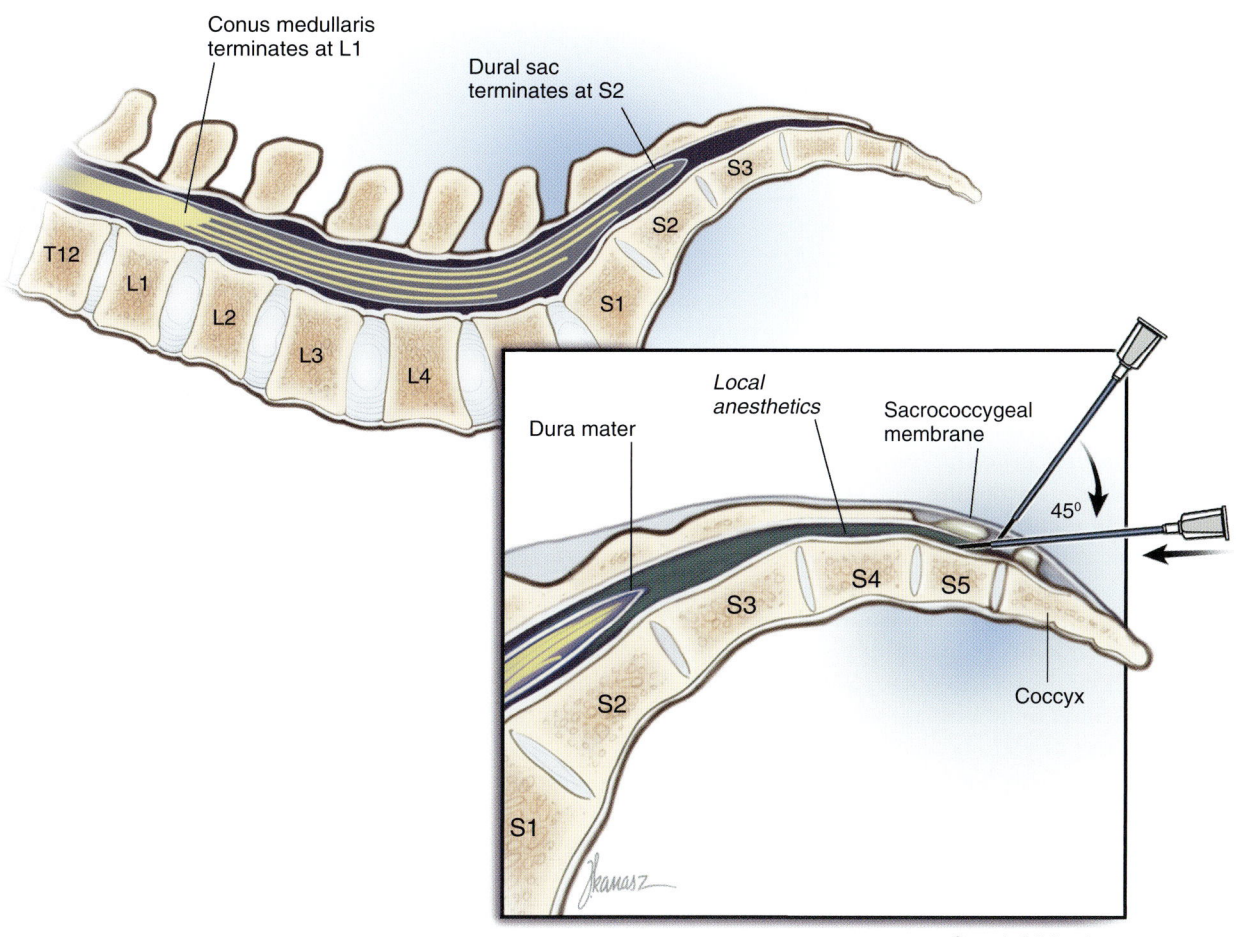

Caudal block

Fig. 39.3 Anatomy of the caudal block with median approach. Note the in-plane position of the needle and its direction from caudal to cephalad position.

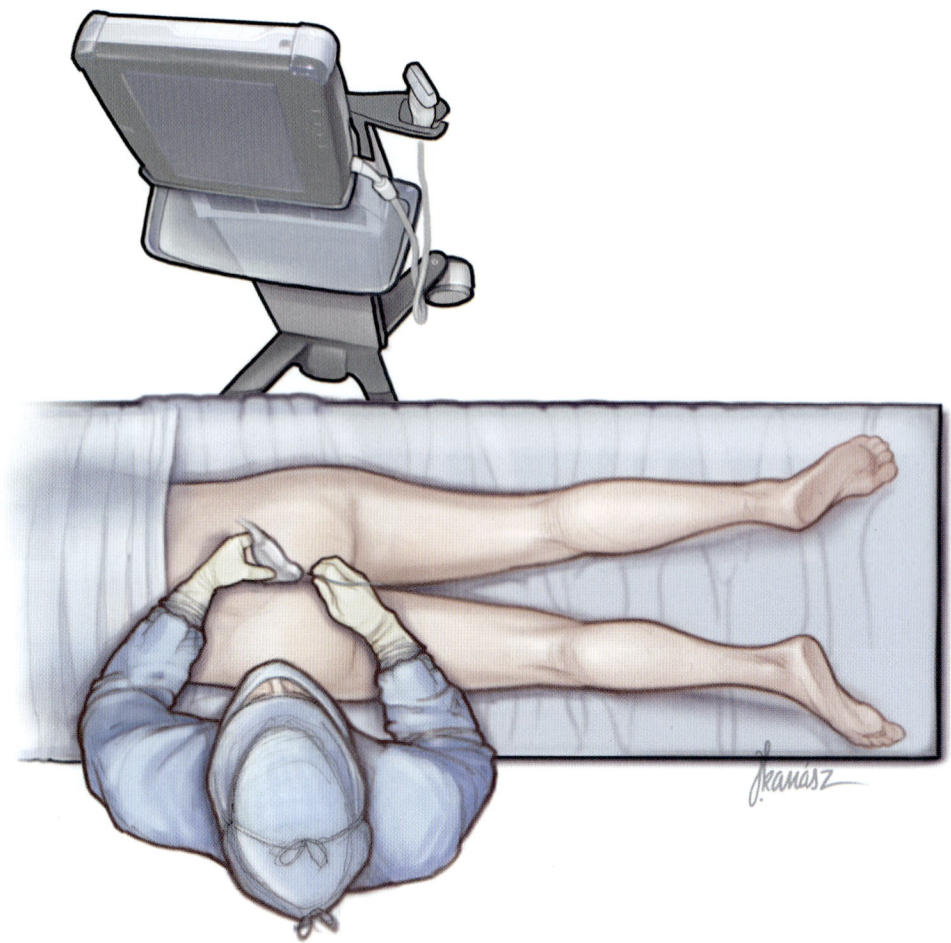

Fig. 39.4 Ultrasound machine position during caudal block performance. Note the probe is in long-axis view of the spine.

LUMBAR NEURAXIAL BLOCKS

The lumbar epidural space can be scanned in the sitting, lateral, or prone position. The author's preference is to perform the scan in the sitting position to allow for maximum flexion of the spine (similar to the familiar landmark technique). Identification of the desired level for the procedure starts by placing the ultrasound probe parallel to the long axis of the sacrum in the midline to identify its flat surface. The probe is moved cephalad slowly to identify the intervertebral space between L5 and S1 as an interruption of the continuity of the sacral line. The ultrasound probe can be advanced longitudinally cephalad along this midline plane or turned 90 degrees to obtain a transverse view of the L5 to S1 interspinous space and then advanced cephalad, keeping the transverse orientation of the probe. Counting the spinous processes (hyperechoic shadows) and the interspinous spaces (hypoechoic windows) will help identify the desired level for the block.

Transverse Axial View The ligamentous structure on the interspinous space is identified at the desired level by its characteristic echogenic appearance (as discussed previously), as well as the ability to see the deeper spinal canal. The needle is usually advanced from lateral to medial, parallel to the ultrasound beam (in-plane approach) until the tip of the needle is engaged in the ligamentum flavum. The epidural space is usually identified by the traditional loss of resistance technique by putting the ultrasound probe down (single operator) or through a second operator.

Tip: The lateral edge of the ultrasound probe can be lifted off the skin to obtain a needle insertion point closer to the midline (Figs. 39.5 and 39.6).

Paramedian Sagittal Oblique View After identifying the appropriate level (as described earlier), the probe is oriented in a paramedian sagittal oblique view (discussed earlier) to allow identification of the epidural space through the interlaminar acoustic window. The epidural space shows as a hypoechoic space between two hyperechoic lines: the ligamentum flavum (posteriorly) and posterior dura (anteriorly). The spinal canal (intrathecal space) can be seen as an anechoic space anterior to the posterior dura, separating it from the anterior complex that appears as a hyperechoic structure.

The needle can be approached through either an in-plane technique from the caudad side of the probe or an out-of-plane technique from the medial side (midline) of the middle of the probe (Fig. 39.7).

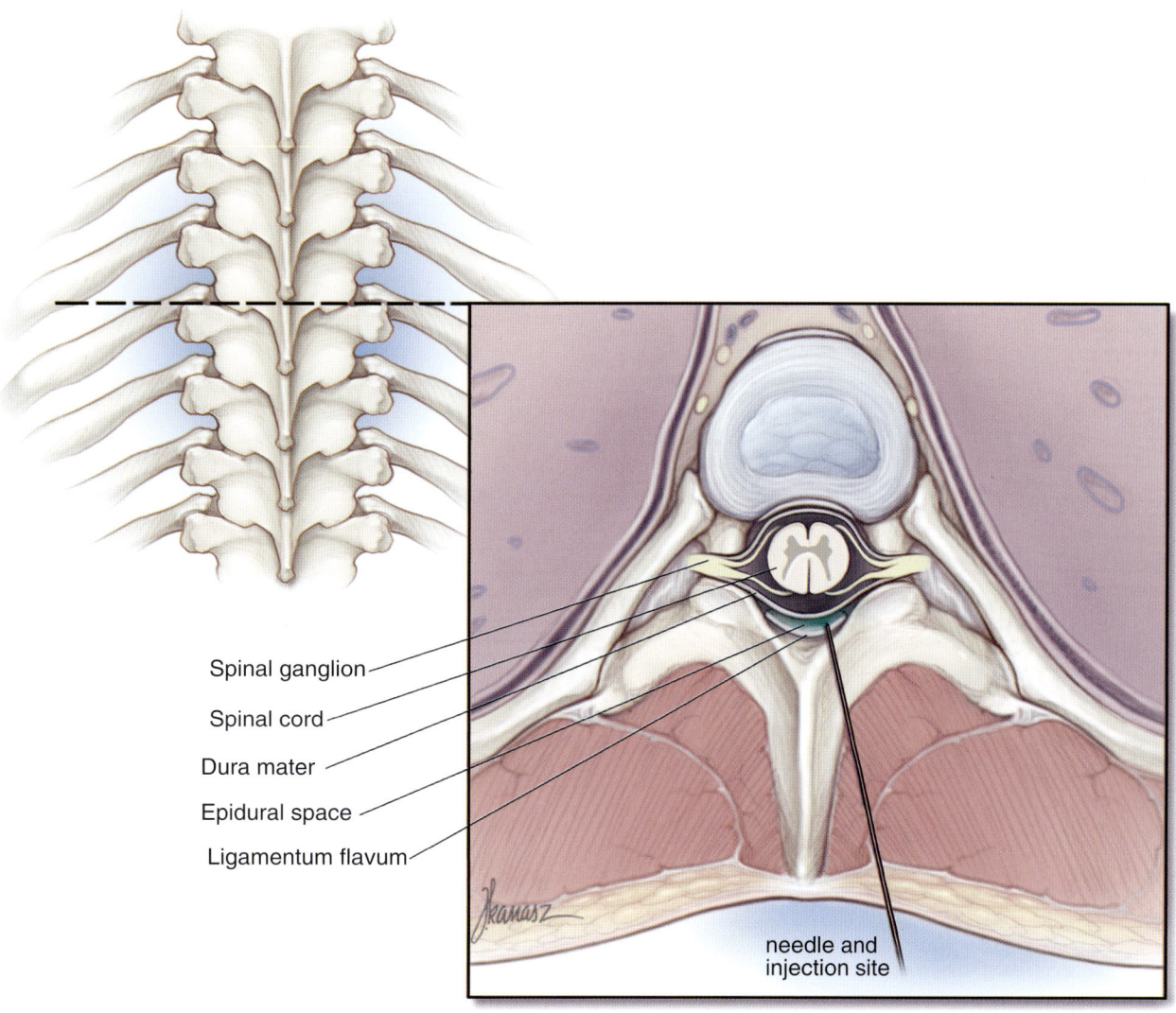

Fig. 39.5 Transverse axial view for lumbar neuraxial block.

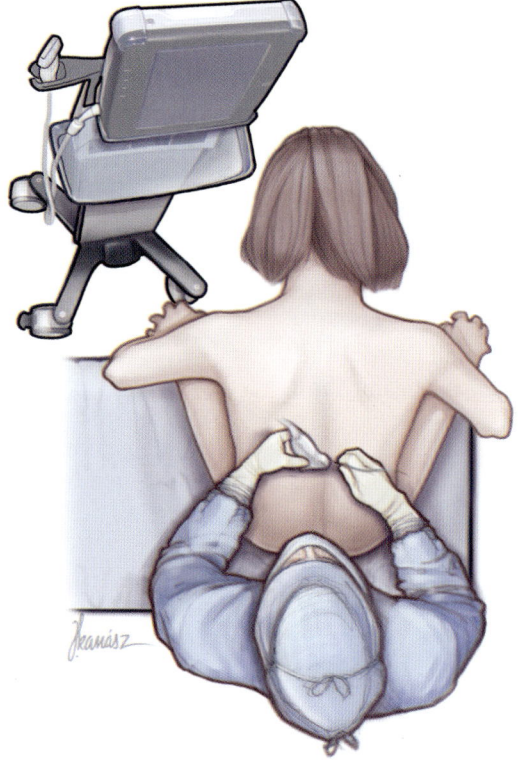

Fig. 39.6 Patient and ultrasound machine position for lumbar neuraxial block using the transverse axial view.

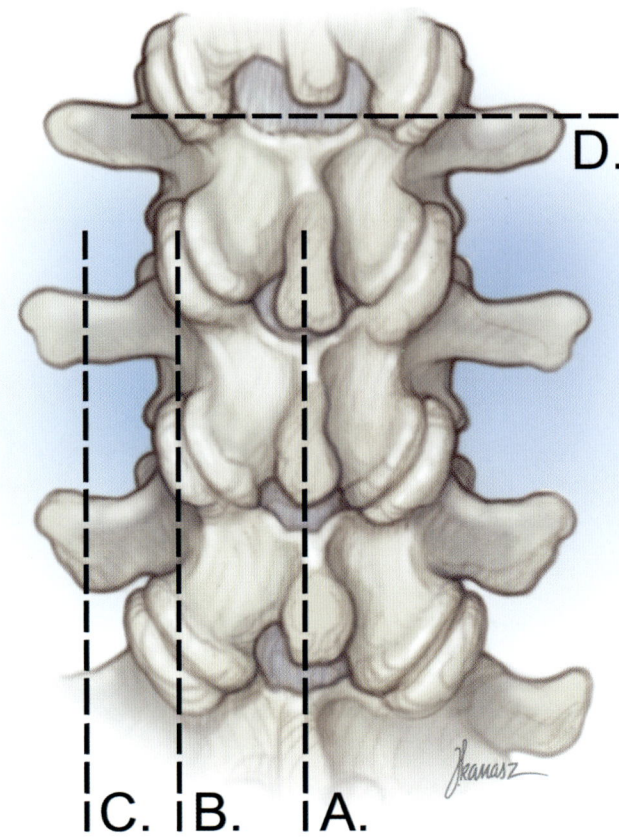

Fig. 39.7 Paramedian sagittal oblique view for lumbar neuraxial block. (A) Midline longitudinal view: Spinous process level. (B) Paramedian longitudinal view: Lamina and articular process level. (C) Paramedian longitudinal view: transverse process level. (D) Transverse axial view: transverse process level.

THORACIC NEURAXIAL BLOCKS

The same concepts and ultrasound techniques are used for scanning the thoracic spine. However, due to the acute angulation and narrower interspinous and interlaminar spaces, the echogenic windows are more challenging to identify and the neuraxial structures are less visible. Paramedian scanning is the only relevant technique for approaching the thoracic epidural space (especially the midthoracic segments with the maximum angulation). Usually, the ultrasound is used to guide the needle to the upper edge of the corresponding lamina, and loss of resistance is used to guide the needle through the ligamentum flavum and epidural space.

PEARLS

- Echogenic Tuohy needles can be helpful to identify the tip of the needle.
- Usually, loss of resistance is needed to confirm the position of the needle tip within the epidural space.
- In pediatric patients and thin patients, some changes can be identified with loss of resistance to saline, a characteristic of correct needle placement, mainly:
  - Widening of the epidural space with anterior displacement of the posterior dura.
  - Compression of the thecal sac can be seen occasionally.
  - Doppler flow of the injected fluid (mainly in small children).
  - Spring-loaded syringes have been recently introduced to the market. They make it possible to perform real-time ultrasound-guided access to the epidural space with loss of resistance confirmed by a single operator.

Spinal Block 40

David L. Brown

Key Points

- Spinal anesthesia is unparalleled in that a small mass of local anesthetic can produce dense surgical anesthesia.
- Bupivacaine is the ideal drug for spinal anesthesia.
- Identification of the lamina at 1 cm lateral to the spinous process is very crucial for a successful paramedian approach.
- The use of a 25-gauge spinal needle is very helpful to avoid postdural puncture spinal headache.
- Taylor technique is a paramedian approach that is performed at L5-S1 interspace, the largest interlaminar interspace of the vertebral column.

PERSPECTIVE

Spinal anesthesia is unparalleled in that a small mass of drug, virtually devoid of systemic pharmacologic effect, can produce profound, reproducible surgical anesthesia. Further, by altering the small mass of drug, very different types of spinal anesthesia can be produced. Low spinal anesthesia, a block below T10, has a different physiologic impact than does a block performed to produce higher spinal anesthesia (above T5). The block is unexcelled for lower abdominal or lower extremity surgical procedures. However, for operations in the midabdomen to upper abdomen, light general anesthesia may have to supplement the spinal block because stimulation of the diaphragm during upper abdominal procedures often causes some discomfort. This area is difficult to block completely through high spinal anesthesia because to do so requires blockade of the phrenic nerve.

Patient Selection. Patient selection for spinal anesthesia often places too much emphasis on a side effect of the technique—namely, spinal headache—than on the applicability of the technique in a given patient. It is clear that the incidence of spinal headache increases with decreasing age and female sex; however, with proper technique and selection of needle size and tip configuration, the incidence of headache should not preclude the use of spinal anesthesia in young, healthy patients if the block has advantages over epidural anesthesia. Almost any patient who is to have a lower extremity operation is a candidate for spinal anesthesia, as are most patients scheduled for lower abdominal surgery, such as inguinal herniorrhaphy and gynecologic, urologic, and obstetric procedures.

Pharmacologic Choice. In the United States, three local anesthetics are commonly used to produce spinal anesthesia: lidocaine, tetracaine, and bupivacaine. Lidocaine is a short-acting to intermediate-acting spinal drug; tetracaine and bupivacaine provide intermediate- to long-acting block. Lidocaine, without epinephrine, is often chosen for procedures that can be completed in 1 hour or less. It is likely that the lidocaine mixture most commonly used is still a 5% solution in 7.5% dextrose, although increasingly anesthesiologists are using 1.5%–2% concentrations of lidocaine without dextrose as alternatives. When epinephrine (0.2 mg) is added to lidocaine, the useful length of clinical anesthesia in the lower abdomen and lower extremities is approximately 90 minutes. Tetracaine is packaged both as niphanoid crystals (20 mg) and as a 1% solution (2 mL total). When dextrose is added to make tetracaine hyperbaric, the drug generally produces effective clinical anesthesia for procedures of up to 1.5–2 hours in the plain form, for up to 2–3 hours when epinephrine (0.2 mg) is added, and for up to 5 hours for lower extremity procedures when phenylephrine (5 mg) is added as a vasoconstrictor. Bupivacaine spinal anesthesia is commonly carried out with 0.5% or 0.75% solution, either plain or in 8.25% dextrose. My impression is that the clinical difference between 0.5% tetracaine and 0.75% bupivacaine as a hyperbaric solution is minimal. Bupivacaine is appropriate for procedures lasting up to 2 or 3 hours.

In addition, local anesthetics can be mixed to produce hypobaric spinal anesthesia. A common method of formulating a hypobaric solution is to mix tetracaine in a 0.1% to 0.33% solution with sterile water. Also, lidocaine can be mixed to provide useful hypobaric spinal anesthesia. This drug is diluted from a 2% solution with sterile water to make a 0.5% solution using a total of 30–40mg.

Many anesthesiologists avoid vasoconstrictors for fear of somehow increasing the risk with spinal anesthesia. These anesthesiologists believe that phenylephrine or epinephrine has such potent vasoconstrictive action that it puts the blood supply of the spinal cord at risk. There are no human data supporting this theory. In fact, because most local anesthetics are vasodilators, the addition of these vasoconstrictors does little more than maintain spinal cord blood flow at a basal level. Commonly used doses of vasoconstrictors are 0.2 to 0.3 mg of epinephrine and 5 mg of phenylephrine added to the spinal anesthetic.

PLACEMENT

Anatomy. As outlined in Chapter 39, Neuraxial Block Anatomy, the spinous processes of the lumbar vertebrae have an almost horizontal orientation in relation to the long axis of their respective vertebral bodies (Fig. 40.1). When a midline needle is inserted between the lumbar vertebral spinous processes, it is most effective if it is placed almost perpendicularly in relation to the long axis of the back. To facilitate spinal anesthesia, the anesthesiologist must constantly keep in mind the midline of the patient's body and the neuraxis in relation to the needle. As illustrated in Fig. 40.1, as a midline needle is inserted into the cerebrospinal fluid (CSF), it logically must puncture the skin, subcutaneous tissue, supraspinous ligament, interspinous ligament, ligamentum flavum, epidural space, and finally the dura mater and arachnoid mater to reach the CSF.

Position. Spinal anesthesia is carried out in three principal positions: lateral decubitus (Fig. 40.2), sitting (Fig. 40.3), and prone jackknife (Fig. 40.4). In both the lateral decubitus and sitting positions, a well-trained assistant is essential if the block is to be easily and efficiently administered by the anesthesiologist. As illustrated in Fig. 40.2, the assistant can help the patient assume the position of legs flexed on the abdomen and chin flexed on the chest. This is most easily

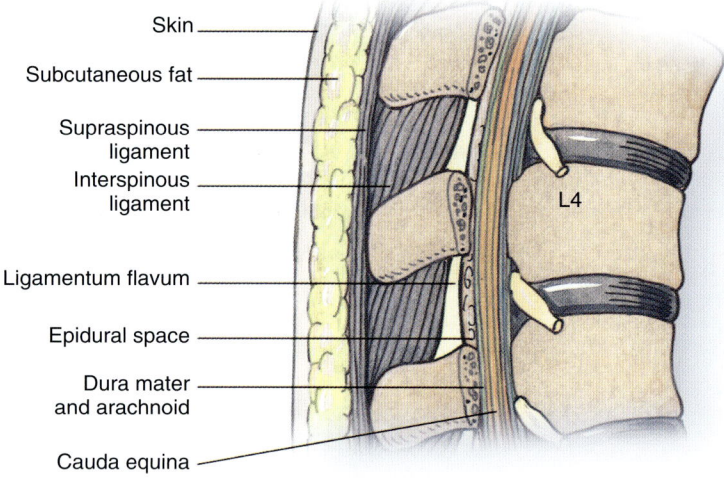

Fig. 40.1 Spinal block: functional lumbar anatomy.

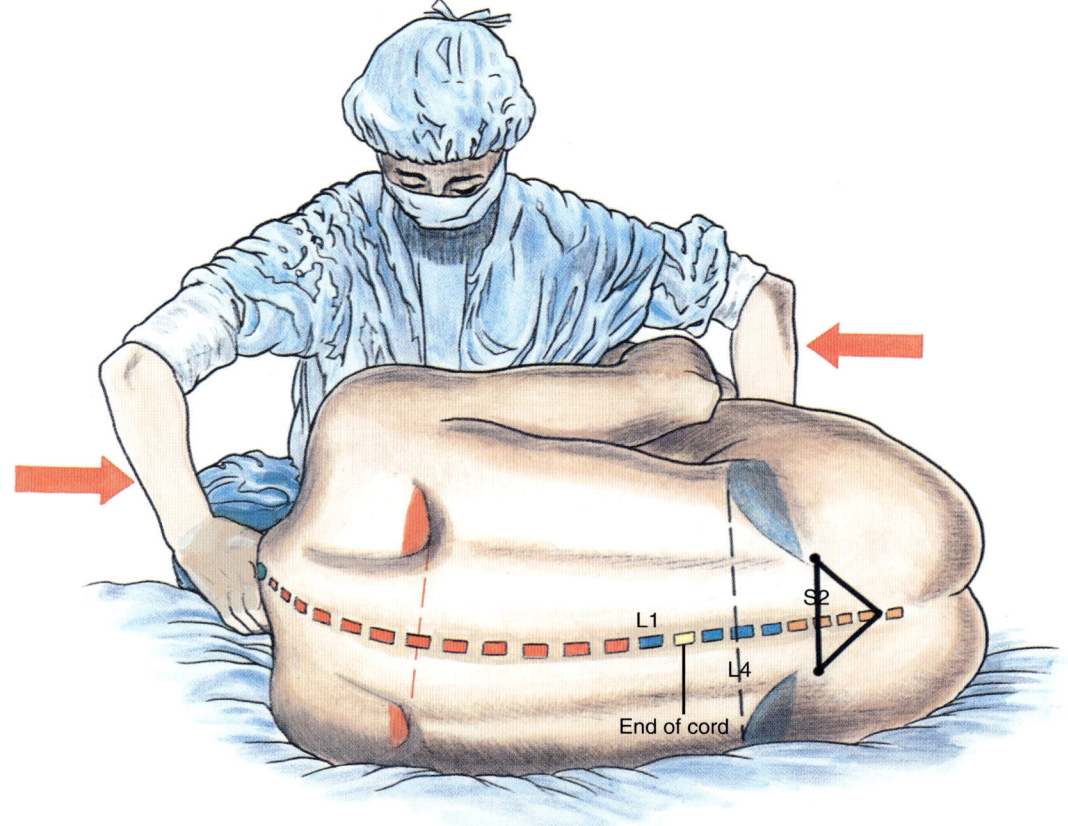

Fig. 40.2 Spinal block: lateral decubitus position.

accomplished by having the assistant pull the head toward the chest, place an arm behind the patient's knees, and push the head and knees together. The position can also be facilitated by using an appropriate amount of sedation that allows the patient to be relaxed yet cooperative.

In some patients, the sitting position can facilitate location of the midline, especially in obese patients or in those with some scoliosis that makes midline identification more difficult. As illustrated in Fig. 40.3A, the patient should assume a comfortable sitting position, with the legs placed over the edge of the operating table and the feet supported by a stool. A pillow should be placed in the patient's lap and the patient's arms allowed to drape over the pillow, resting on the flexed lower extremities. The assistant should be positioned immediately in front of the patient, supporting the shoulders and allowing the patient to minimize lumbar lordosis, while ensuring that the vertebral midline remains in a vertical position (see Fig. 40.3B).

Sometimes it is more efficient to place the patient in a prone jackknife position before administering the spinal anesthetic (see Fig. 40.4). An assistant is not as essential for this technique as for the lateral decubitus and sitting positions, although to make the most efficient use of operating room block time, it is often helpful for the assistant to position the patient in the prone jackknife position while the anesthesiologist readies the spinal anesthesia tray and drugs.

In all three positions, the goal is to place the patient so that the midline is readily identifiable and lumbar lordosis is reduced. Fig. 40.5 shows what the lumbar anatomy looks like when the patient's lumbar lordosis has been ineffectively reduced by poor positioning. As illustrated, the intralaminar space is small and difficult to enter with a needle in the midline. In contrast, Fig. 40.6 illustrates how effective positioning can open the intralaminar space to allow easy access for subarachnoid puncture.

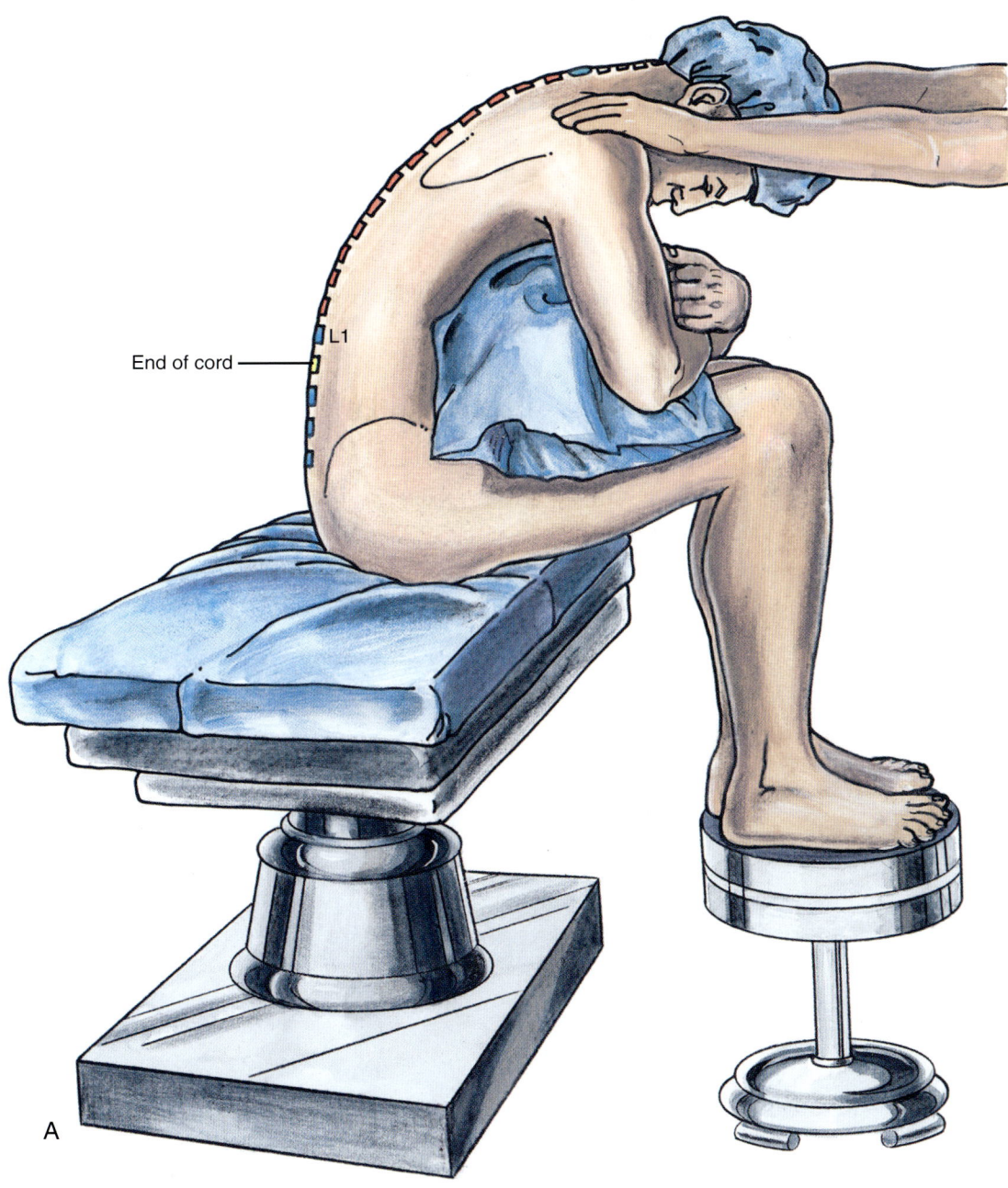

Fig. 40.3 Spinal block: sitting position. **(A)** Lateral view.

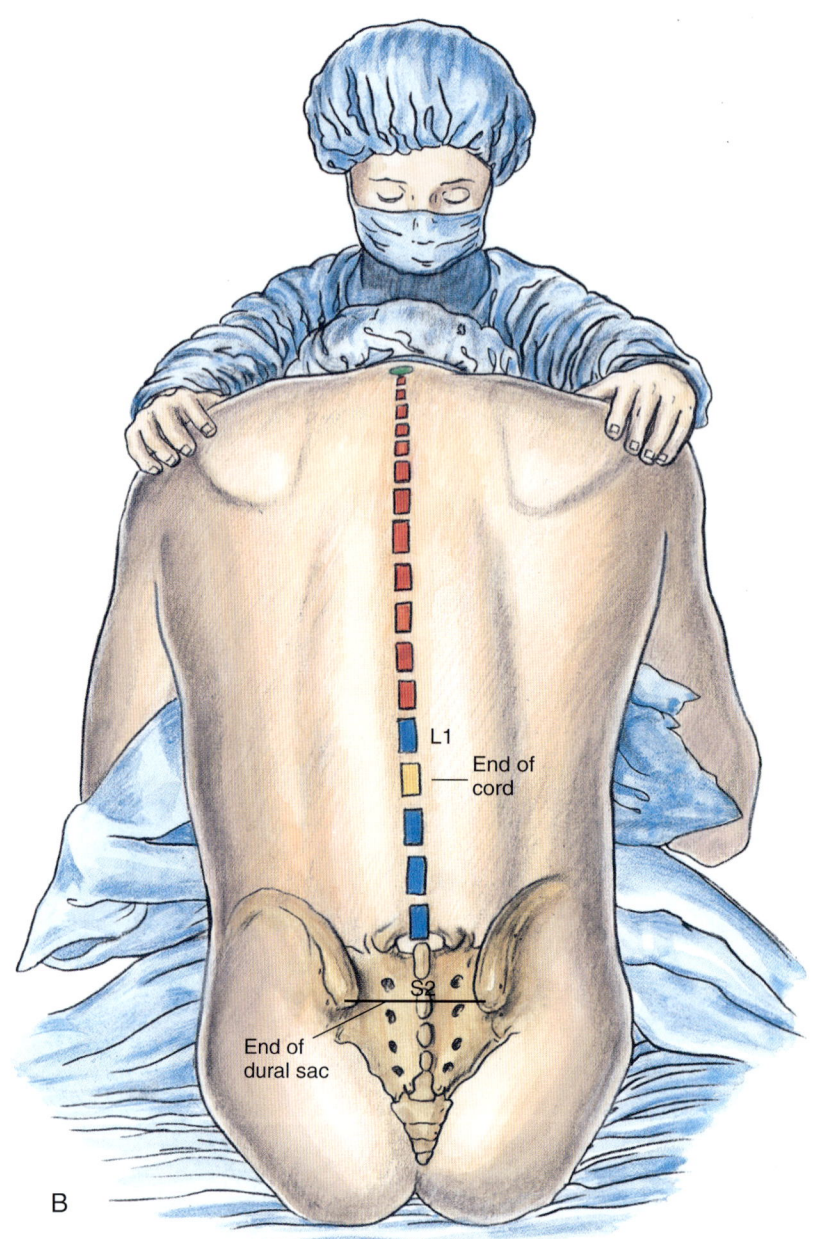

Fig. 40.3 cont'd (B) Posterior view.

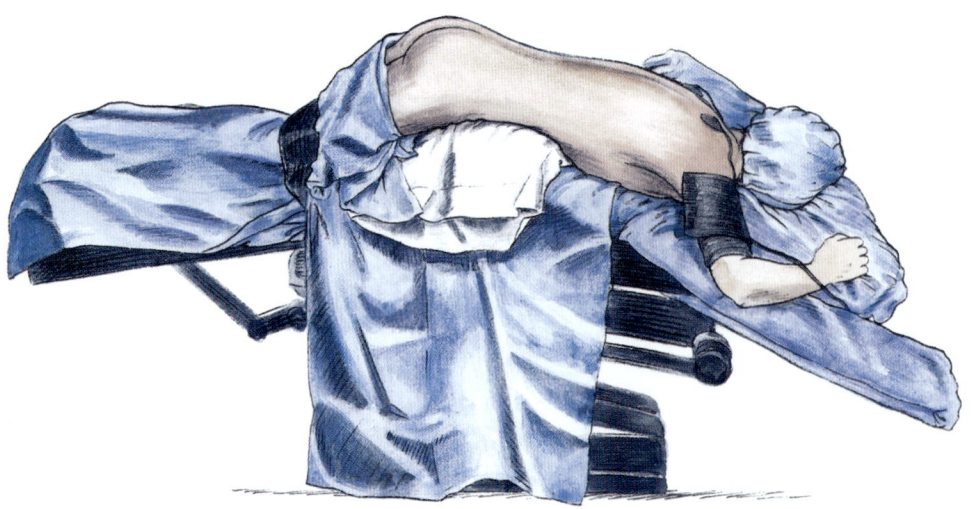

Fig. 40.4 Spinal block: prone jackknife position.

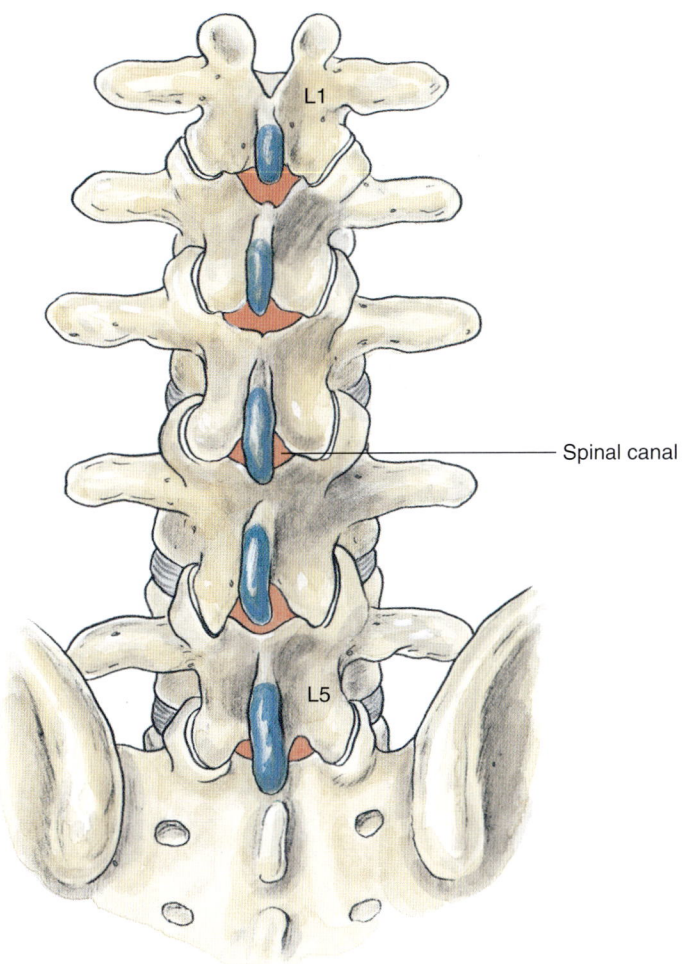

Fig. 40.5 Spinal block: lumbar vertebra. Lumbar lordosis is present because the positioning is inadequate.

Needle Puncture. One of the first decisions to be made in considering spinal anesthesia is what kind of needle to use. Although there are many eponyms for spinal needles, they fall into two main categories: those that cut the dura sharply and those that disrupt the dural fibers by spreading with a cone-shaped tip. The former category includes the traditional disposable spinal needle, the Quincke–Babcock needle; the latter category comprises the Greene, Whitacre, and Sprotte needles. If a continuous spinal technique is chosen, the use of a Tuohy or other thin-walled, curve-tipped needle will facilitate passage of the catheter. To make a logical choice of a spinal needle, the risks and benefits of each must be understood. The use of small needles reduces the incidence of postdural puncture headache; the use of larger needles improves the tactile sense of needle placement, thus increasing operator confidence.

Probably the risk–benefit calculation is not as simple as this. For example, the use of a small needle, such as a 27-gauge needle, will not decrease the incidence of headache in younger patients if a number of "passes" through the dura are required before CSF flow is recognized. Likewise, a larger needle, such as a 22-gauge Whitacre needle, may result in a lower incidence of postdural puncture headache if the subarachnoid needle location is recognized on the first pass. Different needle tip designs result in differences in the incidence of postdural puncture headache even when needle sizes are comparable.

With the patient in the proper position, the anesthesiologist uses the palpating hand to clearly identify the patient's intervertebral space and midline. As illustrated in Fig. 40.7 (*Step 1*), the anesthesiologist can effectively carry out this important maneuver by moving the fingers of the palpating hand alternately cephalocaudad and rolling them from side to side. When the appropriate intervertebral space has been clearly identified, a skin wheal is raised over the space. Next, an introducer is inserted into the substance of the interspinous ligament, taking care to firmly seat it in the midline (Fig. 40.7, *Step 2*). The introducer is grasped with the palpating fingers and steadied while the other hand holds the spinal needle, somewhat like a dart, as illustrated in Fig. 40.7 (*Step 3*). With the fifth finger of the needle hand used as a tripod against the patient's back, the needle, with bevel (if present) parallel to the long axis of the spine, is advanced slowly to heighten the sense of tissue planes traversed, as well as to avoid skewing the nerve roots, until a characteristic change in resistance is noted as the needle passes through the ligamentum flavum and dura. The stylet is then removed, and CSF should appear at the needle hub. If it does not, the needle is rotated in 90-degree increments until CSF appears. If CSF does not appear in any quadrant, the needle should be advanced a few millimeters and rechecked in all four quadrants. If CSF still has not appeared and the needle is at a depth appropriate for the patient, the needle

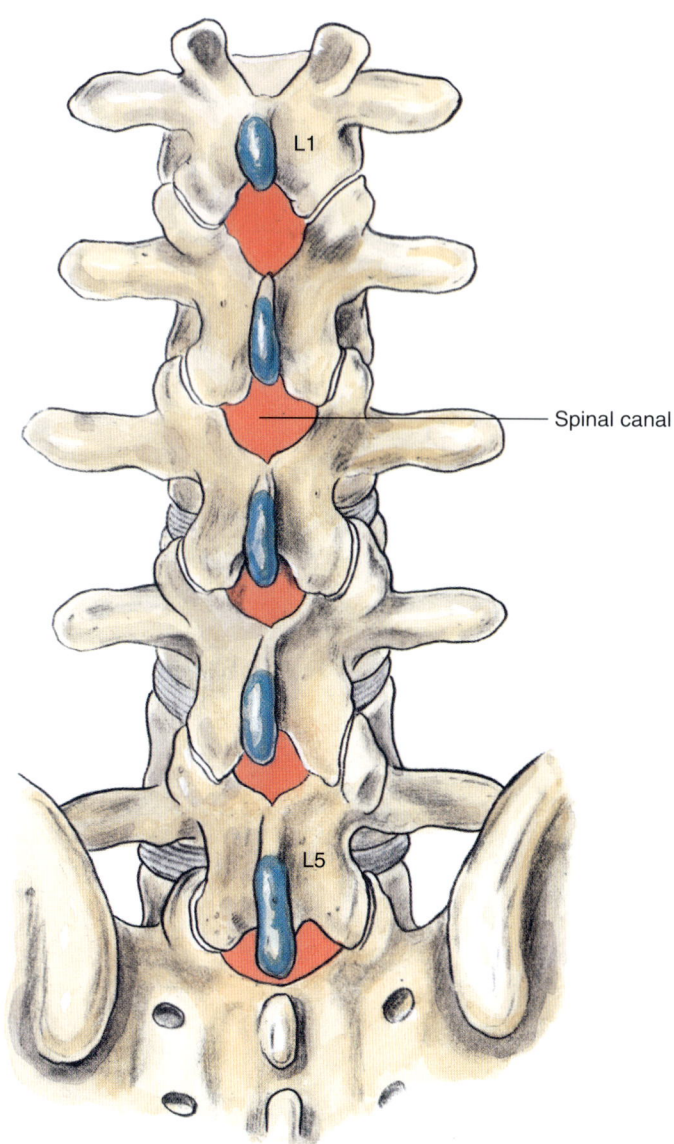

Fig. 40.6 Spinal block: lumbar vertebra. Lumbar lordosis is reversed with ideal spinal positioning.

and introducer should be withdrawn and the insertion steps repeated because the most common reason for lack of CSF return is that the needle was inserted off the midline. Another common error preventing subarachnoid placement is insertion of the needle with too great a cephalad angle on the initial insertion (Fig. 40.8).

Once CSF is freely obtained, the dorsum of the anesthesiologist's nondominant hand steadies the spinal needle against the patient's back while the syringe containing the therapeutic dose is attached to the needle. CSF is again freely aspirated into the syringe, and the dose is injected. Sometimes, when the syringe has been attached to a needle from which CSF was clearly previously dripping, aspiration of additional CSF becomes impossible. As illustrated in Fig. 40.9, one technique that can be used to facilitate CSF aspiration is to "unscrew" the syringe plunger (see Fig. 40.9A) rather than providing constant steady pressure (see Fig. 40.9B).

After the local anesthetic has been injected, the patient and the operating table should be placed in the position appropriate for the surgical procedure and the drugs being used. The midline approach to subarachnoid block is the technique of first choice because it requires anatomic projection in only two planes, and the needle insertion plane is a relatively avascular one. When difficulties with needle insertion are encountered with the midline approach, an option is to use the paramedian route, which does not require the same level of patient cooperation or reversal of lumbar lordosis to be successful. As illustrated in Fig. 40.10, the paramedian approach exploits the larger "subarachnoid target" that exists if a needle is inserted slightly lateral to the midline. In the paramedian approach, the palpating fingers should identify the caudal edge of the cephalad spinous process of the intervertebral space chosen, and a skin wheal should be raised 1 cm lateral and 1 cm caudal to this point. A longer needle, such as a 4-cm, 22-gauge, short-beveled needle, is then used to infiltrate the deeper tissues in a cephalomedial plane. The spinal introducer and needle are then inserted 10–15 degrees off the sagittal plane in a cephalomedial plane, as noted in Fig. 40.10. As with the midline approach, the most common error made with this technique is to angle the needle too far cephalad in its

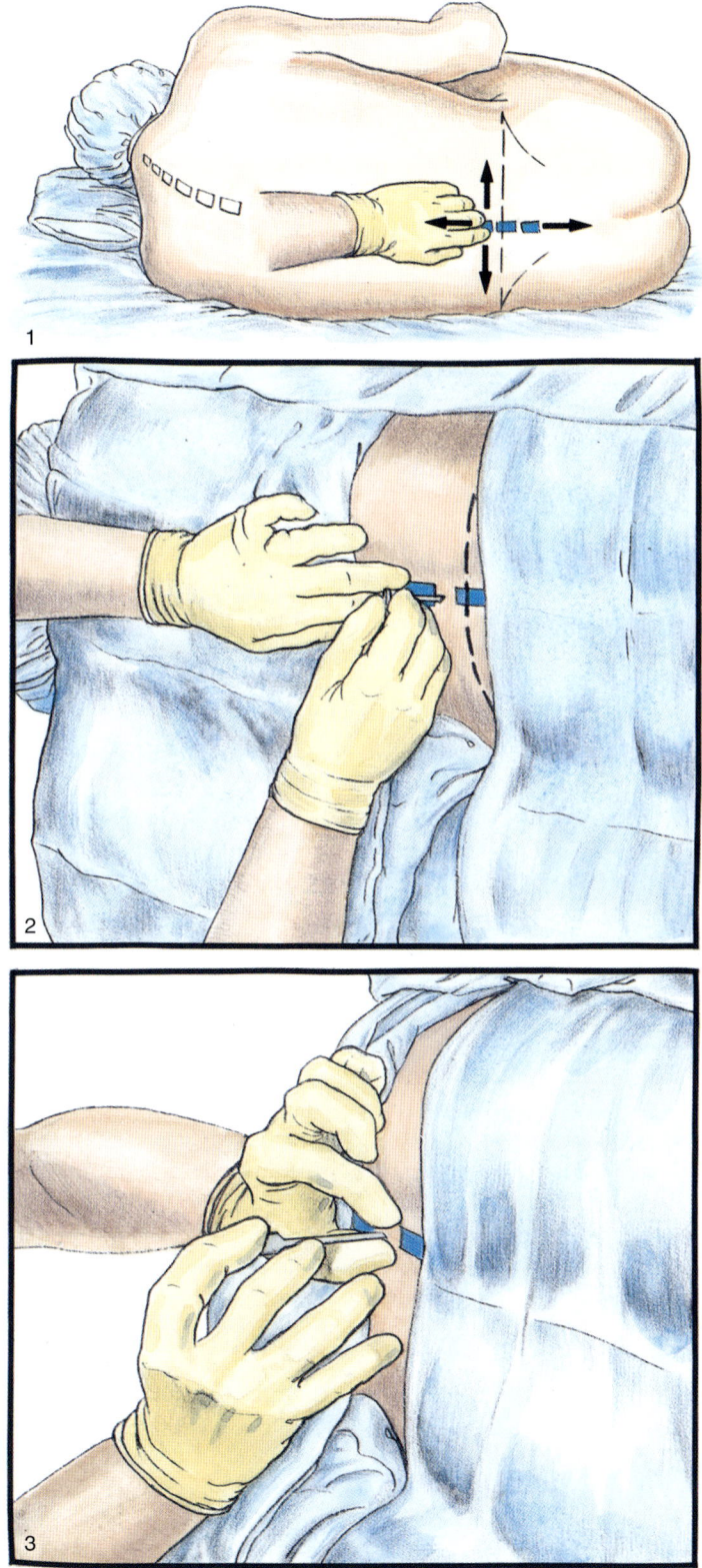

Fig. 40.7 Spinal block: technique.

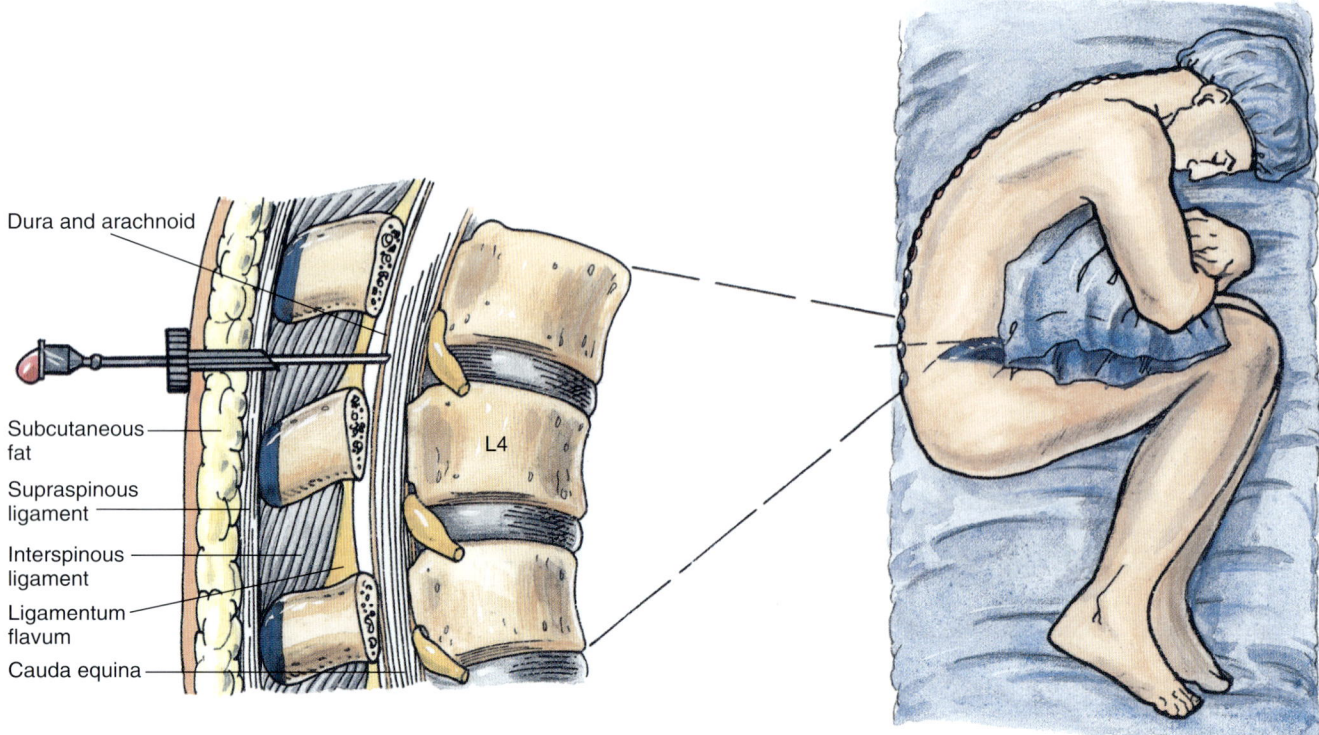

Fig. 40.8 Spinal block: avoiding too large a cephalad angle on insertion.

initial insertion. Once the needle contacts bone with this approach, it is redirected in, slightly cephalad. If bone is again contacted after the needle has been redirected, but at a deeper level, this needle redirection is continued because it is likely that the needle is being "walked up" the lamina toward the intervertebral space. After CSF is obtained, the block continues in the same way as that described for the midline approach.

A variation of the paramedian approach is the lumbosacral approach of Taylor. The technique is carried out at the L5 to S1 interspace, the largest interlaminar interspace of the vertebral column. As illustrated in Fig. 40.11, the skin insertion site is 1 cm medial and 1 cm caudal to the ipsilateral posterosuperior iliac spine. Through this point, a 12- to 15-cm spinal needle is inserted in a cephalomedial direction toward the midline. If bone is encountered on the first needle insertion, the needle is "walked off" the sacrum into the subarachnoid space, as in the method used for a lumbar paramedian approach. Once CSF is obtained, the steps are similar to those previously outlined.

POTENTIAL PROBLEMS

The complication most feared by patients and many anesthesiologists after spinal anesthesia is neurologic injury. However, the risk–benefit calculation of neurologic injury after anesthesia must include those cases that are possible after general anesthesia. These comparisons may show that the incidence of neurologic injury after spinal anesthesia is in fact lower than that after general anesthesia. However, this statement must remain speculative.

In patients in whom the spinal block level has to be precisely controlled or in whom the operation is expected to outlast the usual duration of the anesthetic drugs, a continuous spinal catheter may be used. However, when using a continuous spinal technique, one should be cautious about repeating local anesthetic injections if the block height does not reach the predicted levels. Neurotoxicity (cauda equina syndrome) is hypothetically possible when the spinal catheter position allows local anesthetic concentrations to reach higher-than-expected levels.

A more common complication of spinal anesthesia is postoperative headache. Factors that influence the incidence of postdural puncture headache are age (more frequent in younger patients), sex (more likely in female patients), needle size (more frequent with larger needles), needle bevel orientation (increased incidence when dural fibers are cut transversely), pregnancy (incidence increased), and number of dural punctures necessary to obtain CSF (more likely with multiple punctures). Perhaps more important to physicians than knowing the factors resulting in an increased incidence of postdural puncture headache is the knowledge of how and when to carry out definitive therapy—that is, an epidural blood patch. To use spinal anesthesia effectively, epidural blood patching, when indicated, must be used early. The success rate from a single epidural blood patch should be in the 90% to 95% range, and if a second patch is required, a similar percentage should be obtainable.

One other common side effect of spinal anesthesia is the appearance of a backache in approximately 25% of patients. Patients often blame "the spinal" for backache, but, when looked at systematically, it appears that just as many patients have backaches after general anesthesia as after spinal anesthesia. Thus backache after neuraxial block should not be attributed immediately to "needling" of the back.

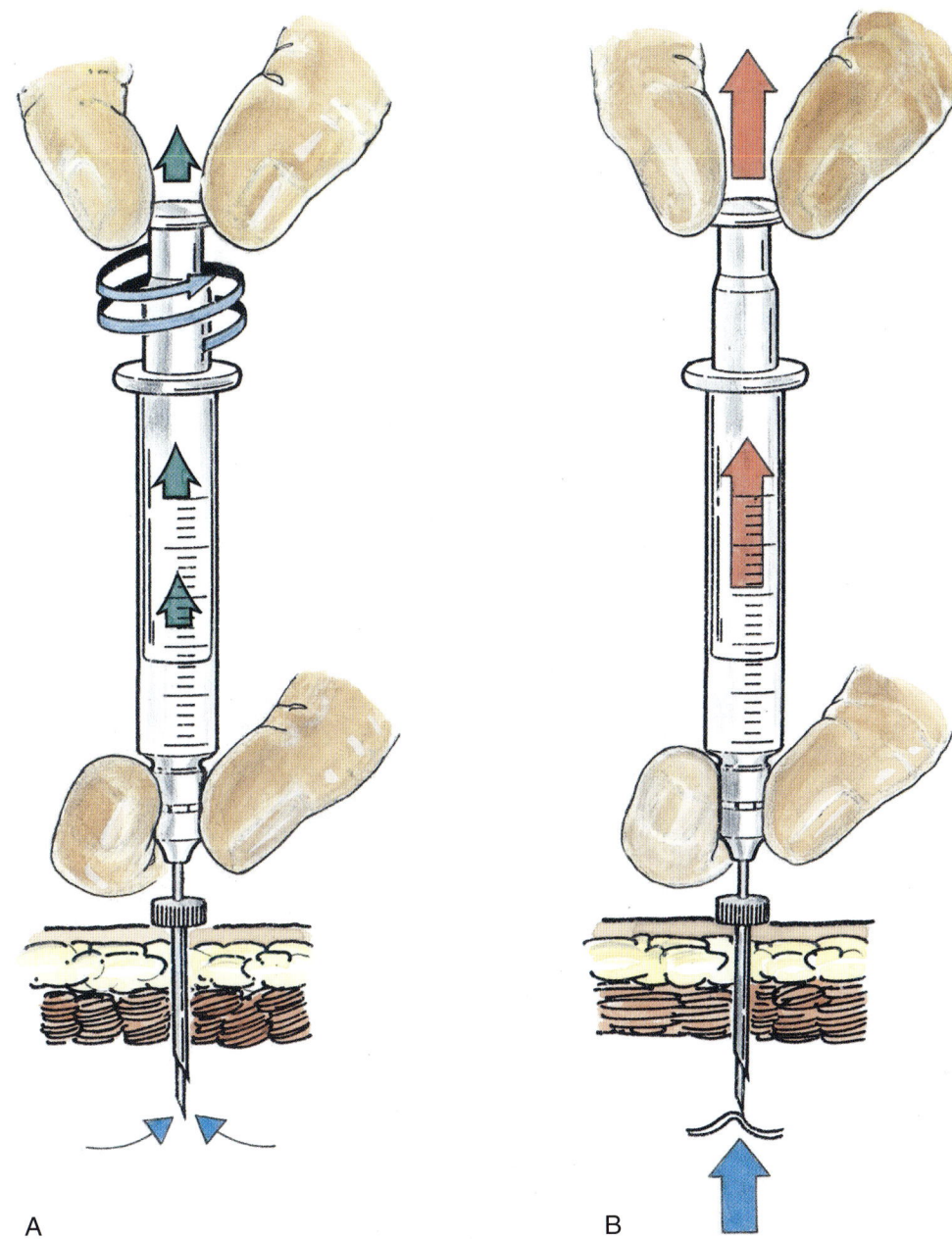

Fig. 40.9 Spinal block: syringe technique to facilitate aspiration of cerebrospinal fluid. (A) Unscrew syringe plunger. (B) Avoid applying constant aspiration.

PEARLS

Probably the most important factor contributing to success with spinal anesthesia in the day-to-day life of an anesthesiologist is the efficiency of the technique. If nurses and surgeons are to be advocates of spinal anesthesia, its use cannot measurably add time to the surgical day. Thus one should plan ahead to maximize efficiency. Often overlooked in this maxim is the fact that patient preparation for operation can begin almost as soon as the block is administered if the patient is properly sedated.

Intraoperatively during high spinal anesthesia (often during cesarean section) patients occasionally complain of dyspnea. This often appears to be a result of loss of chest wall sensation rather than of significantly decreased inspiratory capacity. The loss of chest wall sensation does not allow the patient to experience the reassurance of a deep breath. This impediment to patient acceptance can often be overcome simply by asking the patient to raise a hand in front of his or her mouth and exhale forcefully. The tactile appreciation of a deep exhalation often seems to provide the needed reassurance.

If spinal anesthesia has been used and a neurologic complication is noted after surgery, it is essential to obtain neurologic consultation early. In this way, an unbiased consultant can examine the patient and determine whether the "new" neurologic finding preexisted, is related to a peripheral neuropathy, or, more rarely, is potentially related to the spinal anesthetic. Latent electromyographic alterations associated with denervation due to neurologic injury take time to develop in the lower extremities (14–21 days). Therefore after a potentially spinal anesthesia–related lesion has been identified, electromyographic studies should be obtained early to establish a preblock baseline and allow serial comparison.

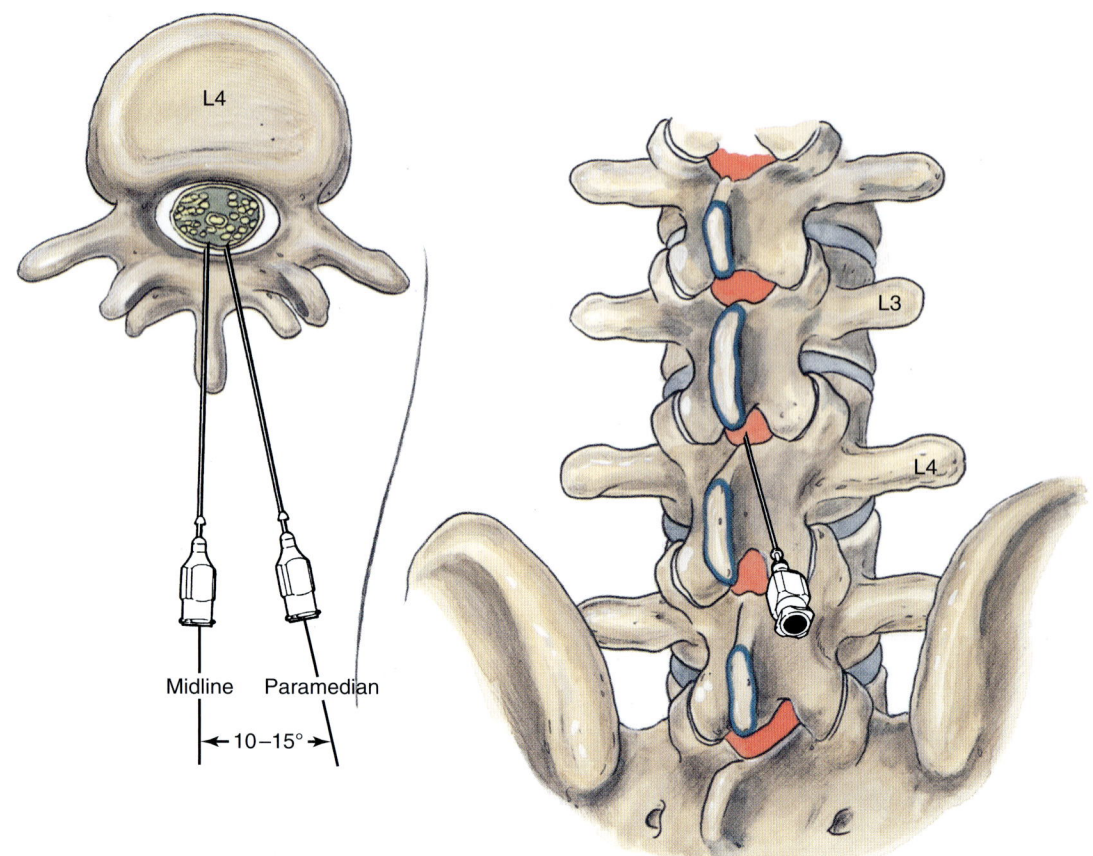

Fig. 40.10 Spinal block: paramedian technique.

It is also useful to consider adding fentanyl (15–25 μg) rather than epinephrine to some shorter-acting spinal local anesthetic mixtures (e.g., lidocaine) because it prolongs the effective sensory block without measurably prolonging the motor block or the time to voiding. This is especially useful in selected surgical outpatients.

Another way to titrate spinal anesthesia for outpatients, or any surgical procedure in which the length of surgery is difficult to predict, is to use a combined spinal–epidural technique. In this technique an epidural needle is placed in the epidural space in a standard fashion, and then a small-gauge spinal needle is advanced through the epidural needle into the CSF. A spinal local anesthetic mixture is then injected and matched to the projected length of the shortest surgical procedure planned. After removal of the spinal needle, an epidural catheter is inserted into the epidural space. At this point, if the surgical procedure lasts longer than anticipated, the epidural catheter can be injected with a local anesthetic appropriate for the anticipated surgical needs. This combined spinal–epidural technique provides the flexibility for both spinal and epidural anesthesia in selected patients.

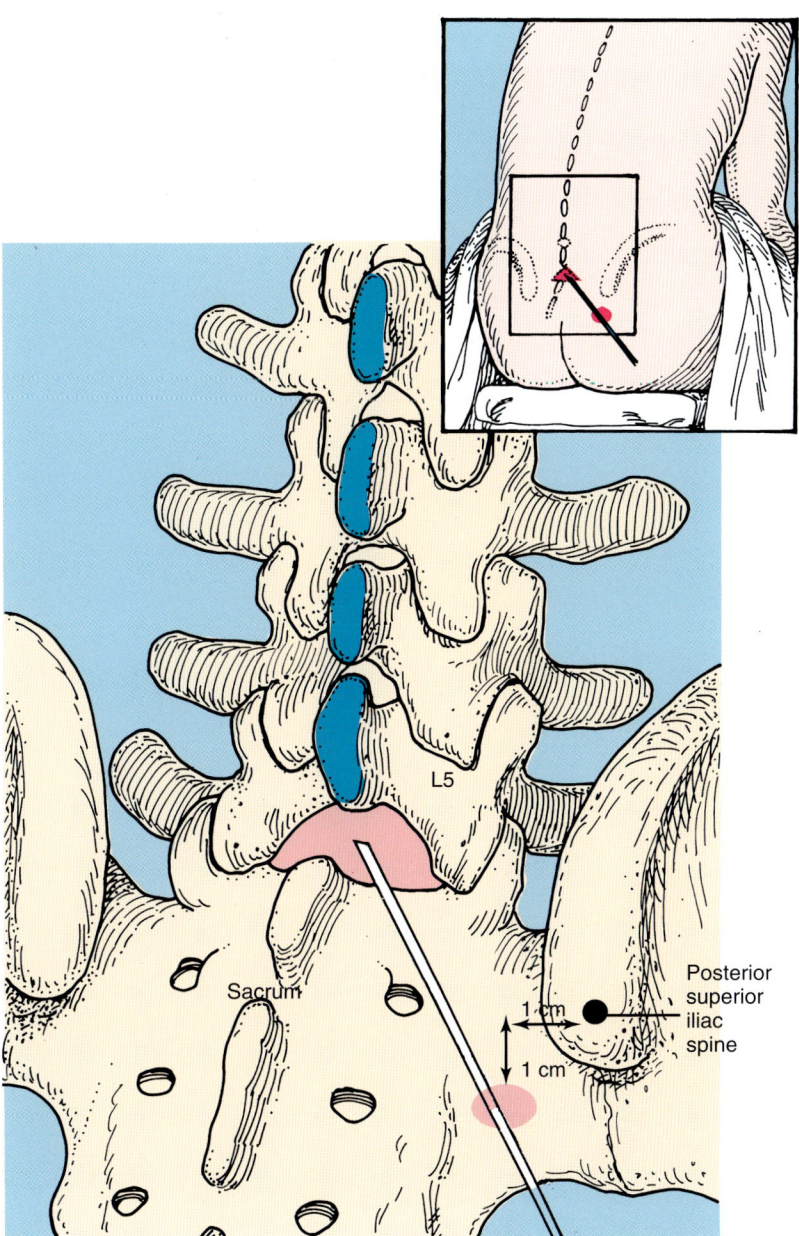

Fig. 40.11 Spinal block: L5 to S1 paramedian technique (Taylor's approach).

Epidural Block 41

David L. Brown

Key Points

- Epidural block can be performed in cervical, thoracic, and lumbar regions of the vertebral column.
- Paramedian approach is the preferred technique for thoracic epidural, while median and paramedian approaches are suitable for lumbar epidural.
- T5–T6 interspace is the preferred position for thoracic epidural catheter insertion.
- The ligamentum flavum is congenitally absent in the midline in some people, which makes them prone to the dural puncture during epidural block.
- Checking for the coagulation status of the patients is very crucial before attempting the epidural block.
- Early diagnosis and management for epidural hematoma are crucial to avoid permanent neural damage.

PERSPECTIVE

Epidural anesthesia is the second primary method of neuraxial block. In contrast to spinal anesthesia, epidural block requires pharmacologic doses of local anesthetics, making systemic toxicity a concern. In skilled hands, the incidence of postdural puncture headache should be lower with epidural anesthesia than with spinal anesthesia. Nevertheless, as outlined in Chapter 40, Spinal Block, I do not believe this should be the major differentiating point between the two techniques. Spinal anesthesia is typically a single-shot technique, whereas frequently intermittent injections are given through an epidural catheter, thus allowing reinjection and prolongation of epidural block. Another difference is that epidural block allows production of segmental anesthesia. Thus if a thoracic injection is made and an appropriate amount of local anesthetic is injected, a band of anesthesia that does not block the lower extremities can be produced.

Patient Selection. Epidural block is appropriate for virtually the same patients who are candidates for spinal anesthesia, except that epidural anesthesia can be used in the cervical and thoracic areas as well—levels at which spinal anesthesia is not advised. As with spinal anesthesia, if epidural block is to be used for intraabdominal procedures involving the upper abdomen, it is advisable to combine this technique with a light general anesthetic because diaphragmatic irritation can make the patient, surgeon, and anesthesiologist uncomfortable. Other candidates for epidural anesthesia are patients in whom a continuous technique has increasingly been found to be helpful in providing epidural local anesthesia or opioid analgesia after major surgical procedures. This clinical application likely explains the increased interest in epidural block over the last 20 years.

Pharmacologic Choice. To use epidural local anesthetics effectively, one must combine an understanding of the potency and duration of local anesthetics with estimates of the length of the operation and the postoperative analgesia requirements. Drugs available for epidural use can be categorized as short-acting, intermediate-acting, and long-acting agents; with the addition of epinephrine to these agents, surgical anesthesia ranging from 45–240 minutes after a single injection is possible.

Chloroprocaine, an amino ester local anesthetic, is a short-acting agent that allows efficient matching of the length of the surgical procedure and the duration of epidural analgesia, even in outpatients. 2-Chloroprocaine is available in 2% and 3% concentrations; the latter is preferable for surgical anesthesia and the former for techniques not requiring muscle relaxation.

Lidocaine is the prototypical amino amide local anesthetic and is used in 1.5% and 2% concentrations epidurally. Concentrations of mepivacaine necessary for epidural anesthesia are similar to those of lidocaine; however, mepivacaine lasts from 15–30 minutes longer at equivalent dosages. Epinephrine significantly prolongs (i.e., by approximately 50%) the duration of surgical anesthesia with 2-chloroprocaine and either lidocaine and mepivacaine. Plain lidocaine produces surgical anesthesia that lasts from 60–100 minutes.

Bupivacaine, an amino amide, is a widely used long-acting local anesthetic for epidural anesthesia. It is used in 0.5% and 0.75% concentrations, but analgesic techniques can be performed with concentrations ranging from 0.125%–0.25%. Its duration of action is not prolonged as consistently by the addition of epinephrine, although up to 240 minutes of surgical anesthesia can be obtained when epinephrine is added.

Ropivacaine, another long-acting amino amide, is also used for regional and epidural anesthesia. For surgical anesthesia, it is used in 0.5%, 0.75%, and 1% concentrations. Analgesia can be obtained with concentrations of 0.2%. Its duration of action is slightly less than that of bupivacaine in the epidural technique, and it appears to produce slightly less motor blockade than a comparable concentration of bupivacaine.

In addition to the use of epinephrine as an epidural additive, some anesthesiologists recommend modifying epidural local anesthetic solutions to increase both the speed of onset and the quality of the block produced. One recommendation is to alkalinize the local anesthetic solution by adding bicarbonate to it to achieve both these purposes. Nevertheless, the clinical advisability of routinely adding bicarbonate to local anesthetic solutions should be determined by local practice protocols.

PLACEMENT

Anatomy. As with spinal anesthesia, the key to carrying out successful epidural anesthesia is understanding the three-dimensional midline neuraxial anatomy that underlies the palpating fingers (Fig. 41.1). When a lumbar approach to the epidural space is used in adults, the depth from the skin to the ligamentum flavum is commonly near 4 cm; in 80% of patients the epidural space is cannulated at a distance of 3.5–6 cm from the skin. In a small number of patients the lumbar epidural space is as near as 2 cm from the skin. In the lumbar region, the ligamentum flavum is 5–6 mm thick in the midline, whereas in the thoracic region it is 3–5 mm thick. In the thoracic region, the depth from the skin to the epidural space depends on the degree of cephalad angulation used for the paramedian approach, as well as the body habitus of the patient (Fig. 41.2). In the cervical region the depth to the ligamentum flavum is approximately the same as that in the lumbar region, 4–6 cm.

The ligamentum flavum will be perceived as a thicker ligament if the needle is kept in the midline than if the needle is inserted off the midline and enters the lateral extension of the ligamentum flavum. Fig. 41.3 illustrates how important it is to maintain the midline position of the epidural needle (*needle A*) during lumbar epidural techniques. If an oblique approach is taken, a "false release" can be produced (*needle C*) or the perception of a thin ligament can be reinforced (*needle B*).

Position. Patient positioning for epidural anesthesia is similar to that for spinal anesthesia, with lateral decubitus, sitting, and prone jackknife positions all applicable. The lateral decubitus position is applicable for both lumbar and thoracic epidural techniques, and the sitting position allows the administration of lumbar, thoracic, and cervical epidural anesthetics. The prone jackknife position allows access to the caudal epidural space.

Needle Puncture: Lumbar Epidural. A technique similar to that used for spinal anesthesia should be carried out to identify the midline structures; and the bony landmarks should be used to determine the vertebral level appropriate for needle insertion (Fig. 41.4). When choosing a needle for epidural anesthesia, one must decide whether a continuous or single-shot technique is desired. This is the principal determinant of needle selection. If a single-shot epidural technique is chosen, a Crawford needle is appropriate; if a continuous catheter technique is indicated, a Tuohy or other needle with a lateral-facing opening is chosen.

The midline approach is most often indicated for a lumbar epidural procedure. The needle is inserted into the midline in the same way as for spinal anesthesia. In the epidural technique, the needle is slowly advanced until the change in tissue resistance is noted as the needle abuts the ligamentum flavum. At this point, a 3- to 5-mL glass syringe is filled with 2 mL of saline solution, and a small (0.25 mL) air bubble is added. The syringe is attached to the needle, and if the needle tip is in the substance of the ligamentum

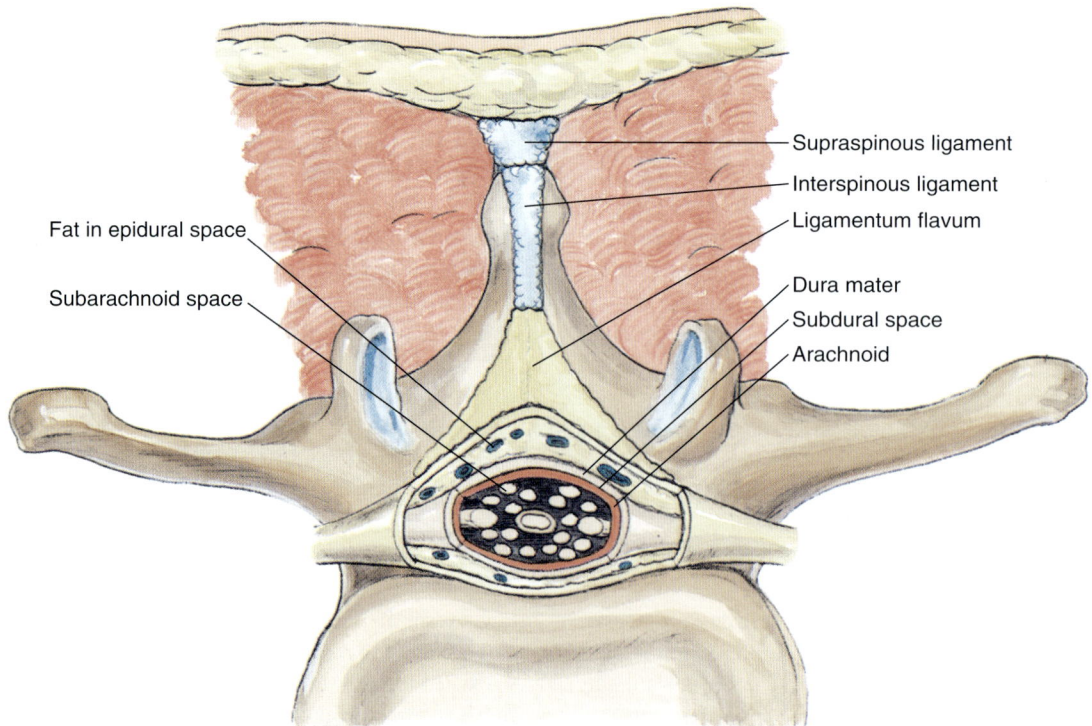

Fig. 41.1 Epidural block: cross-sectional anatomy.

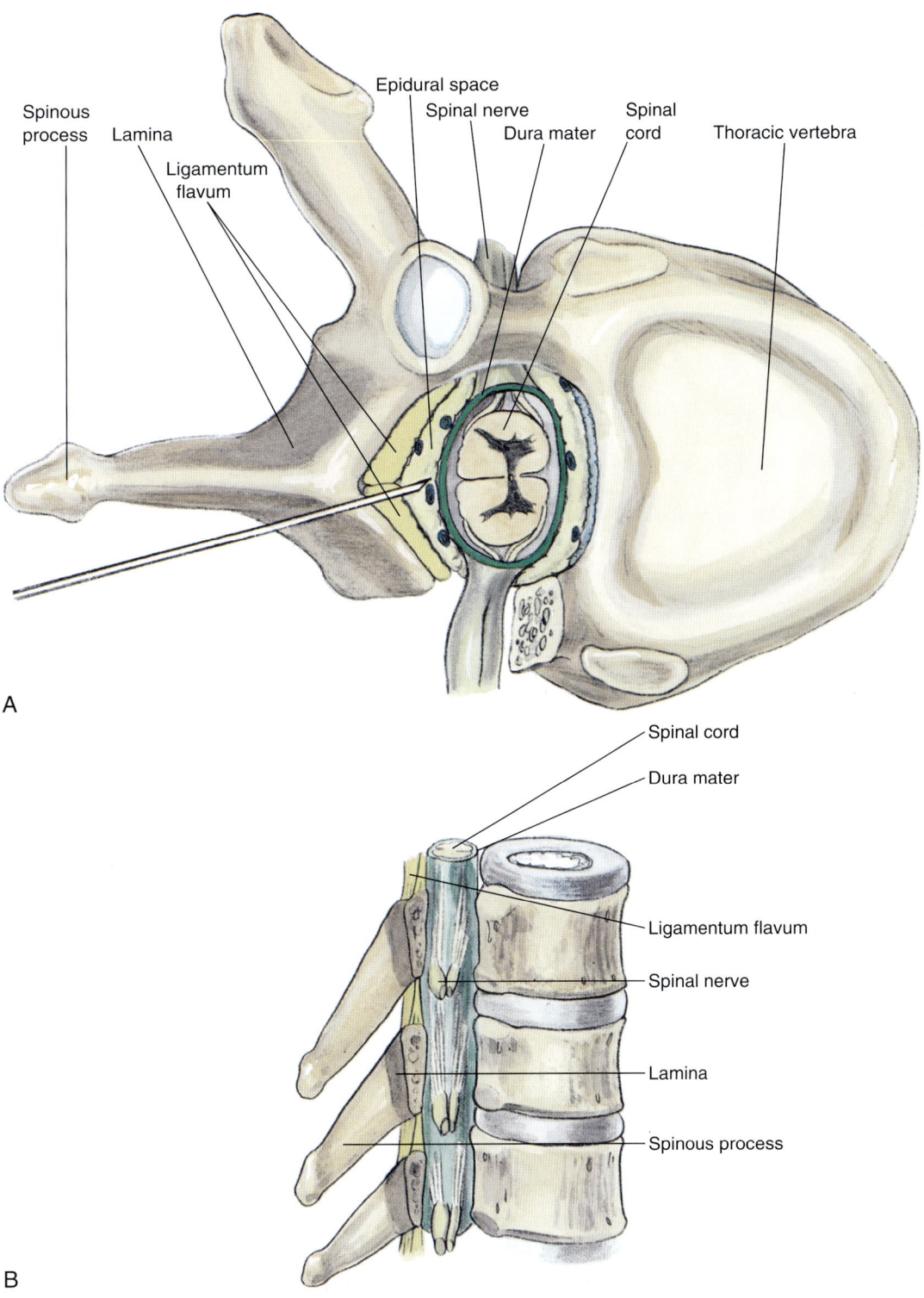

Fig. 41.2 Thoracic epidural block anatomy: overlapping of midthoracic spinous processes requires a paramedian technique. (A) Cross section, superior view. (B) Lateral view, paramedian section.

flavum, the air bubble will be compressible (Fig. 41.5A). If the ligamentum flavum has not yet been reached, pressure on the syringe plunger will not compress the air bubble (Fig. 41.5B). Once compression of the air bubble has been achieved, the needle is grasped with the nondominant hand and pulled toward the epidural space, while the dominant hand (thumb) applies constant steady pressure on the syringe plunger, thus compressing the air bubble. When the epidural space is entered, the pressure applied to the syringe plunger will allow the solution to flow without resistance into the epidural space. An alternative technique, although one that the author believes has a less precise endpoint, is the hanging-drop technique for identifying entry into the epidural space. In this technique, when the needle is placed in the ligamentum flavum, a drop of solution is introduced into the hub of the needle (Fig. 41.6A). No syringe is attached, and when the needle is advanced into the epidural space, the solution should be "sucked into" the space (Fig. 41.6B).

No matter what method is chosen for needle insertion, when the epidural space is cannulated with a catheter, success may be increased by advancing the needle 1–2 mm farther once the space has been identified. In addition, the incidence of unintentional intravenous cannulation

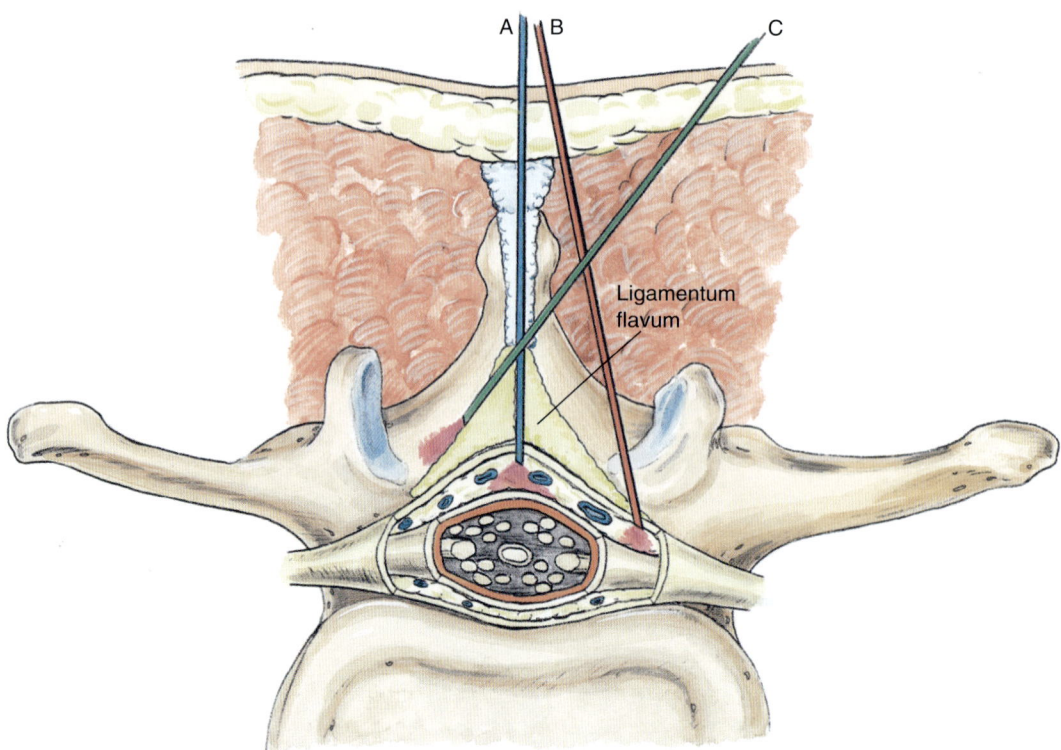

Fig. 41.3 Epidural block: functional anatomy of ligamentum flavum. This figure shows how important it is to maintain the midline position of the epidural needle (*needle A*) during lumbar epidural techniques. If an oblique approach is taken, a "false release" can be produced (*needle C*) or the perception of a thin ligament can be reinforced (*needle B*).

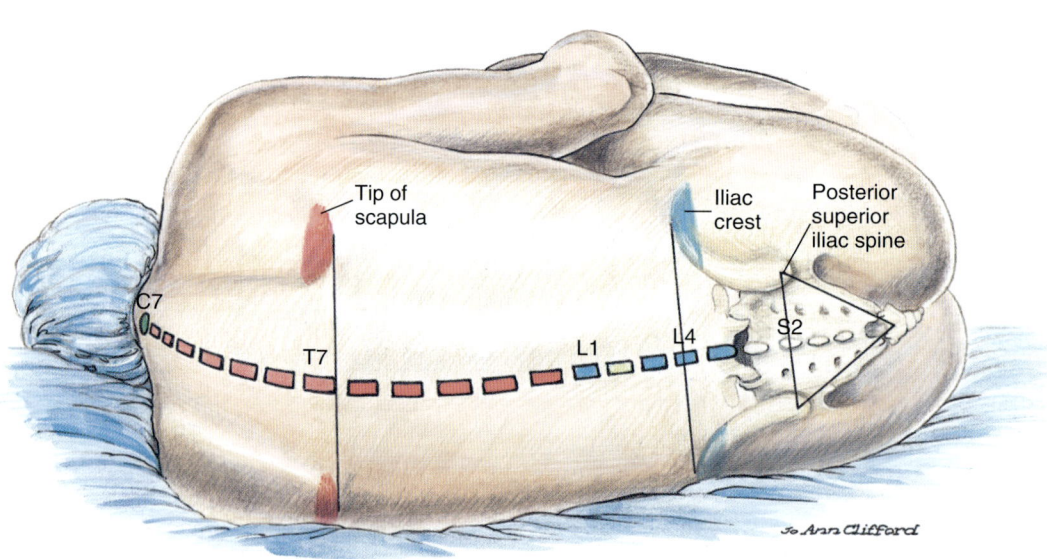

Fig. 41.4 Neuraxial anatomy: surface relationships.

with an epidural catheter may be decreased by injecting 5 to 10 mL of solution before threading the catheter. If a catheter is inserted, it should be inserted only 2–3 cm into the epidural space because threading it farther may increase the likelihood of catheter malposition. Obstetric patients require catheters to be inserted 3–5 cm into the epidural space to minimize dislodgement during labor analgesia.

Needle Puncture: Thoracic Epidural. As with lumbar epidural anesthesia, patients are usually placed into a lateral decubitus position for needle insertion into the thoracic epidural space (Fig. 41.7). In this technique, the paramedian approach is preferred because it allows easier access to the epidural space. This is because the spinous processes in the midthoracic region overlap each other from cephalad to caudad (Fig. 41.8). The paramedian approach is carried out in a manner similar to that used for the lumbar epidural space, although in almost every instance the initial needle insertion will result in contact with the thoracic vertebral lamina by the epidural needle (Fig. 41.9). When this occurs, the needle is withdrawn slightly and the tip redirected cephalad in small incremental steps until the needle is firmly seated in the ligamentum flavum. At this point, the loss-of-resistance technique and insertion of the catheter are carried

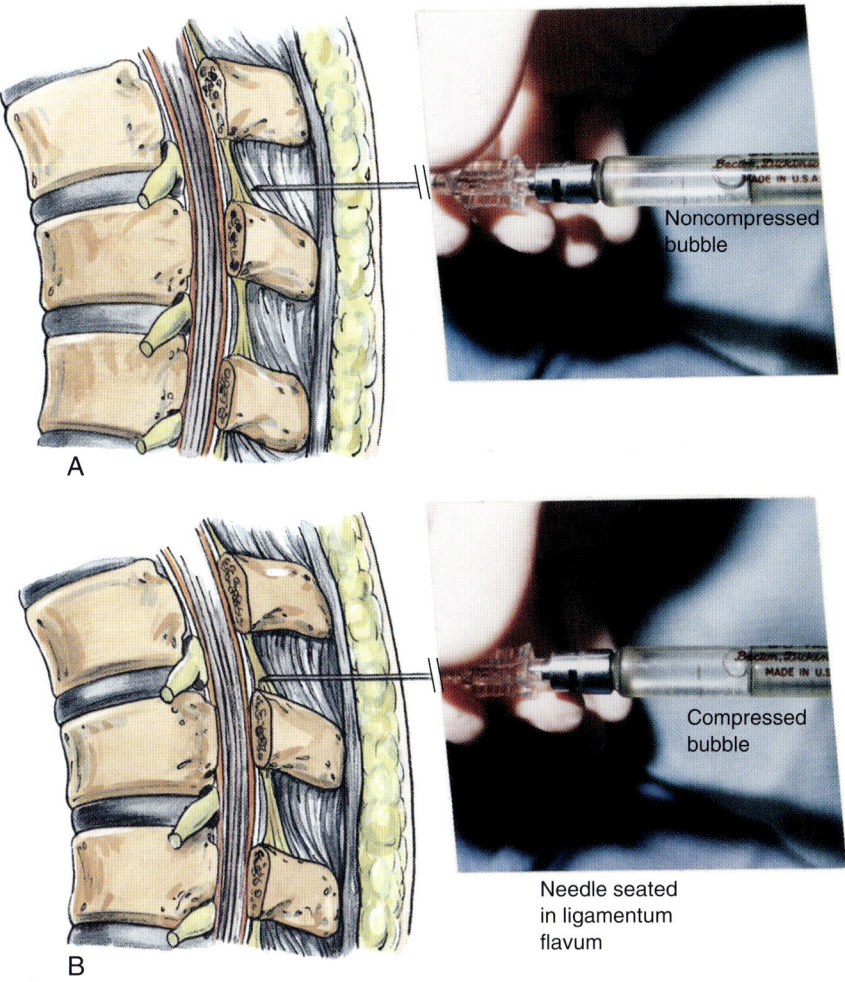

Fig. 41.5 Epidural block: loss-of-resistance technique showing (A) noncompression and (B) bubble compression.

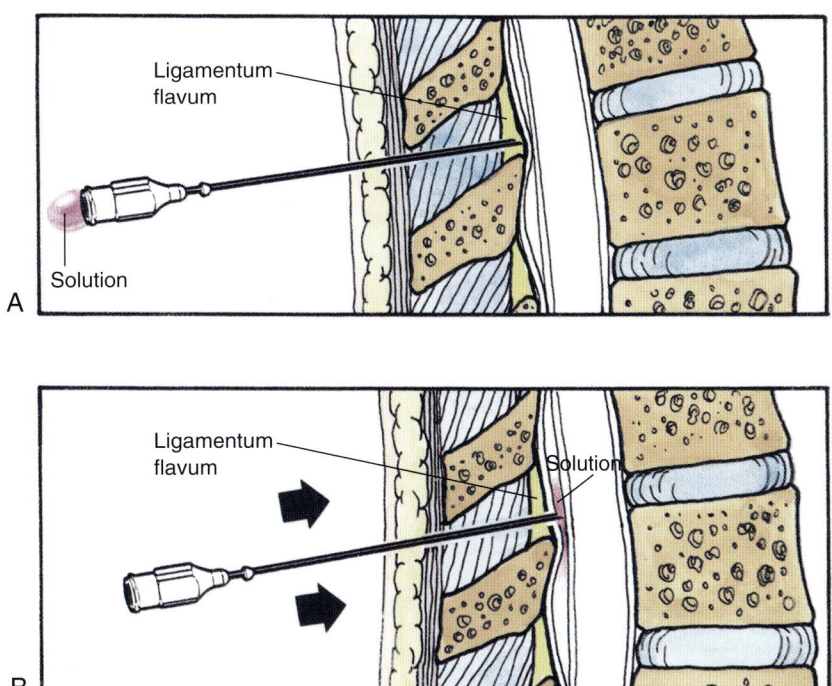

Fig. 41.6 Epidural block: hanging-drop technique. (A) A drop of solution is introduced into the hub of the needle, and when advanced into the epidural space, (B) the solution should be "sucked into" the space.

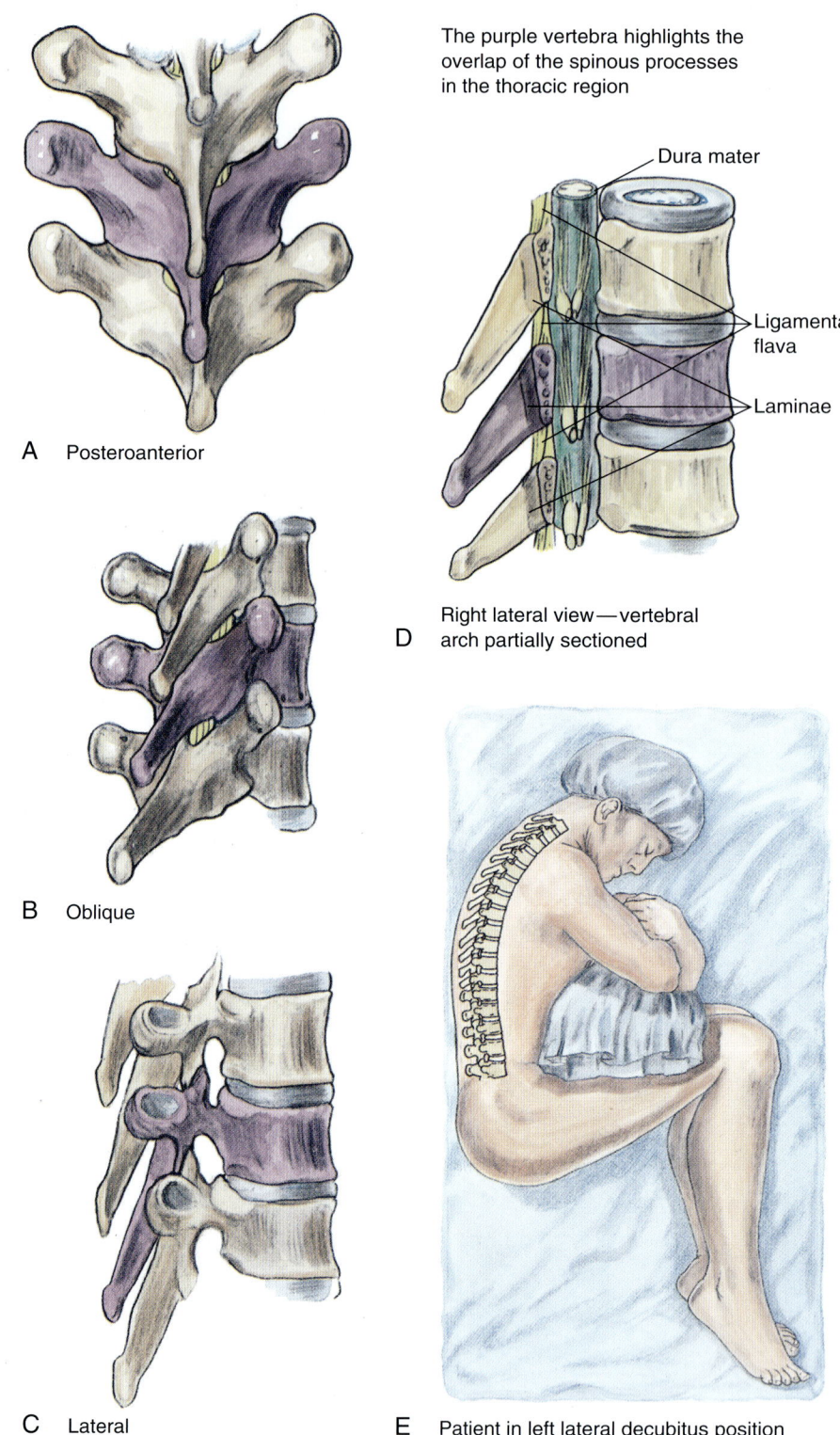

Fig. 41.7 Thoracic epidural block anatomy: midthoracic spine. (A) Posteroanterior view. (B) Oblique view. (C) Lateral view. (D) Lateral view after removal of right vertebral arch. (E) Patient in left lateral decubitus position for thoracic epidural anesthesia.

out in a manner identical to that used for lumbar epidural block. Again, the hanging-drop technique is an alternative method of identifying the thoracic epidural space, although the classic Bromage needle–syringe grip is the author's first choice for the thoracic epidural block (Fig. 41.10).

Needle Puncture: Cervical Epidural. In the cervical epidural technique, the patient is typically in a sitting position with the head bent forward and supported on a table (Fig. 41.11). A comparison of the cervical epidural block with the lumbar epidural block reveals many similarities. The spinous processes of the cervical vertebrae are nearly perpendicular to the long axis of the vertebral column; thus a midline technique is applicable for the cervical epidural block. The most prominent vertebral spinous processes, those of C7 and T1, are identified with the neck flexed (Fig. 41.12). The second (index) and third fingers of the palpating hand straddle the space between C7 and T1, and the epidural needle is slowly inserted in a plane approximately parallel to the floor (or

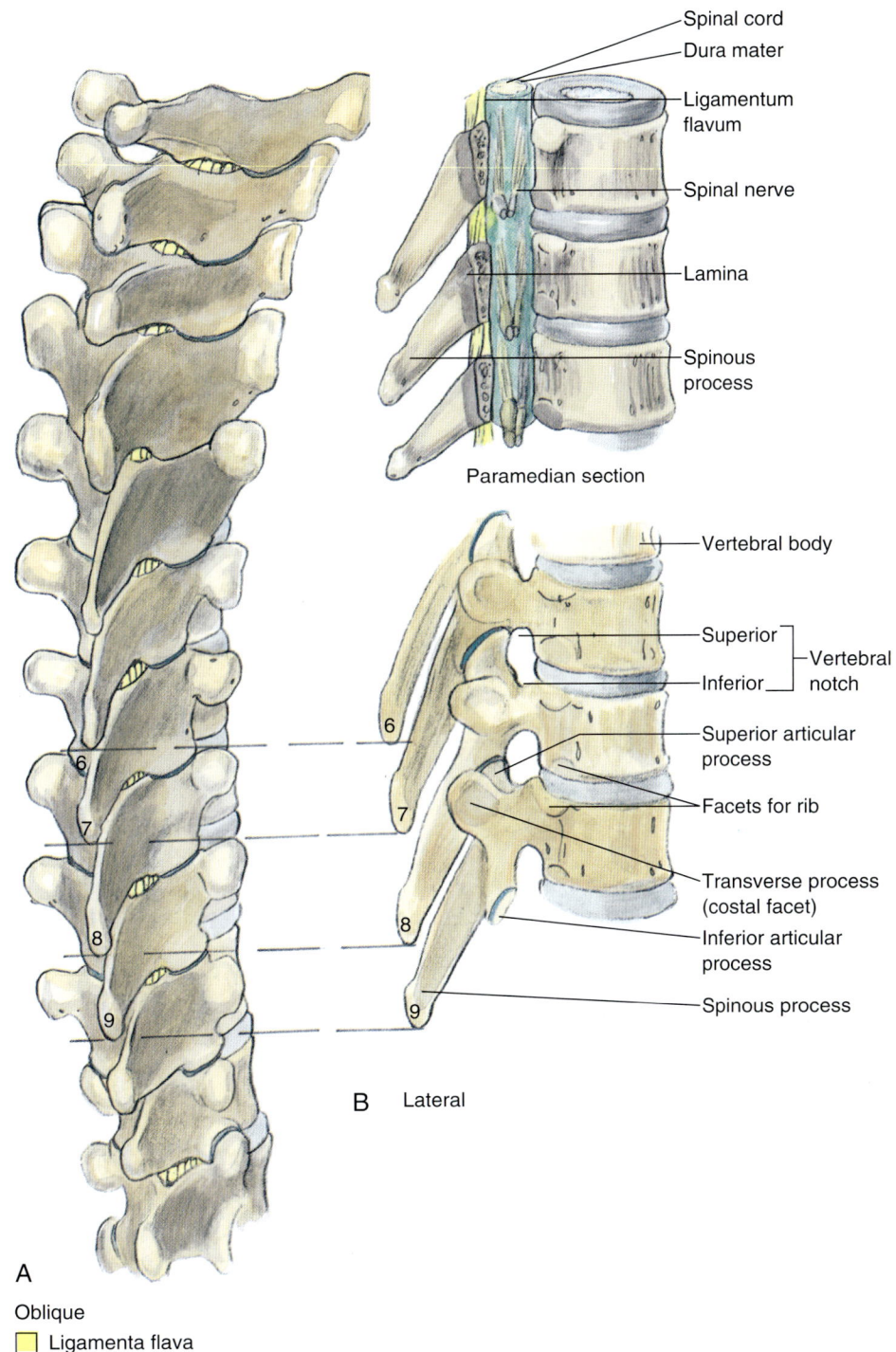

Fig. 41.8 Thoracic vertebral anatomy: degree of spinous process overlap changes from high thoracic to midthoracic to low thoracic. **(A)** Oblique view. **(B)** Lateral view and paramedian section.

parallel to the long axis of the cervical vertebral spinous processes). Abutment of the needle onto the ligamentum flavum will be appreciated at a depth similar to that seen in the lumbar epidural block (i.e., 3.5–5.5 cm), and needle placement is then performed using the loss-of-resistance technique as in the other epidural methods. The hanging-drop method is also an option for identification of the cervical epidural space.

POTENTIAL PROBLEMS

One of the most feared complications of epidural anesthesia is systemic toxicity resulting from intravenous injection of the intended epidural anesthetic (Fig. 41.13). This can occur with either catheter or needle injection. One way to minimize intravenous injection of the pharmacologic doses of local anesthetic needed for epidural anesthesia is to verify needle or catheter placement by administering a test dose before the definitive epidural anesthetic injection. The current recommendation for the test dose is 3 mL of local anesthetic solution containing 1:200,000 epinephrine (15 μg of epinephrine). Even if the test dose is negative, the anesthesiologist should inject the epidural solution incrementally, be vigilant for unintentional intravascular injection, and have all necessary equipment and drugs available to treat local anesthetic-induced systemic toxicity.

Another problem that can occur with epidural anesthesia is the unintentional administration of an epidural

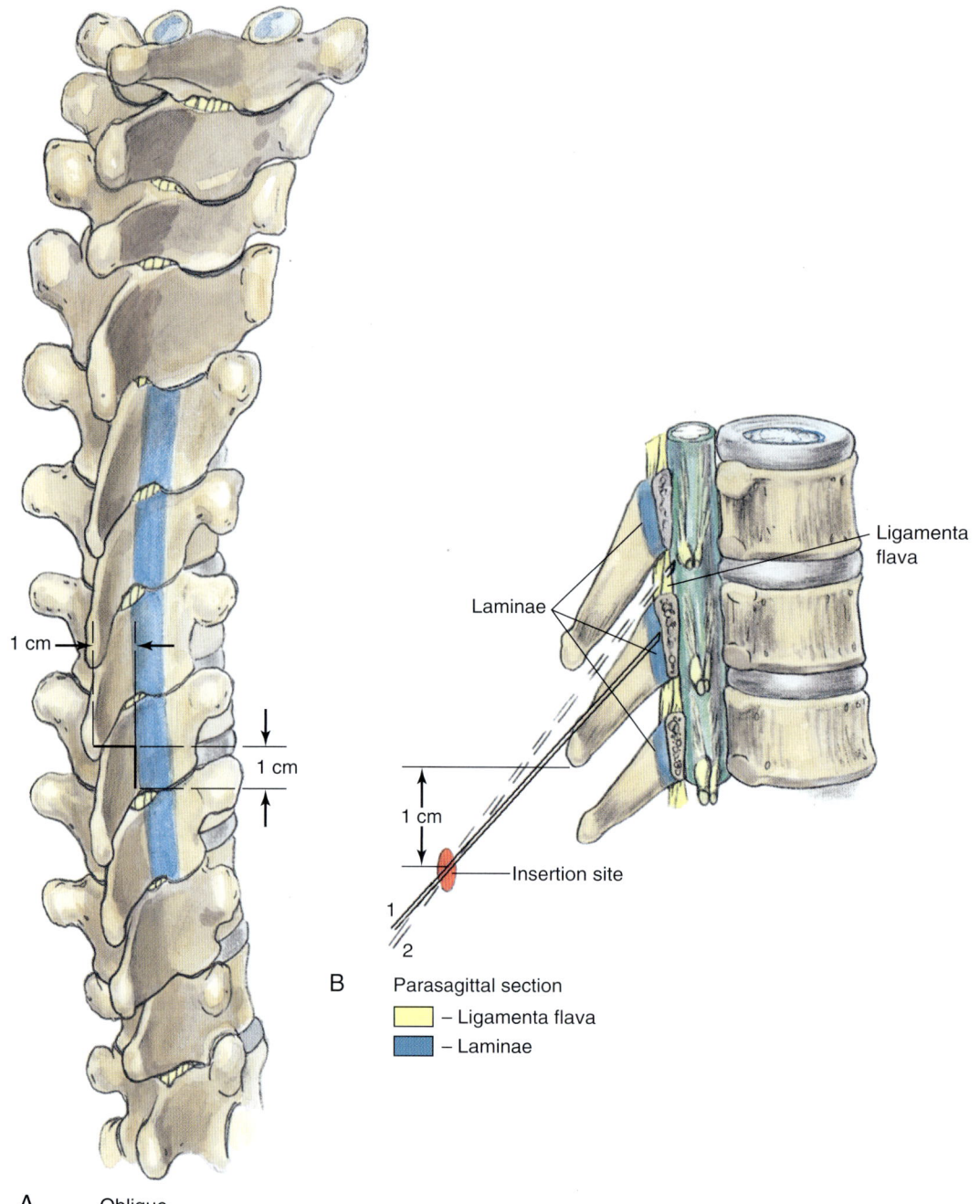

Fig. 41.9 Thoracic epidural block technique. (A) Using the paramedian approach, needle insertion site is 1 cm caudad and 1 cm lateral to the tip of the more cephalad spinous process, similar to the needle insertion used in the lumbar paramedian technique. (B) Parasagittal view of needle insertion and initial contact with lamina *(blue shading)*.

dose into the spinal fluid. In this event, as when any neuraxial block reaches high sensory levels, blood pressure and heart rate should be supported pharmacologically and ventilation should be assisted as indicated. Usually atropine and ephedrine will suffice to manage this situation, or at least will provide time to administer more potent catecholamines. If the entire dose (20–25 mL) of local anesthetic is administered into the cerebrospinal fluid, tracheal intubation and mechanical ventilation are indicated because it will be approximately 1–2 hours before the patient can consistently maintain adequate spontaneous ventilation. When epidural anesthesia is performed and a higher-than-expected block develops after a delay of only 15–30 minutes, subdural placement of the local anesthetic must be considered. Treatment is symptomatic, with the most difficult part involving recognition that a subdural injection is possible.

As with spinal anesthesia, if neurologic injury occurs after epidural anesthesia, a systematic approach to the problem is necessary. No particular local anesthetic, use of needle versus catheter technique, addition or omission of epinephrine, or location of epidural puncture seems to be associated with an increased incidence of neurologic injury. Despite this observation, the performance of cervical or thoracic epidural techniques demands special care with hand and needle control because the spinal cord is immediately deep to the site of both these epidural blocks.

An additional problem with epidural anesthesia is the fear of creating an epidural hematoma with the needles or catheters. This probably happens less frequently than

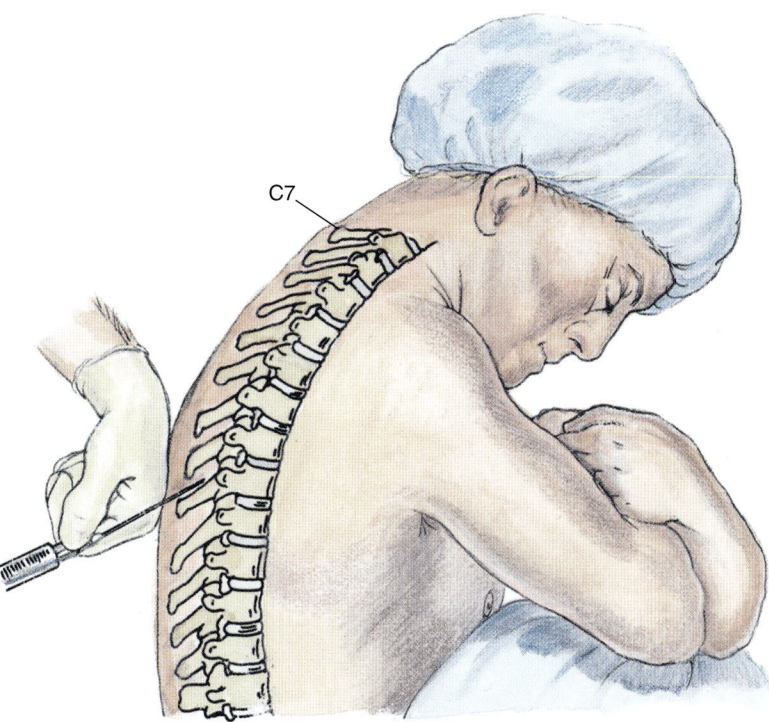

Fig. 41.10 Thoracic epidural block technique: Bromage grip for loss-of-resistance technique in thoracic block.

severe neurologic injury after general anesthesia. Concern about epidural hematoma formation is greater in patients who have been taking antiplatelet drugs such as aspirin or who have been receiving preoperative anticoagulants. The magnitude of an acceptable level of preoperative anticoagulation and the risk–benefit calculation of performing epidural anesthesia in the anticoagulated patient remain indeterminate at this time. The use of epidural techniques in patients receiving subcutaneous heparin therapy is probably acceptable if the block can be performed atraumatically, although the risk–benefit ratio of the technique must be weighed for each patient. Perioperative anticoagulant regimens that demand special consideration are the use of low-molecular-weight heparin (LMWH), or potent antiplatelet drugs concurrently with epidural block. LMWH is used for prophylaxis of deep venous thrombosis and produces more profound effects than other intermittently dosed heparin products. It is currently recommended that no procedure, including withdrawal or manipulation of an epidural catheter, should occur within 12 hours after a dose of LMWH, and the next dose of LMWH should be delayed for at least 2 hours after atraumatic epidural needle or catheter insertion or manipulation. The antiplatelet drugs (e.g., ticlopidine, clopidogrel, and platelet glycoprotein IIb/IIIa receptor antagonists) are sometimes combined with aspirin and other anticoagulants. Expert guidelines need to be consulted when using regional blocks in the increasing number of patients on antiplatelet compounds.

As in spinal anesthesia, postdural puncture headache can result from epidural anesthesia when unintentional subarachnoid puncture accompanies the technique. When using the larger-diameter epidural needles (18 and 19 gauge), it can be expected that at least 50% of patients experiencing unintentional dural puncture will have a postoperative headache.

PEARLS

Avoiding catheters during epidural anesthesia—that is, by selecting an appropriate local anesthetic—can avoid a potential source of difficulty with the technique. Epidural catheters can be malpositioned in a number of ways. If a catheter is inserted too far into the epidural space, it can be routed out of the foramina, resulting in patchy epidural block. The catheter can also be inserted into the subdural or subarachnoid space or into an epidural vein. Similarly, the use of epidural catheters may be complicated by a prominent dorsomedian connective tissue band (epidural septum or fat pad), which is found in some patients.

Another means of facilitating the success of epidural anesthesia is to allow the block enough "soak time" before beginning the surgical procedure. This is most effectively accomplished if the block is carried out in an induction room separate from the operating room. There appears to be a plateau effect in the doses of epidural local anesthetics; that is, once a certain quantity of local anesthetic has been injected, more of the same agent does not significantly increase the block height, but rather may make the block denser, perhaps improving quality.

One observation about epidural anesthesia through a catheter that needs to be emphasized is the often faulty clinical logic that by giving incremental doses through a catheter, the level of sensory anesthesia can be slowly developed, thereby allowing frail and physiologically compromised patients to undergo epidural anesthesia. However, when this approach is taken, anesthesiologists usually do not allow enough time between injections because of the reality of time pressures in the normal operating room. They inject small doses through the catheter, but then do not allow sufficient time to pass before performing the next incremental injection. Often

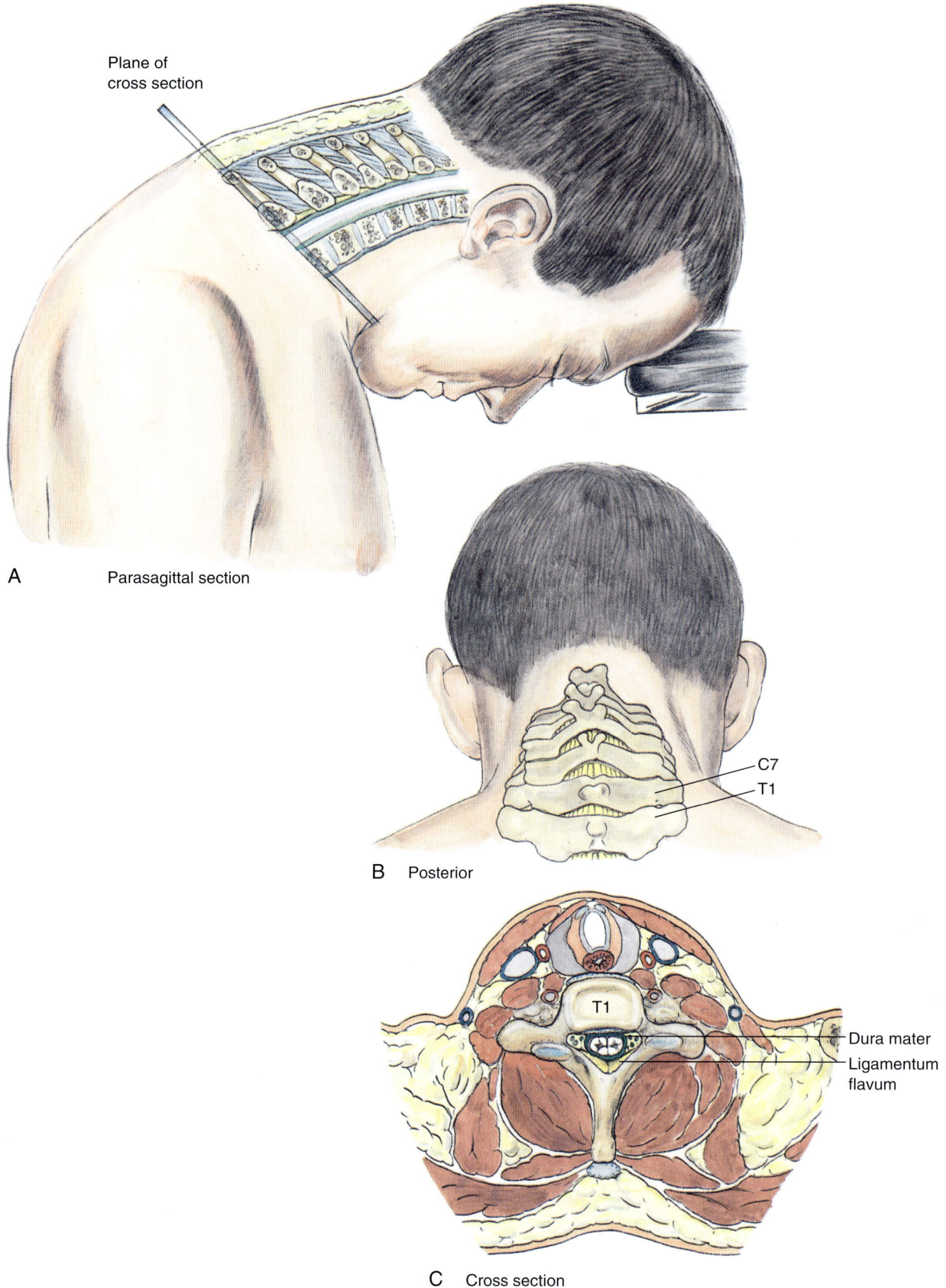

Fig. 41.11 Cervical epidural anatomy. **(A)** Patient sitting with head supported by table, and plane of vertebral cross section. **(B)** Posterior view. **(C)** Vertebral cross section at C7 to T1.

the clinical result is high block levels in just those patients in whom lower levels were the goal. Furthermore, this approach to epidural anesthesia unnecessarily delays preparing the patient for the operation and makes surgical and nursing colleagues less accepting of the technique.

Epidural catheters are indicated in many situations, especially when the technique is used for postoperative analgesia. To place a known length of catheter into the epidural space, either both the catheter and needle must have distance markers, or a way must be found to maintain the catheter position once the needle has been

Epidural Block 271

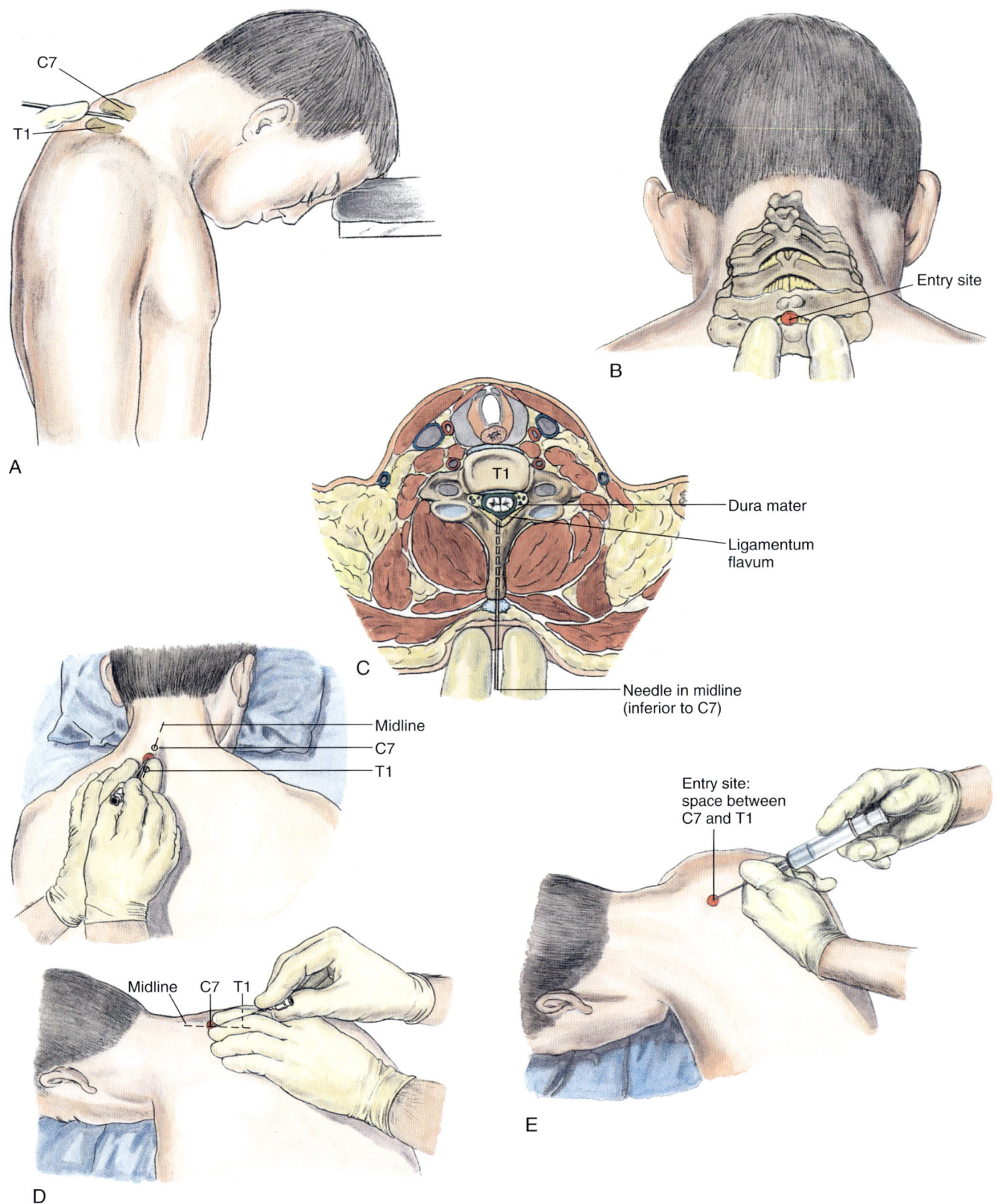

Fig. 41.12 Cervical epidural technique. **(A)** Patient sitting with head supported by table with needle oriented parallel to floor. **(B)** Application of fingers to posterior neck to facilitate cervical epidural block. **(C)** Insertion of needle into ligamentum flavum. **(D)** Insertion of needle during palpation. **(E)** Bromage grip during needle advancement.

withdrawn over the catheter. Because some epidural needles do not have distance markers, a method of maintaining catheter position while the needle is withdrawn over the catheter is required. One technique of positioning the catheter is illustrated in Fig. 41.14. An object of known length, such as a syringe or the anesthesiologist's finger is selected, and that object is placed next to the needle–catheter assembly after the catheter has been inserted 3 cm (or other known distance) into the epidural space. Because the catheter is marked, a known point on the catheter can be related to a known point on either the finger or the syringe. As shown in Fig. 41.14A, the 15-cm mark is opposite the plunger on the syringe or the anesthesiologist's knuckle. Once this relationship has

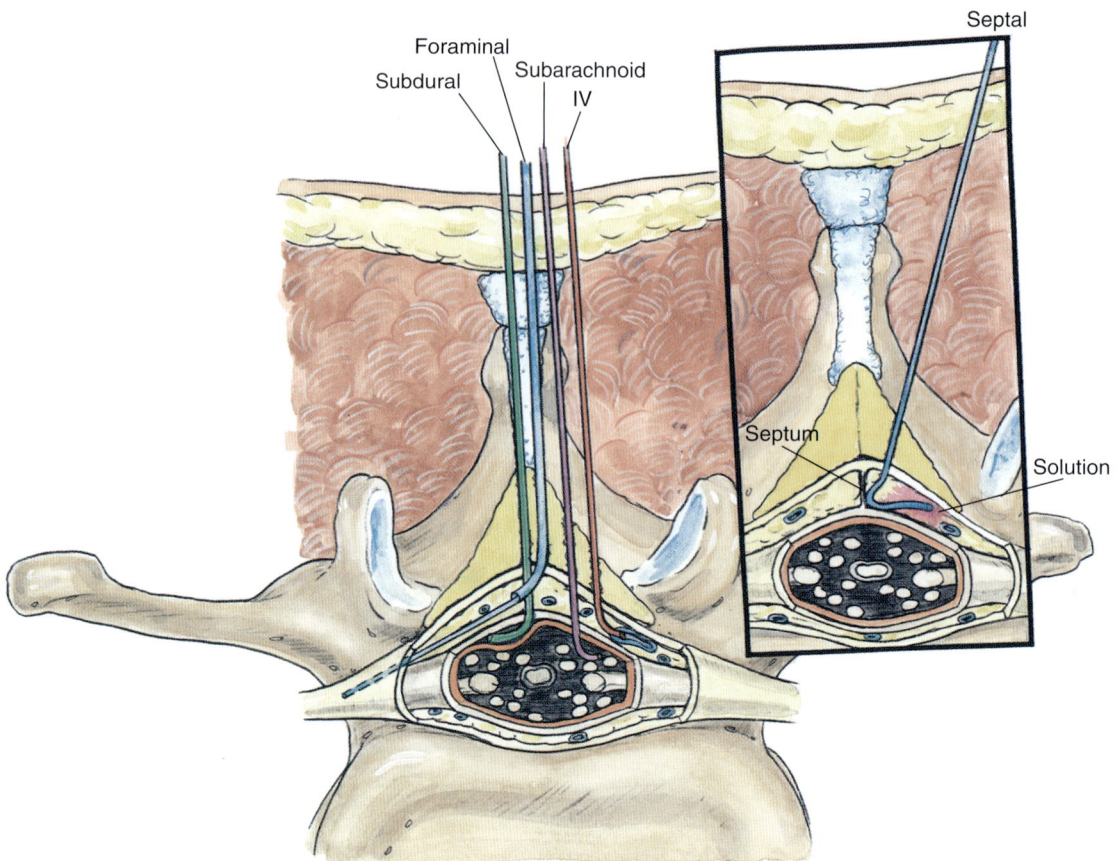

Fig. 41.13 Epidural block: cross-sectional anatomy, showing potential incorrect injection sites. *IV,* intravenous.

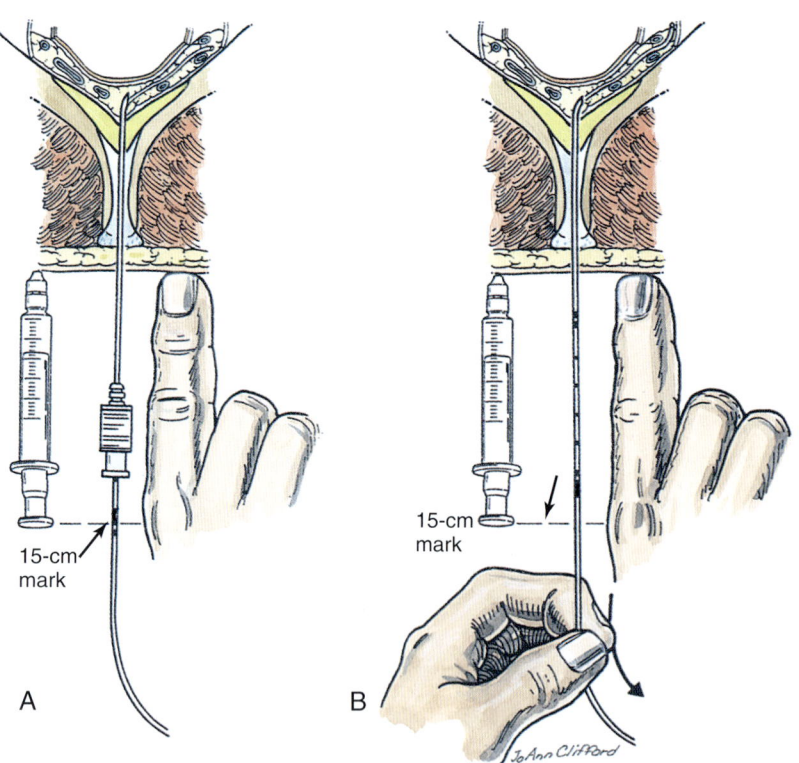

Fig. 41.14 Epidural block: catheter measurement technique. **(A)** The 15-cm mark is opposite the plunger on the syringe or the anesthesiologist's knuckle. **(B)** The measurement object is then placed next to the catheter.

been noted, the needle is removed while the catheter position is maintained. The measurement object is then placed next to the catheter, as illustrated in Fig. 41.14B, and the catheter is withdrawn to the point at which the distance marker on the catheter relates to the previously identified point. In this example, the 15-cm mark on the catheter is placed opposite the plunger of the syringe or the anesthesiologist's knuckle. By using this technique, the epidural catheter can be accurately placed without the need for either a marked needle or a ruler.

Caudal Block 42

David L. Brown

Key Points

- In approximately 5% of adult patients, the sacral hiatus is nearly impossible to cannulate with needle or catheter.
- The tissue mass overlying the sacrum in some patients makes the technique difficult.
- The sacral hiatus lies at the tip of equilateral triangle that joins the poster superior iliac spines bilaterally.
- Caudal block can be performed in a lateral decubitus or a prone position.
- Volumes of local anesthetic in the 25- to 35-mL range can be injected in adult patients to reach a sensory level of T12 to T10 with caudal block.

PERSPECTIVE

With advances in lumbar epidural anesthesia, caudal anesthesia has become an infrequently used and taught technique. Nevertheless, caudal anesthesia can be effectively used for anorectal and perineal procedures, as well as some lower extremity operations.

Patient Selection. Patient selection for caudal anesthesia should be determined by examining the anatomy of the sacral hiatus. In approximately 5% of adult patients, the sacral hiatus is nearly impossible to cannulate with needle or catheter; thus in 1 of 20 patients the technique is clinically unusable. Likewise, there are patients in whom the tissue mass overlying the sacrum makes the technique difficult, and if another technique is applicable, caudal anesthesia should be avoided. Probably more so than for any other block, experience and confidence on the anesthesiologist's part are necessary to carry out the technique effectively.

Pharmacologic Choice. When choosing local anesthetics for caudal anesthesia, the same considerations as those applied to epidural anesthesia are needed. Volumes of local anesthetic in the 25- to 35-mL range are necessary to predictably provide a sensory level of T12 to T10 with caudal injection for adults.

PLACEMENT

Anatomy. Anatomy pertinent to caudal anesthesia centers on the sacral hiatus (Fig. 42.1). This can be most effectively localized by finding the posterosuperior iliac spines bilaterally, drawing a line to join them, and then completing an equilateral triangle caudad. The tip of the equilateral triangle will overlie the sacral hiatus (Fig. 42.2). The caudal tip of the triangle will rest near the sacral cornua, which are unfused remnants of the spinous processes of the fifth sacral vertebra. Overlying the sacral hiatus is a fibroelastic membrane, which is the functional counterpart of the ligamentum flavum. Perhaps more than with any other sex difference found in regional anesthesia, the sacrum is distinctly different in men and women. In men, the cavity of the sacrum has a smooth curve from S1 to S5. Conversely, in women, the sacrum is quite flat from S1 to S3, with a more pronounced curve in the S4 to S5 region (Fig. 42.3).

Position. Caudal block can be carried out in a lateral decubitus position or a prone position. In adults, the author finds the prone position with a pillow placed beneath the lower abdomen most effective. In this position, patients can be sufficiently sedated to make the block comfortable, and it makes the midline more easily identifiable than in the lateral position. As illustrated in Fig. 42.4, pediatric caudal anesthesia is commonly carried out with the child in the lateral decubitus position. Because most pediatric caudal blocks are performed after induction with general anesthesia, the lateral position is almost mandatory. Identification of the midline and performance of the block are less complicated in the pediatric patient, thus making the lateral position clinically practical. To optimize identification of the sacral hiatus, the prone patient should have the legs abducted to a 20-degree angle with the toes rotated inward and the heels outward. This helps relax the gluteal muscles, making it easier to identify the sacral hiatus (Fig. 42.5).

Needle Puncture. As with lumbar epidural anesthesia, caudal anesthesia requires a decision about the use of a single-injection or a catheter technique. If a single-shot caudal block is to be performed, almost any needle of sufficient length to reach the caudal canal is acceptable. In adults, a needle of at least 22 gauge is recommended because it is large enough to allow sufficiently rapid injection of solution to help detect misplaced local anesthetic injections. If a catheter is to be used, a needle that is large enough to allow passage of the catheter is required. As illustrated in Fig. 42.6, after the sacral hiatus is identified, the index and middle fingers of the palpating hand are each placed on the sacral cornua, and the caudal needle is inserted at an angle of approximately 45 degrees to the

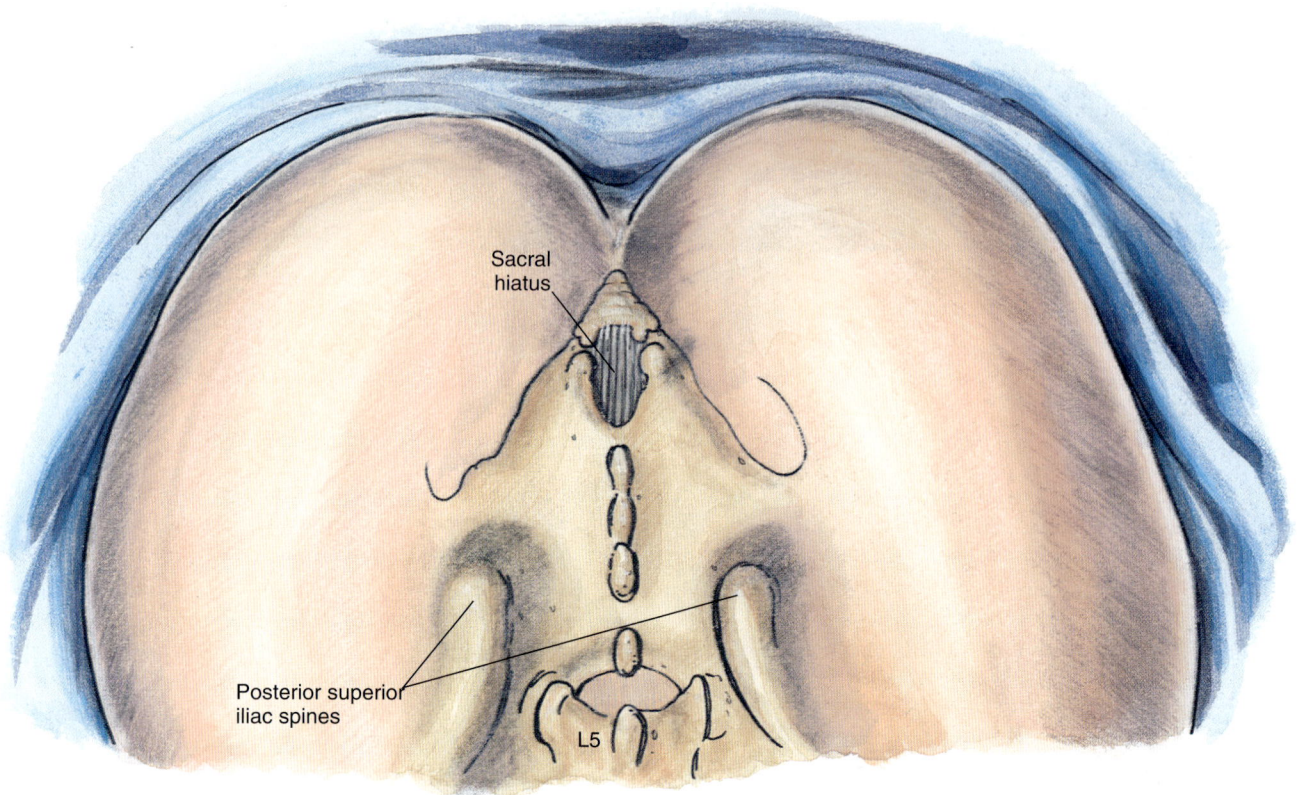

Fig. 42.1 Caudal block: surface anatomy.

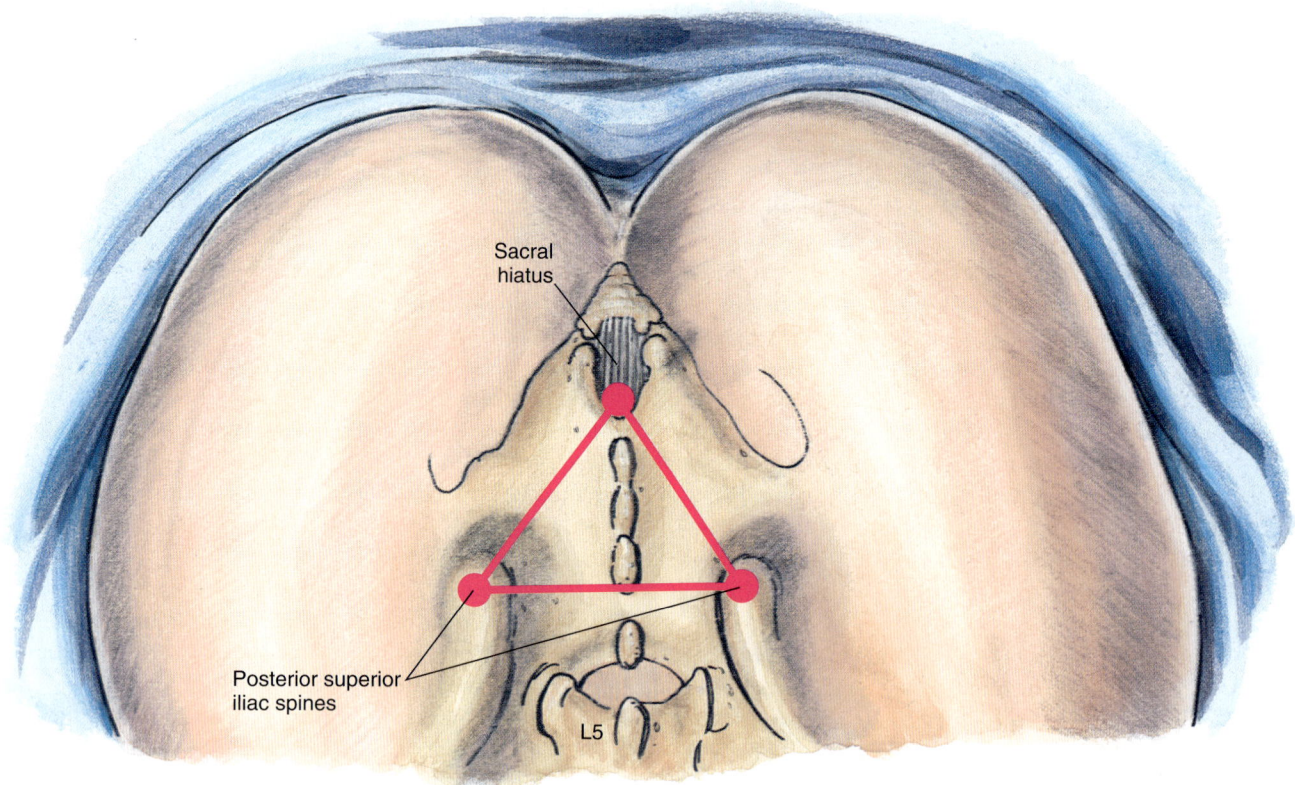

Fig. 42.2 Caudal block: surface anatomy showing sacral hiatus localization.

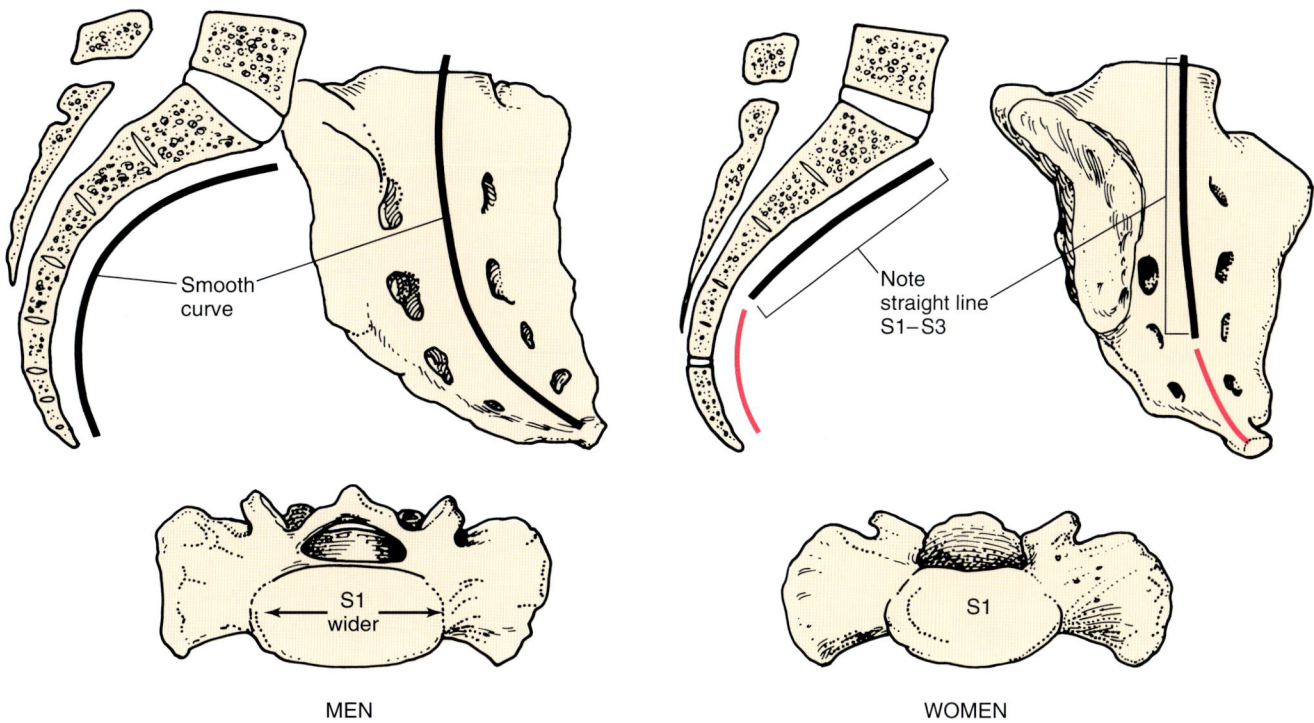

Fig. 42.3 Caudal block: relationship of sacral anatomy to sex.

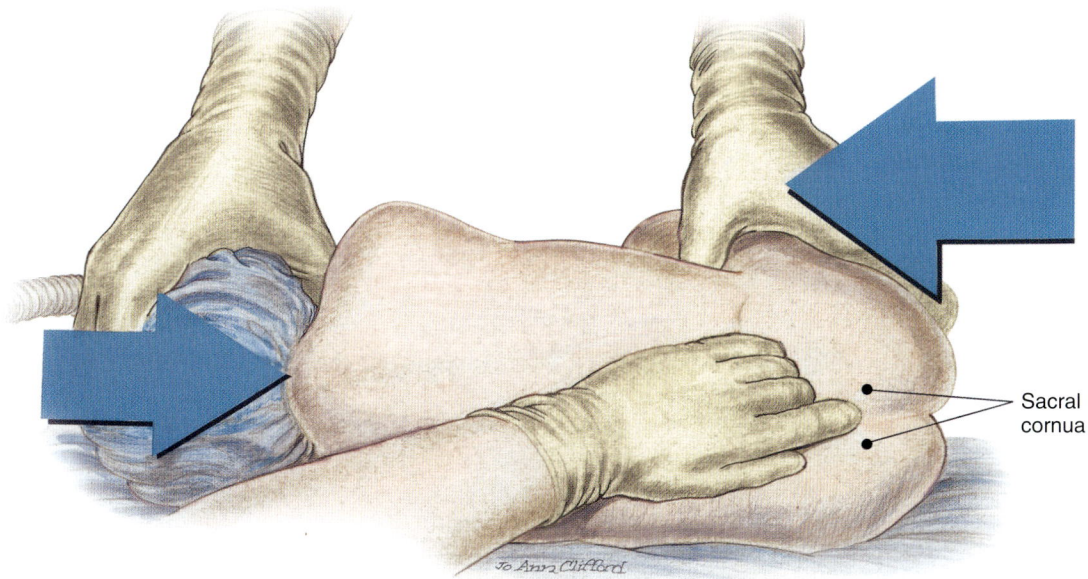

Fig. 42.4 Caudal block: pediatric position.

sacrum. As the anesthesiologist advances the needle, he or she will become aware of a decrease in resistance as the needle enters the caudal canal (*needle position 1*). The needle is then advanced until it contacts bone; this should be the dorsal aspect of the ventral plate of the sacrum. The needle is then withdrawn slightly and redirected so that the angle of insertion relative to the skin surface is decreased. In male patients, this angle will be almost parallel with the tabletop, whereas in female patients, a slightly steeper angle will be necessary (*needle position 2*).

During the redirection of the needle and after noting loss of resistance, the needle should be advanced approximately 1–1.5 cm into the caudal canal. Further advance is not advised because dural puncture and unintentional intravascular cannulation become more likely. Before the injection of the therapeutic dose of local anesthetic, aspiration should be performed and a test dose administered because a vein or the subarachnoid space can be entered unintentionally, as is the case in lumbar epidural anesthesia.

POTENTIAL PROBLEMS

Caudal anesthesia entails most of the same complications that can accompany lumbar epidural anesthesia, although there are some differences. The frequency of local anesthetic

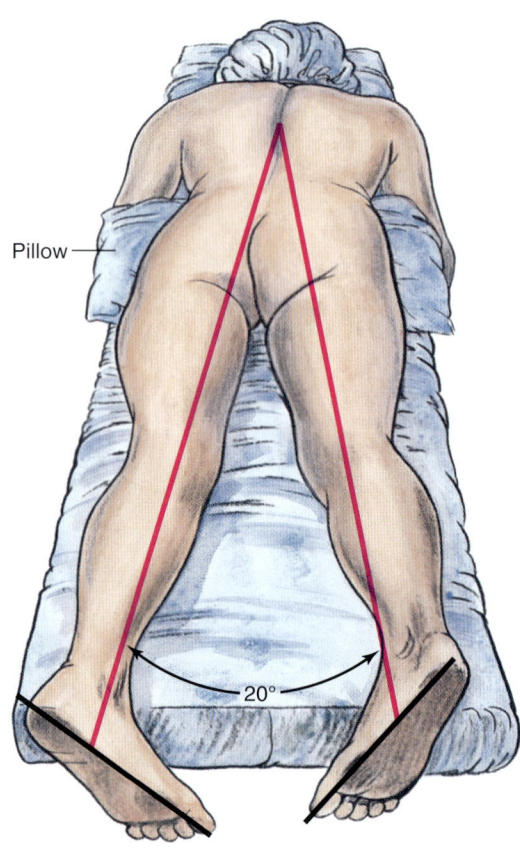

Fig. 42.5 Caudal block: prone position.

anesthesiologists are unfamiliar with the caudal technique and the needle passes anterior to the ventral plate of the sacrum, puncture of the rectum or, in obstetric anesthesia, of fetal parts is possible. As illustrated in Fig. 42.7, the area surrounding the sacral hiatus can be imagined as a potential "circle of errors." The practitioner may be faced with a slitlike hiatus that does not allow easy needle insertion; the hiatus may be located more cephalad than anticipated or, in fact, may be closed. Likewise, loss of resistance may be encountered as the needle is inserted into one of the sacral foramina rather than the hiatus. In the lateral view, it is obvious that needles may be misdirected into subcutaneous or periosteal locations as well as into the marrow of sacral bones.

PEARLS

To produce effective caudal anesthesia, anesthesiologists should be selective about the patients in whom it is attempted. It makes no sense to use the technique in a patient whose anatomy is unfavorable. Because of the anatomic variations in the area around the sacral hiatus, this block seems to require more operator experience and a longer time to attain proficiency than many other regional blocks. As a result, anesthesiologists should develop their technique in patients whose anatomy is favorable.

One helpful hint that will confirm needle location when carrying out caudal anesthesia is illustrated in Fig. 42.8. Once the needle has entered what is thought to be the caudal canal, the anesthesiologist should place a palpating hand across the sacral region dorsally. Then 5 mL of saline solution should be rapidly injected through the caudal needle. By placing the hand as shown, the anesthesiologist should be immediately aware of the subcutaneous needle position overlying the sacrum. If the needle is mispositioned subcutaneously, a bulge during injection will develop in the midline. If the needle is correctly positioned in the caudal canal, no midline bulge should be palpable. In thin individuals, accurate needle placement in the caudal canal and rapid injection of solution may allow the anesthesiologist to feel small pressure waves more laterally overlying the sacral foramina. These smaller pressure waves should not be confused with those associated with a misplaced subcutaneous needle.

toxicity after caudal anesthesia appears to be higher than it is with lumbar epidural block. Another distinct difference is that the incidence of subarachnoid puncture is exceedingly low with the caudal technique. The dural sac ends at approximately the level of S2; thus unless a needle is inserted deeply within the caudal canal, subarachnoid puncture is unlikely. In children, the dural sac is more distally placed in the caudal canal, and this should be considered when carrying out pediatric caudal anesthesia.

Perhaps the most frequent problem with caudal anesthesia is ineffective blockade, which results from the considerable variation in the anatomy of the sacral hiatus. If

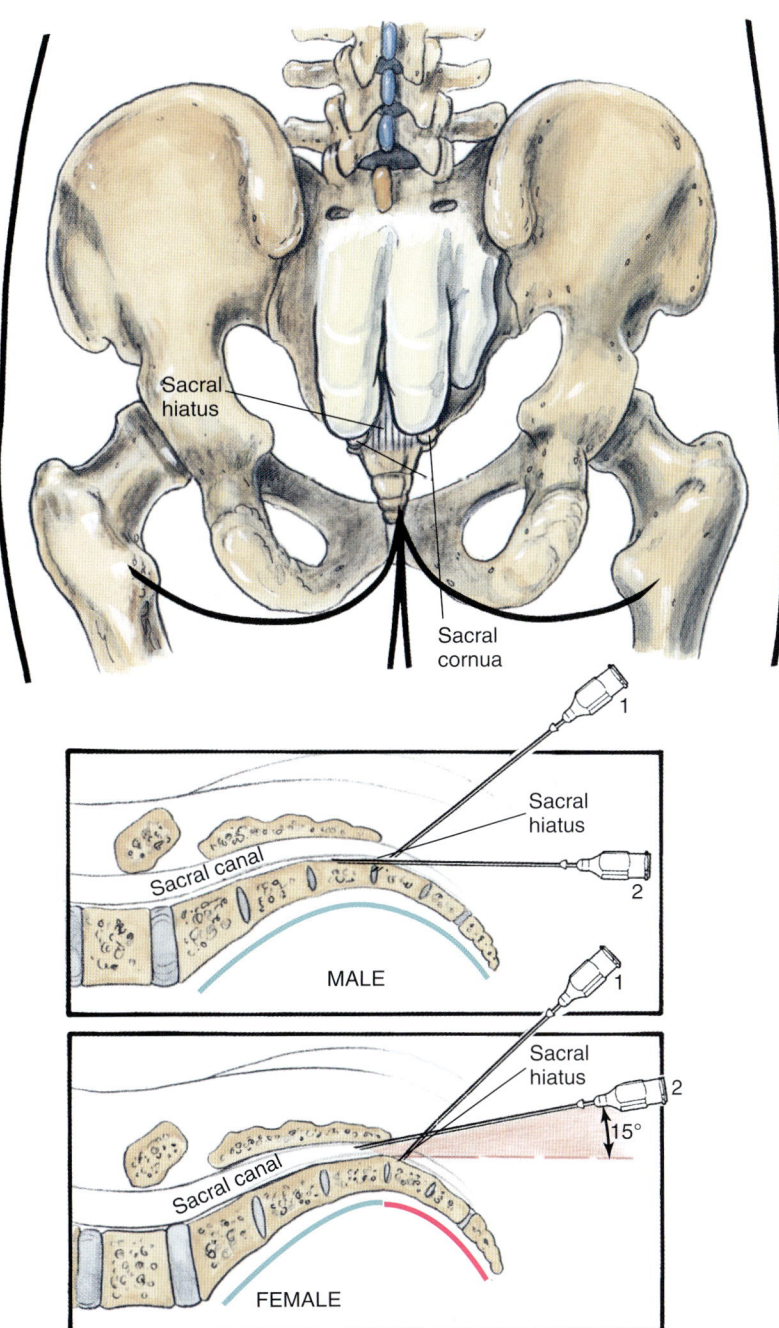

Fig. 42.6 Caudal block: technique.

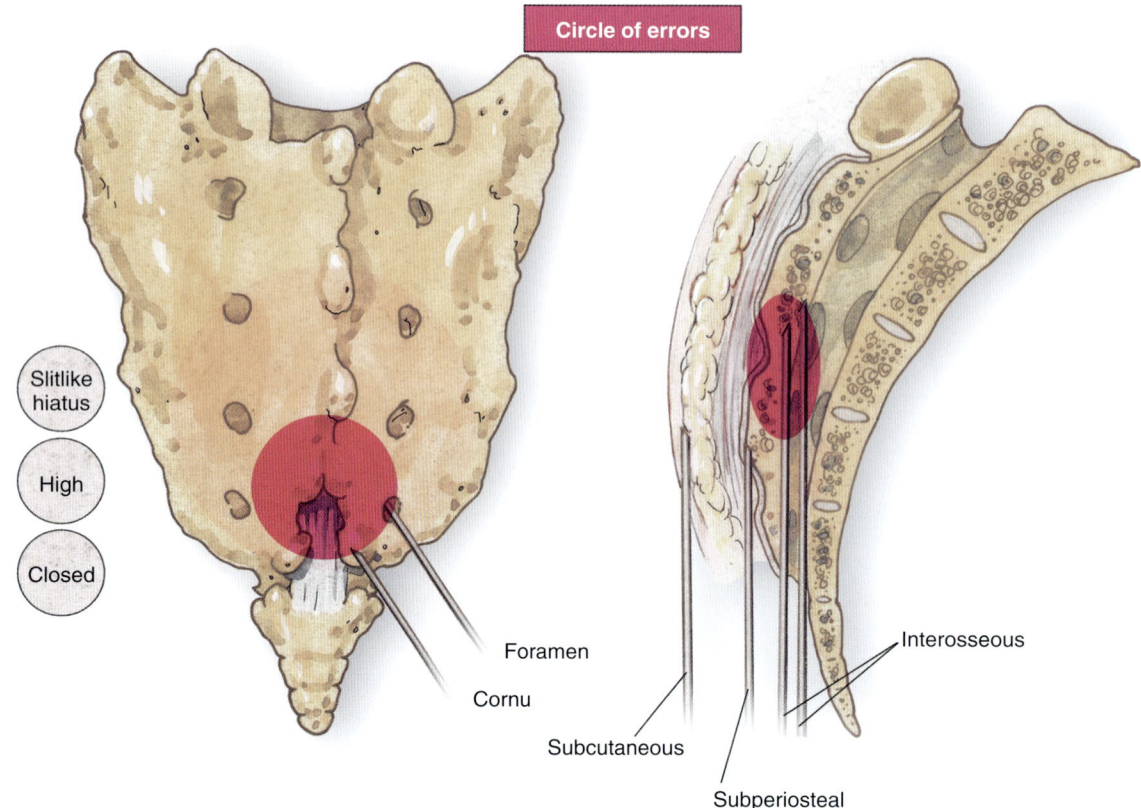

Fig. 42.7 Caudal block: circle of errors.

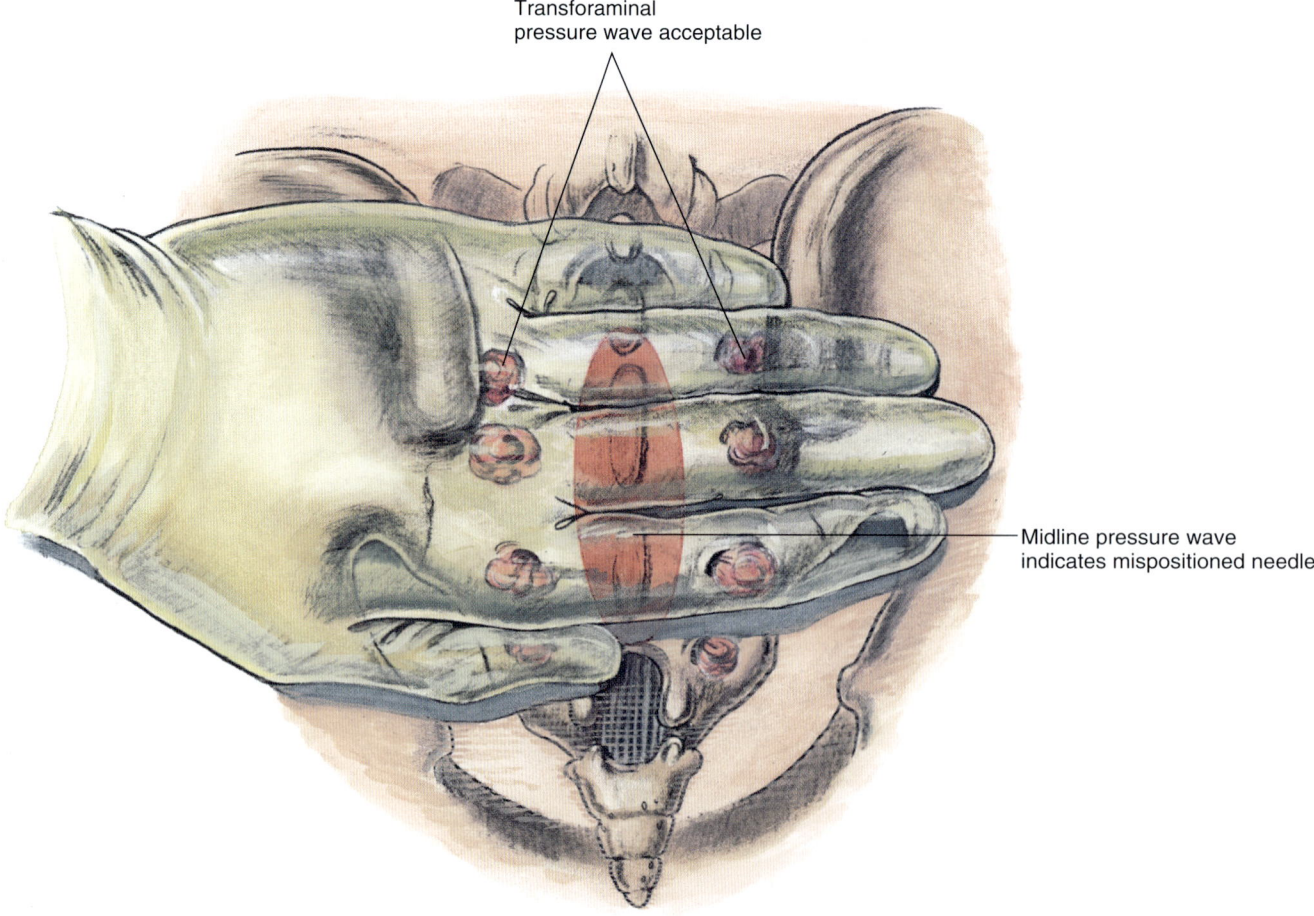

Fig. 42.8 Caudal block: palpation technique.

Section 8
Pediatric Regional Using Ultrasound

Caudal Block in Pediatrics

43

John Seif

Key Points

- Checking the anatomy with ultrasound before and during the procedure assures success. Because the sacrum is not fully ossified, it can still be penetrated by the ultrasound beams.
- Loss of resistance is not significant when placing an epidural because the sacrococcygeal ligament is softer in the pediatric population.
- The needle may be misplaced in the subcutaneous periosteal location or in the dural sac.

POSITION

After induction with general anesthesia, the lateral decubitus position is the most optimum position for full exposure of the sacral hiatus. Flex both knees to the abdomen and identify the mid line above the gluteal crease, where the sacral hiatus can be palpated.

ANATOMY

Draw a triangle with the base line between the two posterosuperior iliac spines (PSIS) and the apex at the sacral hiatus. The caudal tip will lie between the two sacral cornua of the fifth sacral vertebrae. The sacrococcygeal ligament, which resembles the ligamentum flavum, lies between the two sacral cornua (Fig. 43.1).

SONOANATOMY

This technique becomes even more complex when considering variation in patient age, weight, and varying levels of bone ossification. Ultrasound guidance for this procedure is helpful in identifying the underlying anatomic structures. The ones most commonly of interest include the sacral hiatus, sacral cornua, coccyx, and sacrococcygeal ligament. Although probe orientation can be done using either a transverse or longitudinal view of the midline, it is typically best to orient and assess landmarks before performing the procedure. Placing the probe's transverse plane at the coccyx, the sacral cornua are viewed laterally as humps. The sacral hiatus is located between an upper hyperechoic line, representing the sacrococcygeal membrane or ligament, and an inferior hyperechoic line, representing the dorsum of the pelvic surface of the sacrum (Figs. 43.2 and 43.3).

TECHNIQUE

If single-shot analgesia is required, a 22-gauge Angiocath is used, and if an epidural catheter is required, then a larger Angiocath—for example, 20- or 18-gauge—is the appropriate choice. After identifying the anatomy, palpate the sacral cornua with the index finger. Advance the needle at a 45-degree angle to the skin, distal to the index finger. A doughy sensation is felt as the needle is advanced. Then the angle of the Angiocath is dropped to 15 degrees and advanced until a loss of resistance is felt (a light "pop" in the pediatric population). Before injecting the local anesthetic, aspiration and a test dose should be performed.

PEARLS

- Check the block with normal saline first before injecting the local anesthetic, and palpate the sacrum for any subcutaneous injection.
- Patient selection and experience play a big role in the success of the block.

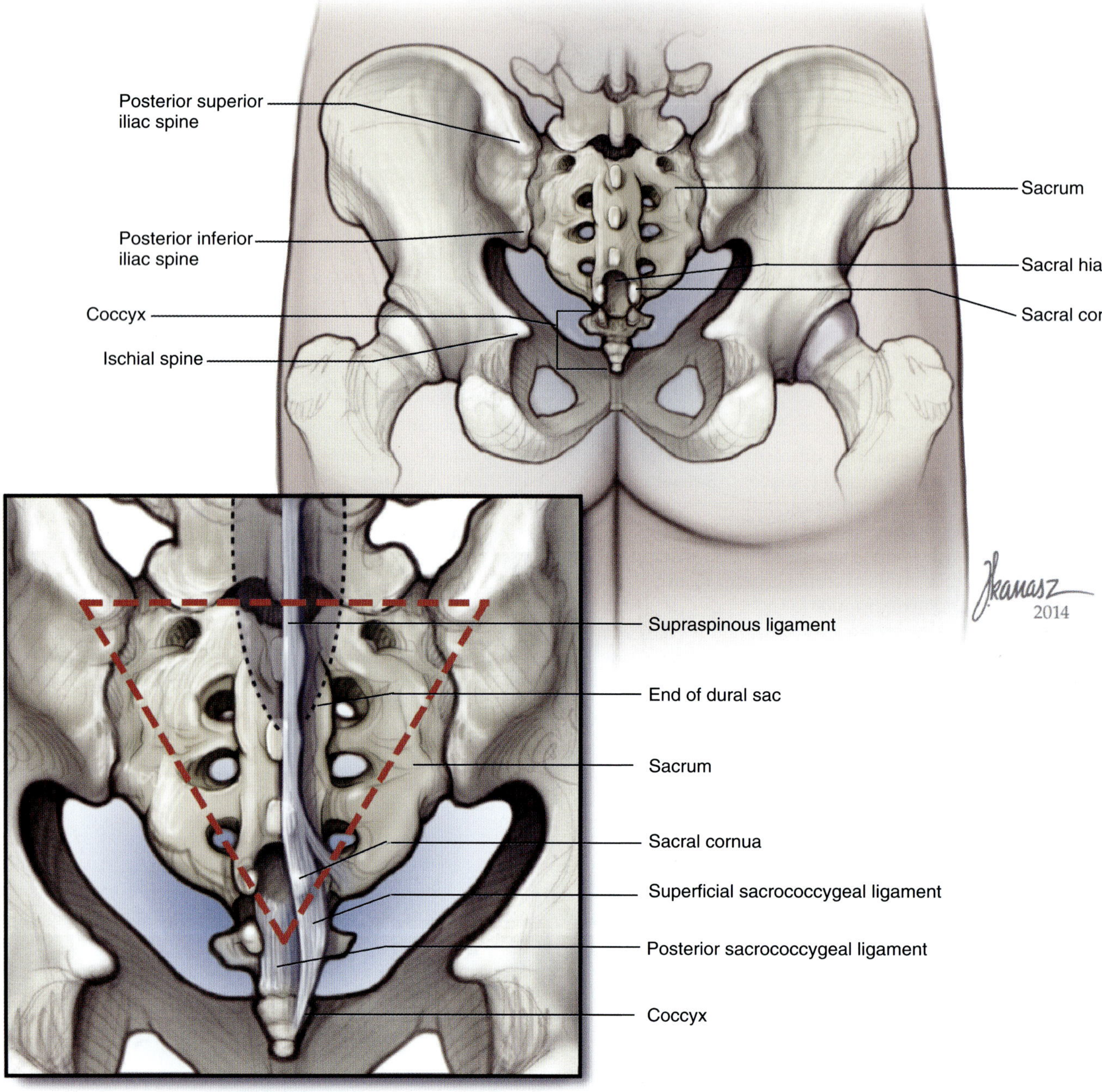

Fig. 43.1 Surface anatomy of caudal space; PSIS and sacral hiatus.

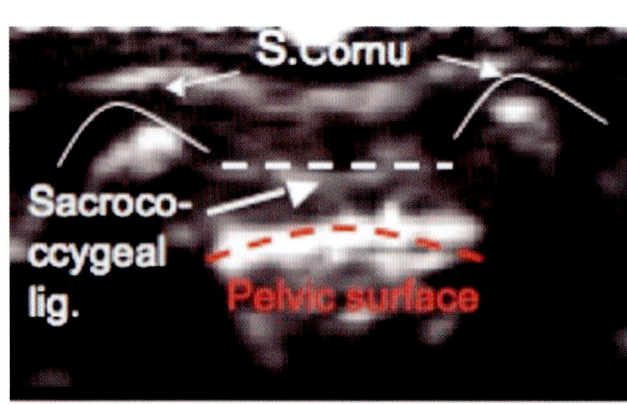

Fig. 43.2 Ultrasound still of anatomy of caudal block in pediatrics.

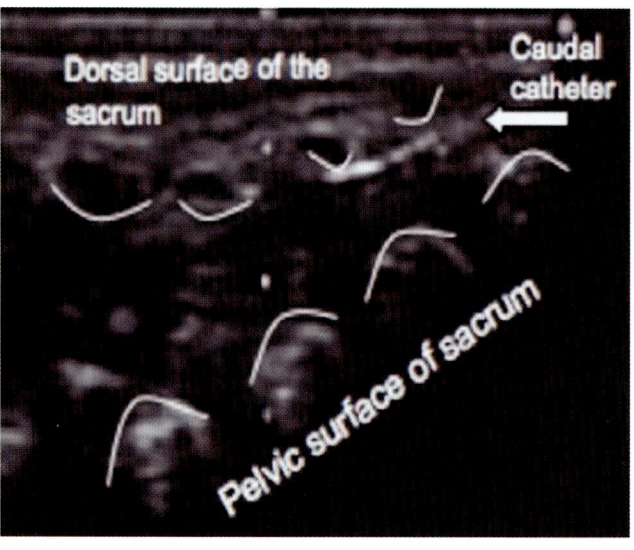

Fig. 43.3 Ultrasound still of anatomy of caudal block in pediatrics.

44 Ilioinguinal and Iliohypogastric Block

John Seif

Key Points

- Identifying the different layers of the muscles is crucial because the peritoneum is the shiniest layer under the transversus abdominis muscle. When the bowels are seen under the peritoneum under ultrasound, the sliding sign appears in response to breathing.
- Loss of resistance when penetrating the different muscle layers can be felt as a pop. Extra caution is needed because the needle could advance accidentally into the peritoneum and perforate the bowel.
- Avoid puncturing the blood vessels, especially the inferior epigastric vessels, because they sometimes accompany the ilioinguinal and iliohypogastric nerves along their path. Ultrasound aids in visualizing these small vessels, especially if using Doppler mode.

POSITION

The patient is placed in the supine position with exposure of the abdominal and pelvic areas (Fig. 44.1).

ANATOMY

Identify the anterosuperior iliac spine (ASIS) and the umbilicus, and draw a line between these two points. Divide this line into three equal distances at the point where the outer one-third meets the inner two-thirds. This is the point of the needle entry. This point is about 2 cm medial and cephalad to the ASIS (Fig. 44.2).

The ilioinguinal and iliohypogastric nerves are formed by branches from T12 to L1, which pass between the internal oblique and transversalis muscles. Performing this block provides good analgesia for most operations of the inguinal regions.

SONOANATOMY AND TECHNIQUE

Place the ultrasound probe on the line connecting the umbilicus to the ASIS. A transverse longitudinal view will reveal the underlying muscles: the external oblique, internal oblique, and transversus abdominis muscle (Fig. 44.3). Advance the blunt injecting needle in-plane with the ultrasound probe until two "pops" are felt. The first pop occurs between the external oblique and the internal oblique muscles. The second pop occurs between the internal oblique and the transversus abdominis muscle (Fig. 44.4A)—this is where the local anesthetic is injected (Fig. 44.4B).

PEARLS

- Visualizing the spread of local anesthetic in the plane between the internal oblique muscle and the transversus abdominis muscle can help ensure excellent results.
- Tenting the muscles is common when using the blunt needle, so a more perpendicular angle needle entrance technique is used.

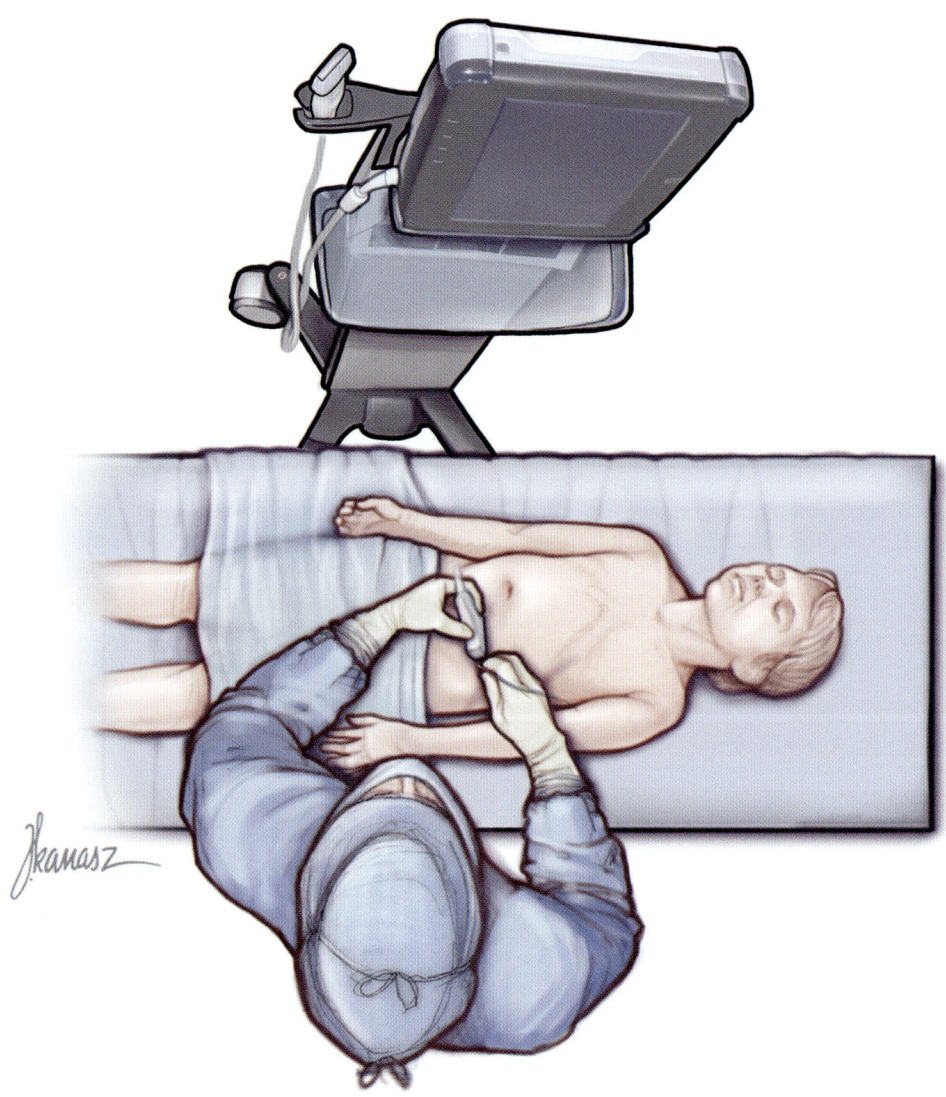

Fig. 44.1 The inguinal and the abdominal areas are exposed and the ultrasound is on the opposite side of the block.

Ilioinguinal and Iliohypogastric Block 285

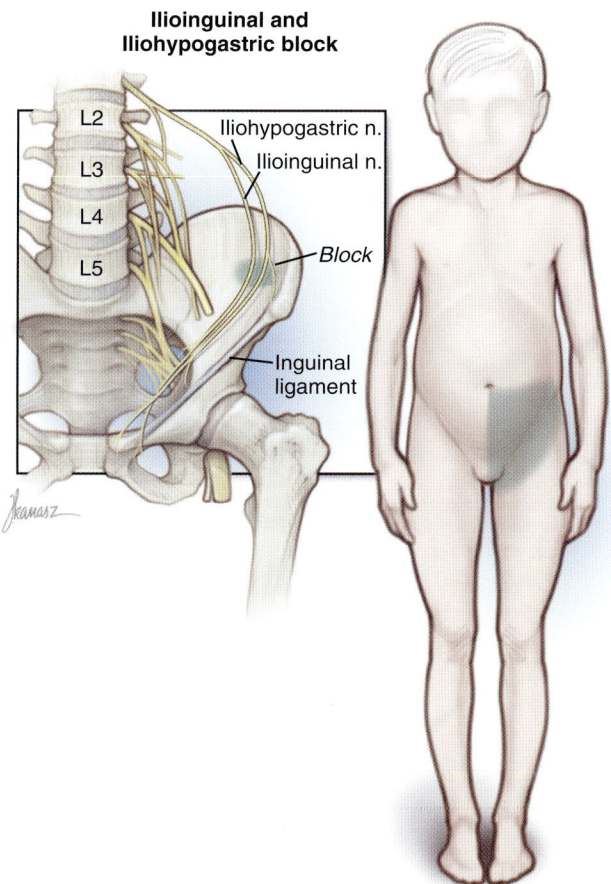

Fig. 44.2 Identify the anterosuperior iliac spine and the umbilicus and draw a line connecting these two points. Apply the ultrasound probe on this line and the needle entrance point will be at the outer third junction of the line.

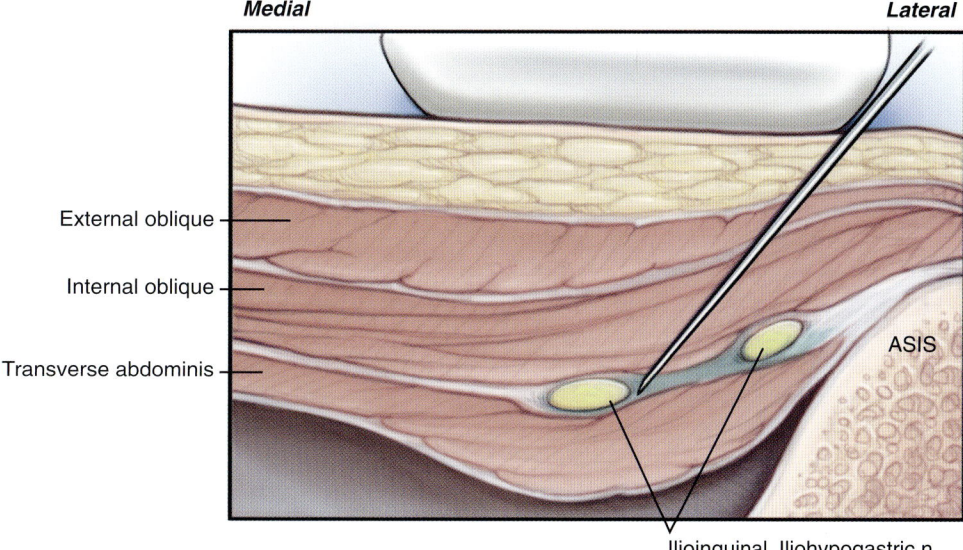

Fig. 44.3 The needle is advanced under ultrasound in-plane approach, penetrating the external and internal oblique muscles targeting the ilioinguinal and iliohypogastric nerves lying in the plane between the internal oblique and the transverse abdominus muscles.

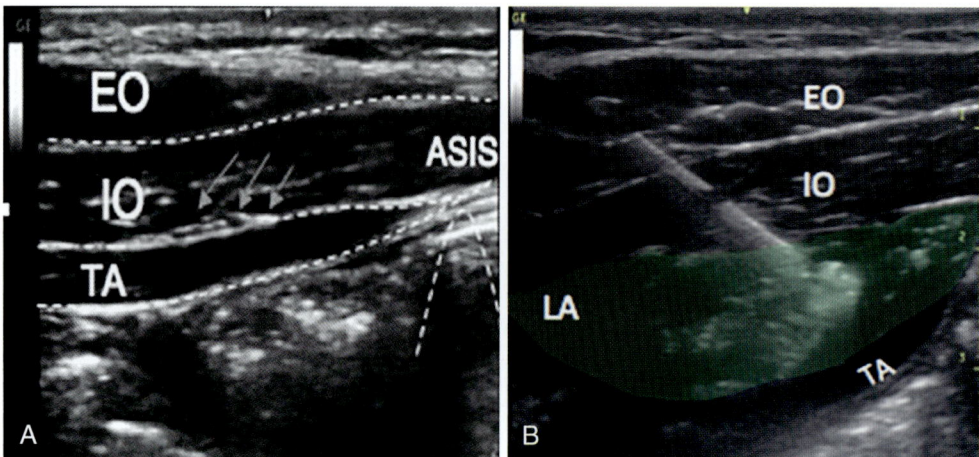

Fig. 44.4 (A) The three muscles under ultrasound, visualizing the ilioinguinal and iliohypogastric nerves (arrows). (B) Local anesthetic spread between the internal oblique and transverse abdominus muscles as shown on the image. *ASIS*, Anterosuperior iliac spine; *EO*, external oblique; *IO*, internal oblique; *LA*, local anesthetic; *TA*, transverse abdominus.

Superficial Cervical Plexus Block

45

John Seif

Key Points

- Stabilize the neck position, and identify the sternocleidomastoid muscle.
- If not using the ultrasound, always feel for the infiltration with the other hand to avoid injecting the local anesthetic in any vascular structure.
- Infiltrate along the posterior border of the sternocleidomastoid muscle superior and inferior to the point of needle entry.

POSITION

Place the patient in the supine position without a pillow. The head is turned to the opposite side of the one being blocked (Fig. 45.1).

ANATOMY AND TECHNIQUE

The superficial cervical plexus provides cutaneous innervation to the ventral rami of C1 to C4 (Fig. 45.2). It includes the lesser occipital, greater auricular, transverse cervical, and supraclavicular nerves (Fig. 45.3). At the midpoint on the posterior border of the sternocleidomastoid muscle is the point of needle entry. The needle is inserted, and local anesthetic is injected behind and along the posterior border of the clavicular head of the sternocleidomastoid muscle.

Under ultrasound, use the linear probe and place it in a transverse position at the needle entry point over the sternocleidomastoid muscle. The needle is aligned with the ultrasound probe in the in-plane position. Visualizing the local anesthetic spread on the posterior border of the sternocleidomastoid muscle is the key to a successful block (Fig. 45.4).

PEARLS

- If deep injection occurs, it could lead to deep cervical plexus block and partial phrenic nerve block. Hoarseness and an inability to clear secretions may occur.
- Superficial injection of local anesthetic with a 22-gauge needle is recommended.
- This block covers only cutaneous sensation and could be used in mastoidectomy and in clavicular bone fracture, especially in the lateral one-third of the clavicle, for postoperative pain control (see Fig. 45.4).

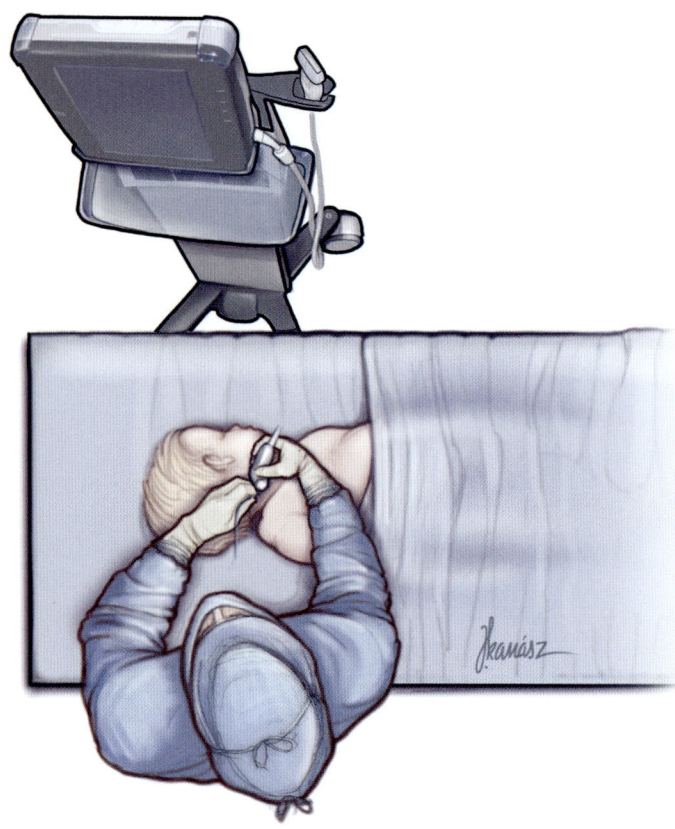

Fig. 45.1 Supine position turning the head to the opposite side of the block and ultrasound position on the opposite side of the block facing the physician.

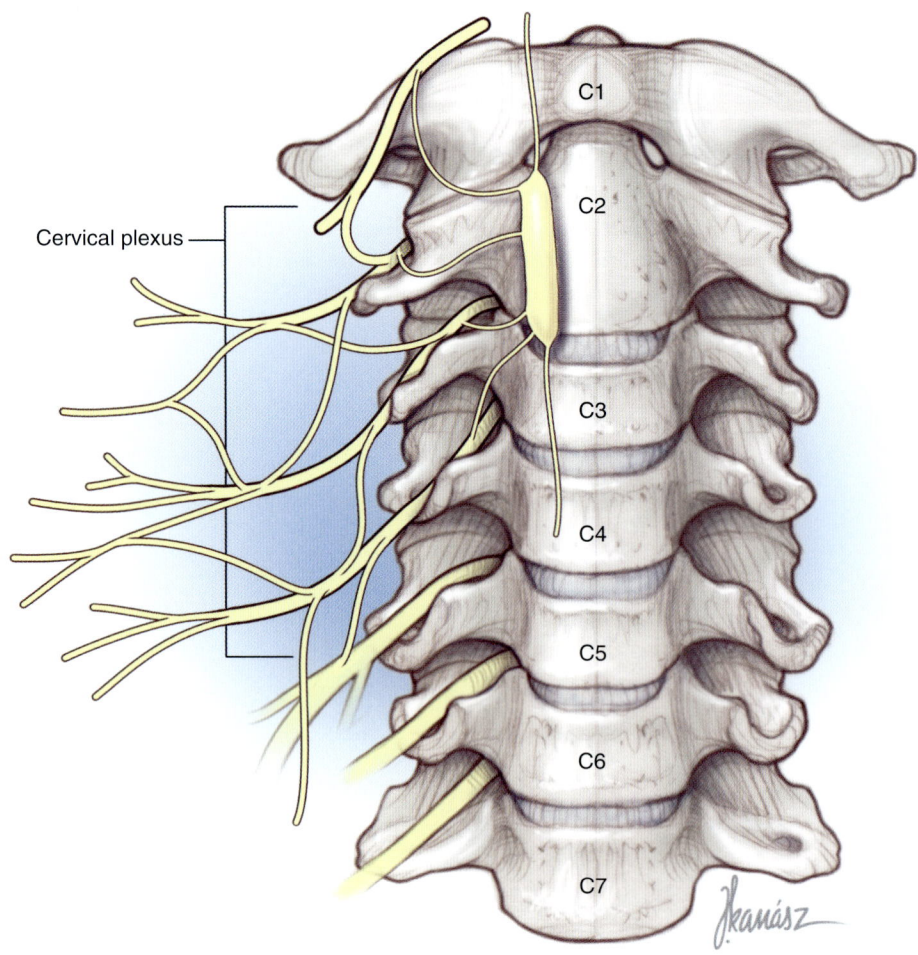

Fig. 45.2 Superficial plexus block provides cutaneous innervation of C1 to C4.

Superficial Cervical Plexus Block   289

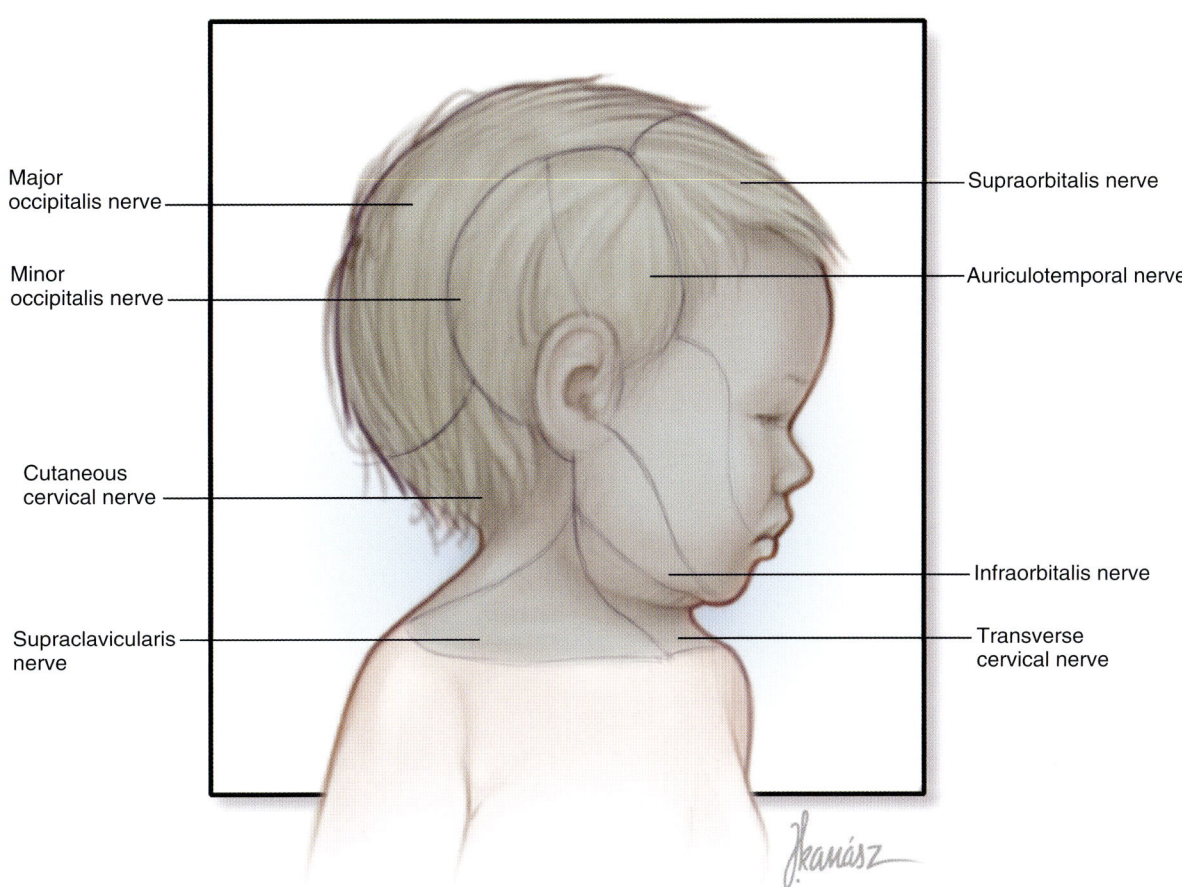

Fig. 45.3 The superficial plexus block will cover the following: lesser occipital, greater auricular, transverse cervical, and Medial and lateral supraclavicular nerves, Accessory nerve.

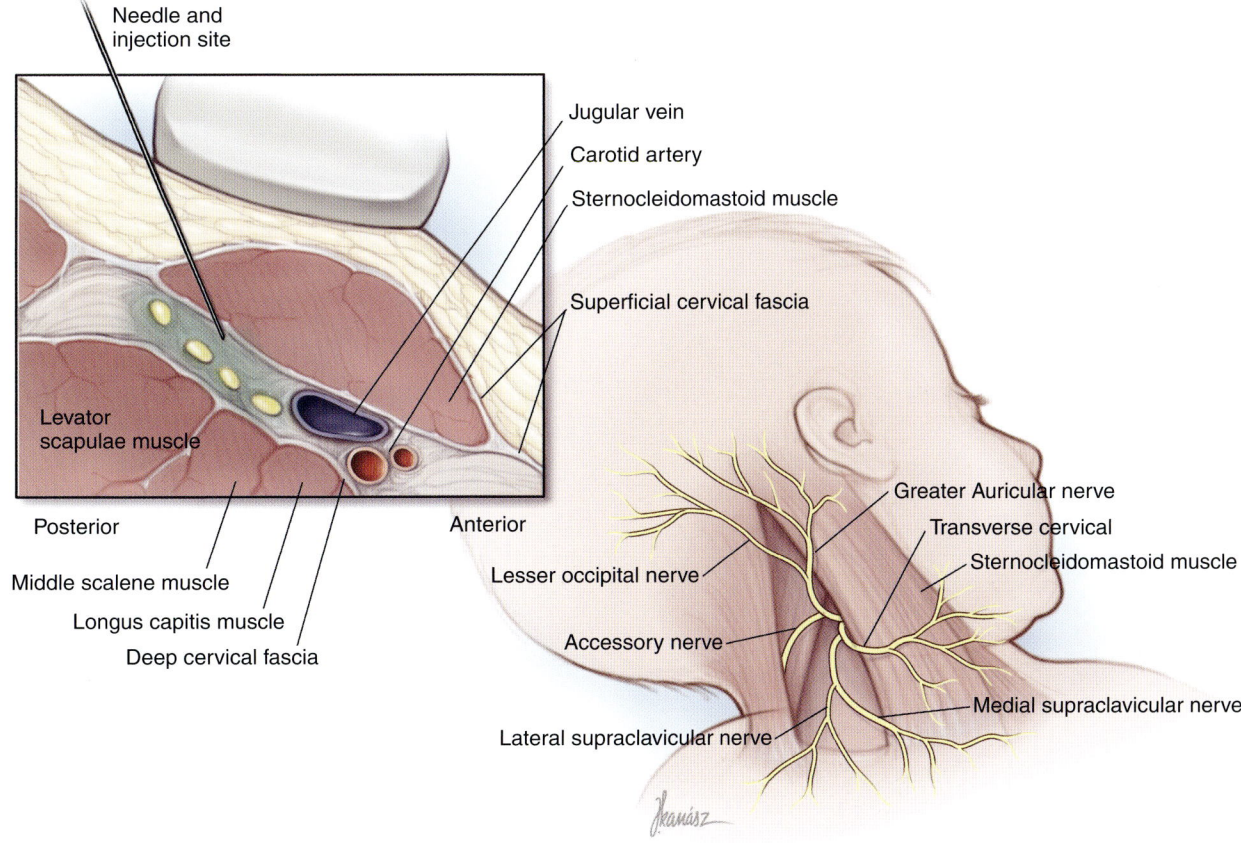

Fig. 45.4 Visualizing the needle advancement in linear approach, targeting the posterior border of the sternocleidomastoid muscle, and infiltrating the area with local anesthetic.

Pudendal Nerve Block   46

John Seif

Key Points

- Patient selection plays a major role in performing the block; it is challenging with obese patients.
- Ultrasound experience is required to maximize the success rate of the block.
- Vascular injection is a risk if no spread is visualized with deposition of local anesthetics under ultrasound.
- Avoid contamination as the area of injection is close to the perianal area.

INDICATIONS

- Perineal operations in both sexes.
- Hypospadias and circumcision are the most common surgeries.
- Scrotal and testicular surgeries with a supplementation of ilioinguinal blockade.

CONTRAINDICATIONS

- Infection or presence of perianal inflammation.

SONOANATOMY

- The pudendal nerve derives its fibers from the ventral branches of the second, third, and fourth sacral nerves. It leaves the pelvis through the lower part of the greater sciatic foramen, passes behind the spine of the ischium, and reenters the pelvis through the lesser sciatic foramen. It accompanies the internal pudendal vessels along the medial border of the ischial tuberosity (Fig. 46.1).
- Placing the patient in a frog-like or lithotomy position helps to expose the area and identify the underlying structures. The linear ultrasound transducer probe is placed on the perineum lateral to the anus at 3 to 9 o'clock and overlies the ischial tuberosity (Fig. 46.2).
- The pudendal artery can be visualized medial to the ischial tuberosity.

TECHNIQUE

- The ischial tuberosity is visualized and the needle is introduced out-of-plane at a 45-degree angle to the skin. The needle is advanced in an anterior to posterior direction in the middle of the ultrasound probe just medial to the ischial tuberosity where the local anesthetic solution is deposited (Fig. 46.3).
- Little resistance will be experienced by passing through the sacrotuberous ligament.
- A nerve stimulator is used 0.3mA to 1.0 mA beside the ultrasound where penile and anal contractions are observed, and this also confirms the pudendal nerve. Sometimes it is challenging to find the nerve under ultrasound.
- Bupivacaine 0.25% up to 1mL/kg in pediatric populations.
- This block is performed bilaterally to reach maximum pain relief.

PEARLS

- Positioning in lithotomy/frog-like position facilitates the block performance.
- Use color Doppler ultrasound to visualize the pudendal artery medial to the ischial tuberosity where the pudendal nerve is located.
- Visualizing the local anesthetic spread medial to the ischial tuberosity increases the success rate of the block.

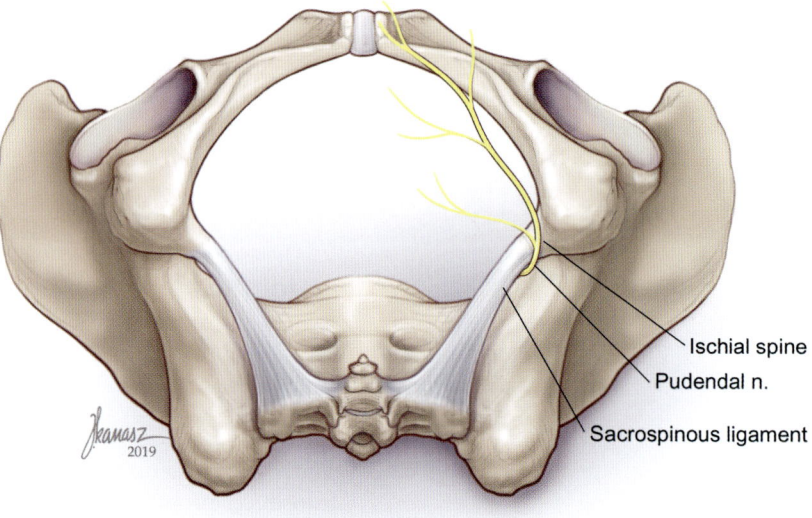

Fig. 46.1 Pudendal nerve is located medial to the ischial tuberosity under the ischial spine ligament.

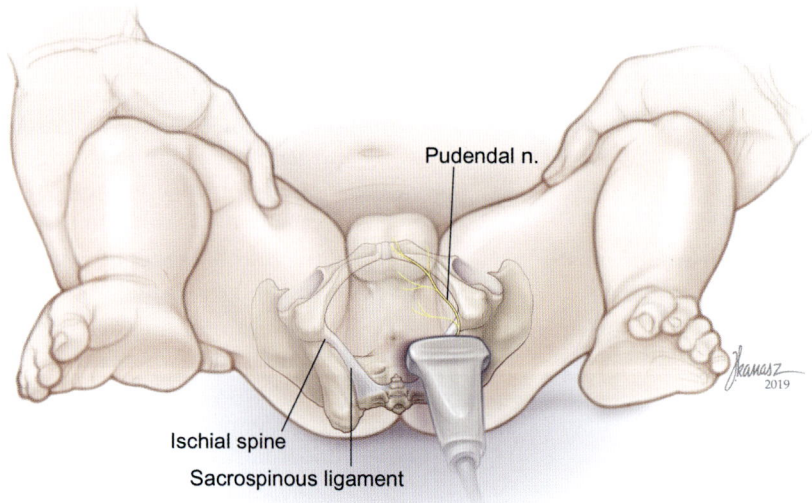

Fig. 46.2 In lithotomy/frog-like position, the ischial tuberosity is the most medial bony prominence. Linear ultrasound probe overlies the ischial tuberosity.

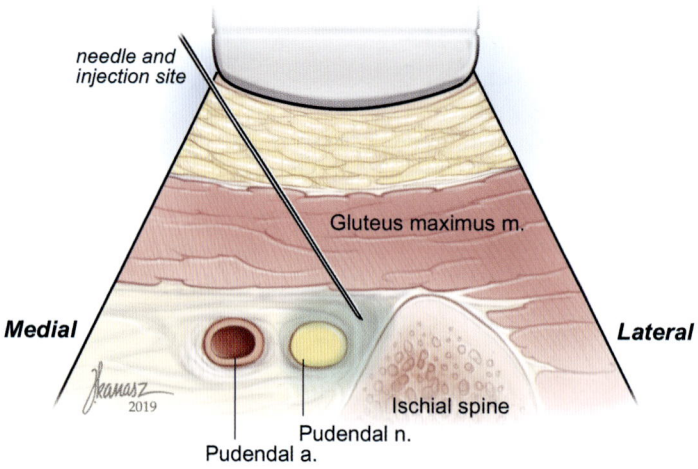

Fig. 46.3 Needle-tip target is medial to the ischial tuberosity, where the local anesthetic is deposited.

Paravertebral Catheters in Pediatrics

47

John Seif

Key Points

- Performing this block requires ultrasound experience.
- Needle visualization plays a major role in achieving a successful block.
- Epidural spread can occur from a unilateral injection.

INDICATIONS

- Patients who undergo operative procedures of the chest and upper abdomen.
- Unilateral coverage as thoracotomies, cholecystectomy, mastectomies, and other urological procedures with preservation of the pulmonary functions.
- Inadequate or unsuccessful epidural placement where bilateral catheters are placed.

CONTRAINDICATIONS

- Caution with populations using anticoagulation and antiplatelet therapy.

SONOANATOMY

- The thoracic paravertebral space is a small triangular space lateral to the vertebral column.
- Bounded posteriorly by superior costotransverse ligament, anteriorly by the parietal pleura, and superiorly and inferiorly by the adjacent head and neck of the adjacent rib.
- The paravertebral space can be scanned in both the transverse and paramedian approach.
- In the transverse approach (short access) the ultrasound probe is aligned in the space between the two adjacent ribs overlying the transverse process. In this approach the space can be identified between the external intercostal muscle and intercostal membrane superiorly, and parietal pleura inferiorly.
- In the paramedian approach (long access) the probe lies in the paramedian plane of the transverse process. The external intercostal muscle and costotransverse ligament lie between the transverse process and deeper to it is the parietal pleura. The area between is the paravertebral space.

TECHNIQUE

- In the transverse approach, the linear ultrasound probe is aligned over the long axis of the rib. Identifying the transverse process medially and the intercostal muscles and deep to it is the parietal pleura (sliding sign) (Fig. 47.1).
  - The needle, 18-gauge Tuohy, is introduced in line with the linear ultrasound probe from lateral to medial under direct visualization. The needle tip ends in the paravertebral space deep to the costotransverse ligament and just above the parietal pleura where the local anesthetic is deposited. Then a 19-gauge paravertebral catheter is inserted thorough the Tuohy needle up to 5 cm beyond the length of the needle.
- Local anesthetic used is ropivacaine 0.2% (1mL/kg) bolus up to 10 mL followed by a continuous infusion (max 0.4 mg/kg/hour).
- In the paramedian approach a linear ultrasound probe is used (short access) visualizing the transverse process and the intercostal muscles and identifying the lung pleura deeper. The local anesthetic is deposited above the pleura and underneath the internal intercostal membrane.

PEARLS

- Placing the patient in a lateral position is the best option in the pediatric population.
- Identify the parietal pleura from the costotransverse ligament by visualizing the sliding sign where the parietal and visceral layer of the lung rub against each other.
- The presence of the lung sliding sign before and after the procedure is important as it rules out pneumothorax.
- Pneumothorax, complete spinal blockade, and local anesthetic toxicity are common complications for this block, which can be avoided when performed by experienced practioners.

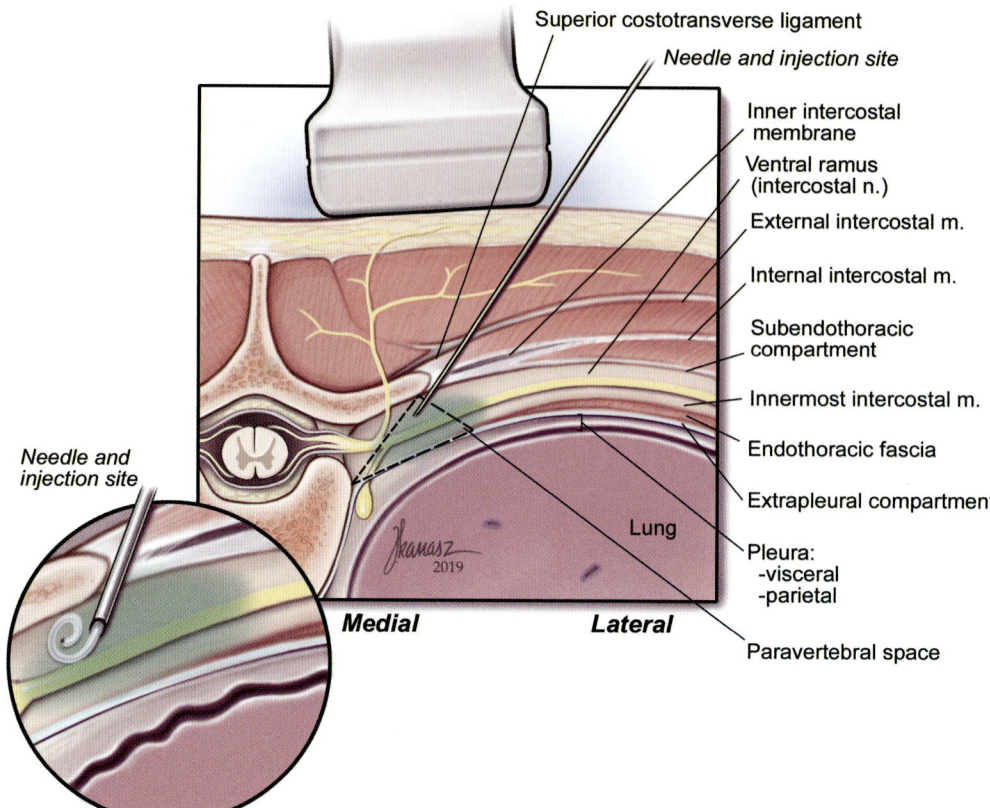

Fig. 47.1 Ultrasound probe in a transverse approach with needle advancement from lateral to medial approaching the paravertebral space.

Section 9
Obstetrics Regional Anesthesia

Regional Techniques During Pregnancy and Delivery

48

Cynthia A. Wong

Key Points

- Neuraxial analgesia/anesthesia (spinal, epidural, combined spinal-epidural) are mainstays of safe anesthesia care of the obstetric patient. The anesthesia provider is caring for the mother, and by extension, the fetus.
- Hormonal and anatomic changes during pregnancy influence neuraxial technique and drug administration.
- Neuraxial analgesia (usually epidural or combined spinal-epidural) is the only analgesic technique that provides complete analgesia for labor and vaginal delivery.
- Neuraxial labor analgesia is usually initiated in a midlumbar interspace; a sensory block from T10 to S4 is necessary for complete labor analgesia.
- During cesarean delivery, a dense block to T6 is necessary to block afferent nerves innervating pelvic and abdominal organs. The addition of lipid-soluble opioids to neuraxial local anesthetics potentiates the density of the block.

PERSPECTIVES

The anesthesia care of obstetric patients is dominated by regional anesthesia and analgesia, primarily neuraxial techniques (spinal, epidural, combined spinal-epidural). The anesthetic care of the obstetric patient must also consider effects on the fetus/neonate. In general, neuraxial compared to systemic analgesia/anesthesia results in less drug transfer across the placenta to the fetus.

Neuraxial analgesia is the only analgesic technique that can provide complete analgesia for labor and vaginal delivery. Given that labor lasts a variable duration (less than an hour to several days), a continuous technique is optimal. Neuraxial labor analgesia is typically initiated with a bolus injection of local anesthetic combined with a lipid-soluble opioid into the subarachnoid or epidural space. An epidural catheter (rarely a spinal catheter) is sited and used to maintain analgesia throughout labor and delivery. Other regional techniques and nerve blocks may be performed, often by the obstetrician (bilateral paracervical blocks, bilateral pudendal nerve blocks), but these techniques are not continuous and do not provide complete analgesia. Paracervical blocks provide analgesia for the first stage of labor, when pain impulses originate from the cervix and lower uterine segment. Pudendal nerve blocks are useful for the second stage of labor as the fetus descends in the birth canal, when pain originates from the vagina and perineum. Only neuraxial analgesia can block these pain impulses simultaneously.

Neuraxial anesthesia is considered the optimal technique for cesarean delivery, both scheduled and intrapartum deliveries. Advantages compared with general anesthesia include: 1) it is safer for the mother (no need to manipulate the airway), 2) less drug(s) crosses the placenta and depresses the fetus/neonate, and 3) it allows the mother to be awake and father to be present for the delivery of their child. Single-shot spinal anesthesia is frequently used for elective procedures. Combined spinal-epidural anesthesia is used when long case duration is anticipated (e.g., repeat procedure, obese body habitus). Epidural anesthesia is a common technique for intrapartum cesarean delivery in women who have an indwelling epidural catheter sited for labor analgesia; epidural *analgesia* is transitioned to epidural *anesthesia*.

Postcesarean delivery analgesia is most often provided using multimodal analgesia—a common component of multimodal analgesia is single-shot neuraxial morphine analgesia. In women who are not able to receive neuraxial morphine (e.g., general anesthesia is used), the transversus abdominal plane block (see Chapter 36), and the quadratus lumborum block (see Chapter 38) have been shown to supplement systemic analgesia. However, these blocks do not improve the analgesia provided by neuraxial morphine and are therefore not indicated in women who receive spinal or epidural morphine.

PATIENT SELECTION

Most obstetric patients are candidates for neuraxial analgesia/anesthesia. Contraindications mimic those for nonpregnant patients. Absolute contraindications include patient refusal, coagulopathy, infection at the site of needle placement, and uncorrected maternal hypotension (e.g., in the setting of hemorrhage). Systemic infection is a relative contraindication, although most clinicians will proceed with a neuraxial technique once antibiotics have been administered and the patient is not exhibiting signs of frank septicemia. Thromboembolic disease is a major cause of maternal morbidity and mortality; thus many pregnant women receive pharmacologic anticoagulation. Guidelines for the initiation of neuraxial procedures in women who have received pharmacologic anticoagulation generally mimic those for the nonobstetric population, although a thorough risk-benefit analysis should be individualized to each patient. Several obstetric conditions are associated with a frank consumptive coagulopathy, including placental abruption and amniotic fluid embolism. Coagulopathy should be ruled out in these women before proceeding with a neuraxial procedure.

PHARMACOLOGIC CHOICE

In the United States, four local anesthetics are commonly used for obstetric neuraxial analgesia/anesthesia. Bupivacaine (0.0625%–0.125%) and ropivacaine (0.1%–0.2%) are commonly used for epidural labor analgesia. Spinal anesthesia for cesarean delivery is usually initiated with 0.75% bupivacaine with dextrose (hyperbaric bupivacaine), although some clinicians use plain bupivacaine. In most patients this formulation is slightly hypobaric. Epidural anesthesia is commonly initiated with 2% lidocaine plus epinephrine 1:200,000, or 3% 2-chloroprocaine (useful for emergency procedures when short latency to onset of anesthesia is critical). Typically, 18–25 mL of a local anesthetic solution is required for epidural anesthesia for cesarean delivery. Neuraxial anesthesia is also indicated for cervical cerclage placement (both elective and rescue procedures) and postpartum tubal ligation surgery, although these are usually short-duration procedures and use of short-acting local anesthetic agents may be appropriate.

In almost all cases, a lipid-soluble opioid (fentanyl or sufentanil) is added to the local anesthetic. The opioid and local anesthetic work synergistically, thus lower doses of both drugs are needed, contributing to decreased side effects from both the local anesthetic and opioid. Fentanyl 10–25 µg and sufentanil 1.5–5 µg are common spinal adjuvants for initiation of combined spinal-epidural labor analgesia and spinal anesthesia for cesarean delivery. Fentanyl 1.5–3 µg/mL or sufentanil 0.2–0.4 µg/mL is often combined with a low-concentration local anesthetic solution to maintain epidural labor analgesia. Neuraxial morphine is commonly used as part of a multimodal technique for post-cesarean delivery analgesia (spinal dose 0.050–0.150 mg, epidural dose 2–4 mg).

Epinephrine (0.2 mg) may be added to spinal bupivacaine to prolong the duration of anesthesia. Spinal and epidural clonidine may enhance analgesia and anesthesia, although the use is off-label in the United States for obstetric patients, because it may cause hypotension and sedation.

PLACEMENT

ANATOMY

During labor, painful impulses from the uterus and cervix are transmitted by visceral afferent nerve fibers that travel with sympathetic nerve fibers and enter the spinal cord at the low thoracic and high lumber (T10 through L1) spinal segments. As labor progresses and the fetus descends in the birth canal, distention of the vagina and stretching of the perineum results in pain impulses that are transmitted via the pudendal nerves to the S2 to S4 spinal segments. Epidural catheters are commonly sited in the midlumbar epidural space. Early in labor, the sensory block must extend cephalad to T10 to block labor pain. Later in labor, sensory blockade must also extend caudad to the sacral dermatomes to provide complete analgesia as the fetus descents in the birth canal.

During cesarean delivery, afferent nerves innervating the abdominal and pelvic organs must be blocked. These nerves travel with sympathetic nerves fibers from the T5 through L1 spinal segments. Therefore dense motor and sensory block, which extends from the sacral dermatomes to T6, is necessary to provide satisfactory cesarean delivery anesthesia. Because of differential sensory blockade (i.e., block to touch occurs at a lower dermatome than block to temperature), most clinicians aim for a sensory block to a cold stimulus at the T4 dermatome. Inadequate extent and density of anesthesia during cesarean delivery—which is more common with epidural than spinal anesthesia—will contribute to intraoperative nausea, vomiting, and pain.

Anatomic and hormonal changes during pregnancy contribute to progressively lower anesthetic requirements as gestation advances. Elevated progesterone levels, among other hormonal changes, contribute to altered pharmacodynamics during pregnancy. Progressive lumbar lordosis during pregnancy alters the relationship of the vertebral column to surface anatomy. The imaginary line joining the posterior superior iliac crests (Tuffier's line) crosses the vertebral column at a higher (more cephalad) position in pregnancy. This may increase the risk of misidentifying the actual lumbar interspace (i.e., anesthesia providers using landmark techniques may identify an interspace that is one or two levels higher than the intended interspace). The space between adjacent spinous processes is narrower and it may be harder for pregnant women to assume the flexed position that facilitates needle access to the neuraxial canal. Ligaments become more "lax," causing the ligamentum flavum to feel less "dense" during advancement of the spinal or epidural needle. Blood volume increases and by midgestation the enlarging uterus compresses the inferior vena cava and impedes venous return from the lower extremities, and along with an increase in intraabdominal pressure, this results in the shunting of blood from the inferior vena cava to the azygous system. The expanded blood volume in the lumbar neuraxial canal, along with the increasing fat volume that accompanies pregnancy, causes a decrease in lumbar cerebrospinal fluid (CSF) volume as the dural sac is compressed and lumbar CSF is translocated cephalad. Additionally, the apex of the normal lumbar lordosis shifts caudad and the normal thoracic kyphosis is reduced and shifts cephalad. Finally, CSF specific gravity decreases during pregnancy. These changes contribute to altered distribution of subarachnoid hyperbaric (or hypobaric) anesthetic solutions. At term, the local anesthetic dose required for neuraxial anesthesia is reduced by 25%–30% compared to nonpregnant patients.

The enlarged epidural veins may increase the risk of unintentional cannulation of epidural veins by a needle or catheter. Additionally, engorgement of the foraminal veins may block egress of anesthetic solution injected into the epidural space and contribute to the lower epidural anesthetic requirement observed during pregnancy.

POSITION

Patient positioning for the initiation of neuraxial analgesia does not differ in the pregnant patient (see Chapters 40 and 41). Laboring patients may prefer the lateral or sitting position, and clinicians may have a preference for one position. Occasionally, patient comorbidities may dictate patient position (for example, a patient with a dilated cervix and fetus with a footling breech presentation should be placed in the lateral position to decrease the risk of umbilical cord prolapse). Patient position should be considered when initiating spinal anesthesia with a hyperbaric (or less commonly, hypobaric) anesthetic solution. Monitoring during the initiation of anesthesia mimics that for nonpregnant patients, with the addition of fetal heart rate monitoring. The anesthesia provider may need to collaborate with the nurse or midwife to optimally position the patient for neuraxial anesthesia and fetal monitoring.

Increasingly more common, preprocedure ultrasonography is used to facilitate identification of lumbar vertebral anatomy (see Chapter 39). It is particularly useful for obese parturients in identifying the midline, the interspinous space, and the estimated depth to the epidural space. Two views are typically obtained with a low frequency (2–5 MHz) curved array probe, the parasagittal oblique (PSO) view, and the transverse median (TM) view. The acoustic window may be larger using the PSO view, especially in women with narrow interspaces. The depth to the epidural space is estimated by obtaining an image of the posterior complex (the ligamentum flavum, the epidural space, and the posterior dura-arachnoid) using the PSO or TM view. The estimation of the depth to the epidural space may underestimate the actual depth measured by the neuraxial needle by as much as 1 cm, especially in obese women. This underestimation is attributable to soft tissue compression by the ultrasound probe, which is often necessary to obtain a satisfactory view.

Spinal anesthesia is initiated in a midlumbar interspace (L2–L3 or lower). Epidural analgesia/anesthesia is also usually initiated in a midlumber interspace because of the need for both a thoracic and sacral anesthesia. Rarely, a two-epidural catheter technique is used in which one catheter is placed at a low-thoracic interspace to provide analgesia for the first stage of labor, and a second caudal catheter is placed to provide sacral analgesia. Like spinal anesthesia, combined spinal-epidural analgesia/anesthesia is initiated at the L2–L3 interspace or lower because of the need to avoid trauma to the conus medullaris.

Use of sterile technique during the initiation of neuraxial anesthesia is critical to the safety of the parturient. When in the sitting position, the mother should don a surgical hat to keep hair and scalp skin flakes from falling onto the sterile field. All individuals in the labor room should don a face mask, and commonly, only one support person is allowed to stay in the labor room during the procedure. The skin over the needle puncture site is usually decontaminated with chlorhexidine in alcohol. The proceduralist should wash their hands with an alcohol-based antiseptic solution and all hand and wrist jewelry and watches should be removed before donning sterile gloves.

NEEDLE PUNCTURE

Young women of childbearing age are at increased risk for postdural puncture headache, therefore subarachnoid puncture should be performed with a small-gauge (usually 25- to 27-gauge) pencil-point needle.

Epidural analgesia/anesthesia is usually initiated with a 17-gauge Tuohy or other epidural needle appropriate for catheter insertion. In virtually all cases, a single or multiorifice epidural catheter (19- or 20-gauge) is passed through the epidural needle and secured for the duration of labor and delivery. A midline approach is common—obstetric patients are young and the interspinous ligament is rarely calcified. The depth to the epidural space is increased in pregnancy because of an increase in subcutaneous fat. Loss-of-residence to saline is a common technique to identify the epidural space; the hanging-drop method is less reliable during pregnancy because of increased intraabdominal, and therefore epidural-space pressure. A small bolus dose of anesthetic solution may be injected through the epidural needle before the epidural catheter is passed though the needle. More commonly, the epidural catheter is threaded into the epidural space and the anesthetic solution necessary to establish analgesia/anesthesia is injected incrementally through the catheter.

Combined spinal-epidural analgesia/anesthesia combines the advantages of both spinal and epidural anesthesia: rapid onset of analgesia with a low dose of drug(s), followed by the ability to provide continuous analgesia/anesthesia. It may be used for both labor analgesia and cesarean delivery anesthesia. It is most common to use a needle-through-needle technique in which the epidural needle is advanced into the epidural space (Fig. 48.1). The epidural needle then acts as an "introducer" for a long spinal needle (25- to 27-gauge). The spinal needle is advanced through the epidural needle using the anesthesia provider's dominant hand while the nondominant hand anchors the epidural needle by grasping the epidural needle hub between the thumb and first finger and placing the back of the hand against the patient's back. This technique is similar to spinal anesthesia when the nondominant hand steadies the introducer needle as the spinal needle is advanced with the dominant hand. As the spinal needle tip passes the tip of the epidural needle, a small increase in resistance to advancement is usually noted. As soon as the anesthesia provider perceives the "pop" indicating puncture of the dura-arachnoid with the tip of the spinal needle, spinal needle advancement should stop. The hubs of the spinal needle and epidural needle are then firmly grasped together between the thumb and first finger of the nondominant hand and the spinal needle stylet is removed. After verifying backflow of CSF through the spinal needle, the syringe with the prepared spinal anesthetic solution is attached to the spinal needle hub and injected, and the empty syringe and spinal needle are removed together. The epidural catheter is then sited in the epidural space, exactly as if initiating continuous epidural anesthesia.

POTENTIAL PROBLEMS

Adverse effects and complications of neuraxial anesthesia in obstetric patients mimic those observed on nonpregnant

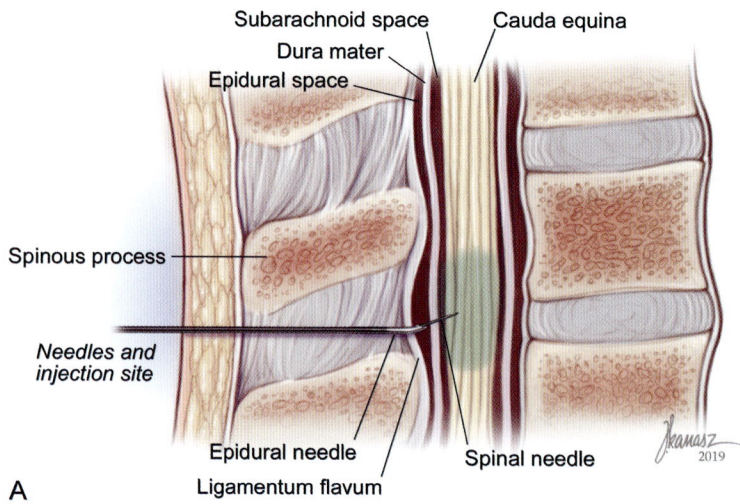

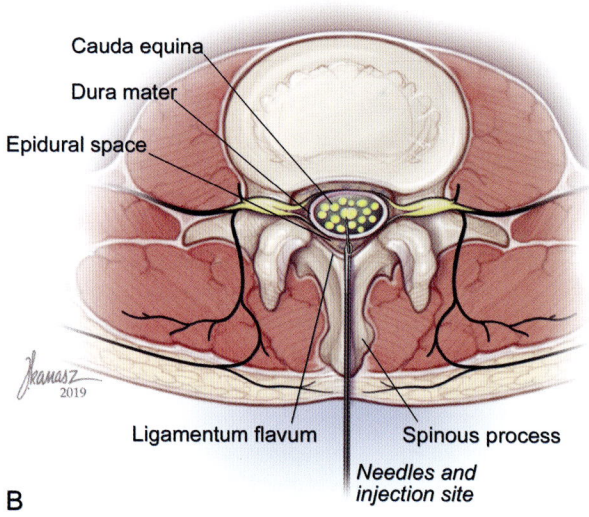

Fig. 48.1 Combined spinal-epidural block. The epidural needle is sited in the normal fashion and a long spinal needle is passed through the epidural needle to puncture the dura. (A) Sagittal view. (B) Transverse view.

patients. The neuraxial injection of local anesthetic agents results in sympathetic blockade. This blockade is extensive when anesthesia for cesarean delivery is initiated; neuraxial anesthesia to the midthoracic dermatomes results in a significant decrease in systemic vascular resistance as a result of arterial vasodilation. Cardiac output increases and blood pressure decreases, sometimes profoundly. Uteroplacental perfusion is not autoregulated; therefore perfusion is directly related to maternal blood pressure. A decrease in uteroplacental perfusion results in a decrease in oxygen delivery to the fetus. Although there is significant margin of safety in oxygen delivery to the healthy placenta and fetus, this margin is reduced in some women (e.g., those with preeclampsia). Maternal hypotension is associated with low neonatal Apgar scores and acidemia. Thus it is critical that the anesthesia provider maintain maternal blood pressure close to baseline during neuraxial analgesia/anesthesia. Blood pressure should be carefully monitored after the initiation of anesthesia. A patient complaint of shortness of breath, nausea, or just "not feeling well" within 15 minutes of initiating neuraxial anesthesia is caused by hypotension until proven otherwise. Often the hypotension is preceded by an increase in heart rate. A combination of a rapidly administered intravenous fluid bolus, beginning at the time of initiation of anesthesia (so-called coload), and administration of a prophylactic vasopressor (e.g., phenylephrine), is the best method for maintaining blood pressure; hypotension should be treated with additional bolus doses of a vasopressor.

Other adverse effects of neuraxial analgesia/anesthesia include pruritus (from neuraxial opioid administration), urinary retention, and shivering. Low-grade fever occurs in approximately 15% of parturients with neuraxial analgesia—the mechanism is currently not known but is likely related to noninfectious inflammation.

Neuraxial analgesia/anesthesia may fail for a number of reasons. The most obvious cause is failure to inject the drugs into the intended space. Women in advanced labor may complain of pain because of "sacral sparing." Anesthesia solution injected into the lumbar epidural space preferentially distributes cephalad rather than caudad. Therefore the low-thoracic sensory block established early in labor may provide satisfactory analgesia early in labor, but as labor progresses and sacral dermatome blockade is necessary, breakthrough pain may result. The injection of a large volume of dilute local anesthetic solution (10–15 mL) may facilitate local anesthetic distribution to the sacral canal.

Complications of neuraxial anesthesia in obstetric patients mirror those in nonobstetric patients and are discussed in Chapters 40 and 41. These include the unintended injection of the local anesthetic solution into an epidural vein, resulting in local anesthetic systemic toxicity, or into the subarachnoid space, resulting in high or total spinal anesthesia. Occasionally, the epidural needle tip or catheter is unintentionally sited in the subdural "space" (a potential space between the dura and arachnoid membranes). The injection of local anesthetic solution into this space results in a characteristically patchy block; onset time is similar to epidural anesthesia, but the cephalad extension of the block may be higher than expected.

Multiple drug errors have been reported—care must be taken to correctly identify all drugs prepared for neuraxial injection, particularly those injected into the subarachnoid space. Permanent cauda equina syndrome may result from the unintentional injection of neurotoxic substances.

Neuraxial damage may result from direct trauma to the spinal cord, conus medullaris, cauda equina, or spinal nerves. Indirect nerve tissue damage may result from ischemia or compression injury from a neuraxial hematoma or abscess. Obstetric patients are at increased risk for thromboembolic disease and death from pulmonary embolism; thus many patients receive prophylactic pharmacologic anticoagulation therapy. A thorough drug history is necessary before planning a neuraxial technique.

Neuraxial infection is a rare but feared iatrogenic complication of neuraxial analgesia/anesthesia. Epidural abscesses are usually caused by skin contaminants—thorough skin decontamination is indicated before initiating neuraxial techniques, particularly in the labor and delivery room, which is not a clean/sterile environment compared to an operating room. Meningitis after neuraxial procedures is almost always associated with a break in sterile technique. Streptococcus viridans species, which thrive in a watery medium (e.g., CSF), may be transmitted from the oropharynx of the proceduralist to the needles, catheters, and drugs used for neuraxial anesthesia.

Postdural puncture headache is a complication of neuraxial procedures. Young women are at higher risk than other patient populations. The unintentional puncture of the dura-arachnoid with a large-bore epidural needle can cause a debilitating headache in the postpartum period that interferes with maternal-neonatal bonding.

Short-term backache after an obstetric neuraxial procedure may be due to local tissue trauma. There is no evidence that obstetric neuraxial procedures are associated with long-term backache, although many women suffer musculoskeletal back pain in the postpartum period.

PEARLS

- Preprocedural ultrasound-facilitated identification of neuraxial anatomy is particularly helpful for obese parturients; however, the posterior complex may be difficult to visualize. In the TM view, the depth from the skin to a line drawn between the transverse processes approximates the depth to the epidural space. It may not be possible to accurately identify the interspace in morbidly obese women, but it is almost always possible to identify the tip of the spinous process. It is useful to remember that the length (posterior to anterior) of the typical adult lumbar spinous process is 3–3.5 cm. An estimate of the depth to the epidural space can be obtained by adding this value to ultrasound-measured distance from the skin to the tip of the spinous process. Finally, an ultrasound-assisted paraspinous approach has been described in which the hyperechoic tips of adjacent spinous processes are identified and marked on the skin in the TM view. The needle is introduced 1 cm lateral and 1 cm superior to the tip of the spinous process, and advanced using a classical paraspinous approach to the interlaminar space (the needle is angled slightly cephalad [5–10 degrees] and slightly toward the midline [5–10 degrees], and walked off the lamina if bone is encountered).
- When caring for obese patients, longer needles (e.g., 10–13 cm) may be necessary to reach the neuraxial canal and use of a larger gauge needle (e.g., 24-gauge spinal needle) mitigates the tendency of small gauge needles to veer off to the side as they are advanced. Alternatively, a combined spinal-epidural technique can be considered because it is easier to advance the larger gauge epidural needle through the spinal ligaments into the epidural space.
- Laboring patients may have difficulty maintaining a still position. Patients may reflexively move and rotate their spine during painful contractions. If difficulty advancing the neuraxial needle is encountered (e.g., repeatedly contacting the vertebra), reassessment of body position may be helpful. Additionally, most patients are readily able to differentiate needle movement to the left or right side of the sagittal midline plane; when difficulty is encountered, it may be helpful to query the patient, "Do you feel this on the left or right side, or in the middle?" Assessment of shoulder height may help identify axial rotation (the shoulders should be level if the spine is not rotated). Continuous, reassuring verbal communication with the patient is critical to success.
- When using the combined spinal-epidural technique, the spinal needle tip must extend 12–17 mm beyond the epidural needle tip when the spinal needle is fully advanced through the epidural needle (Fig. 48.2), or the spinal needle tip may not reliably reach the subarachnoid space when the epidural needle tip is sited in the epidural space. A 127-mm spinal needle is commonly used with a standard 9-mm epidural needle. However, because of differences in hub configurations among needle manufacturers,

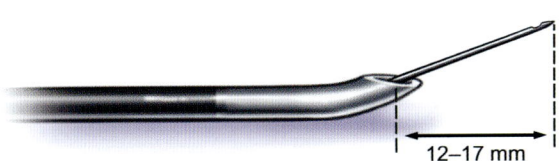

Fig. 48.2 Combined spinal-epidural needle configuration. The spinal needle extends beyond the tip of the epidural needle 12–17 mm.

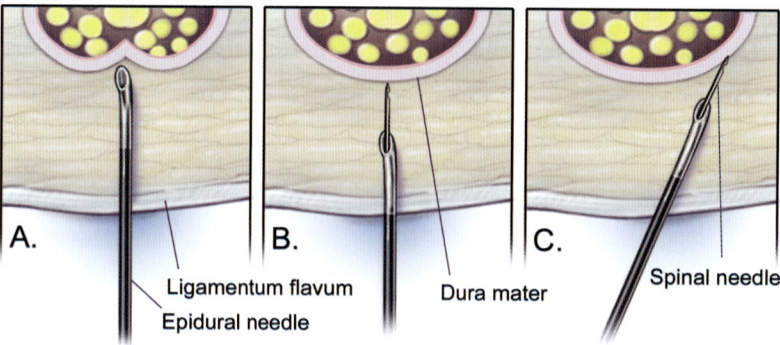

Fig. 48.3 Possible causes of failure of the combined spinal-epidural block—the spinal needle does not puncture the dura-arachnoid membrane. (A) The pencil-point spinal needle displaces, but does not puncture the dura. (B) The spinal needle does not extend far enough past the tip of the epidural needle to reach the dura-arachnoid membrane. (C) The epidural needle is directed obliquely into the epidural space and the spinal needle passes to the side of the dural sac.

some spinal and epidural needles may not be compatible for combined spinal-epidural anesthesia; the spinal needle tip may not extend far enough beyond the epidural needle tip. Some manufactures provide combined spinal-epidural anesthesia "kits" in which both the spinal and epidural needle are packaged together.

- Failure of the spinal needle to puncture the dura-arachnoid after advancement through the epidural needle sited in the epidural space has several causes (Fig. 48.3). If the clinician is very confident that the tip of the epidural needle is sited in the epidural space, they may choose to abandon the combined spinal-epidural technique and proceed with epidural analgesia/anesthesia. However, epidural anesthesia is more likely to fail in this scenario, presumably because the epidural needle tip is not correctly sited in the epidural space, or it is sited off the midline and may contribute to one-sided anesthesia.
- During labor, especially late labor, a block that extends from T10 to the sacral dermatomes is necessary to block the pain of labor. A large *volume* of local anesthetic/opioid solution injected into the lumbar epidural space is required to establish the block. The median effective dose (ED_{50}) of local anesthetic is lower when a high-volume of low-concentration local anesthetic solution is used (e.g., 0.125% bupivacaine), rather than a low-volume, higher-concentration solution (e.g., 0.25% bupivacaine).
- Epidural anesthesia results in a block that is less "dense" than spinal anesthesia. Patients often complain of nausea and vomiting during surgical manipulation of the viscera, especially after delivery of the fetus if the obstetrician exteriorizes the uterus during repair, and during closure of the fascia. The density of the epidural block can be improved by "repainting the fence." Approximately 20 minutes after the initial local anesthetic bolus dose, an additional dose (20%–25% of the initial dose) is injected into the epidural space. This serves to "reinforce" the sensory/motor block, rather than extend it. Administration of neuraxial (or systemic) opioids also serves to treat the nausea caused by visceral stimulation. Used for this purpose, opioid administration treats nausea and vomiting, rather than causing it.

Index

Page numbers followed by "f" indicate figures, "b" indicate boxes, and "t" indicate tables.

A

Abdominal wall
  anterior, anatomy of, in subcostal transversus abdominal plane block, 233f
  muscle layers of, anatomy of, in transversus abdominis plane block, 231
Accessory nerve, anatomy of
  in glossopharyngeal block, 190f, 192f
  in superficial cervical plexus block, 289f
Accessory phrenic nerve, anatomy of, in supraclavicular block, 30f
Achilles tendon, anatomy of, in ankle block, 160f
Acromion, anatomy of, in infraclavicular block, 64f
Adductor brevis muscle, anatomy of, in adductor canal block, 151f
Adductor canal, anatomy of, 151, 151f, 152f, 154f
Adductor canal block, 151, 152
  local anesthetics for, 154f
  position for, 153f
  sonoanatomy for, 151
  technique for, 152, 154f
Adductor longus muscle, anatomy of
  in adductor canal block, 151f, 152f
  in femoral block, 122f
Adductor magnus muscle, anatomy of
  in adductor canal block, 151f
  in popliteal block, 149f, 150f
Adductor muscles
  anatomy of, 151f
  cross-sectional magnetic resonance images of, 98f
Airway block
  anatomy for, 183, 184, 183f, 184f, 185f, 186f, 187f
  glossopharyngeal, 189, 190f, 191f, 192f
  magnetic resonance imaging in, 187f
  superior laryngeal, 193, 194f
  translaryngeal, 195, 196f
American Society of Regional Anesthesiologists (ASRA), 15b
Amide local anesthetics, 7
Amino amides, 4, 4f, 5f
Amino esters, 3, 3f, 4f
Anatomical landmark technique, 129
Anesthetics, local. *see* Local anesthetics
Anisotropy, 20, 21f
Ankle block, 157, 159
  anatomy for, 157, 158f, 159f, 160f, 161f
  indications, 159
  needle puncture for, 157, 160f, 161f
  patient selection for, 157
  pharmacologic choice for, 157
  sonoanatomy, 159
  technique, 159

Anterior cutaneous nerve, anatomy of
  in paravertebral block, 216f
  in superficial cervical plexus block, 289f
Anterior scalene muscle, anatomy of
  in infraclavicular block, 60f, 61f
  in interscalene block, 33, 34f, 35f, 37f, 38f, 40f
  in supraclavicular block, 30f, 31f, 46f, 48f, 50f, 54f
Anterior subcostal quadratus lumborum (QL) block, 238, 239f
Anterior superior iliac spine, anatomy of
  in femoral block, 117f, 118f
  in ilioinguinal and iliohypogastric block, 283, 285f
  in sciatic block, 112f
Anticoagulants, with epidural block, 268
Antiplatelet drugs, with epidural block, 268
Arachnoid mater, anatomy of
  in epidural block, 262f
  in spinal block, 250f, 256f
Arm
  dermatomes of, 27f, 28f
  innervation of
    with pronation, 27f
    with supination, 27f
  osteotomes of, 28f
Armpit, anatomy of, in infraclavicular block, 60f
ASRA. *see* American Society of Regional Anesthesiologists (ASRA)
Attenuation, 16
Axilla
  anatomy of, in infraclavicular block, 59
  proximal, anatomy of, in infraclavicular block, 31, 31f
Axillary artery, anatomy of
  in axillary block, 69, 70f, 71f
  in infraclavicular block, 31f, 61f, 64f, 67f
Axillary block, 69
  anatomy for, 69, 70f
  continuous catheter technique for, 71, 72f
  indications for, 72
  in-plane technique, 75f
  local anesthetic for, 69
  needle puncture for, 70, 71f
  neuropathy with, 71
  patient selection for, 69
  pharmacologic choice for, 69
  position for, 69, 70f
  potential problems with, 71
  sonoanatomy for, 72, 73f
  systemic toxicity with, 71
  technique for, 72, 74f, 75f
  traditional block technique of, 69
  ultrasonography-guided, 72
Axillary catheter
  complications for, 75
  indications for, 74
  technique, 73

Axillary nerve, anatomy of, 26f
  in infraclavicular block, 60f, 61f
  in interscalene block, 42f, 43f
  in pronated arm, 27f
  in supinated arm, 27f
  in supraclavicular block, 51f, 52f
Axillary sheath, anatomy of, in infraclavicular block, 59
Axillary vein, anatomy of, in infraclavicular block, 31f, 67f
AXIS block *vs.* supraclavicular block, 50

B

Backache. *see* Back pain
Back pain, with spinal block, 256
Bicarbonate, local anesthetic with, for epidural block, 262
Biceps femoris muscle
  anatomy of, in popliteal and saphenous block, 142f, 144f, 149f, 150f
  cross-sectional magnetic resonance images of, 98f
Bier block, 85f
Brachial artery, anatomy of, in axillary block, 72f
Brachial cutaneous nerve, anatomy of
  in pronated arm, 27f
  in supinated arm, 27f
Brachial plexus
  anatomy of, 26, 26f
  dermatomes in, 27f, 28f
  at first rib, 30
  in infraclavicular block, 31, 27f, 28f, 31f
  in interscalene block, 34f, 35f, 38f, 40f, 42f
  osteotomes in, 28f
  peripheral nerves in, 25, 27f
  prevertebral fascia in, 26
  in supraclavicular block, 30, 26f, 30f, 31f, 48f, 49f, 50f, 52f, 54f
  cords of, 25, 26f
  divisions of, 25, 26f
  roots of, 25, 26f
  trunks of, 25, 26f
Brachial plexus block
  anatomy for, 25
  axillary, 69, 73f. *see also* Axillary block
  infraclavicular, 59. *see also* Infraclavicular block
  interscalene, 33. *see also* Interscalene block
  "push, pull, pinch, pinch" mnemonic in, 29f
  supraclavicular, 45. *see also* Supraclavicular block
Brachial vessels, anatomy of, in infraclavicular block, 61f
Bromage needle-syringe grip, in thoracic epidural block, 264, 269f

Bupivacaine, 4f, 5, 5f, 7
   for ankle block, 157
   for axillary block, 69
   cardiotoxicity of, 5
   for epidural block, 261
   for epidural labor analgesia, 298
   for erector spinae plane block, 221
   for femoral block, 115
   for infraclavicular block, 59
   for interscalene block, 33, 36
   liposomal, 8
   maximum recommended doses of, 11t
   for obturator block, 135
   for popliteal block, 141, 150
   for pudendal nerve block, 291
   for sciatic block, 107
   single-shot caudal epidural dose of, 8t
   for spinal block, 249
   for stellate ganglion block, 177
   suggested epidural infusion concentrations and rates for, 8t
   for supraclavicular block, 45

C

Calcaneal nerve, anatomy of, 95f, 96f
   in ankle block, 159f
Calcaneus, cross-sectional magnetic resonance images of, 98f
Cardiopulmonary resuscitation (CPR), for local anesthetic toxicity, 11
Carotid artery, anatomy of
   in glossopharyngeal block, 189, 190f, 192f
   in interscalene block, 40f
   in stellate ganglion block, 177, 178f
   in superficial cervical plexus block, 289f
Catheters, 13
   for continuous nerve block
     in axillary block, 71, 72f
     in femoral block, 115, 120f
   epidural, 269, 272f
Cauda equina, anatomy of, in spinal block, 250f, 256f
Cauda equina syndrome, with spinal block, 256
Caudal block, 273
   anatomy for, 273
   circle of errors in, 276, 278f
   ineffective, 276, 278f
   local anesthetics for, 273
   needle puncture for, 273, 277f
   palpation technique in, 276, 278f
   patient selection for, 273
   in pediatrics, 281
     anatomy for, 281, 282f
     position for, 281
     sonoanatomy for, 281
     technique for, 281
   position for, 273, 275f, 276f
   potential problems in, 275, 278f
Caudal epidural block, 244, 244f, 245f, 246f
Cephalocaudal arc of needle redirection, in infraclavicular block, 63f
Cephalolateral quadrant, anatomy of, in popliteal and saphenous block, 141, 142f
Cerebrospinal fluid aspiration, in spinal block, 254, 257f

Cervical epidural block
   anatomy for, 270f
   needle puncture for, 266, 270f, 271f
Cervical fascia, anatomy of, in cervical plexus block, 171, 175f
Cervical pleura, anatomy of, in supraclavicular block, 52f
Cervical plexus
   anatomy of, 171
   cutaneous branches, 171
   sensory distribution of, 172f
   in superficial cervical plexus block, 288f
Cervical plexus block
   position for, 174f
   sonoanatomy, 171
   technique, 171
   ultrasound technique, 171, 175f
Cervical sympathetic ganglion, anatomy of, in airway block, 184f, 185f
Cervicothoracic ganglion. see Stellate ganglion block
Chassaignac's tubercle, anatomy of, in infraclavicular block, 63f
Chloroprocaine, 3, 10, 3f
   for epidural block, 261, 298
   maximum recommended doses of, 11t
   suggested epidural infusion concentrations and rates for, 8t
Ciliary ganglion, anatomy of, in retrobulbar (peribulbar) block, 167, 168f, 170f
Ciliary nerve, anatomy of, in retrobulbar (peribulbar) block, 167, 170f
Circulation, support, for local anesthetic toxicity, 12
Clavicle, anatomy of
   in brachial plexus block, 73f
   in infraclavicular block, 31f, 60f, 61f, 64f
   in interscalene block, 34f, 35f, 38f, 40f, 42f
   in supraclavicular block, 30f, 31f, 46f, 47f, 48f, 49f, 50f, 51f
   in suprascapular block, 56f
Cluneal nerve, anatomy of, 96f
Cocaine, 3, 3f
Coccyx, anatomy of
   in caudal epidural block, 244f, 245f
   in pediatric caudal block, 282f
Color Doppler ultrasonography. see Ultrasonography
Color-flow Doppler ultrasonography, 18
Combined spinal-epidural block, 300f, 302f
Combined spinal-epidural technique, 301, 301f
Common continuous nerve blocks, dosage chart for, 15t
Common fibular nerve, anatomy of
   in popliteal block, 144f, 145f
   in subgluteal sciatic nerve block, 114f
Common peroneal nerve, anatomy of, 93f
   in popliteal and saphenous block, 141, 142f
Continuous infusion dosage, 13
Conus medullaris, anatomy of, in caudal epidural block, 245f
Coracoid process, anatomy of
   in axillary block, 72f
   in infraclavicular block, 31f

Costoclavicular block, 65, 67f, 68f
Crawford needle, for lumbar epidural block, 262
Cricoid cartilage, anatomy of
   in airway block, 185f, 186f, 187f
   in interscalene block, 33, 34f, 35f, 36f
   in superior laryngeal block, 194f
   in supraclavicular block, 46f
   in translaryngeal block, 195, 196f
Cricothyroid membrane, anatomy of
   in airway block, 185f, 186f
   in translaryngeal block, 195, 196f
Cupola, of lung, anatomy of, in supraclavicular block, 46f
Curvilinear probe, 20, 21f
Cutaneous cervical nerve, anatomy of, in superficial cervical plexus block, 289f
Cutaneous nerve
   anterior, anatomy of
     in paravertebral block, 216f
     in superficial cervical plexus block, 289f
   brachial, anatomy of
     in pronated arm, 27f
     in supinated arm, 27f
   lateral, anatomy of, in paravertebral block, 216f
   lateral femoral. see Lateral femoral cutaneous nerve
   median, anatomy of, 26f
   posterior, anatomy of, in sciatic block, 114f

D

Deep cervical fascia, anatomy of, in superficial cervical plexus block, 289f
Deep peroneal nerve
   anatomy of, 93f, 96f
   in ankle block, 160, 159f, 160f, 162f
   needle puncture at, for ankle block, 157
Dermatomes
   of lower extremity, 96f
   in truncal block, 200f
   of upper extremity, 27f, 28f
Descending genicular artery, anatomy of, in saphenous block, 143f
Digital block, of distal upper extremity block, 82, 83f
Distal upper extremity block, 77
   digital block, 82, 83f
   median nerve, 77, 78f
   radial nerve, 79, 81f
   sonoanatomy, 77, 78f
   ulnar nerve, 79, 80f, 81f
   wrist block, 81, 81t, 82f
Doppler shift, 18
Drugs, for regional anesthesia, 3. see also Local anesthetics; Vasoconstrictors
Dural puncture
   headache after, 253, 256
   with epidural block, 269
   with spinal block, 253, 256
Dural sac, anatomy of, in caudal epidural block, 245f
Dura mater, anatomy of
   in caudal epidural block, 245f
   in epidural block, 262f, 263f, 266f, 267f, 270f, 271f

Dura mater, anatomy of *(Continued)*
   in interscalene block, 37f
   in spinal block, 250f, 256f
   in thoracic neuraxial blocks, 247f
Dysesthesias, with sciatic block, 109
Dyspnea, with high spinal block, 257

E
EMLA cream, 9
   recommended doses and application areas for, 9t
Endothoracic fascia, anatomy of, in paravertebral block, 218f
Epidural anesthesia, 297
Epidural block, 261
   anatomy for, 262, 262f, 263f, 264f
   anticoagulation with, 268
   catheter in, 269, 272f
   cervical
      anatomy for, 270f
      needle puncture for, 266, 270f, 271f
   headache with, 269
   hematoma with, 268
   incorrect injection sites in, 267, 272f
   local anesthetics for, 261, 272f
   lumbar, needle puncture for, 262, 264f, 265f
   neurologic injury after, 268
   patient selection for, 261
   position for, 262
   potential problems with, 267, 272f
   thoracic
      anatomy of, 263f
      needle puncture for, 264, 266f, 267f, 268f, 269f
Epidural blood patch, for post-dural puncture headache, 256
Epidural catheters, 269, 297, 298, 272f
Epidural space, anatomy of
   in epidural block, 262f, 263f
   in spinal block, 250f
   in thoracic neuraxial block, 247f
Epidural veins, 298
Epiglottis, anatomy of
   in airway block, 183, 184, 185f, 186f
   in translaryngeal block, 195, 196f
Epinephrine, 6, 6f
   for epidural anesthesia, 298
   for epidural block, 261
   for erector spinae plane block, 221
   for infraclavicular block, 59
   for interscalene block, 33
   for spinal block, 249
   for stellate ganglion block, 177
Erector spinae muscle, anatomy of
   in erector spinae plane block, 222, 222f
   in lumbar plexus block, 104f
   in quadratus lumborum block, 238, 237f, 239f, 240f
Erector spinae plane block
   anatomy, 222
   cranial-caudal in-plane approach, 222
   indications, 221t
   local anesthetics, 221
   pharmacologic choice, 221
   position, 222
   potential complications, 226
   sonoanatomy, 224f

Erector spinae plane block *(Continued)*
   thorax, posterior wall of, 223f
   ultrasound guided injection technique, 222, 224f, 226f
Esmarch bandage, venous exsanguination with, 85, 87f
Esophagus, anatomy of, in stellate ganglion block, 177, 178f
Ester local anesthetics, 9
Etidocaine, 5, 4f, 5f
Exparel, 6
Exsanguination, venous, in intravenous regional block, 85, 87f
Extensor hallucis longus tendon
   anatomy of, in ankle block, 160f
   cross-sectional magnetic resonance images of, 98f
External intercostal muscle, anatomy of, in paravertebral block, 215, 218f
External jugular vein, anatomy of
   in interscalene block, 33, 34f, 38f
   in supraclavicular block, 46f
External laryngeal nerve/branch, anatomy of, in airway block, 184, 184f, 185f
External oblique muscle, anatomy of
   in quadratus lumborum block, 237f
   in subcostal transversus abdominal plane block, 233f, 235f
   in transversus abdominis plane block, 231
Extrapleural compartment, anatomy of, in paravertebral block, 218f
Extrinsic back muscles, anatomy of, in erector spinae plane block, 222, 222f

F
Fascia iliaca, anatomy of, in femoral block, 125f
Fascia iliaca compartmental block (FICB), 127, 128f
   anatomy of, 127
   sonoanatomy of, 127, 128f
   technique of, 127
Fascia lata, anatomy of, in femoral block, 125f
Femoral artery, anatomy of
   in adductor canal block, 151f, 152f, 154f
   in femoral block, 117f, 118f, 122f, 125f
   in popliteal and saphenous block, 144f, 149f, 150f
Femoral block, 115
   continuous catheter technique for, 115, 120f
   indication for, 120
   local anesthetic for, 115, 119f, 125f
   needle puncture for, 115, 118f, 124f, 125f
   patient selection for, 115
   pharmacologic choice for, 115
   position for, 123f
   potential problems with, 115
   sonoanatomy for, 120
   technique for, 122
   ultrasonography-guided, 120
Femoral canal, anatomy of, in femoral block, 125f
Femoral cutaneous nerve
   lateral. *see* Lateral femoral cutaneous nerve
   posterior, anatomy of, 95f, 96f

Femoral nerve, anatomy of, 91, 92f, 93f, 94f, 95f, 96f
   in adductor canal block, 151
   in femoral block, 115, 116f, 117f, 118f, 119f, 121f, 122f, 125f
   in lumbar plexus block, 100f, 105f
   in sciatic block, 108f, 109f, 110f, 112f
Femoral neurovascular bundle, cross-sectional magnetic resonance images of, 98f
Femoral sheath, anatomy of, in femoral block, 125f
Femoral vein, anatomy of
   in adductor canal block, 151f, 152f
   in femoral block, 117f, 118f, 125f
Femoral vessels, on magnetic resonance imaging, 112f
Femur
   distal, cross-sectional magnetic resonance images of, 98f
   greater trochanter of, anatomy of, in sciatic block, 109f, 110f, 111f, 112f, 113f, 114f
   proximal, cross-sectional magnetic resonance images of, 98f
Fentanyl
   for combined spinal-epidural labor analgesia, 298
   in spinal block, 258
Flexor digitorum longus tendon, cross-sectional magnetic resonance images of, 98f
Flexor hallucis longus muscle and tendon, cross-sectional magnetic resonance images of, 98f
Flexor hallucis muscle, anatomy of, in ankle block, 160f
Forearm surgery
   axillary block for, 69
   interscalene block for, 34

G
Gag reflex, eliminating, glossopharyngeal block for, 189
Gastrocnemius muscle, anatomy of, in popliteal and saphenous block, 142f, 144f
Genicular artery, anatomy of, in saphenous block, 143f
Genitofemoral nerve, anatomy of, 91, 92f, 93f, 94f, 95f, 96f
"Gentle pressure", anatomy of, in axillary block, 70f
Glossopharyngeal block, 189, 190f, 191f, 192f
   anatomy for, 189, 190f
   intraoral, 189, 191f
   local anesthetic for, 189
   needle puncture for, 189
   patient selection for, 189
   peristyloid approach, 189, 192f
   position for, 189
   potential problems with, 189
Glossopharyngeal nerve, anatomy of
   in airway block, 183, 183f, 187f
   in glossopharyngeal block, 189, 190f, 191f

Gluteus maximus muscle
  anatomy of, in sciatic block, 112f, 114f
  cross-sectional magnetic resonance
    images of, 98f
Gracilis muscle, anatomy of
  in adductor canal block, 151f, 152f
  in femoral block, 122f
  in saphenous block, 143f
Gravity, venous exsanguination by, 85, 87f
Great auricular nerve, anatomy of
  in cervical plexus block, 171, 173f
  in superficial cervical plexus block, 289f
Greater saphenous vein, cross-sectional
  magnetic resonance images of, 98f
Greene needle, for spinal block, 253

H
Hand surgery
  axillary block for, 69
  interscalene block for, 34
  supraclavicular block for, 49
Hanging-drop technique, in epidural
  block, 262, 265f
Headache, post-dural puncture, 253, 256
  with epidural block, 269
  with spinal block, 253, 256
Hematoma
  with epidural block, 268
  with retrobulbar (peribulbar) block,
    167, 170
  with supraclavicular block, 49
Heparin, low-molecular-weight, epidural
  block and, 268
Hip pain, diagnosis of, obturator block
  for, 135
Humerus, anatomy of
  in axillary block, 70f, 71f
  in infraclavicular block, 60f, 64f
  in suprascapular block, 56f
Hunter's canal, 151. see also Adductor canal
Hyoid bone
  anatomy of
    in airway block, 184, 185f, 186f
    in superior laryngeal block, 193, 194f
    in translaryngeal block, 196f
  displacement of, in superior laryngeal
    block, 193, 194f
Hypoglossal nerve, anatomy of, in
  glossopharyngeal block, 190f, 192f

I
Iliac crest, anatomy of, in epidural block,
  264f
Iliac spine
  anatomy of, in pediatric caudal block,
    282f
  anterior superior, anatomy of
    in femoral block, 117f, 118f
    in ilioinguinal and iliohypogastric
      block, 283, 285f
    in sciatic block, 112f
  posterior superior, anatomy of
    in caudal block, 273, 274f
    in epidural block, 264f
    in sciatic block, 110f, 111f
    in subgluteal sciatic nerve block, 113f
Iliacus fascia, anatomy of, in femoral
  block, 125f

Iliacus muscle, anatomy of
  in femoral block, 116f, 122f
  in lumbar plexus block, 100f
  in obturator block, 136f
Iliocostalis muscle, anatomy of, in erector
  spinae plane block, 222, 222f, 223f
Iliohypogastric block, 283
  anatomy for, 283
  position for, 283
  sonoanatomy and technique for, 283
Iliohypogastric nerve, anatomy of, 91,
  283, 92f, 93f, 94f, 95f, 96f, 285f, 286f
Ilioinguinal block, 283
  anatomy for, 283
  position for, 283
  sonoanatomy and technique for, 283
Ilioinguinal-iliohypogastric block, 130f
Ilioinguinal nerve, anatomy of, 91, 283,
  92f, 93f, 94f, 285f, 286f
  in lumbar plexus block, 105f
Iliopectineal fascia, anatomy of, in
  femoral block, 125f
Iliopsoas muscle
  anatomy of, in femoral block, 125f
  cross-sectional magnetic resonance
    images of, 98f
"Immigrant" muscles, 222
Inferior articular process, anatomy of, in
  epidural block, 267f
Inferior cervical ganglion, anatomy of, in
  stellate ganglion block, 177, 178f
Inferior ganglion of vagus nerve, anatomy
  of
  in airway block, 184f, 185f
  in superior laryngeal block, 194f
Inferior lateral brachial cutaneous nerve,
  anatomy of
  in pronated arm, 27f
  in supinated arm, 27f
Infraclavicular block, 59
  anatomy for, 31, 59, 31f, 60f, 61f, 62f
  continuous catheter technique
    for, 63
  indications for, 64
  in-plane technique of, 67f
  lateral approach for, 66f
  local anesthetics for, 64
  medial approach for, 65f
  patient selection for, 59
  pharmacologic choice for, 59
  position for, 62
  potential problems with, 63
  sonoanatomy for, 63
  technique for, 64
  traditional block technique of, 59, 63f
  ultrasonography-guided, 63, 64f
Infraorbital nerve, anatomy of, in
  superficial cervical plexus
    block, 289f
Infraspinatus muscle, anatomy of, in
  suprascapular block, 56f
Inguinal ligament
  anatomy of
    in adductor canal block, 151f
    in femoral block, 116f, 122f, 125f
    in lumbar plexus block, 105f
    femoral nerve anatomy at, 117f, 121f,
      122f

Inguinal perivascular block, 99, 100f
Inguinal region blocks, 129
  anatomical landmark technique, 129
  anatomy, 129
  complications, 130
  indication, 129
  medication, 129
  ultrasound-guided, 129, 130f
Inner intercostal membrane, anatomy of,
  in paravertebral block, 218f
Innermost intercostal muscle, anatomy of,
  in paravertebral block, 218f
Innominate artery, anatomy of, in airway
  block, 185f
In-plane technique, axillary block
  of, 75f
Intercostal blocks
  PECS 1, 203
  PECS 2, 203
  pecto-intercostal block, 203
  potential complications, 205
  ultrasound-guided injection technique,
    203
Intercostal muscle, anatomy of, 211, 201f,
  212f
Intercostal nerve, anatomy of, 201f
  in intercostal block, 203
  in paravertebral block, 216f, 218f
Intercostal nerve blocks
  analgesia after, 214f
  needle position and injection, 211, 213f
  rib, angle of, 211, 212f
  sonoanatomy, 211
  technique, 211
  ultrasound for, 211, 212f, 213f
Intercostal nerves, 227
Intercostobrachial cutaneous nerve,
  anatomy of
  in pronated arm, 27f
  in supinated arm, 27f
  in supraclavicular block, 52f
Intercostobrachial nerve, anatomy of, in
  intercostal block, 203
Interfascial injection technique, 138
Intermesenteric aortic plexus, anatomy
  of, 93f
Internal carotid artery, anatomy of, in
  glossopharyngeal block, 189, 192f
Internal intercostal muscle, anatomy of, in
  paravertebral block, 218f
Internal jugular vein, anatomy of, in
  glossopharyngeal block, 189, 190f,
    192f
Internal laryngeal nerve/branch, anatomy
  of, in airway block, 184, 184f, 185f
Internal oblique aponeurosis, anatomy of,
  in subcostal transversus abdominal
    plane block, 233f
Internal oblique muscle, anatomy of
  in quadratus lumborum block, 237f
  in subcostal transversus abdominal
    plane block, 233f, 235f
  in transversus abdominis plane block,
    231
Interosseous nerve, of leg, in popliteal
  block, 142f
Interpleural space, anatomy of, in
  paravertebral block, 218f

Interscalene block, 33, 38f
   anatomy for, 33, 34f, 35f, 39f, 40f
   indications for, 37
   local anesthetic for, 33, 34
   needle puncture for, 34, 36f, 37f
   patient selection for, 33
   phrenic block with, 36
   position for, 33, 35f, 41f
   potential problems in, 36
   sonoanatomy for, 37, 37f
   technique for, 38, 42f
   ulnar nerve block with, 36
   ultrasound for, 36, 37f
Interscalene groove, identification of, 33
Interspinous ligament, anatomy of
   in epidural block, 262f
   in spinal block, 250f, 256f
Intertransverse ligament, anatomy of, in paravertebral block, 218f
Intervertebral space, identification of, for spinal block, 253, 255f
Intralipid 20%, for local anesthetic toxicity, 12
Intravenous regional block, 85
   anatomy for, 85
   distal IV site for, 86f
   early Bier block technique for, 85f
   equipment for, 86f
   local anesthetic for, 88
   mechanisms of action of, 88f
   needle puncture for, 85, 86f
   patient selection for, 85
   pharmacologic choice for, 85
   position for, 85, 86f
   potential problems with, 88
   tourniquet inflation pressures for, 85
   venous exsanguination in, 87f
Intrinsic back muscles, anatomy of, in erector spinae plane block, 222, 222f
Intubation
   glossopharyngeal block for, 189, 190
   superior laryngeal block for, 193
   translaryngeal block for, 195
Ischial spine, anatomy of
   in caudal epidural block, 244f
   in pediatric caudal block, 282f
Ischial spine ligament, anatomy of, in pudendal nerve block, 292f
Ischial tuberosity
   cross-sectional magnetic resonance images of, 98f
   in pudendal nerve block, 291, 292f
   in sciatic block, 109f, 110f, 111f, 112f, 114f

J
Jugular vein, anatomy of
   in glossopharyngeal block, 189, 190f, 192f
   in interscalene block, 33, 34f, 38f, 40f
   in stellate ganglion block, 177, 178f
   in superficial cervical plexus block, 289f
   in supraclavicular block, 46f

K
Knee surgery, femoral block in, 120
Kulenkampff supraclavicular block, 45

L
Lacrimal artery, anatomy of, in retrobulbar (peribulbar) block, 168f
Lamina, anatomy of, in epidural block, 263f, 266f, 267f, 268f
Laryngeal nerve, anatomy of
   in airway block, 184, 184f, 185f, 186f
   in superior laryngeal block, 193, 194f
Lateral antebrachial cutaneous nerve, anatomy of
   in interscalene block, 42f, 43f
   in pronated arm, 27f
   in supinated arm, 27f
   in supraclavicular block, 52f
Lateral cutaneous nerves, anatomy of, in serratus anterior muscles, 207, 208f
Lateral decubitus position
   for epidural block, 262
   for quadratus lumborum block, 237f, 238f
   for spinal block, 250, 250f
Lateral femoral cutaneous nerve, anatomy of, 91, 92f, 93f, 94f, 95f, 96f
   in femoral block, 117f, 118f, 121f
   in lumbar plexus block, 100f
   in sciatic block, 108f, 109f, 110f
Lateral femoral cutaneous nerve of the thigh (LFCN), 131
   anatomy of, 131, 132f
   sonoanatomy of, 131
   technique of, 131, 132f
   ultrasound-guided, 131, 133f
Lateral malleolus, cross-sectional magnetic resonance images of, 98f
Lateral rectus muscle, anatomy of, in retrobulbar (peribulbar) block, 167, 168f, 169f, 170f
Lateral supraclavicular nerve, anatomy of, in superficial cervical plexus block, 289f
Latissimus dorsi muscle, anatomy of, 201f
   in erector spinae plane block, 222, 222f
   in quadratus lumborum block, 237f, 239f, 240f
   in serratus anterior muscles, 207, 208f
Leg. *see* Lower extremity
Lesser occipital nerve, anatomy of
   in cervical plexus block, 171, 173f
   in superficial cervical plexus block, 289f
Levator scapulae muscle, anatomy of, in superficial cervical plexus block, 289f
Levobupivacaine, 6, 8
   for erector spinae plane block, 221
   maximum recommended doses of, 11t
Lidocaine, 4–5, 94f,
   for ankle block, 157
   for axillary block, 69
   for epidural anesthesia, 298
   for epidural block, 261
   for glossopharyngeal block, 189
   for infraclavicular block, 59
   for interscalene block, 33, 36
   for intravenous regional block, 85
   for obturator block, 135
   for popliteal and saphenous block, 141
   for sciatic block, 107
   for spinal block, 249
   subarachnoid, 4

Lidocaine *(Continued)*
   for superior laryngeal block, 193
   for supraclavicular block, 45
   and tetracaine transdermal patch, 9
   for translaryngeal block, 195
Ligamentum flavum, anatomy of
   in epidural block, 262, 262f, 263f, 264f, 265f, 266f, 267f, 268f, 270f, 271f
   in spinal block, 250f, 256f
   in thoracic neuraxial block, 247f
Linear probe, 20
Lithotomy position, anatomy of, 96f
Local anesthetics, 3, 4f
   amino amides as, 4, 4f, 5f
   amino esters as, 3, 3f, 4f
   for caudal epidural block, 244f, 245f
   in pediatrics, 7
      amide, 7
      ester, 9
      maximum recommended doses of, 11t
      toxicity of, 10
   structure of, 3, 4f
   timeline of, 3, 4f
   toxicity of, 6, 6t
      with axillary block, 71
      with epidural block, 261, 272f
   vasoconstrictors with, 6
Long ciliary nerve, anatomy of, in retrobulbar (peribulbar) block, 167, 170f
Longissimus muscle, anatomy of, in erector spinae plane block, 222, 222f, 223f
Long thoracic nerve, anatomy of, 207, 26f, 208f
Longus capitis muscle, anatomy of, in superficial cervical plexus block, 289f
Longus colli muscle, anatomy of, in stellate ganglion block, 177, 178f
Loss-of-resistance technique
   in lumbar epidural block, 265f
   in thoracic epidural block, 264, 269f
Lower extremity
   anatomy of, 92f, 93f, 94f, 95f
      lithotomy position, 96f
   dermatomes, 96f
   osteotomes of, 97f
Lower extremity block, anatomy for, 89, 92f, 93f, 95f, 97f, 98f
Lumbar epidural block, needle puncture for, 262, 264f, 265f
Lumbar lordosis, in spinal block, 251, 253f
Lumbar neuraxial block, 246
   paramedian sagittal oblique view of, 246
   transverse axial view of, 246
Lumbar paravertebral block, 99
Lumbar plexus, anatomy of, 91, 93f
Lumbar plexus block, 99, 103–104f, 105f
   indication for, 104
   inguinal perivascular, 99, 100f
   injection site in, 102f
   paramedial longitudinal scanning technique for, 100, 102f
   psoas compartment block, 99
   relevant anatomy for, 99
   transverse oblique scanning technique for, 101

Lumbosacral (Taylor) approach, to spinal block, 256, 259f
Lumbosacral plexus, anatomy of, 92, 92f, 93f
Lung, anatomy of
 in infraclavicular block, 61f
 in supraclavicular block, 46f, 49f, 54f

M
Magnetic resonance imaging
 in airway block, 187f
 lower extremity anatomy on, 98f
 in sciatic nerve block, 112f
 in supraclavicular block, 49f
Malleolus, cross-sectional magnetic resonance images of, 98f
Mandible, anatomy of in airway block, 187f
Mandibular angle, in glossopharyngeal block, 192f
Mandibular ramus, anatomy of, in glossopharyngeal block, 190f
Mastoid, anatomy of, in glossopharyngeal block, 189, 192f
Maxilla, anatomy of, in glossopharyngeal block, 190f
Medial antebrachial cutaneous nerve, anatomy of, in supraclavicular block, 52f
Medial brachial cutaneous nerve, anatomy of, in supinated arm, 27f
Medial malleolus, cross-sectional magnetic resonance images of, 98f
Medial patellar retinaculum, anatomy of, in saphenous block, 143f
Medial plantar nerve, anatomy of, 95f
Medial supraclavicular nerve, anatomy of, in superficial cervical plexus block, 289f
Median antebrachial cutaneous nerve, anatomy of
 in pronated arm, 27f
 in supinated arm, 27f
Median cutaneous nerve, anatomy of, 26f
Median nerve
 anatomy of, 25, 26f
 in axillary block, 69, 70f, 71f, 72f, 73f
 in brachial plexus block, 73f
 in infraclavicular block, 61f, 62f
 in interscalene block, 42f, 43f
 in supraclavicular block, 51f, 52f
 of distal upper extremity block, 77, 78f
 in pronated arm, 27f
 in supinated arm, 27f
Mepivacaine, 4f, 5, 5f
 for ankle block, 157
 for axillary block, 69
 for epidural block, 261
 for infraclavicular block, 59
 for interscalene block, 33, 36
 for obturator block, 135
 for popliteal and saphenous block, 141
 for sciatic block, 107
 for supraclavicular block, 45
Middle cervical ganglion, anatomy of, in stellate ganglion block, 177, 178f
Middle scalene muscle, anatomy of
 in infraclavicular block, 60f
 in interscalene block, 34f, 35f, 37f, 38f, 40f

Middle scalene muscle, anatomy of *(Continued)*
 in superficial cervical plexus block, 289f
 in supraclavicular block, 30f, 46f, 48f, 50f, 54f
Midline approach
 to lumbar epidural block, 262
 to spinal block, 254, 258f
Midline incisions, bilateral blocks for, 231
Musculocutaneous nerve
 anatomy of, 25, 26f
 in axillary block, 69, 70f, 71f, 72f
 in brachial plexus block, 73f
 in infraclavicular block, 60, 61f, 62f
 in supraclavicular block, 51f
 block of, 69
Myotome innervation, of upper limb, 37f, 43f

N
Needles, 13, 14f, 15f
Nerve block, ultrasonography-guided, 19, 19f, 20f
Nerve root, anatomy of, in interscalene block, 40f
Nerve stimulators, 13, 16f
Neuraxial analgesia, pregnancy and delivery
 anatomy, 298
 needle puncture, 299
 patient selection, 297
 pharmacologic choice, 298
 position, 299
 potential problems, 299
Neuraxial anatomy, surface relationships in, 264f
Neuraxial block
 caudal, 273
 epidural, 261
 spinal, 250, 256
 ultrasound-assisted, 243
  caudal epidural block, 244, 244f, 245f, 246f
  lumbar, 246
  sonoanatomy for, 243
  thoracic, 248, 247f, 248f
Neuraxial damage, 301
Neuraxial infection, 301
Neuraxial labor analgesia, 297
Neurologic injury
 with epidural block, 268
 with spinal block, 256
Neurotoxicity, direct, of local anesthetics, in pediatrics, 10

O
Oblique muscle, anatomy of
 in retrobulbar (peribulbar) block, 170f
 in subcostal transversus abdominal plane block, 235f
 in transversus abdominis plane block, 231
Obturator block, 135
 indications for, 136
 needle puncture for, 135
 patient selection for, 135
 pharmacologic choice for, 135
 position for, 135

Obturator block *(Continued)*
 sonoanatomy for, 136
 technique for, 138, 137f,
Obturator foramen, anatomy of, in obturator block, 136f, 137f
Obturator nerve, anatomy of, 91, 92f, 93f, 95f, 96f
 in femoral block, 118f
 in lumbar plexus block, 100f, 105f
 in obturator block, 135, 136f, 137f
 in sciatic block, 108f, 109f, 110f
Occipitalis nerve
 major, anatomy of, in superficial cervical plexus block, 289f
 minor, anatomy of, in superficial cervical plexus block, 289f
Ophthalmic artery, anatomy of, in retrobulbar (peribulbar) block, 167, 168f, 169f, 170f
Optic nerve, anatomy of, in retrobulbar (peribulbar) block, 167, 168f, 169f, 170f
Orbicularis oculi muscle block, Van Lint method, 167, 169f
Orbit, anatomy of, 167, 168f, 170f
Osteotomes
 of lower extremity, 97f
 of upper extremity, 28f

P
Paramedian approach
 to spinal block, 256, 258f, 259f
 to thoracic epidural block, 264, 263f, 268f
Paraspinous muscle, anatomy of, 201f
 in paravertebral block, 218f
Paravertebral block, 215
 contraindications to, 215
 indications for, 215
 patient positioning for, 217f
 sonoanatomy for, 215
 technique for, 215
Paravertebral catheters, in pediatrics
 contraindications, 293
 indications, 293
 local anesthetics, 293
 paramedian approach, 293
 sonoanatomy, 293
 technique, 293
 transverse approach, 293, 294f
Paravertebral space, anatomy of, in paravertebral block, 216f, 218f
Parietal pleura, anatomy of, in paravertebral block, 218f
Parsonage-Turner syndrome, 54
PART, 20, 22f
Patellar ligament, anatomy of, in saphenous block, 143f
PECS 1 block, intercostal, 203, 204f, 205f
PECS 2 block, intercostal, 203, 204f, 205f
Pectineus muscle, anatomy of, in femoral block, 125f
Pecto-intercostal block, 203, 206f
Pectoralis major muscle, anatomy of, in infraclavicular block, 31f, 61f, 62f
Pectoralis minor muscle, anatomy of, in infraclavicular block, 61f, 64f, 67f

Pectoralis muscles
    in infraclavicular block, 60f
    in serratus anterior muscles, 207, 208f
Pediatric position, for caudal block, 273, 275f
Pediatrics, caudal block in, 281
Peribulbar block. *see* Retrobulbar (peribulbar) block
Peripheral nerve block, 88f
Peroneal nerve, anatomy of, 95f
    in popliteal and saphenous block, 141
Peroneus brevis muscle, anatomy of, in ankle block, 160f
Peroneus brevis tendon, cross-sectional magnetic resonance images of, 98f
Peroneus longus tendon, cross-sectional magnetic resonance images of, 98f
Pharmacology, 3
Pharyngeal nerve, anatomy of, in airway block, 183, 184f
Phenylephrine, 6, 6f
    for spinal block, 249
Phrenic block, interscalene block with, 36
Phrenic nerve, anatomy of, 30
    in interscalene block, 34f
    in supraclavicular block, 30f, 46f
Phrenic nerve block, with supraclavicular block, 49
Piriformis muscle, anatomy of, in sciatic block, 109f, 110f
Plantar nerve, anatomy of, in ankle block, 159f
Pleura, anatomy of
    in interscalene block, 35f
    in supraclavicular block, 52f
Plumb bob supraclavicular block
    needle puncture for, 48, 48f, 49f, 50f
    position for, 48
Pneumothorax, with supraclavicular block, 45
Popliteal artery, anatomy of, in popliteal block, 144f
Popliteal block, 141, 143
    anatomy for, 141
    indications for, 143
    needle angle for, 143f
    needle puncture for, 141
    patient selection for, 141
    pharmacologic choice for, 141
    position for, 141, 146f, 147f
    potential problems with, 141
    sonoanatomy for, 143
    technique for, 144, 148f, 149f, 150f
Popliteal fossa, anatomy of, in popliteal and saphenous block, 141, 142f, 144f
Popliteal neurovascular bundle, cross-sectional magnetic resonance images of, 98f
Postcesarean delivery analgesia, 297
Posterior antebrachial cutaneous nerve, anatomy of, in pronated arm, 27f
Posterior brachial cutaneous nerve, anatomy of, in pronated arm, 27f
Posterior cutaneous nerve, anatomy of
    in popliteal block, 145f
    in sciatic block, 109f
    in serratus anterior muscles, 207, 208f
Posterior femoral cutaneous nerve, anatomy of, 95f, 96f

Posterior sacrococcygeal ligament, anatomy of, in pediatric caudal block, 282f
Posterior scalene muscle, anatomy of, in interscalene block, 37f
Posterior superior iliac spine, anatomy of, 273, 274f
    in epidural block, 264f
    in sciatic block, 110f
    in subgluteal sciatic nerve block, 114f
Posterior tibial artery, anatomy of, in ankle block, 160f
Posterior tibial nerve
    anatomy of, in ankle block, 160f
    needle puncture at, for ankle block, 157
Prevertebral fascia, anatomy of
    in brachial plexus, 26
    in cervical plexus block, 171, 175f
Prilocaine, 5, 85, 5f
    for intravenous regional block, 85
Procaine, 3, 3f, 4f
Prone jackknife position
    for epidural block, 262
    for spinal block, 250, 252f
Prone position, for caudal block, 273, 276f
Psoas compartment block, 99
Psoas major muscle, anatomy of
    in femoral block, 122f
    in lumbar plexus block, 104f
    in quadratus lumborum block, 237f, 239f
Psoas minor tendon, anatomy of, in femoral block, 125f
Psoas muscle, anatomy of
    in femoral block, 116f
    in lumbar plexus block, 100, 100f
    in obturator block, 136f
Pubic tubercle, anatomy of
    in femoral block, 117f, 118f
    in obturator block, 136f, 137f
    in sciatic block, 112f
Pudendal nerve, anatomy of, 291, 94f, 292f
Pudendal nerve block, 291
    contraindications, 291
    indications, 291
    position, 291, 292f
    sonoanatomy, 291
    technique, 291
"Push, pull, pinch, pinch" mnemonic, in brachial plexus block, 29f

Q

Quadratus femoris muscle
    anatomy of, in sciatic block, 112f, 114f
    cross-sectional magnetic resonance images of, 98f
Quadratus lumborum block, 237
    anterior, 238, 238f
    lateral, 238, 238f
    posterior, 238, 238f
    sonoanatomy for, 237, 237f
    subcostal, 238, 239f
    suprailiac anterior, 239, 240f
    technique for, 238, 239f
Quadratus lumborum muscle, anatomy of
    in femoral block, 116f
    in lumbar plexus block, 100f
    in quadratus lumborum block, 237, 237f, 238f

Quincke-Babcock needle, for spinal block, 253

R

Radial nerve, anatomy of, 25, 26f
    in axillary block, 69, 70f, 71f, 72f
    in brachial plexus block, 73f
    in distal upper extremity block, 77, 79, 81f
    in infraclavicular block, 61f, 62f
    in interscalene block, 42f, 43f
    in pronated arm, 27f
    in supinated arm, 27f
    in supraclavicular block, 51f, 52f
Rami communicantes, anatomy of, 199, 201f
Ramus
    dorsal, 204f
        in paravertebral block, 216f, 218f
        in truncal block, 199, 201f
    ventral, 203, 204f
        in paravertebral block, 216f, 218f
        in transversus abdominis plane block, 231
        in truncal block, 199, 201f
Rectus abdominis muscle, anatomy of
    in rectus sheath block, 227, 228f
    in subcostal transversus abdominal plane block, 233, 233f, 235f
Rectus muscle, anatomy of, in retrobulbar (peribulbar) block, 167, 168f, 169f, 170f
Rectus sheath, 227
Rectus sheath block, 227, 229
    and catheter in adults, 227, 229
    sonoanatomy, 227, 228f
    technique, 227, 228f, 229f
Recurrent laryngeal nerve, anatomy of, in airway block, 184, 184f, 185f, 186f
Reflection, 18
Regional anesthesia
    drugs for, 3. *see also* Local anesthetics
    ultrasonography-guided. *see* Ultrasonography
    vasoconstrictors in, 6
Resolution, 16
Retrobulbar (peribulbar) block, 167
    anatomy for, 167, 168f, 170f
    hematoma with, 167, 170
    needle puncture for, 167, 169f
    patient selection for, 167
    position for, 167, 168f
    potential problems with, 170
    Van Lint method for, 167, 169f
Retroclavicular block, 65
Rhomboid muscle, anatomy of, in erector spinae plane block, 222, 222f, 223f
Rib
    facets for, anatomy of, in epidural block, 267f
    first
        anatomy of
            in infraclavicular block, 60f, 61f
            in interscalene block, 34f, 38f
            in supraclavicular block, 30f, 31f, 46f, 47f, 48f, 49f, 50f, 54f
        brachial plexus anatomy at, 30, 31f
        neck of, anatomy of, in paravertebral block, 218f

Ropivacaine, 4f, 5–6, 5f, 8
  for ankle block, 157
  for axillary block, 69
  for epidural block, 261
  for epidural labor analgesia, 298
  for erector spinae plane block, 221
  for femoral block, 115
  for infraclavicular block, 59
  for interscalene block, 33, 36
  for obturator block, 135
  for paravertebral block, 216
  for popliteal block, 141, 150
  for sciatic block, 107
  single-shot caudal epidural dose of, 8t
  for stellate ganglion block, 177
  suggested epidural infusion concentrations and rates for, 8t
  for supraclavicular block, 45
Rotator cuff, anatomy of, in suprascapular block, 56f

S
Sacral anatomy, sex of patient and, 273, 274f, 275f
Sacral canal, anatomy of, in caudal block, 244f, 277f
Sacral cornua, anatomy of, in caudal block, 244f, 275f, 277f
  pediatric, 281, 282f
Sacral hiatus, anatomy of
  in caudal block, 273, 244f, 274f, 277f
  pediatric, 281, 282f
  in sciatic block, 111f
Sacrococcygeal membrane, anatomy of, in caudal epidural block, 244f, 245f
Sacrospinous ligament, anatomy of, in pudendal nerve block, 292f
Sacrotuberous ligament, anatomy of, in sciatic block, 114f
Sacrum, anatomy of, in caudal block, 244f
  pediatric, 282f
Saphenous block
  local anesthetics for, 141
  needle puncture for, 141, 143f
  patient selection for, 141
  pharmacologic choice for, 141
  with popliteal block, 141
  position for, 141
  potential problems with, 141
Saphenous nerve
  anatomy of, 93f, 95f, 96f
    in adductor canal block, 151f, 152f, 154f
    in ankle block, 162, 159f, 160f, 163f
    in saphenous block, 143f
  needle puncture at, for ankle block, 157
  sonoanatomy of, 151
Sartorius muscle
  anatomy of
    in adductor canal block, 152f, 154f
    in femoral block, 122f
    in saphenous block, 143f
  cross-sectional magnetic resonance images of, 98f
Scalene muscle, anatomy of
  in infraclavicular block, 60f, 61f
  in interscalene block, 33, 34f, 35f, 37f, 38f, 40f

Scalene muscle, anatomy of *(Continued)*
  in supraclavicular block, 30f, 46f, 48f, 50f, 54f
Scapula, anatomy of
  in epidural block, 264f
  in infraclavicular block, 60f
  in suprascapular block, 56f
Scapular ligament, anatomy of, in suprascapular block, 56f
Scapular notch, anatomy of, in suprascapular block, 56f
Sciatic block
  anatomy for, 107, 108f, 109f, 110f
  anterior approach to, 108
    needle puncture for, 108, 112f
    position for, 108
  classic approach to, 107
    needle puncture for, 107, 111f
    position for, 107, 110f
  local anesthetic solution for, 107
  patient selection for, 107
  pharmacologic choice for, 107
  potential problems with, 109
  sonoanatomy for, 110
  surface marking technique for, 111f
  technique for, 110, 113f
  traditional block technique of, 107
  ultrasonography-guided, 110, 112f
Sciatic nerve
  anatomy of, 107, 108f, 109f, 110f
    in popliteal block, 144f, 145f, 149f
    in subgluteal sciatic nerve block, 113f
  on magnetic resonance imaging, 112f
Sclerotome innervation, of upper limb, 38f, 42f
Seizure, from local anesthetic toxicity, prevention and treatment of, 12
Semimembranosus muscle and tendon
  anatomy of, in popliteal and saphenous block, 142f, 143f, 144f, 149f, 150f
  cross-sectional magnetic resonance images of, 98f
Semitendinosus muscle and tendon
  anatomy of, in popliteal and saphenous block, 142f, 143f, 144f, 149f, 150f
  cross-sectional magnetic resonance images of, 98f
Serratus posterior inferior muscles, anatomy of, in erector spinae plane block, 222, 222f
Serratus anterior block
  anatomy, 207, 208f
  potential complications, 208
  sensory distribution of, 208f
  ultrasound-guided injection technique, 207, 209f
Serratus anterior muscle
  anatomy of, in infraclavicular block, 59, 60f
Serratus anterior muscle, anatomy of, 207, 201f, 208f
Short ciliary nerve, anatomy of, in retrobulbar (peribulbar) block, 167, 170f
Shoulder surgery, interscalene block for, 34
Single-shot technique, serratus anterior muscles, 208, 209f

Sitting position
  for epidural block, 262
  for spinal block, 251, 252f
Skin, anatomy of, in spinal block, 250f
Soleus muscle, cross-sectional magnetic resonance images of, 98f
Specular reflection, 18
Spinal anesthesia, 299
Spinal block, 249, 250
  anatomy for, 250, 250f
  backache with, 256
  cerebrospinal fluid aspiration in, 254, 257f
  combined spinal-epidural technique in, 258
  continuous, 256
  fentanyl in, 258
  headache with, 249, 253, 256
  high, dyspnea with, 257
  hyperbaric, 249
  hypobaric, 249
  local anesthetics for, 249
  lumbosacral (Taylor) approach to, 256, 259f
  midline approach to, 254, 258f
  needle puncture for, 253, 255f, 256f, 257f, 258f, 259f
  neurologic injury with, 256
  paramedian approach to, 254, 258f, 259f
  patient selection for, 249
  position for, 250, 250f, 252f, 253f, 254f
  potential problems with, 256
  vasoconstrictors for, 249
Spinal canal, anatomy of, in spinal block, 253f, 254f
Spinal cord, anatomy of
  in epidural block, 263f, 267f
  in thoracic neuraxial blocks, 247f
Spinal fluid, in epidural block, 267
Spinal ganglion, anatomy of, 201f
  in thoracic neuraxial blocks, 247f
Spinalis muscle, anatomy of, in erector spinae plane block, 222, 222f, 223f
Spinal needles, for glossopharyngeal block, 189
Spinal nerve, anatomy of
  in epidural block, 263f, 267f
  in intercostal block, 203
  in paravertebral block, 216f
  in supraclavicular block, 51f
Spinous process, anatomy of, in epidural block, 263f, 267f
Sprotte needles, for spinal block, 253
Stellate ganglion block, 177–178, 180
  anatomy, 177, 178f
  indications, 177t
  palpation, 177
  pharmacologic choice, 177
  position, 177
  potential complications, 180
  ultrasound-guided injection technique, 177, 179f
Sternocleidomastoid muscle, anatomy of
  in cervical plexus block, 171, 173f
  in infraclavicular block, 61f
  in interscalene block, 33, 34f, 35f, 37f, 38f, 40f
  in superficial cervical plexus block, 289f
  in supraclavicular block, 46f, 48f, 49f, 50f, 54f

Sternum, anatomy of, in infraclavicular block, 61f
Styloid process, anatomy of, in glossopharyngeal block, 189, 190f, 192f
Subarachnoid puncture, with caudal block, 275
Subarachnoid space, anatomy of, in epidural block, 262f
Subclavian artery
  anatomy of
    in infraclavicular block, 62f
    in interscalene block, 34f, 38f
    in supraclavicular block, 30, 31f, 46f, 47f, 48f, 49f, 50f, 54f
  puncture of, during supraclavicular block, 45
Subclavian vein, anatomy of
  in infraclavicular block, 61f
  in interscalene block, 34f, 38f
  in supraclavicular block, 46f, 48f, 49f, 50f
Subcostal nerve, anatomy of, 94f
Subcostal transversus abdominal plane block, 233, 234
  indication for, 234
  position of patient and ultrasound machine for, 234f
  sonoanatomy for, 233
  technique for, 234
Subcutaneous fat, anatomy of, in spinal block, 250f, 256f
Subdural injection, in epidural block, 267, 272f
Subdural space, anatomy of, in epidural block, 262f
Subendothoracic compartment, anatomy of, in paravertebral block, 218f
Subgluteal approach, to ultrasonography-guided sciatic block, 114f
Subscapular nerve, anatomy of, 26f
Sufentanil, for combined spinal-epidural labor analgesia, 298
Superficial cervical fascia, anatomy of, in superficial cervical plexus block, 289f
Superficial cervical plexus, anatomy of, 287
Superficial cervical plexus block, 287, 288f, 289f
  anatomy and technique for, 287
  position for, 287
Superficial peroneal nerve
  anatomy of, 93f, 96f
    in ankle block, 161, 159f, 160f, 163f
  needle puncture at, for ankle block, 157
Superficial sacrococcygeal ligament, anatomy of, in pediatric caudal block, 282f
Superior articular process, anatomy of, in epidural block, 267f
Superior cervical ganglion, anatomy of, in stellate ganglion block, 177, 178f
Superior costotransverse ligament, anatomy of, in paravertebral block, 218f
Superior gluteal nerve, anatomy of, in popliteal block, 145f

Superior laryngeal block, 193, 194f
Superior laryngeal nerve, anatomy of
  in airway block, 184, 184f, 185f, 186f
  in superior laryngeal block, 193, 194f
Superior oblique muscle, anatomy of, in retrobulbar (peribulbar) block, 170f
Superior rectus muscle, anatomy of, in retrobulbar (peribulbar) block, 168f, 170f
Supraclavicular block, 45
  anatomy for, 30, 45, 30f, 31f, 46f
  AXIS block vs., 50
  classic
    needle puncture for, 45, 47f
    position for, 45
  indications for, 51
  patient selection for, 45
  pharmacologic choice for, 45
  pneumothorax with, 49
  potential problems with, 49
  sonoanatomy for, 50, 51f, 52f
  ultrasonography-guided, 50, 53f, 54f
  vertical (plumb bob)
    needle puncture for, 48, 48f, 49f, 50f
    position for, 48
Supraclavicularis nerve, anatomy of, in superficial cervical plexus block, 289f
Supraclavicular nerve, anatomy of
  in cervical plexus block, 171, 173f
  in pronated arm, 27f
  in supinated arm, 27f
  in supraclavicular block, 52f
Suprailiac anterior quadratus lumborum (QL) block, 240f
Supraorbitalis nerve, anatomy of, in superficial cervical plexus block, 289f
Suprascapular artery, anatomy of, in suprascapular block, 56f
Suprascapular block, 55
  indications for, 55
  sonoanatomy for, 55, 56f
  technique for, 55, 56f, 57f
Suprascapular nerve, anatomy of, 26f
  in suprascapular block, 55, 56f
Supraspinatus muscle, anatomy of, in suprascapular block, 56f
Supraspinous ligament, anatomy of
  in epidural block, 262f
  in pediatric caudal block, 282f
  in spinal block, 250f, 256f
Sural nerve
  anatomy of, 95f, 96f
    in ankle block, 159f, 160f, 162, 163f
  cross-sectional magnetic resonance images of, 98f
  needle puncture at, for ankle block, 157
  in popliteal and saphenous block, 142f, 144f
Sympathetic chain, anatomy of, in stellate ganglion block, 177, 178f
Sympathetic nerve fibers, 298
Sympathetic trunk, anatomy of, 93f, 201f
  in glossopharyngeal block, 190f, 192f
Syringes, 13
Syringe technique, for cerebrospinal fluid aspiration, 254, 257f

Systemic toxicity, of local anesthetics, in pediatrics, 10
  clinical picture of, 10
  predisposing factors in, 10
  prevention/reducing risk of, 11

T

TAP block. *see* Transversus abdominis plane (TAP) block
Taylor's (lumbosacral) approach, to spinal block, 256, 259f
Tendocalcaneus, anatomy of, in ankle block, 160f
Teres major muscle, anatomy of, in suprascapular block, 56f
Teres minor muscle, anatomy of, in suprascapular block, 56f
Tetracaine, 4, 4f, 9
  dose of, for spinal anesthesia for inguinal hernia repair, 10t
  lidocaine and, transdermal patch, 9
  for spinal block, 249
Thoracic epidural block
  anatomy of, 263f
  needle puncture for, 264, 266f, 267f, 268f, 269f
Thoracic neuraxial block, 248, 247f, 248f
Thoracic spinal nerve, anatomy of, in subcostal transversus abdominal plane block
  T10, 233f
  T11, 233f
  T12, 233f
Thoracic vertebra, anatomy of, 263f
Thoracoabdominal nerves, 229f
Thoracodorsal nerve, anatomy of, 26f
Thoracolumbar fascia, deep, anatomy of, in quadratus lumborum block, 237f
Thoracolumbar spinal nerves, anatomy of, 227, 228f
Three-in-one block, 99, 100f
Thromboembolic disease, 297
Thyroepiglottic ligament, anatomy of, in airway block, 186f
Thyrohyoid membrane, anatomy of
  in airway block, 184, 186f
  in superior laryngeal block, 193, 194f
  in translaryngeal block, 196f
Thyroid cartilage, anatomy of
  in airway block, 185f, 186f, 187f
  in interscalene block, 34f
  in superior laryngeal block, 194f
  in supraclavicular block, 46f
Thyroid gland, anatomy of, in stellate ganglion block, 177, 178f
Tibia, anatomy of, in saphenous block, 143f
Tibial collateral ligament, anatomy of, in saphenous block, 143f
Tibialis anterior tendon
  anatomy of, in ankle block, 160f
  cross-sectional magnetic resonance images of, 98f
Tibialis posterior tendon, cross-sectional magnetic resonance images of, 98f

Tibial nerve
  anatomy of, 93f
    in ankle block, 159, 160f, 162f
    in popliteal and saphenous block, 141, 142f, 144f, 145f
    in sciatic block, 108f, 113f
  cross-sectional magnetic resonance images of, 98f
Time gain compensation (TGC), 18
Tongue, anatomy of, in airway block, 187f
Tonsillar nerves, anatomy of, in airway block, 183
Tourniquet inflation pressure, for intravenous regional block, 85
Trachea, anatomy of
  in airway block, 184, 186f
  in stellate ganglion block, 177, 178f
  in translaryngeal block, 196f
Tracheal intubation
  glossopharyngeal block for, 189, 190
  superior laryngeal block for, 193
  translaryngeal block for, 195
Transdermal patch, lidocaine and tetracaine, 9
Translaryngeal block, 195, 196f
Transversalis fascia, anatomy of, in quadratus lumborum block, 237f
Transverse abdominis muscle, anatomy of, in subcostal transversus abdominal plane block, 233f, 235f
Transverse cervical nerve, anatomy of
  in cervical plexus block, 171, 173f
  in superficial cervical plexus block, 289f
Transverse oblique scanning technique, for lumbar plexus block, 101
Transverse process, anatomy of
  in epidural block, 267f
  in lumbar plexus block, 104f
  in paravertebral block, 218f
Transversus abdominis muscle, anatomy of
  in quadratus lumborum block, 237f
  in transversus abdominis plane block, 231
Transversus abdominis plane (TAP) block
  anatomy for, 231
  classic approach of, 231, 232
  indications for, 232
  technique for, 231
Trapezius muscle, anatomy of
  in erector spinae plane block, 222, 222f, 223f
  in infraclavicular block, 61f

Trapezius muscle, anatomy of *(Continued)*
  in interscalene block, 37f
  in suprascapular block, 56f
Trigeminal nerve, anatomy of, in airway block, 183, 183f, 187f
Truncal anatomy
  cross-section of, 201f
  dermatomes in, 200f
Truncal block, anatomy for, 199, 200f, 201f
Tuohy needles
  epidural analgesia/anesthesia, 299
  for lumbar epidural block, 262
  for spinal block, 253

U
Ulnar nerve, anatomy of, 25, 26f
  in axillary block, 69, 70f, 71f, 72f
  in brachial plexus block, 73f
  in infraclavicular block, 61f, 62f
  in interscalene block, 42f, 43f
  in pronated arm, 27f
  in supinated arm, 27f
Ulnar nerve block, interscalene approach to, 36
Ulnar nerve, of distal upper extremity block, 77, 79, 80f, 81f
Ultrasonography
  for axillary block, 72
  for femoral block, 120
  for infraclavicular block, 63, 64f
  for interscalene block, 36, 37f
  for neuraxial block, 243
  for sciatic block, 110, 112f
  for supraclavicular block, 50, 53f, 54f
Ultrasound, 14. *see also* Ultrasonography
  generation, 16
  wavelength and frequency, 16, 17f
Upper extremity
  cutaneous innervation of, 52f
  dermatomes of, 27f, 28f
  myotome innervation of, 37f, 43f
  osteotomes of, 28f
  sclerotome innervation of, 38f, 42f
Upper extremity block. *see also* Brachial plexus block
  anatomy for, 23. *see also* Brachial plexus, anatomy of
  intravenous regional, 85. *see also* Intravenous regional block
Upper limb. *see* Upper extremity
Uteroplacental perfusion, 299

V
Vagus nerve, anatomy of
  in airway block, 183, 183f, 184, 184f, 185f, 187f
  in glossopharyngeal block, 189, 190f, 192f
  in superior laryngeal block, 193, 194f
Van Lint block, of orbicularis oculi muscle, 167, 169f
Vasoconstrictors, 6
  for spinal block, 249
Vastus intermedius muscle, anatomy of, in adductor canal block, 151f
Vastus lateralis muscle, cross-sectional magnetic resonance images of, 98f
Vastus medialis muscle
  anatomy of
    in adductor canal block, 151f, 152f
    in saphenous block, 143f
  cross-sectional magnetic resonance images of, 98f
Venous exsanguination, with Esmarch bandage, 86f
Ventricle, anatomy of
  in airway block, 186f
  in translaryngeal block, 196f
Vertebral artery, anatomy of
  in interscalene block, 33, 35f
  in supraclavicular block, 30, 30f, 46f
Vertebral body, anatomy of, in epidural block, 267f
Vertebral notch, anatomy of, in epidural block, 267f
Vertebra, thoracic, anatomy of, 263f
Vestibular fold, anatomy of
  in airway block, 186f
  in translaryngeal block, 196f
Visceral afferent nerve fibers, 298
Visceral pleura, anatomy of, in paravertebral block, 218f
Vocal ligament, anatomy of
  in airway block, 186f
  in translaryngeal block, 196f

W
Whitacre needles, for spinal block, 253
Wrist block, of distal upper extremity block, 81, 81t, 82f